Handbook of
Behavioral Neurobiology

Volume 1
Sensory Integration

HANDBOOK OF BEHAVIORAL NEUROBIOLOGY

General Editor:
Frederick A. King
University of Florida College of Medicine, Gainesville, Florida

Editorial Board:
Vincent G. Dethier
Robert W. Goy
David A. Hamburg
Peter Marler
James L. McGaugh
William D. Neff
Eliot Stellar

Volume 1   Sensory Integration
            Edited by R. Bruce Masterton

Volume 2   Neuropsychology
            Edited by Michael Gazzaniga

A Continuation Order Plan is available for this series. A continuation order will bring delivery of each new volume immediately upon publication. Volumes are billed only upon actual shipment. For further information please contact the publisher.

Handbook of
Behavioral Neurobiology

Volume 1
Sensory Integration

Edited by

R. Bruce Masterton
The Florida State University
Tallahassee, Florida

PLENUM PRESS · NEW YORK AND LONDON

Library of Congress Cataloging in Publication Data

Main entry under title:

Sensory integration.

   (Handbook of behavioral neurobiology; v. 1)
   Includes bibliographies and index.
   1. Senses and sensation. 2. Sense-organs. 3. Physiology, Comparative. I. Masterton, R.
Bruce. II. Series [DNLM: 1. Behavior. 2. Neurophysiology. 3. Psychophysics. WL102.3
H236]
QP431.S4515   596'.01'82   78-17238
ISBN 0-306-35191-9

© 1978 Plenum Press, New York
A Division of Plenum Publishing Corporation
227 West 17th Street, New York, N.Y. 10011

Printed in the United States of America

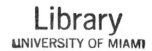

Contributors

LINDA M. BARTOSHUK, *John B. Pierce Foundation and Yale University, New Haven, Connecticut*

MARK BERKLEY, *Department of Psychology, Florida State University, Tallahassee, Florida*

SUSAN M. BELMORE, *Department of Psychology, University of Kentucky, Lexington, Kentucky*

MANNING J. CORREIA, *Departments of Otolaryngology, Physiology, and Biophysics, University of Texas Medical Branch, Galveston, Texas*

TIMOTHY J. CUNNINGHAM, *Department of Anatomy, Medical College of Pennsylvania, Philadelphia, Pennsylvania*

ROBERT P. ERICKSON, *Departments of Psychology and Physiology, Duke University, Durham, North Carolina*

K. K. GLENDENNING, *Department of Psychology, Florida State University, Tallahassee, Florida*

MICHAEL E. GOLDBERG, *Neurobiology Department, Armed Forces Radiobiology Research Institute, Bethesda, Maryland*

FRED E. GUEDRY, JR., *Naval Aerospace Medical Research Laboratory, Naval Air Station, Pensacola, Florida*

J. M. HARRISON, *Department of Psychology, Boston University, Boston, Massachusetts, and New England Regional Primate Research Center, Harvard Medical School, Southborough, Massachusetts*

R. BRUCE MASTERTON, *Department of Psychology, Florida State University, Tallahassee, Florida*

D. G. MOULTON, *Monell Chemical Senses Center and Department of Physiology, University of Pennsylvania, and Veterans Administration Hospital, Philadelphia, Pennsylvania*

E. HAZEL MURPHY, *Department of Anatomy, Medical College of Pennsylvania, Philadelphia, Pennsylvania*

RICHARD J. RAVIZZA, *Psychology Department, Pennsylvania State University, University Park, Pennsylvania*

DAVID LEE ROBINSON, *Neurobiology Department, Armed Forces Radiobiology Research Institute, Bethesda, Maryland*

C. VIERCK, *Department of Neuroscience, University of Florida College of Medicine, Gainesville, Florida*

MARTHA WILSON, *Department of Psychology, University of Connecticut, Storrs, Connecticut*

Preface

The principal goal of the *Handbook of Behavioral Neurobiology* is a systematic, critical, and timely exposition of those aspects of neuroscience that have direct and immediate bearing on overt behavior. In this first volume, subtitled "Sensory Integration," the subject matter has been subdivided and the authors selected with this particular goal in mind. Although the early chapters (on the phylogeny and ontogeny of sensory systems, and on the common properties of sensory systems) are somewhat too abstract to permit many direct behavioral inferences, the focus on behavior has been maintained there too as closely as is now possible. A behavioral orientation is most obvious in the remaining chapters, which lay out for each sensory modality in turn what is now known about structure–behavior relationships.

The handbook is primarily intended to serve as a ready reference for two types of readers: first, practicing neuroscientists looking for a concise and authoritative treatment of developments outside of their particular specialities; and second, students of one or another branch of neuroscience who need an overview of the persistent questions and current problems surrounding the relation of the perceptual systems to behavior. The requirements imposed by the decision to address these particular audiences are reflected in the scope and style of the chapters as well as in their content.

To begin with, the difficult task of weighing and editing, which was needed to distill the myriad of facts into a single volume of reasonable length, has been accomplished by the contributing authors instead of the editors. Thus, the integrity of the individual chapters has been preserved in spite of the limitations of space required by the handbook format.

Another decision dictated by the intended audience was that the level and style of presentation of the subject matter should address the pedagogical aims of the handbook. This decision was made by the editors to help resolve the dilemma of authors who are asked to contribute a "concise overview" of developments in their speciality areas. For, if authors decide to be both concise and comprehensive, the result can be an abbreviated, almost mathematical, style so cryptic and compact as to be comprehensible only to those already well versed in the subject. On the other hand, if authors decide to be both unequivocal and readable, the result can be a discursive style which places them in jeopardy among their scientific colleagues who recognize the exceptions to the truncated array of general principles, or who generate counter-examples or question the selection of subtopics, etc.

Therefore, the editors of this volume made the decision that pedagogical usefulness should supersede blind encyclopedic completeness, and this requirement was imposed on the individual authors. From the outset, the authors were asked to sacrifice comprehensiveness for illumination, in spite of any natural inclination to the contrary. Thus, the editors take the responsibility for the omission of some topics and the expansion of others.

The reader of several chapters of this volume will soon notice that the scope of treatment for the several modalities varies considerably. The reason for this variation is that inquiry into the behavioral roles of sensory structures has progressed at widely differing rates in the several modalities. For example, it has been necessary to allot three chapters to the visual system and two chapters each to the auditory and vestibular systems in order to provide reasonably complete coverage for these very active or highly sophisticated lines of inquiry. Each of these chapters could be easily expanded into an entire volume or even a set of volumes. At the other extreme, the olfactory and gustatory systems are technically more difficult areas in which to experiment, and have only recently gained the concentrated attention that they deserve. Thus, there are only single chapters on olfaction and gustation, and these deal more with receptor processes and their psychophysical counterparts rather than with the more subtle contributions of central sensory structures as seen in the chapters on vision or audition. Therefore, though the lack of uniformity among the chapters may be regretted, it cannot be seriously faulted. The current level of knowledge and, consequently, the focus of current research into the behavioral contributions of the several sensory modalities are simply too different to permit a single, fixed format of presentation.

Finally, it has been said that one of the less obvious but perhaps more lasting measures of any scientific book is whether or not the currency and clarity of its specific examples succeed in provoking its readers to make them obsolete. Using this yardstick, each of us who have played some part in the preparation of this volume join in wishing it an active but reasonably short life.

R. BRUCE MASTERTON

Contents

CHAPTER 10

Vestibular Function in Normal and in Exceptional Conditions 353

Fred E. Guedry, Jr., and Manning J. Correia

Chapter 11

Functional Properties of the Auditory System of the Brain Stem 409

J. M. Harrison

Chapter 12

Auditory Forebrain: Evidence from Anatomical and Behavioral
Experiments Involving Human and Animal Subjects 459

Richard J. Ravizza and Susan M. Belmore

Phylogeny of the Vertebrate Sensory Systems

R. Bruce Masterton and K. K. Glendenning

Introduction

Most of the sensory systems of vertebrates have an evolutionary history that stretches back to before the origin of the vertebrates themselves. If this long history were available for close inspection, a number of fundamental questions about the physiology of the senses and their primary behavioral contributions could be quickly answered and these answers could be expected to bring with them a kind of insight into sensory system function not possible to gain by experiment alone. Even as incompletely known as it now is, the evolutionary history of the sensory systems remains a source of new and relatively independent ideas about structure-function relationships that serve to augment the range of plausible hypotheses fueling direct physiological and behavioral experimentation (Tucker and Smith, 1976; Wever, 1976; Stebbins, 1970; Glickstein, 1976; Berkley, 1976). It is for this reason that the conclusions of the comparative and paleontological sciences are of particular value to those interested in the neural mechanisms of sensory integration.

Since the 1960s, knowledge about the structural evolution of the sensory systems has expanded rapidly as a result mostly of advances in the techniques that allow the tracing of pathways within the central nervous system of lower vertebrates (e.g., Nauta and Gygax, 1954; Fink and Heimer, 1967; La Vail *et al.*, 1973; Cowan *et al.*, 1972). Similarly, advances in behavioral technique now allow the

R. Bruce Masterton and K. K. Glendenning   Department of Psychology, Florida State University, Tallahassee, Florida 32306.

R. BRUCE MASTERTON
AND K. K.
GLENDENNING

precise determination of sensory limitations in previously intractable species (Stebbins, 1970; Masterton *et al.*, 1969). In general, both neuroanatomical and behavioral techniques have almost caught up with electrophysiological techniques in their adaptability to any vertebrate species regardless of peculiarities in its nervous system or behavior, and already they have led to a wide array of new knowledge concerning the evolution and probable selective pressures exerted on the sensory systems (Masterton *et al.*, 1976*a,b*).

As it has turned out, this new knowledge has helped to simplify the picture of sensory evolution (Nauta and Karten, 1970). For example, it is now known that there are many more structural homologies among vertebrate species than was ever previously supposed (cf. Ariëns Kappers *et al.*, 1936). This means that the structural arrangement of each sensory system is sufficiently similar throughout vertebrates that it is now possible to derive a plan that is common to all vertebrates except possibly an aberrant few. Although common plans are valuable in their own right, more importantly they allow ready recognition of variations from the plans in specialized species. That is, knowledge of the common plan of a sensory system makes aberrations from the plan in one or other species recognizable for the peculiarities that they are and allows them to be either correlated with behavioral peculiarities or exploited for experimental purposes. Therefore, the common plan and chief variations of a sensory system usually are as interesting and useful as the system's evolutionary history, and these topics are also included in the sections that follow.

This chapter is divided into six sections corresponding to six chief sensory systems: olfactory, visual, somatosensory, gustatory, vestibular, and auditory. In each section three questions are discussed: first, what is the structural plan of the system common to vertebrates; second, what are the more striking variations in this plan; and, third, what were the most notable changes in the system that probably took place along mankind's particular lineage.

Olfactory System

Since the most generalized and neurologically primitive of vertebrates (the jawless hagfish and lampreys) have an olfactory system similar to that of other vertebrates, the origin of the olfactory system probably predates the origin of the vertebrates themselves (Allison, 1953; Parsons, 1967; Bertmar, 1969). Although the chief behavioral contribution of this system is usually presumed to be its role in food-seeking, the fact has become increasingly apparent in recent years that it serves most vertebrates in a much wider role. In fishes its sensitivity to a wide range of amino acids indicates that it is probably a generalized detector of living things, whether they are to be avoided for safety or to be sought for food or for mating (Suzuki and Tucker, 1971; Tucker and Suzuki, 1972). Its reproductive and social roles, in particular, have recently gained considerable attention with the discovery that many odors ("pheromones") are used as a means of intraspecies communication (e.g., Doty, 1976; Shorey, 1976; see Chapter 4).

The common plan of the vertebrate olfactory system is shown in Fig. 1. The cell bodies of the first-order neurons are part of a mucous-covered *olfactory epithelium.* The peripheral processes of these neurons serve as receptors, and their axons make up the *olfactory nerve,* which passes upward into the cranial cavity to terminate in the *olfactory bulb.* Just before termination, the first-order axons divide into dense glomeruli which give the bulb a corticoid appearance when it is viewed in cross-section (Graziadei, 1974; Shepherd, 1972).

The cell bodies of the second-order neurons, or *mitral cells,* reside in a thin layer below the glomeruli. These cells have dendritic processes that extend radially toward the bulb's surface and make contact with the glomerular complex of the first-order cells. Although the projection of the first-order neurons on the mitral cells of the bulb is orderly, there is a good deal of convergence. In rabbits, for example, 26,000 first-order neurons synapse on only 100 mitral cells (Allison and Warwick, 1949).

The first-order, second-order synapse at the glomeruli is complicated by the presence of other cell types. Most of these periglomerular cells are reminiscent of the horizontal and amacrine cells in the retina in that they are axonless and apparently allow lateral interaction between the terminal glomeruli of the first-order neurons. In general, the ultrastructure of the glomerular complex seems to be quite similar in all classes of vertebrates (Andres, 1970).

The axons of the mitral cells collect in the center of the olfactory bulb and project into the forebrain as the *olfactory tract.* The axons of the olfactory tract

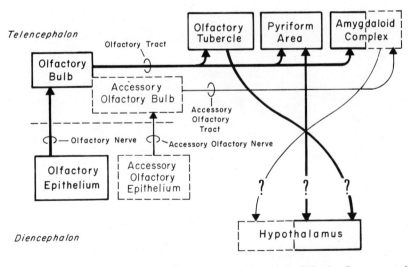

Fig. 1. Common plan of the vertebrate olfactory system. This and the following figures are schematic diagrams illustrating the common plan of each of the sensory systems. In each, the dashed line indicates the division between the peripheral and central nervous system; solid lines indicate known projections common to all but aberrant vertebrate species; solid lines interrupted by question marks indicate projections probably common to all but aberrant species, although not yet as firmly established.

terminate in one of three (third-order) targets: the olfactory tubercle, the pyriform area, or the amygdaloid complex (e.g., Skeen and Hall, 1977; Scalia and Winans, 1975; Broadwell, 1975; Heimer, 1969).

The *olfactory tubercle* is composed of several cell types of which large pyramidal cells with long apical dendrites are predominant. In mammals, the axons from some of these third-order neurons terminate in the *hypothalamus* and in the *dorsal thalamus,* the latter serving as an olfactory link to *prefrontal neocortex* (Heimer, 1972; Krettek and Price, 1974; Scott and Leonard, 1971). The targets of these cells in nonmammals have not yet been unequivocally demonstrated, but it appears that at least some of them also project to the hypothalamus and possibly the thalamus (Scalia and Winans, 1975).

The fiber projections from the olfactory tract to the pyriform area fan out over its surface and then penetrate a short way to terminate mainly in superficial pyramidal cells. Axons of many of these pyriform cells give off collaterals to other cells within the area. However, those leaving the area join the deep white matter directed, at least in mammals, to the hypothalamus (Heimer, 1968; Price and Powell, 1971).

The third target of the olfactory tract is the *amygdaloid complex.* The further projections of this division are known only in mammals (Scott and Leonard, 1971).

VARIATIONS IN THE VERTEBRATE OLFACTORY SYSTEM

The greatest and most obvious variation in the common plan of the olfactory system is the presence of a second or *accessory olfactory system* in some vertebrates. This system parallels the main olfactory system in most respects, but is quite separate from it. It is present in amphibians, reptiles, and mammals, but not in fish or birds. Therefore, it is almost certainly of later origin than the main olfactory system—probably arising with amphibians and undergoing secondary atrophy in birds.

The plan of the accessory olfactory system is also shown in Fig. 1. It originates in neurons whose cell bodies are embedded in sensory epithelium at the roof of the mouth, or in the floor of the nasal cavity, the vomeronasal organ (Allison, 1953; Negus, 1958). Although there exists a great deal of variation among species in the structure of the vomeronasal organ, the sensory neurons themselves, although lacking cilia, are similar to those of the main olfactory system. Their peripheral processes serve as receptors and their axons terminate in glomeruli in a restricted part of the olfactory bulb. The area of the olfactory bulb which receives axons from the accessory olfactory epithelium is called the *accessory olfactory bulb,* although it is a part of the main olfactory bulb rather than being a physically separate bulb.

The mitral cells of the accessory olfactory bulb are the second-order neurons. Their axons pass out of the bulb into the forebrain in the *accessory olfactory tract.* Unlike the main olfactory system, the accessory olfactory tract does *not* terminate in either the olfactory tubercle or the pyriform area, but continues to the *amygdala.* At this structure it terminates in the medial and the posteromedial cortical divisions and does *not* overlap with the projections of the main olfactory system which terminate in the anterior and posterolateral cortical divisions (Scalia and Winans, 1975: Skeen and Hall, 1977).

This segregation of the two olfactory systems seems to be maintained still further in mammals: the amygdaloid targets of the accessory system project to the anteromedial hypothalamus, while the amygdaloid targets of the main system seem to project to the posterolateral hypothalamus (Scalia and Winans, 1976). Therefore, despite the obvious structural similarities in the first- and second-order neurons and the similarity in function that this implies, the main and accessory olfactory systems remain segregated over at least their first three synapses. The significance of this segregation is not presently known.

In addition to the presence of an accessory olfactory system and its own variation among tetrapods, the main olfactory system shows considerable quantitative variation among vertebrates. One of these variations that has proved to be very useful for experimental purposes is in the relative lengths of the olfactory nerve and the olfactory tract. In most vertebrates with long snouts, the olfactory bulb remains close to the sensory epithelium so that the olfactory nerve is very short and the olfactory tract is long. In the garfish, however, the olfactory bulb remains close to the forebrain so that the olfactory tract is short and the olfactory nerve is long. Thus for many experiments on olfactory nerve the garfish makes a convenient preparation (Easton, 1971; Gross and Beidler, 1973).

The olfactory epithelium and olfactory bulb also vary greatly in size. They range from massive (in animals such as bottom-feeding fishes) to very large (in sharks or dogs) to meager (in seed-eating birds) to none at all (in marine mammals such as porpoises and toothed whales). Although this variation can be seen to correspond closely with the feeding tactics of the animals involved, the correlation is not perfect. For example, the persistence of an olfactory system in birds and many herbivorous mammals which rely mostly on vision for food suggests that food-seeking does not exhaust the contributions of the system. Even in the totally anosmic whale without an olfactory nerve, bulb, or tract, it is noteworthy that the third-order neurons of the olfactory system still persist. Apparently, the higher-order neurons make contributions beyond the mere ability for olfactory sensation (Nachman and Ashe, 1974; Eleftheriou, 1972).

TRENDS IN THE EVOLUTION OF THE HUMAN OLFACTORY SYSTEM

The evolution of the olfactory system in mankind's lineage has been conservative (Tucker and Smith, 1976). To begin with, the great number of homologues in the system throughout vertebrates, the general plan of the system, and, in particular, the constancy of the chief targets of the olfactory tract (i.e., olfactory tubercle, pyriform area, and amygdala) makes evident that each part was probably present at the origin of vertebrates.

The first obvious modification of the system seems to have come about when man's amphibian ancestors invaded land and took up a life in air. This shift in medium can be expected to have placed particularly great selective pressure on the olfactory system. To begin with, the gustatory system could no longer aid in odor detection as it probably did (and does now) for water-dwelling fish. Second,

R. BRUCE MASTERTON
AND K. K.
GLENDENNING

the class of adequate stimuli for the olfactory system must have changed dramatically in that a much lesser variety of molecules can be borne by air than by water. For example, heavy and nonvolatile molecules were no longer available for the detection of friend, foe, or food. Third, apparently to protect the olfactory epithelium from drying out, it became covered by a thick mucus and this covering added another barrier to potential odorants: they had to be lipid soluble in order to reach the receptor surface. Therefore, olfactory stimuli had only to be water soluble to be usable by the preamphibians, but to be usable by the tetrapods, they had to be soluble both in air and in lipids.

It was at this time that the accessory olfactory system developed. Although the exact nature of the stimuli activating this system is still a matter of dispute (Tucker, 1971), it is difficult to avoid the notion that its development was a response to the unavailability of once important olfactory stimuli resulting from the shift from water to air. It is not impossible that the accessory system allowed the transduction of odorants incapable of stimulating the main olfactory system by providing a more watery, less lipid medium on the tongue and in the mouth to help bypass the lipid barrier of the main system (Parsons, 1970). Quite independent of any difference in chemical sensitivity, however, the obvious difference in the central projections of the two systems suggests an equally obvious difference in their behavioral contributions.

At a still later time, the main olfactory system underwent another change: the pyriform area became corticalized. In fish and amphibians the pyriform area has no apparent cortical structure, while in reptiles, mammals, and birds the area is clearly cortical in appearance, with three conspicuous layers. Although the significance of this change is not clear, it apparently took place sometime near the origin of repitles. Later, with the appearance of neocortex in mammals, the pyriform cortex became sharply delimited by the *rhinal fissure,* which separates neocortex above and pyriform cortex below on the ventrolateral surface of the cerebral hemispheres of most mammals.

With the origin of man's mammalian ancestors both the main and accessory olfactory systems were retained and possibly expanded throughout the long period when carnivorous reptiles held them to a nocturnal and semisubterranean life (Elliot Smith, 1910; Le Gros Clark, 1959). At this stage the mammalian system , in addition to the targets common to other vertebrates, had acquired primary ipsilateral projections to the tenia tecta, the nucleus of the lateral olfactory tract, and the entorhinal cortex; secondary projections to the contralateral olfactory bulb, the anterior olfactory nucleus, and the pyriform cortex; a wealth of ipsilateral interconnections among the several targets of the olfactory tract; and descending fibers back to the olfactory bulb (Skeen and Hall, 1977). The accessory olfactory bulb also had acquired projections to the bed nucleus of the accessory olfactory tract and the bed nucleus of the stria terminalis as well as interconnections of the medial amygdala, the posteromedial cortical amygdala, and the bed nucleus and fibers descending from the amygdala to the accessory olfactory bulb (Raisman, 1972).

Still later as the predatory pressure of the reptiles was relieved, the daytime was reopened to mammals as a viable niche, vision redeveloped (see below), and the expansion of the olfactory system seems to have been arrested. Although it is often stated that after the origin of Primates the olfactory system became reduced, this is not altogether true. It is true that the accessory olfactory system has become vestigial in man (it is present in human embryos, not in adults), but the main olfactory system in man and other anthropoids is far from vestigial. In absolute size the olfactory bulbs of man are as large as in many of the most macrosmotic and neurologically primitive insectivores. Only insofar as the system has become dwarfed by the vast expansion of man's forebrain can it be said to be reduced. Thus the oft-repeated claim that in man olfaction is almost vestigial may be more a product of introspection through smog-polluted noses than of fact (see Cain, 1977).

VISUAL SYSTEM

Since even the most generalized and neurologically primitive vertebrates now extant have eyes and visual systems essentially similar to those of every other vertebrate, it can be concluded that the visual system arose before the origin of the vertebrates. Although many invertebrates before them had rhodopsin and some probably had eyes, they did not have eyes in any way homologous with those that were to arise in vertebrates. As far as is now known, the vertebrate eye is structurally unique and without homologue outside of vertebrates, although functionally it is far from unique since analogues exist throughout the animal kingdom.

Because of this structural uniqueness and because of a lack of clues to the formative stages from either comparative or paleontological materials, the sequence of changes that eventuated in the origin of the vertebrate eye and visual system cannot be documented. Consequently, all past and present theories of the origin of eye and visual system are almost entirely speculative despite their often uncritical repetition in several generations of texts (Sarnat and Netsky, 1974). Most of these theories differ only in their emphasis on one or another feature of the visual system such as the energy demands of photosensitive cells, the reversed retina, or the decussation of the optic tract at the chiasm (e.g., Walls, 1939; Polyak, 1957; Dowling, 1970; Rodieck, 1973). It can be anticipated that until more comparative material is discovered, or the physiology of the system is better understood so that the present material can be reinterpreted in a more productive way, our ignorance of the origin of the visual system will not change appreciably.

COMMON PLAN

The organization of the common elements of the visual system of vertebrates is illustrated in Fig. 2. For convenience in the discussion that follows, the terminology used for Mammalia will be used for vertebrates in general.

The axons of the retinal ganglion cells leave the eye in the *optic tract* and distribute directly to six major targets: the hypothalamus, ventral lateral geniculate nucleus, dorsal lateral geniculate nucleus, accessory optic nuclei, pretectal complex, and superior colliculus. In each of these targets, except possibly the hypothalamic and accessory optic nuclei, retinotopic relationships are faithfully preserved.

The *suprachiasmatic nucleus of the hypothalamus* receives optic projections and not coincidentally has been implicated in the mechanism for timing circadian rhythms (e.g., Stephan and Nunez, 1977).

The *ventral lateral geniculate nucleus* of the thalamus receives both retinal and tectal projections and itself projects to the hypothalamus, pons, and tectal and pretectal nuclei (e.g., Edwards *et al.,* 1974; Swanson *et al.,* 1974; Graybiel, 1974).

The *accessory optic nuclei* receive retinal projections via the *accessory optic tract,* which leaves the main optic tract in the region of the chiasm and courses through the hypothalamus without terminating. The projections to the accessory optic nuclei are usually, if not always, contralateral despite any bilaterality that might exist in the main optic tract (Hayhow, 1958).

In all vertebrate classes, the *superior colliculus* (or *optic tectum*) receives a substantial portion of retinal projections and distributes most of its efferents caudally in multisynaptic pathways toward motor mechanisms in the brain stem and spinal cord for eye, head, and body orientation (see Chapter 5 for a discussion of this system). Many of its efferents also project rostrally to the *pulvinar nucleus* of the thalamus and from there to the telencephalon. The function and significance of this pathway from eye to colliculus to pulvinar to telencephalon are discussed in Chapter 7.

Another major diencephalic target of retinal ganglion cells is the *dorsal lateral geniculate nucleus,* which in turn projects to the telencephalon in every vertebrate species. However, this nucleus gains predominance only in mammals where its telencephalic target is striate or visual cortex (for further discussion of this system, see Chapter 6).

Although the efferents of the several targets of the optic tract combine to form several circuits and reciprocal connections, the most notable circuit is formed by third-order fibers running from the telencephalic target of the dorsal lateral

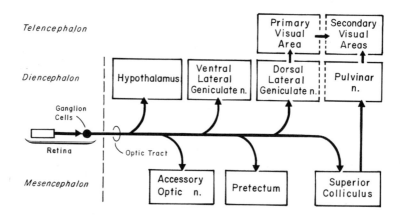

Fig. 2. Common plan of the vertebrate visual system. The dashed lines between two thalamic and telencephalic structures indicate that in some species these areas are not clearly differentiable. Terms used here are typical for mammalian species, but see Ebbesson (1972) for several other terminologies.

geniculate (i.e., striate cortex in mammals) to the superior colliculus. This pathway completes a retinal-diencephalic-telencephalic-mesencephalic pathway that converges with the direct projections from the retina to the mesencephalon.

Variations in the Vertebrate Visual System

Although there is considerable variation in the eye and retina of vertebrates, the variation in the central visual system is relatively modest. In general, there seem to be four ways in which this variation is expressed: (1) in the degree of bilaterality of the central projections, (2) in the differentiation of the visual centers from their surround, (3) in the degree of integration of stimuli accomplished at the retina, and (4) in the relative size and intrinsic differentiation of the various central structures.

Bilaterality of Optic Projections. In all vertebrates the central visual projections are mainly contralateral. However, the amount of ipsilateral projections varies widely. The number of fibers that do *not* cross at the optic chiasm varies from practically none at all in animals such as most fish, amphibians, and birds to nearly 50% in humans and other primates. It has long been noticed that the degree of bilaterality in the visual system corresponds to the degree of overlap of the two visual fields: animals with front-set eyes have more ipsilateral projections than animals with side-set eyes and more panoramic vision (Walls, 1939; Tansley, 1950, 1965). This observation leads to the idea that the bilateral projections are the substrate of stereoscopic vision and depth perception through the neural analysis of retinal disparities (see Chapter 7).

Although there are few, if any, animals with side-set eyes that have strongly bilateral visual systems, there are many animals with front-set eyes (owls and hawks, for example) that have essentially complete crossing of fibers at the chiasm. Until recently these exceptions seemed to contraindicate the idea that front-set eyes suggest stereopsis and that stereopsis requires bilateral projections. However, it is now known that at least the telencephalic visual area of these animals has bilateral input (Karten and Nauta, 1968). This bilaterality is not accomplished at the chiasm as it is in mammals, but in the geniculotelencephalic projections themselves. That is, the projection from the lateral geniculate to the visual Wulst in birds is bilateral and not wholly ipsilateral as are the geniculostriate radiations in mammals. The result is that input to the main telencephalic visual center is bilateral in birds even though the lower targets of the optic tract are contralateral. A recent demonstration of true stereopsis in a falcon suggests that bilateral projections to the telencephalon may be sufficient for stereopsis (Fox *et al.*, 1976*b*).

Sharks also have a crossed geniculotelencephalic pathway, but in this case it is predominantly contralateral, instead of bilateral as it is in birds. Therefore, in sharks the input to the telencephalic target of the visual system is almost entirely unilateral, as it is in most animals with panoramic vision, but it is ipsilateral instead of contralateral—the crossover at the chiasm being almost completely negated by the crossover in the thalamotelencephalic projections (Ebbesson and Schroeder, 1971). The origin, significance, and function of the double crossover in sharks remain a puzzle.

R. BRUCE MASTERTON
AND K. K.
GLENDENNING

DEGREE OF DIFFERENTIATION OF VISUAL CENTERS. A second way in which the central visual system varies among vertebrates is in its degree of differentiation. In most animals with a modest visual system because of either a nocturnal life or a life in a turbid medium, the central visual system is poorly differentiated from surrounding structures. Indeed, in many of these animals, structures such as the lateral geniculate nucleus cannot be identified without prior knowledge of the locus of terminations of the optic tract (e.g., Hall and Ebner, 1969; Gulley *et al.,* 1975). On the other hand, in primate species the dorsal lateral geniculate not only stands out clearly from surrounding structures but also has itself undergone profound internal differentiation.

For years this difference in degree of differentiation was considered a main trend in the evolution of the primate visual system so that it was believed that those animals with a more recent common ancestry with Primates had a better-differentiated system than those with more remote common ancestry. However, with the discovery of well-differentiated systems among lower vertebrates that have good vision, it now seems likely that the degree of differentiation is more an indication of the degree of selective pressure on vision in the life of the species than a long-term evolutionary trend unique to mankind's lineage. It now seems probable that vision has waxed and waned in importance in many phylogenetic lineages, mankind's included, and the degree of differentiation of the central visual system has waxed and waned in parallel.

INTEGRATION AT THE RETINAL LEVEL. The third way in which the visual system of vertebrates varies is in the degree of integration achieved in the retina. The receptive fields of retinal ganglion cells show more specificity and hence more integrative capacity in nonmammalian species than in most mammals. In almost all mammals the receptive fields of the retinal ganglion cells are "center-surround" in configuration without orientation or directional selectivity (see Chapter 6). However, in some animals, such as frogs, birds, and rabbits, retinal ganglion cells have receptive fields that are directionally selective—responding to a stimulus passing over them in one direction but not in the opposite direction (Lettvin *et al.,* 1959; Miles, 1972; Barlow *et al.,* 1964). Therefore, in these animals, retinal cells are more like the "simple" cortical cells of mammals (see Chapter 6).

The higher degree of specificity in nonmammalian retinas is paralleled by a higher degree of structural complexity. Animals that have directionally selective ganglion cells in their retinas also have more conventional synapses in the inner plexiform layer of their retinas than animals without such retinal selectivity (Dubin, 1970). Whether there exist still more examples of even more specific and hence more integrative retinas is not now known. But the further possibility is opened that varying degrees of integrative capacity may occur at each of the higher visual centers, too.

QUANTITATIVE VARIATION. The final general way in which the visual system of vertebrates varies is in the relative size and intrinsic differentiation of its central structures. Quite apart from the extrinsic differentiation of visual structures from their nonvisual surround, they also vary enormously in their internal differentiation and relative size. For example, even among mammals, the dorsal lateral geniculate nucleus varies from a small homogeneous nucleus in animals such as the opossum, rat, or hedgehog, to a large many-layered structure in animals such as cats, raccoons, tree shrews, and primates. Similarly, the superior colliculus in vertebrates varies from a relatively small and apparently five-layered structure in frogs to an enormous 14-layered structure in some birds (Cajal, 1911; Karten *et al.*, 1973; Ariëns Kappers *et al.*, 1936).

Most of this type of variation is obviously related to the importance of vision in the life of the animal, but not all of it. The two most obvious variations that are not clearly related to the overall size (and importance) of the animal's visual system are the size of the retinogeniculate projection and the size of the tectal-pulvinar-extrastriate system.

The first of these variations can be seen in a comparison of mammals to nonmammals. In all mammals, regardless of the overall size and importance of their visual system, the retinogeniculate projection is much larger than the retino-tectal projection. In nonmammals the reverse occurs. The second of these variations can be seen in a comparison of primates with nonprimates. In all primates the pulvinar-extrastriate system is very large; in nonprimates it is small, even in species such as squirrels, phalangers, and carnivores where the rest of the visual system is substantial (e.g., Masterton *et al.*, 1974).

The variation in size of the retinogeniculate and pulvinar-extrastriate systems does not correspond so well with the animal's present habitat as it does with successive grades in mankind's phylogenetic lineage. This point is discussed in the following section.

TRENDS IN THE EVOLUTION OF THE HUMAN VISUAL SYSTEM

Although many evolutionary trends in vision have been suggested in the past (e.g., toward greater acuity, toward better color vision, toward better depth perception), recent discoveries of keen visual abilities in lower vertebrates have rendered most, if not all, of these suggestions untenable (e.g., Ingle, 1976; Fox *et al.*, 1976*a*). Although the visual abilities of man are excellent by any standard, there are many nonprimate mammals and nonmammalian vertebrates whose visual ability exceeds that of man along almost every single dimension. For example, there are animals with all-rod retinas, such as hedgehogs and rodents, that are as sensitive as man's (Walls, 1942). There are other animals with all-cone retinas, such as birds, tree shrews, and squirrels, that probably have color vision equal to that of man (Grether, 1939; Duke-Elder, 1961; Tigges, 1963; Crescitellia and Pollack, 1965). And there are still other animals, such as eagles, that have visual acuity which is better than that of man (Walls, 1942; Schlaer, 1972; Fox *et al.*, 1976*a*; Warkentin, 1937). Therefore, despite the adaptive strategy of Primates toward excellent vision, the evolution of mankind's visual system is not describable as an improvement in merely optical or psychophysical factors. Indeed, the vision of many lower vertebrates may be equally as good as man's at least along most usual dimensions of comparison.

It is most likely that the evolution of mankind's particular kind of vision has resulted in a change in what can be done with what is seen, rather than in what can be seen (e.g., Masterton *et al.*, 1974). For this contribution we look to the central visual system.

R. BRUCE MASTERTON
AND K. K.
GLENDENNING

The evolution of mankind's central visual system seems to have occurred in four great steps separated by relatively long periods of only slight change. The first step, at or before the origin of vertebrates, was the origin of the visual system itself. This dramatic occurrence led to the organization we have described as the common plan and forms the basis for all the variations due to later specializations.

Few changes large enough to be considered qualitative occurred until the origin of Mammalia and with it the relatively sudden expansion of the geniculo-cortical system. This second change established the mammalian form of the visual system, and little more than modifications in the relative size and degree of differentiation of its constituent structures (accompanying the specializations in the various mammalian lineages) occurred until the origin of Primates. With Primates came a third change—an elaboration of the geniculostriate system—and still later the fourth change—an elaboration of the pulvinar-extrastriate system (Allman, 1977). Since little is known about the origin of the visual system, the following discussion is confined to the last three of these modifications: the one that occurred with the origin of mammals and the later two with the origin of primates.

DEVELOPMENT OF THE MAMMALIAN GENICULOCORTICAL SYSTEM. The most notable contrast among the visual systems of the several classes of vertebrates, other than those merely quantitative or differentiative, is that between mammals and nonmammals. In the past most views of the evolution of the visual system at this stage have leaned heavily on the idea that the superior colliculus is the principal visual center in nonmammalian vertebrates while striate cortex seems to be principal in mammals. Thus the idea arose that the evolution of the visual system can be characterized as a progressive shift of function from tectum to cortex, and the phrase "the corticalization of vision" became popular (Elliot Smith, 1910; Marquis, 1935; Noback, 1959). The theory of corticalization is based on three observations. First, in nonmammalian vertebrates most optic nerve fibers terminate in the optic tectum, while in mammals most terminate in the dorsal lateral geniculate nucleus. Second, in nonmammalian forms, lesions of the optic tectum seemed to have more devastating effects on visual abilities than did lesions of the forebrain. In mammals the reverse seemed to be the case. Finally, the trend toward a dependence of mammalian vision on the forebrain instead of the midbrain seemed to continue even within mammalian species themselves. For example, after lesions of the striate cortex, human patients seemed to be worse off than monkeys, monkeys worse off than cats, and rats hardly affected at all. Thus corticalization of vision seemed obvious and most of the inconsistencies among vision experiments were interpreted as due to the differing degrees of corticalization among the animal subjects that were used.

However, with the advent of modern neuroanatomical and behavioral techniques, the idea of a progressive change in visual function from midbrain to forebrain has suffered some severe setbacks. In general, the most difficult contradictions to absorb are the results of ablation-behavior experiments on the tectum of mammals and on the forebrain of sharks and birds. Where it was once thought that damage to the superior colliculus of mammals resulted mostly in deficits in eye orientation and not in vision itself (depending on the degree of corticalization, of course), it is now known that tectal lesions in mammals may result in severe visual deficits—resulting in a kind of behavioral unawareness of visual stimuli reminiscent of blindness in many respects (see Chapter 6; Sprague and Meikle, 1965; Sprague *et al.*, 1970; Casagrande *et al.*, 1972; Schneider, 1969).

Conversely, damage to the forebrain of nonmammals, once thought to be without serious visual effect, is now known to result in visual deficits similar to those suffered by mammals with striate cortex lesions. For example, sharks and birds lose the ability to discriminate patterns of equal luminous flux after fore-brain lesions (Graeber *et al.*, 1972; Hodos and Karten, 1970; Hodos *et al.*, 1973). Therefore, the question of the corticalization of vision is far from settled. Certainly, evidence for it is far from unequivocal (Ward and Masterton, 1970).

Nevertheless, there is a good deal of difference between mammals and nonmammals in the size and degree of development of the retinogeniculotelencephalic pathway. In all nonmammals the retinogeniculate pathway to telencephalon is a very modest one, while in mammals it is the largest visual pathway to telencephalon. Therefore, an important structural change in the visual system and presumably, an equally important functional change must have taken place during or shortly before the origin of mammals. Perhaps the best explanation of this change is embodied in the so-called bottleneck theory of the origin of mammals (e.g., Polyak, 1957).

According to this view, mammals arose while the earth was still dominated by predatory reptiles. The presence of the carnivorous reptiles kept the newly evolved mammals in a nocturnal or virtually subterranean way of life (much like shrews and other insectivores lead today). This relatively lightless habitat resulted in a severe reduction of the retinotectal type of visual system they had inherited from their reptilian forebears: the visual system became almost vestigial. Before it was lost entirely, however, the predatory reptiles became extinct and the "bottleneck" was passed. With reduced predatory pressure, the ancient mammals increased rapidly and refilled the previously forbidden diurnal landscape. The result of this sudden release of selective pressure against a daytime existence was a return of pressure for good vision, and, in response, the visual system began to expand once again. But since neocortex with its potentialities for more complex adaptations had already appeared in the forebrain of mammals, the visual system expanded toward this new telencephalic target, rather than simply reexpanding its old connections with the tectum. Thus, according to this theory, the mammalian form replaced the reptilian form not as the result of a gradual and prolonged competition between tectum and cortex extending into modern mammalian lineages but rather as a result of there being little more than a vestige of the retinotectal system remaining before the retinogeniculate system developed.

Although this theory was intended to provide an explanation of the obvious difference in the visual system of mammals and nonmammals, it also serves to explain the similarity in the visual system of reptiles and birds. Birds arose after mammals. However, because of their ability to fly, they escaped the predatory pressure of the ruling reptiles and thereby escaped commitment to a nocturnal life and the consequent reduction of the visual system. Without losing and rebuilding their visual system, birds merely expanded the retinotectal form that they had

R. BRUCE MASTERTON
AND K. K.
GLENDENNING

inherited from the reptiles, with the result that the visual system in modern birds is little more than a superreptilian system.

Because most of the necessary elements of the "bottleneck" theory (i.e., the nocturnality of ancient mammals and the timing of the successive events) are based on evidence entirely independent from the comparative neurological data on the visual system, it has a reasonably good chance of being substantially true. Whether or not it can explain all of the anatomical differences between the visual systems of mammals and nonmammals remains to be seen. In either event, the question remains whether the geniculocortical system took over the functions of the earlier retinotectal system or whether the mammalian geniculocortical system added entirely new functions quite beyond those of the premammalian retinotectal system. Certainly, an expanded geniculocortical system is not necessary for good vision (witness the hawk) and, certainly, the mammalian system does not necessarily bestow good vision on mammals (witness rodents). Therefore, the question of the possible transfer of tectal functions to the cortex is still open. The significance of the partial dependence of nonmammals on their forebrain and of mammals on their tectum for visual functions is an important question in any account of the evolution of vision.

DEVELOPMENT OF THE PRIMATE VISUAL SYSTEM.   Many millions of years after the origin of mammals and the blossoming of the geniculocortical visual system, some ground-dwelling insectivores followed their insect prey into the recently evolved flowering bushes and trees. Some of these enterprising insectivores eventually gave rise to the primate lineage, and, as it evolved, a second noteworthy change in the visual system took place. This second expansion remains etched in the brains of the tree-dwelling insectivores (tree shrews) and the most remote primate relatives of mankind, the prosimians (bushbabies, lemurs, lorises, etc.) (Masterton *et al.,* 1974; Allman, 1977).

This later modification began with a further expansion of the dorsal lateral geniculate and striate cortex. Even today, tree shrews and prosimians have peculiarly elongated cerebrums due almost entirely to the expansion of their occipital lobes to accommodate more striate cortex (Le Gros Clark,1959).

After this second expansion of the geniculocortical system still another modification began. This elaboration occurred in the tectal-pulvinar-extrastriate system and it seems to have continued throughout the remainder of primate evolution. The most obvious evidence for the expansion of this system can be seen in the great increase in size of the temporal lobe in a series of primates with successively more recent common ancestry with mankind. It can also be seen in the increase in the size and degree of differentiation in the pulvinar itself (Masterton *et al.,* 1974).

In nonprimates, the pulvinar is an inconspicuous nucleus (often called "lateralis posterior"), and the extrastriate visual cortex occupies a very small area of the cerebral surface. In tree shrews, however, both the pulvinar and extrastriate cortex are large and are well differentiated from surrounding structures (Diamond *et al.,* 1970; Kaas *et al.,* 1972). In prosimian primates, these structures are larger still. The pulvinar is differentiated into at least two subdivisions (only one of which receives direct tectal projections), and several subdivisions of extrastriate cortex are discernible, each with its own retinotopic map (Glendenning *et al.,*

1975; Allman *et al.*, 1973, 1977; Harting *et al.*, 1973). In anthropoid primates, this process has continued still further, the pulvinar now having at least four subdivisions (still only one with direct tectal input) and extrastriate cortex having at least eight distinct subdivisions each with its own retinotopic map (e.g., Allman and Kaas, 1971, 1974; Zeki, 1969; Allman, 1977).

Obviously, this tremendous expansion of the targets of an old, indirect, and formerly inconspicuous visual pathway to the telencephalon must have brought with it a new kind of adaptation to the visual world. But other than its correlation with an animal's ability to make visual abstractions (Mishkin, 1966; Masterton *et al.*, 1974) little is known of its significance (see Chapter 7).

In summary, mankind's visual system seems to have evolved spasmodically, with four relatively quick leaps separated by long periods of little significant change. The first leap was at or before the origin of vertebrates with the "sudden" appearance of the eye and basic plan of the visual system. Thereafter followed a long period of relatively little substantial change through fish, amphibian and reptilian stages. This period ended with the first mammals suffering a severe reduction of the system. The second major step took place after the extinction of the dominant reptiles: the geniculocortical system expanded rapidly, giving the system the form now typical of mammals. Again, relatively little change occurred until the origin of primates; then the geniculocortical system expanded once more and the occipital lobe to accommodate it. Finally, the expansion and elaboration of the pulvinar-extrastriate system began. This expansion was slower than the previous three (or perhaps its recency and more easy documentation make it appear slower) and has continued until the appearance of hominoids. It has resulted in the characteristically large and complex pulvinar and temporal lobe of anthropoids and is probably the substrate of the special kind of visual adaptation peculiar to anthropoids.

Somatosensory System

Any member of the animal kingdom can respond to mechanical stimuli applied directly to its body. Moreover, any animal with a central nervous system possesses a network of nerves functionally analogous to the vertebrate somatosensory system. Nevertheless, true homologues of the structures in the vertebrate version of the somatosensory system can be traced back with a reasonable degree of certainty only as far as nonvertebrate Chordates, such as *Amphioxus*.

The cord of *Amphioxus*, like that of vertebrates, consists of a central gray reticulum surrounded by white matter containing ascending and descending tracts. And even at this primitive stage, a quasisegmental relationship exists between levels of the cord and levels of the body. However, *Amphioxus* has no dorsal root ganglia and the emerging nerves are not paired but rather alternate along the cord (Barrington and Jefferies, 1975). Furthermore, specific homologues of the higher-order somatosensory structures of vertebrates have not been identified in *Amphioxus* or any other nonvertebrate (Barrington and Jefferies, 1975). Therefore, the origin of the vertebrate version of a somatosensory system can probably be dated to the period after the divergence of the vertebrate lineage from nonvertebrate chordates. Since the somatosensory system in lower vertebrates, such as lampreys or sharks, is essentially similar in organization to that found in mammals (Ebbesson, 1972; Nieuwenhuys, 1972), the origin of the system probably can be narrowed further, to the time period before the origin of the vertebrates themselves.

Among vertebrates the somatosensory system has very many points of similarity. However, there are considerable differences in the relative size and degree of differentiation of the constituent nuclei and tracts. Most of these differences seem to be relatively superficial variations reflecting the differences in body form or the varying sensitivity of particular regions of the body, but some variations are not so easily explained. These latter variations include modifications in the basic relationship between somatosensory and motor neurons and therefore are of paramount importance in understanding the evolution and function of sensory-motor mechanisms (see Chapter 8).

COMMON PLAN

The organization of the somatosensory system of vertebrates is illustrated in Fig. 3. In all vertebrates the system consists of at least two divisions each with three components. The *spinal division* includes the anterolateral column system, the

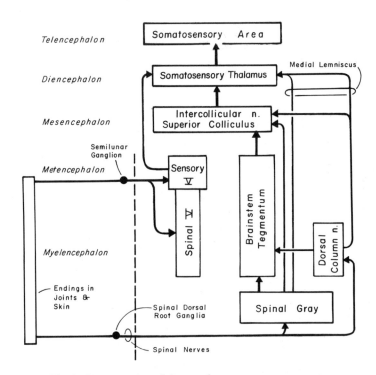

Fig. 3. Common plan of the vertebrate somatosensory system.

dorsal column system, and the spinocerebellar system. The *trigeminal division* includes the main sensory, the spinal, and the mesencephalic systems of cranial nerve V.

With one exception, the cell bodies of the primary somatosensory neurons lie outside the CNS in peripheral sensory ganglia: the spinal dorsal root ganglia for the spinal division and the semilunar ganglion for the trigeminal division. The one exception is the mesencephalic component of the trigeminal nerve, whose cell bodies surround the periaqueductal gray in the midbrain.

The axons from the primary neurons enter the CNS either via the dorsal roots of the spinal cord or via the trigeminal root in the pons (Liu and Chambers, 1957). After entrance they separate into their subsidiary components.

SPINAL DIVISION. The majority of fibers in the *anterolateral column* component of the spinal division synapse in the ipsilateral substantia gelatinosa or nucleus proprius of the spinal gray. Most of the second-order fibers of this component cross to the opposite anterolateral column and ascend to a variety of structures in the brain stem (such as the brain stem tegmentum and intercollicular nucleus) and via the medial lemniscus to the thalamus as the spinothalamic tract (Mehler *et al.*, 1960; Fuller and Ebbesson, 1973*b*; Joseph and Whitlock, 1968*a*).

Most of the primary fibers in the *dorsal column* component pass without synapse into the ipsilateral dorsal column and ascend to the dorsal column nuclei at the spinal-medullary junction. Some of the second-order fibers arising there decussate and project to several brain stem targets including the brain stem tegmentum and intercollicular nucleus, while most course to the thalamus via the medial lemniscus (Schroeder and Jane, 1976; Norton and Kruger, 1973; Groenewegem *et al.*, 1975; Robards *et al.*, 1976).

The third component of the spinal somatosensory system carries mostly proprioceptive information from the muscles and joints to the cerebellum as the *spinocerebellar* system. Some of the fibers in this component follow the same route as those already described while others project directly to the cerebellum and other motor structures. These sensorimotor pathways are not included in Fig. 3 and will not be mentioned further. Finally, still other fibers of this division synapse within the spinal cord after ascending or descending several segments (Hayle, 1973).

Before leaving the spinal division, it is worth noting that still another and possibly common component has been discovered in recent years—the so-called *lateral cervical* pathway. It consists of fibers originating in the middle lamina of the spinal gray and terminating in a nucleus located in the dorsal lateral column at the cervical levels of the spinal cord. Fibers arising from this lateral cervical nucleus project in turn to the somatosensory thalamus. Among mammals the lateral cervical nucleus is present in rat, guinea pig, ferret, rabbit, cat, dog, sheep, seal, and whale (Rexed and Brodal, 1951; Gwyn and Waldron, 1968, 1969; Hagg and Ha, 1970; Ha, 1971). However, it appears to be lacking in humans and some monkeys (Truex *et al.*, 1970). In reptiles it is also only sometimes present (Ebbesson, 1967, 1969). Therefore, at present, it is difficult to decide whether it should be included in the vertebrate common plan (and its absence viewed as aberrant) or whether it is a specialization of only a few genera, orders, or subclasses. In either case, many of the properties of this system seem to be similar to the dorsal column system.

TRIGEMINAL DIVISION. In the trigeminal division, the *main sensory* component synapses in the pons—in the principal sensory trigeminal nucleus (i.e., sensory V). This component seems to subserve somatosensory functions for the head similar to those served by the dorsal column system for the body. Axons of neurons in the main sensory nucleus project contralaterally to the somatosensory thalamus and ipsilaterally to the cerebellum (Darian-Smith, 1973).

The spinal component of the trigeminal division synapses in the spinal trigeminal nucleus (i.e., spinal V), which extends from the pons to the cervical levels of the spinal cord. This component subserves somatosensory functions most similar to those served by the anterolateral component of the spinal division. The second-order axons from neurons in the spinal nucleus of the trigeminal project to the somatosensory thalamus, brain stem tegmentum (Stewart and King, 1963; Dunn and Matze, 1968); and thalamic intralaminar nuclei (Mehler, 1966).

The third component of the trigeminal nerve, the *mesencephalic* component, receives proprioceptive stimuli directly from the jaw muscles and sends its axons directly to motor centers.

HIGHER-ORDER SOMATOSENSORY STRUCTURES. As noted above, several structures in the brain stem and thalamus gain converging projections from second-order neurons of both the dorsal and anterolateral column components of the spinal division and possibly some second-order neurons from the main sensory and spinal trigeminal components as well. These third-order structures (the brain stem tegmentum, the intercollicular nucleus, the deep layers of the superior colliculus, and the somatosensory nuclei of the dorsal thalamus) project, in turn, either to motor centers or, in the case of the thalamic neurons, to the telencephalon.

The telencephalic targets of the somatosensory system include cerebral cortex in those animals that possess it (reptiles, birds, and mammals) and dorsal telencephalon in those animals that do not have cerebral cortex (fish and amphibians) (Kruger and Berkowitz, 1960; Ebbesson, 1969; Ebbesson and Northcutt, 1976; Northcutt, 1970; Vesselkin *et al.,* 1971). In addition to these more obvious telencephalic projections, there are probably still others, but as yet these remain undemonstrated in lower vertebrates and therefore cannot yet be included as part of the common plan.

VARIATIONS IN THE VERTEBRATE SOMATOSENSORY SYSTEM

As in each of the other sensory systems, most of the variation in the central somatosensory system among vertebrates consists of differences in the size and degree of differentiation of the constituent nuclei and their connecting tracts. In the somatosensory system the most notable variations of this kind correspond closely to variations in the relative density of the sensory endings over the body's surface. As was noted by Adrian (1940), there is a close correspondence between the density of sensory endings in a patch of skin and the amount of central nervous system tissue representing that patch of skin. For example, the snout of a pig is represented by a greater number of neurons at each synapse in the central somatosensory system than is its forefoot, while in raccoon the reverse is true (Adrian, 1940; Welker and Seidenstein, 1959). Similarly in man, the hands and face, particularly the lips and tongue, are represented by many more neurons than are the feet or trunk. Of course, this is the reason that the sensory "homunculus" contained in each nucleus appears to be a grotesque caricature of the body's surface (Woolsey and Fairman, 1946; Bombardieri *et al.*, 1975; Woolsey *et al.*, 1975).

In addition to the variation among vertebrates resulting from "Adrian's Rule," vertebrate somatosensory systems also vary widely because of differences in body size. For example, in some short-spined animals (such as frogs) there may be only 10 or 11 pairs of spinal nerves, while in long-spined animals (such as some sharks) the number of spinal roots can reach 100 (Ariëns Kappers *et al.*, 1936). This variation is related to the number of vertebrae, and, consequently, the number of access points to the spinal cord.

The somatosensory system also varies among vertebrates according to peculiarities of their skin. For example, the sensitive and hairy skin of mammals contains many more sensory nerve endings than the scaly skin of fish. In correspondence, mammals also have larger spinal roots, larger tracts ascending to the brain, and more neurons involved at each synapse (Bishop *et al.*, 1971; Rushton, 1951). Similarly, the shrunken dorsal column system in birds is related to the evolution of feathers and consequent reduction in the role of the skin as a sensory organ (Papez, 1929; Ariëns Kappers *et al.*, 1936). Clearly, this sort of variation is little more than another expression of Adrian's Rule.

Changes in body form have also been accompanied by variation in the somatosensory system. For example, the development of legs in the tetrapods is associated with an increase in size and differentiation in the somatosensory system, particularly in the prominence of the dorsal column system. This relationship can be seen by comparing snakes with other reptiles. Without legs and feet, the snake has its spinal nerves in the cervical and lumbar regions reduced in size with consequent reduction in the dorsal columns (Ebbesson, 1969). In contrast, the cervical and lumbar nerves and spinal segments are greatly expanded in large-legged animals—the so-called cervical and lumbar enlargements. In an extreme case, such as the extinct *Tyrannosaurus,* the massive hindlegs resulted in a lumbar enlargement large enough to be mistaken for a displaced or subsidiary brain (Elliot Smith, 1910). Obviously, these relationships are still another expression of Adrian's Rule.

In general, then, most of the variation in the somatosensory system of vertebrates conforms to Adrian's Rule in its widest sense, whether due to increased density of nerve endings or to increased body area: the greater the number of peripheral somatosensory nerves, the greater is their central representation. In the discussion of evolutionary trends in the somatosensory system that follows, this sweeping rule must be kept in mind, for many of the trends in mankind's lineage

R. BRUCE MASTERTON
AND K. K.
GLENDENNING

once thought to be indicative of some especially important rearrangement or reparcellation of central somatosensory pathways and connections are now known to be little more than the sort of variation expected from changes in body form and size, in the sensitivity of the skin, or in the use of the limbs and hands.

TRENDS IN THE EVOLUTION OF THE HUMAN SOMATOSENSORY SYSTEM

Although most of the differences in the central somatosensory system can be traced to differences in the number or density of sensory endings in the skin and therefore are merely an expression of Adrian's Rule, there have been some changes in the somatosensory system that are not so directly related. Most of these latter changes are in the relationship between the somatosensory and motor systems and have been discovered in the spinal cord. But it can be anticipated that as higher-level somatosensory structures become better understood, significant evolutionary modifications will probably be found there, too.

Quite beyond the changes in the spinal cord to accommodate large peripheral nerves, there are also a number of evolutionary changes that have taken place at the cytoarchitectonic level. To begin with, the motoneurons in lower vertebrates have much more widespread dendritic fields than they do in mammals (Joseph and Whitlock, 1968b). For example, in cyclostomes, motoneuron dendrites extend into the lateral column and their dorsal extension toward the dorsal horn is much more limited. Furthermore, in lower vertebrates (such as frogs) the incoming sensory fibers end in more dorsal laminae while in higher forms (such as monkeys) the sensory fibers descend to deeper levels, synapsing closer to the motoneuron cell bodies. As guessed by Herrick (1948), one result of this modification is that local reflex arcs have become more secure in higher vertebrates.

A second major evolutionary trend that seems too marked to be completely explained by Adrian's Rule is the progressive increase in the size of the somatosensory tracts ascending to the brain. This trend can be seen by comparing the relative amounts of white matter in the cervical segments of the cords of lower vs. higher vertebrates. For example, in cartilaginous fish the dorsal columns make up only 6% of the total white matter of the spinal cord compared to 39% in man (Ariëns Kappers et al., 1936).

This increase in the size of the ascending tracts has also resulted in a greater ratio between total white matter and total gray matter in the spinal cord of higher vertebrates. Since the number of *descending* motor fibers has increased as well, evidence for the concept of "encephalization" is obvious. There seems little question that along mankind's lineage the brain has become more and more involved in spinal cord function (Heffner and Masterton, 1975). Along with this trend toward encephalization, the brain stem and telencephalic targets of the ascending somatosensory fibers have become larger, better differentiated, and more clearly related to the variations in the density of sensory endings at the periphery.

For over a hundred years, comparisons of the somatosensory systems of vertebrates have served as the basis of theories of the evolution of the entire central nervous system and have resulted in a number of organizational principles, some true, some false. For example, the idea of progressive encephalization of the somatosensory and motor systems, popularized by Ariëns Kappers, remains uncontradicted by modern neuroanatomical, neurophysiological, and neurobehavioral methods. Higher vertebrates have more long fibers ascending from the spinal cord to the brain, and more long fibers descending from the brain to the spinal cord, and they suffer much more loss after spinal cord transection than do lower vertebrates. Certainly, these facts support the idea of encephalization in the vertebrate lineage leading to mankind.

However, in sharp contrast, the idea, once equally as popular as encephalization, that the "epicritic" dorsal column system is a new functional refinement overlying the older "protopathic" anterolateral column system is probably incorrect. This idea is apparently contradicted by the demonstration of a dorsal column system in the lowest vertebrates with the most generalized spinal cords (Ebbesson, 1976).

Similarly, more sweeping theories of the course of nervous system evolution engendered by comparisons of the somatosensory system in different species have also been contradicted. For example, the idea that the newer "lemniscal" pathways bypass older synaptic sites in order to gain a more direct route to the forebrain (again, based on the idea that the dorsal column system is a more recent development than the anterolateral system) is not a general principle, although it may be true in some limited situations (e.g., Strominger *et al.*, 1977).

In summary, several likely trends in the evolution of the somatosensory system of man can be deduced: throughout mankind's vertebrate lineage, there has been a new increase in the size of the long ascending fiber pathways and their associated nuclei. This increase seems to have depended, primarily, on specific changes in body form suggested by Adrian's Rule. Among these changes are the gradual increase in body size and the evolution of legs, soft skin, hair, and investigatory snouts, mouths, and hands. Accompanying these specific demands on the somatosensory system there seems to have been an additional trend toward encephalization—in the sense that the brain's involvement in spinal cord activity has increased more than would be expected on the basis of Adrian's rule. Beyond these gross changes, more subtle changes in the relationship between sensory and motor structures have also taken place: more and more direct local reflexes seem to have appeared.

GUSTATORY SYSTEM

In many respects the olfactory and gustatory systems have much in common (see Chapter 4). Nevertheless, gustation has been neurologically separate from olfaction since before the origin of vertebrates. Even in the lamprey, where there is no jaw to provide a barrier against more direct entry to the brain, the gustatory nerves follow entirely different paths than the olfactory nerve, entering the cranium far more caudally. Whatever the significance of the similarities and interactions among the two sensory systems, it is now clear that they maintain a distinct anatomical integrity over at least the first two or three synapses in the central nervous system. Therefore, in this chapter we use the term "gustation" to refer to that chemoreceptive sensory sytsem that is connected to the CNS via cranial nerves VII, IX, and X. With this strictly anatomical definition, all vertebrates have homologous gustatory systems (see Chapter 13).

COMMON PLAN

Although the gustatory system of vertebrates has not been investigated in nearly the detail as have most of the other sensory systems, several details of the common plan have already become evident (Fig. 4).

The portion of the *facial nerve* (CN7) concerned with gustation is the *chorda tympani,* which gains its name by passing close to the tympanic membrane on its way to the brain stem. It usually innervates the taste buds on the anterior two-thirds of the tongue. It also innervates the taste buds on the external surface of the body in the fish which have them (Atema, 1971; Todd *et al.,* 1967). The cell bodies of the chorda tympani lie in the *geniculate ganglion* and their axons terminate in the rostral part of *nucleus solitarius*—the site of the second-order gustatory neurons in the brain stem. Some of the neurons constituting the *glossopharyngeal nerve* (CN9) innervate taste buds situated caudally to those innervated by the chorda tympani—usually in the posterior one-third of the tongue. The cell bodies of the gustatory neurons in the glossopharyngeal nerve lie in the *petrosal ganglion* and their axons terminate in nucleus solitarius caudal to the terminations of the chorda

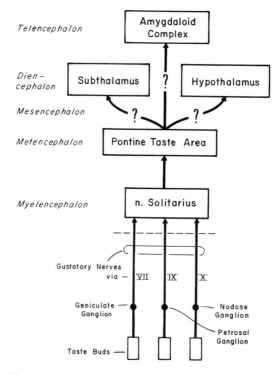

Fig. 4. Common plan of the vertebrate gustatory system.

tympani. Some neurons in the *vagal nerve* (CN10) also innervate taste buds still more caudally situated, i.e., in the esophageal and soft palate region. The cell bodies of the gustatory branch of the vagal nerve lie in the *nodose ganglion* and send their axons to the most caudal region of nucleus solitarius. Therefore, the VIIth, IXth, and Xth cranial nerves innervate successively more caudal receptors in the mouth and terminate in successively more caudal regions of nucleus solitarius.

Nucleus solitarius is the principal second-order gustatory nucleus of the central nervous system. It extends from bulbar levels of the brain stem to the cervical levels of the spinal cord. Both ascending and descending second-order pathways arise from it. The descending fibers terminate ipsilaterally in the medial funicular nucleus and dorsal reticular substance of the spinal cord (Finger, 1976). The ascending pathway follows the medial lemniscus to the so-called *pontine taste area,* which consists of a diffuse population of cells in the pontine tegmentum (Norgren and Leonard, 1973).

Third-order fibers course rostrally from the pontine taste area to the subthalamus, hypothalamus, and amygdaloid complex (Norgren, 1976). It is noteworthy that the gustatory fibers terminate in the central divisions of the amygdaloid complex—those which do *not* receive olfactory or cortical input (see the previous section on olfaction). This gustatory division of the amygdala, in turn, projects back to nucleus solitarius, as well as to the reticular formation and lateral hypothalamus (Hopkins and Holstege, 1976; Lawrence and Kuypers, 1968).

In addition to the projections to subthalamus, hypothalamus, and amygdala, the pontine taste area in mammals projects to the medial division of the ventroposterior nucleus (VPM) of the dorsal thalamus and from there to neocortex. However, a similar projection in nonmammals is yet to be demonstrated.

Variations in the Vertebrate Gustatory System

Too little is known about the gustatory system in nonmammals to allow description of its range of variation. However, at the periphery, there is considerable variation in the number and distribution of taste buds. For example, few taste buds, if any, are present in snakes and sea gulls, a bat has 4 times more than a starling, a human 10 times more than a bat, and a catfish 10 times more than a human (Kare, 1971). Although this wide variation is undoubtedly related to food acquisition, only a loose relationship with an animal's degree of omnivorousness now seems evident.

In the central nervous system there is less variation than at the periphery, but even here nucleus solitarius varies widely in size and form across classes of vertebrates. For example, in fish with a large number of taste buds, an immense n. solitarius clearly worthy of the term "facial lobe" is evident (Herrick, 1944). This kind of variation is reminiscent of that seen in the somatosensory system—the variation in size and elaboration of the central structures following the variation in the number of receptors. However, it is not yet clear whether this kind of variation exists at higher-order gustatory targets (e.g., the pontine taste area).

In general, the lack of information about the taste system in nonmammals renders premature a discussion of the nature of its variation.

R. BRUCE MASTERTON
AND K. K.
GLENDENNING

Although entirely undocumented, the evolution of a generalized chemoreceptive system in marine animals and the advantage of its further differentiation into separate olfactory and gustatory systems seem evident. However, the transition from life in water to life in air undoubtedly brought with it marked changes in the gustatory as well as the olfactory system. Taste buds became completely confined to the mouth so that food had to enter the mouth to be tasted. Certainly, this modification physically separated gustatory and olfactory systems even further and it seems likely that they may have become more psychologically separable, too (Boudreau, 1974).

Centrally, the forebrain maintained direct olfactory input while any gustatory input to the forebrain had to await the evolution of central pathways from hindbrain to forebrain. Although it has not yet been determined whether or not nonmammals possess gustatory pathways and gustatory centers in the telencephalon other than the amygdala, mammals certainly do and this difference may be real (Benjamin, 1963). However, until the higher-order gustatory connections of nonmammals have been adequately investigated, a serious discussion of evolutionary trends is precluded.

Vestibular System

Unlike most of the other sensory systems of vertebrates which originated before the origin of Vertebrates, the evolutionary development of the vestibular system probably began at the time of, or slightly after, the origin of Vertebrates. The probable sequence of its development can be seen in the labyrinth of extant mammals beginning with the jawless hagfish and lamprey, which have only one semicircular canal, progressing through cartilaginous fish, which have two joined canals and a third independent one, and ending in bony fish and amphibians, which have virtually the same complement and arrangement of canals, utricle, and saccule as the remainder of vertebrates. Details of the origin and development of the vertebrate labyrinth can be found in the review by Baird (1974).

Much like other sensory systems, however, the central vestibular system has fewer variations than the peripheral apparatus in the same animals. In lamprey, the general form of the central system is already laid down with mostly ipsilateral projections to the vestibular nuclei and the cerebellum (Rubinson, 1974). The targets of the vestibular nerve in fish remain quite separate from those areas which later, in amphibians, are occupied by auditory projections (Wever, 1976). However, the severe and inescapable selective pressure on the vestibular system to provide positional and gravitational sense despite radical changes in modes of locomotion has resulted in a large degree of differentiation in each class of vertebrates that appeared. For example, in the lamprey, the second-order vestibular-oculomotor connections are already well established but the vestibulocerebellar and vestibulospinal projections are meager (Rubinson, 1974). In jawed fish, and then later in the tetrapods, the spinal and cerebellar targets show a much higher degree of differentiation, and along with them the vestibulocerebellar and vestibulospinal systems are differentiated sufficiently to take on the characteristics of the mammalian system (Gregory, 1972; Larsell, 1967). Thus the functional intimacy of the vestibular and motor systems is manifested throughout vertebrates as a mutual anatomical differentiation. As each motor system developed, the vestibular connections to that system also developed (see Chapter 9).

COMMON PLAN

The plan of the vertebrate vestibular system is shown in Fig. 5. The *vestibular nerve* (or vestibular branch of the VIIIth nerve) consists of first-order fibers whose peripheral processes end at the base of *hair cells* in the labyrinth and whose central processes end either in the vestibular nuclei or the cerebellum.

The second-order fibers which arise from neurons of the vestibular nuclei project either contralaterally to the vestibular nuclei of the other side, bilaterally to the cerebellum (Gregory, 1972; Mehler, 1972), or via the medial longitudinal fasciculus bilaterally to the oculomotor, trochlear, and abducens nuclei (Fuller and Ebbesson, 1973a). Other secondary vestibular fibers descend in the spinal cord as the *vestibulospinal tract*.

Because of the obviously motor nature of most of the targets of the second-order vestibular fibers, third-order fibers are usually subsumed under a motor system rubric.

VARIATIONS IN THE VERTEBRATE VESTIBULAR SYSTEM

The general plan of the vestibular system is common to vertebrates from lamprey to mammal. However, the size and differentiation of various second-order pathways are markedly different in the several classes. Although the vestibular nucleus of adult lampreys and fishes is by no means small relative to the rest of their hindbrain, its homologue in amphibians is much larger, extending caudally to the level of exit of the XIIth nerve (Fuller, 1974). In reptiles, the primary

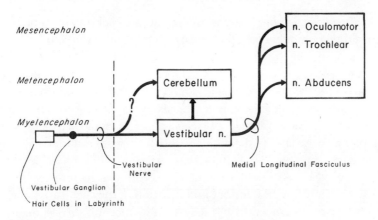

Fig. 5. Common plan of the vertebrate vestibular system.

R. BRUCE MASTERTON
AND K. K.
GLENDENNING

vestibular projections and their targets are still more differentiated so that fibers originating in clearly separate parts of the labyrinth project to clearly different parts of the vestibular nuclei (Leake, 1974). This differential projection is paralleled by distinct differentiation within the vestibular nuclei themselves. From an indistinct three-way subdivision in lampreys and fishes, the vestibular nuclei have a clearly partitioned six-way subdivision in crocodilians and lizards (Leake, 1974; DeFina and Webster, 1974). This differentiation is seen even more clearly in birds (Boord and Karten, 1974), and in mammals. Although further interclass and interorder differences beyond differentiation undoubtedly exist, a clear picture of the vestibular system in nonmammals is only just beginning to emerge.

TRENDS IN THE EVOLUTION OF THE HUMAN VESTIBULAR SYSTEM

Perhaps more than any other vertebrate sensory system, the vestibular system in its evolution is characterized by progressive differentiation. As the motor systems for locomotion evolved first toward the tetrapod form, then the mammalian and finally the upright hominoid form, the demands placed on the vestibular system were severe and direct. As a result, changes in the degree of differentiation of the vestibular system closely parallel changes in the motor systems. Large and intimate connections of the vestibular system to the oculomotor system are as old as the two systems themselves. As tetrapod locomotion evolved, the cerebellum and vestibulocerebellar projections enlarged and differentiated as did the direct vestibulospinal projections for the maintenance of posture. This increase in the motor systems and the vestibular input to them occurred several more times in succession as the demands of a large, upright body and the speed and efficiency of its locomotion were served. Other than this overall trend toward expansion and differentiation that paralleled the development of larger and more differentiated motor systems, not enough is yet known about the comparative anatomy of the system to draw more detailed conclusions.

AUDITORY SYSTEM

Unlike the other sensory systems, the vertebrate cochlea and central auditory system constitute a uniquely tetrapod feature. Therefore, it probably first arose in amphibians as they left the sea to begin a life in air. To be sure, preamphibians, like most fish today, could probably respond to underwater sounds emanating from a nearby source (i.e., near-field sound) through use of their lateral line system for detecting water movement. It is also possible that the preamphibians, like teleosts today, were capable of responding to some far-field sounds by detecting pressure variations through use of their swim bladder. Although the lateral line and swim bladder system have several points of analogy with the tetrapod system, the peripheral structures involved are in no way homologous (Wever, 1976). Therefore, the history and function of the cochlea-type or tetrapodian auditory system begin with amphibians, and hence it is the last major sensory system to have evolved.

The sources of selective pressure on the ear and auditory system of extant tetrapods are probably too numerous and varied to be specified. However, the system's exquisite sensitivity to transient sounds—stimuli generated by transient movements—leads to the idea that before anything else the auditory system is an "event or movement detector." Insofar as most natural sounds are caused by other animals, the system thus serves as an animal detector (Pumphrey, 1950). This fundamental function of the auditory system can be readily seen in the orienting reaction of animals to an unexpected sound, even one of low intensity (e.g., a person's reaction to a faint floorboard squeak in an otherwise empty house) (Masterton and Diamond, 1973).

Since transient sounds are usually perceived as indicating the presence of other animals in the vicinity, the selective pressures on hearing include pressure on the localization and identification of the intruder as well as on more sensitive hearing (Capranica, 1976). These sources of selective pressure, in turn, give rise to pressures for a wider frequency range of hearing and a more refined spectral analysis by the ear and, finally, for communication with conspecifics and for identifying the meaning of messages (Marler, 1957). Presumably, it is these persistent sources of selective pressures that account for most of the transformations of the ear and central auditory system since their origin in the ancient amphibians.

Origins

The origins of the cochlea and its relationship with the lateral line, labyrinth, and ear of fish have been a matter of argument for over a century. However, it is now almost certain that a sound-sensitive inner ear arose not from the lateral line, as was once thought, but as a specialization of the vestibular apparatus (Wever, 1976). Although the very few amphibians still extant have an unusual variant of the cochlea, its continuity at least from the origin of reptiles is readily apparent.

The origin of the central auditory system seems to have occurred as suddenly as the origin of the ear in the sense that the central system of amphibians has clear homologues with that of tetrapods of later origin, at least through the midbrain, which is as high as the central auditory system in amphibians has presently been traced (Capranica, 1976). Although the difference in degree of differentiation between the central system in amphibians and that in the later tetrapods is extreme, homologous structures prevail (Boord, 1969). But because the few amphibians still extant have an unusual cochlea and their central system has not yet been explored in suitable detail, the remainder of this account is based mostly on reptiles, mammals, and birds (*cf.* Karten, 1967, 1968; Boord, 1969; Chapters 12 and 13).

Common Plan

The common plan of the tetrapod auditory system is shown in Fig. 6. The cell bodies of the first-order fibers lie near the cochlea with their distal processes terminating at the base of *hair cells* in the cochlea that serve as receptors. The proximal processes or axons of these cells form the *cochlear division* of the VIIIth cranial nerve and terminate in the cochlear nucleus.

The *cochlear nucleus* is divisible into two major parts in birds and reptiles and into three major parts in mammals. The second-order fibers arising there project to the superior olivary complex, the nuclei of the lateral lemniscus, and the inferior colliculus (see Chapter 11).

The *superior olivary complex* is also divisible into many parts in mammals: superior olivary nuclei, nuclei of the trapezoid body, and periolivary and preolivary nuclei. However, exact nonmammalian homologues of these, and still more refined subdivisions, have not yet been identified. Nevertheless, the three chief nuclei of the superior olivary complex, namely the lateral superior olive, the medial nucleus of the trapezoid body, and the medial superior olive, seem to be homologous, respectively, with the lateral and medial parts of the superior olive and, possibly, nucleus laminaris in reptiles and birds (Parks and Rubel, 1975).

The *nucleus of the lateral lemniscus* is usually divided into a dorsal and a ventral division in mammals, but in most mammals and in all reptiles and birds yet studied it is an almost continuous cluster of cell bodies scattered along the length of the lemniscus from medulla to inferior colliculus.

The mammalian *inferior colliculus* is the homologue of the nonmammalian *torus semicircularis.* In mammals, it is also subdivisible into three or four parts, two of which receive descending fibers from the forebrain en route to the superior olivary complex (Rockel and Jones, 1973*a,b;* Morest, 1966; Diamond *et al.,* 1969; van Noort, 1969). The ascending efferents of the inferior colliculus project to the

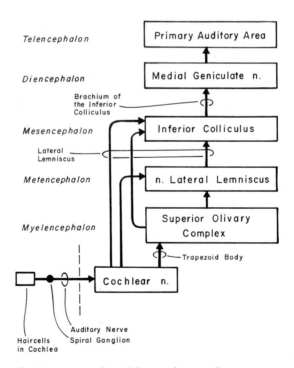

Fig. 6. Common plan of the vertebrate auditory system.

thalamus. In mammals the thalamic target is the medial geniculate body, while in birds and reptiles its homologue is called nucleus ovoidalis and nucleus reuniens, respectively (Karten, 1968; Foster, 1974, 1976). These thalamic targets, in turn, project to the telencephalon (see Chapter 12).

The *medial geniculate* in mammals is divisible into at least three parts (ventral, dorsal, and medial). The ventral division projects to primary or core *auditory cortex,* the other divisions project to a belt of secondary auditory cortex surrounding the core (Raczkowski *et al.,* 1976; see Chapter 12). The mammalian medial geniculate also projects to the putamen, which may provide a more direct line with motor centers. In birds and reptiles, the medial geniculate projects not to neocortex (which is absent in these classes) but to the *dorsal ventricular ridge*—an outcropping of what was once thought to be a homologue of the mammalian basal ganglia but is now thought to be (on the basis of afferents such as these) a precursor of neocortex (e.g., Nauta and Karten, 1970).

In general, then, the ascending auditory system of mammals seems to be mostly a better-differentiated replica of the same system found in birds and reptiles. Although the auditory structures in mammals are much more differentiated than in nonmammals and consequently look quite different under microscopic examination, the similarity of their connections is clear.

Nonmammalian homologues of the mammalian descending auditory system have not yet been extensively studied. However, fibers that originate in the brain stem and terminate in the cochlea are known to exist in reptiles and in birds as well as in mammals. Whether or not this system extends all the way from forebrain to ear, as it does in mammals, remains to be seen.

VARIATIONS IN THE VERTEBRATE AUDITORY SYSTEM

Possibly because the auditory system is a relatively recent acquisition of vertebrates, there appears to be a good deal of variation in the common plan among the tetrapod classes. Most of this variation lies in degree of differentiation, but not all of it. For example, mammals with a medial superior olive are capable of resolving binaural time differences to allow them to localize sounds, while animals lacking a medial superior olive seem to be incapable of detecting binaural time differences (Masterton *et al.,* 1975). Similarly, some reptiles (e.g., caiman) have a nucleus laminaris as part of their hindbrain auditory system while others (e.g., the iguana) do not (Foster, 1976; Leake, 1974).

Despite these examples of apparently qualitative differences, however, the most striking differences in vertebrate auditory systems are in their size and degree of differentiation. For example, we have seen that the cochlear nuclei of mammals have three major subdivisions and those of nonmammals two; but within these major subdivisions, mammals have from seven to thirteen distinctive cell types while nonmammals seem to have but three or four (Brawer *et al.,* 1974; Harrison and Warr, 1962; Harrison and Feldman, 1970; Caspary, 1972).

The superior olivary complex of mammals is also more differentiated than its homologue in nonmammals. The mammalian version is easily divisible into from five to seven discrete nuclei while reptiles and birds have only two or three

R. BRUCE MASTERTON
AND K. K.
GLENDENNING

depending on whether nucleus laminaris is included within it (e.g., see Parks and Rubel, 1975). Similarly, a large number of subparts occur in other structures of the mammalian auditory system. For example, in mammals the inferior colliculus has either three or four subdivisions, the medial geniculate from three to seven, and the auditory cortex from three to six (Rockel and Jones, 1973*a,b*; Morest, 1965; Woolsey, 1960). The homologues of these structures in nonmammals are not easily subdivided at all (Potter, 1965). Although it can be anticipated that the nonmammalian structures may admit some subdivision under closer study, the differences in degree of differentiation between mammals and nonmammals are easily visible even to the untrained eye. In general, therefore, what at first glance seems to be a great deal of variation on the common plan turns out to be mostly accounted for by differences in degree of differentiation.

Trends in the Evolution of the Human Auditory System

The major changes in the auditory system in man's lineage can be subdivided into three subtopics, each of which has become a science in itself: the middle ear, the inner ear, and the central system. The changes in the middle and inner ear and their effect on the sensitivity and range of hearing, particularly the mammalian ability to hear very high frequencies, are well discussed by Manley (1972), by Wever and Werner (1970), and by Masterton *et al.* (1969). Here, only changes in the central system will be discussed.

As has already been described, most of the differences between mammalian and nonmammalian central auditory systems are to be found in the much greater degree of differentiation of the mammalian system. This difference seems to parallel the more dramatic changes in the middle and inner ear.

As the ear transformed and became more sensitive, particularly to high frequencies, the sounds that could be received were amenable to the extraction of more and more useful kinds of information concerning the animals producing them. For example, the localization of a sound source by amphibians is probably confined to scanning for the direction of maximum intensity or homing by proceeding up (or down) the intensity gradient (Feng and Capranica, 1976). This primitive localization technique requires little central analytic apparatus, but it means that for a sound source to be localizable it has to emit continuously or repetitively. Thus it is sufficient for the finding of a noise-making mate or slow-moving prey, but not very good for avoiding predators (see Capranica, 1976).

The avoidance of predators probably provided the selective pressure for the instantaneous localization of brief sounds—sounds too brief to allow localization by homing or by scanning with directionally sensitive ears. For this obviously superior technique of localization, central analytic apparatus is required because only a comparison of the spectrum or timing of the sound arriving at the two ears contains sufficient information. This process probably was the source of selective pressure on the differentiation of the superior olivary complex and the parts of the cochlear nucleus supplying it. It resulted in the differentiation of the lateral and medial superior olive in mammals for the analysis of binaural spectral and time disparities, respectively; and probably it is the pressure behind the differentiation of nucleus laminaris in reptiles and birds, although this function of nucleus laminaris has not yet been confirmed (Masterton *et al.*, 1975; Parks and Rubel, 1975).

The selective pressure for the differentiation of still higher central auditory structures in man's lineage and its effect on hearing are not known because the function of these structures is not yet known in any vertebrate. However, there is one structural trend only recently discovered and that is in the anthropoid segment of mankind's lineage. As has already been described, in mammals and apparently in nonmammals as well the cochlear nucleus (i.e., the second-order auditory neurons) projects only to the hindbrain (e.g., superior olives, nuclei of lateral lemniscus) and midbrain (inferior colliculus or torus semicircularis). However, in chimpanzee (and presumably, then, in man) some of the fibers of the cochlear nucleus bypass these hindbrain and midbrain targets to terminate directly in the medial geniculate nucleus of the thalamus (Strominger *et al.*, 1977). This means that in chimps, at least, cells in the auditory cortex may be fourth-order neurons instead of fifth-, sixth-, or seventh-order as in other mammals. This bypassing of lower cell groups to synapse directly in the thalamus and then cortex is reminiscent of the idea of corticalization because it can be argued that this new acquisition of the auditory system provides an express line to cortex for "conscious appreciation," etc. Although this may be the case, it is more likely that the bypassing of lower auditory centers is not so dramatic in its significance. Since motor activity in man's lineage certainly came to depend more and more on neocortex, as has been described above, the more direct route of auditory fibers to cortex is evidence only of a more direct route to the predominant motor system in anthropoids. Only insofar as one wishes to equate this trend with a trend toward increased consciousness of hearing does the evidence speak to the latter issue at all (see Chapter 12).

In summary, very little is known about the progressive differentiation in the auditory system that took place in man's lineage except for a few nuclei in the superior olivary complex. However, it should be recognized that this progressive differentiation was not confined to man's lineage—every mammal with a well-developed ear and auditory system shows an equally high level of differentiation, and some superauditory orders such as Chiroptera (bats), Cetacea (whales and porpoises), and Carnivora (cats, dogs, raccoons, etc.) have even better-differentiated auditory systems than man. Therefore, man's auditory system, although far from humble, is also far from superior to that of other mammals (Masterton *et al.*, 1969).

REFERENCES

Adrian, E. D. Double representation of the feet in the sensory cortex of the cat. *J. Physiol. (London),* 1940, *98*, 16.
Allison, A. C. The morphology of the olfactory system in the vertebrates. *Biol. Rev.,* 1953, *28*, 195–244.
Allison, A. C., and Warwick, R. T. T. Quantitative observations on the olfactory system of the rabbit. *Brain,* 1949, *72*, 186–197.
Allman, J. Evolution of the visual system in the early primates. In J. M. Sprague and A. N. Epstein

(eds.), *Progress in Psychobiology and Physiological Psychology*. Academic Press, New York, 1977, pp. 1–53.

Allman, J. M., and Kaas, J. H. Representation of the visual field in striate and adjoining cortex of the owl monkey *(Aotus trivirgatus). Brain Res.,* 1971, *35*, 89–106.

Allman, J. M., and Kaas, J. H. The organization of the second visual area (VII) in the owl monkey: A second order transformation of the visual hemifield. *Brain Res.,* 1974, *76*, 247–265.

Allman, J. M., Kaas, J. H., and Lane, R. H. The middle temporal visual area (MT) in the bush baby, *Galago senegalensis. Brain Res.,* 1973, *57*, 197–202.

Andres, K. H. Anatomy and ultra-structure of the olfactory bulb in fish, amphibians, reptiles, birds, and mammals. In G. E. W. Wolstenholme and J. Knight (eds.), *Taste and Smell in Vertebrates.* Churchill, London, 1970.

Ariëns Kappers, C. U., Huber, G. C., and Crosby, E. C. *The Comparative Anatomy of the Nervous System of Vertebrates, Including Man.* Hafner, New York, 1936.

Atema, J. Structure and functions of the sense of taste in the catfish *(Ictalurus natalis). Brain Behav. Evol.,* 1971, *4*, 273–294.

Baird, I. L. Some aspects of the comparative anatomy and evolution of the inner ear in submammalian vertebrates. *Brain Behav. Evol.,* 1974, *10*, 11–36.

Barlow, H. B., Hill, R. M., and Levick, W. R. Retinal ganglion cells responding selectively to direction and speed of image motion in the rabbit. *J. Physiol. (London),* 1964, *173*, 377–407.

Barrington E. J. W., and Jefferies, R. P. S. (eds.). *Protochordates: Symposium of the Zoological Society of London.* Academic Press, London, 1975.

Benjamin, R. M. Some thalamic and cortical mechanisms of taste. In Y. Zotterman (ed.), *Olfaction and Taste.* Macmillan, New York, 1963, pp. 309–329.

Berkley, M. A. Some comments on visual acuity and its relation to eye structure. In R. B. Masterton, M. E. Bitterman, C. B. G. Campbell, and N. Hotten (eds.), *Evolution of Brain and Behavior in Vertebrates.* Lawrence Erlbaum Assoc., Hillsdale, N. J., 1976, pp. 73–88.

Bertmar, G. The vertebrate nose, remarks on its structural and functional adaptation and evolution. *Evolution,* 1969, *23*, 131–152.

Bishop, G. H., Clare, M. H., and Landau, W. M. The relation of axon sheath thickness to fiber size in the central nervous system of vertebrates. *Int. J. Neurosci.,* 1971, *2*, 69–78.

Bombardieri, R. A., Jr., Johnson, J. I., Jr., and Campos, G. B. Species differences in mechanosensory projections from the mouth to the ventrobasal thalamus. *J. Comp. Neurol.,* 1975, *163*, 41–64.

Boord, R. L. The anatomy of the avian auditory system. *Ann. N.Y. Acad. Sci.,* 1969, *167*, 186–198.

Boord, R. L., and Karten, H. J. The distribution of primary lagenar fibers within the vestibular nuclear complex of the pigeon. *Brain Behav. Evol.,* 1974, *10*, 228–235.

Boudreau, J. C. Neural encoding in cat geniculate ganglion tongue units. *Chem. Senses Flavor,* 1974, *1*, 41–51.

Brawer, J. R., Morest, D. K., and Kane, E. C. The neuronal architecture of the cochlear nucleus of the cat. *J. Comp. Neurol.* 1974, *155*, 251–300.

Broadwell, R. D. Olfactory relationships of the telencephalon and diencephalon in the rabbit. I. An autoradiographic study of the efferent connections of the main and accessory olfactory bulbs. *J. Comp. Neurol.,* 1975, *163*, 329–346.

Cain, W. S. Differential sensitivity for smell: "Noise" at the nose. *Science,* 1977, *195*, 796–798.

Cajal, S. R. Y. *Histologie du Système Nerveux de l'Homme et des Vertébrés.* Maloine, Paris, 1911.

Capranica, R. R. Morphology and physiology of the auditory system. In R. Llinás and W. Precht (eds.), *Frog Neurobiology.* Springer-Verlag, New York, 1976, pp. 551–575.

Casagrande, V. A., Harting, J. K., Hall, W. C., Diamond, I. T., and Martin, G. F. Superior colliculus of the tree shrew: A structural and functional subdivision into superficial and deep structures. *Science,* 1972, *177*, 444–447.

Caspary, D. Classification of subpopulations of neurons in the cochlear nuclei of the kangaroo rat. *Exp. Neurol.,* 1972, *37*, 131–151.

Cowan, W. M., Gottlieb, D. I., Hendrickson, A. E., Price, J. L. and Woolsey, T. A. The autoradiographic demonstration of axonal connections in the central nervous system. *Brain Res.,* 1972, *37*, 21–51.

Crescitellia, F., and Pollack, J. D. Color vision in the antelope ground squirrel. *Science,* 1965, *150*, 1316–1318.

Darian-Smith, I. The trigeminal system. In *Handbook of Sensory Physiology,* Vol. II: *Somatosensory System.* Springer-Verlag, New York, 1973, pp. 271–314.

DeFina, A. V., and Webster, D. B. Projections of the intraotic ganglion to the medullary nuclei in the tegu lizard, *Tupinambis nigropunctatus. Brain Behav. Evol.,* 1974, *10*, 197–211.

Diamond, I. T., Jones, E. G., and Powell, T. P. S. The projection of the auditory cortex upon the diencephalon and brainstem in the cat. *Brain Res.*, 1969, *15*, 305–340.

Diamond, I. T., Snyder, M., Killackey, H., Jane, J., and Hall, W. C. Thalamocortical projections in the tree shrew *(Tupaia glis)*. *J. Comp. Neurol.*, 1970, *139*, 273–306.

Doty, R. L. *Mammalian Olfaction, Reproductive Processes and Behavior.* Academic Press, New York, 1976.

Dowling, J. Organization of vertebrate retinas. *Invest. Ophthalmol.*, 1970, *9*, 655–680.

Dubin, M. The inner plexiform layer of the vertebrate retina: A quantitative and comparative study. *J. Comp. Neurol.*, 1970, *140*, 479–505.

Duke-Elder, S. The anatomy of the visual system. In S. Duke-Elder (ed.), *System of Ophthalmology*, Vol. 2. Kimpton, London, 1961.

Dunn, J., and Matze, H. A. Efferent fiber connections of the marmoset *(Oedipomidas oedipus)* trigeminal nucleus caudalis. *J. Comp. Neurol.*, 1968, *133*, 429–438.

Easton, D. M. Garfish olfactory nerve: Easily accessible source of numerous long homogeneous nonmyelinated axons. *Science*, 1971, *172*, 952–955.

Ebbesson, S. O. E. Ascending axon degeneration following hemisection of the spinal cord in the tegu lizard *(Tupinambis nigropunctatus)*. *Brain Res.*, 1967, *5*, 178–206.

Ebbesson, S. O. E. Brain stem afferents from the spinal cord in a sample of reptilian and amphibian species. *Ann. N.Y. Acad. Sci.*, 1969, *167*, 80–101.

Ebbesson, S. O. E. New insights into the organization of the shark brain. *Comp. Biochem. Physiol.*, 1972, *42*, 121–129.

Ebbesson, S. O. E. Morphology of the spinal cord. In R. Llinás and W. Precht (eds.), *Frog Neurobiology.* Springer-Verlag, New York, 1976, pp. 688–706.

Ebbesson, S. O. E., and Northcutt, R. G. Neurology of anamniotic vertebrates. In R. B. Masterton *et al.* (eds.), *Evolution of Brain and Behavior of Vertebrates.* Lawrence Erlbaum Assoc., Hillsdale, New Jersey, 1976, pp. 115–146.

Ebbesson, S. O. E., and Schroeder, D. M. Connections of the nurse shark's telencephalon. *Science*, 1971, *173*, 254–256.

Edwards, S. B., Rosenquist, A. C., and Palmer, L. A. An autoradiographic study of ventral lateral geniculate projections in the cat. *Brain Res.*, 1974, *72*, 282–287.

Eleftheriou, B. E. (ed.). *The Neurobiology of the Amygdala.* Plenum, New York, 1972.

Elliot Smith, G. Some problems relating to the evolution of the brain. *Lancet,* 1910, *1*.

Feng, A. S., and Capranica, R. R. Sound localization in anurans. I. Evidence of binaural interaction in dorsal medullary nucleus of bull frogs *(Rana catesbeiana)*. *J. Neurophysiol.*, 1976, *39*, 871–881.

Finger, T. E. Gustatory pathways in the bullhead catfish. I. Connection of the anterior ganglion. *J. Comp. Neurol.*, 1976, *165*, 513–526.

Fink, R. P., and Heimer, L. Two methods for selective silver impregnation of degenerating axons and their synaptic endings in the central nervous system. *Brain Res.*, 1967, *4*, 369–374.

Foster, R. E. The ascending brainstem auditory pathway in a reptile, *Iguana iguana. Anat. Rec.*, 1974, *178*, 357.

Foster, R. E. The organization of central acoustic pathways in a reptile, *Iguana iguana.* Ph.D. dissertation, Duke University, 1976.

Fox, R., Lehmkuhle, S. W., and Westendorf, D. H. Falcon visual acuity. *Science*, 1976a, *192*, 263–265.

Fox, R., Lehmkuhle, S. W., and Bush, R. C. Stereoscopic vision in the falcon *(Falco sparverius)*. Paper presented at Society for Neuroscience, Toronto, 1976b.

Fuller, P. M. Projections of the vestibular nuclear complex in the bullfrog *(Rana catesbeiana)*. *Brain Behav. Evol.*, 1974, *10*, 157–169.

Fuller, P. M., and Ebbesson, S. O. E. Central connections of the vestibular nuclear complex in the bullfrog *(Rana catesbeiana)*. *Anat. Rec.*, 1973a, *175*, 325.

Fuller, P. M., and Ebbesson, S. O. E. Central projections of the trigeminal nerve in the bullfrog *(Rana catesbeiana)*. *J. Comp. Neurol.*, 1973b, *152*, 193–200.

Glendenning, K. K., Hall, J. A., Diamond, I. T., and Hall, W. C. The pulvinar nucleus of *Galago senegalensis. J. Comp. Neurol.*, 1975, *161*, 419–458.

Glickstein, M. The vertebrate eye. In R. B. Masterton, M. E. Bitterman, C. B. G. Campbell, and N. Hotten (eds.), *Evolution of Brain and Behavior in Vertebrates.* Lawrence Erlbaum Assoc., Hillsdale, N.J., 1976, pp. 53–72.

Graeber, R. C., Schroeder, D. M., Jane, J. A., and Ebbesson, S. O. E. The importance of telencephalic structures in visual discrimination learning in nurse sharks. Society for Neuroscience, Second Annual Meeting, 1972.

Graybiel, A. M. Visuo-cerebellar and cerebello-visual connections involving the ventral lateral geniculate nucleus. *Exp. Brain Res.*, 1974, *20*, 303–306.

Graziadei, P. P. C. The olfactory organ of vertebrates: A survey. In R. Bellairs and E. G. Gray (eds.), *Essays on the Nervous System; a Festschrift for Professor J. Z. Young.* Clarendon Press, Oxford, 1974, pp. 191–222.

Gregory, K. M. Central projections of the eighth nerve in frogs. *Brain Behav. Evol.,* 1972, *5,* 70–88.

Grether, W. F. Color vision and color blindness in monkeys. *Comp. Psychol. Monogr.,* 1939, *15,* 1–38.

Groenewegem, H. J., Boesten, A. J. P., and Voogd, J. The dorsal column nuclear projections to the nucleus ventralis posterior lateralis thalami and the inferior olive in the cat: An autoradiographic study. *J. Comp. Neurol.,* 1975, *162,* 505–518.

Gross, G. W., and Beidler, L. M. Fast axoplasmic transport in the c-fibers of the garfish olfactory nerve. *J. Neurobiol.,* 1973, *4,* 413–428.

Gulley, R. L., Cochran, M., and Ebbesson, S. O. E. The visual connections of the adult flatfish, *Achirus lineatus. J. Comp. Neurol.,* 1975, *162,* 309–320.

Gwyn, D. G., and Waldron, H. A. A nucleus in the dorsolateral funiculus of the spinal cord of the rat. *Brain Res.,* 1968, *10,* 342–351.

Gwyn, D. G., and Waldron, H. A. Observations on the morphology of a nucleus in the dorsolateral funiculus of the spinal cord of the guinea-pig, rabbit, ferret and cat. *J. Comp. Neurol.,* 1969, *136,* 233–236.

Ha, H. Cervicothalamic tract in the rhesus monkey. *Exp. Neurol.,* 1971, *33,* 205–212.

Hagg, S. and Ha, H. Cervicothalamic tract in the dog. *J. Comp. Neurol.,* 1970, *139,* 357–374.

Hall, W. C., and Ebner, F. F. Thalamo-telencephalic projections in a turtle *(Pseudemys scripta). Anat. Rec.,* 1969, *193,* 163.

Harrison, J. M., and Feldman, M. L. Anatomical aspects of the cochlear nucleus and superior olivary complex. In W. D. Neff (ed.), *Contributions to Sensory Physiology,* Vol. IV. Academic Press, New York, 1970, pp. 95–142.

Harrison, J. M., and Warr, W. B. A study of the cochlear nuclei and ascending auditory pathways of the medulla. *J. Comp. Neurol.,* 1962, *119,* 341–380.

Harting, J. K., Glendenning, K. K., Diamond, I. T., and Hall, W. C. Evolution of the primate visual system: Anterograde degeneration studies of the tecto-pulvinar system. *Am. J. Phys. Anthropol.,* 1973, *38,* 383–392.

Hayhow, W. R. The cytoarchitecture of the lateral geniculate body in the cat in relation to the distribution of crossed and uncrossed optic fibers. *J. Comp. Neurol.,* 1958, *1,* 110.

Hayle, T. H. A comparative study of spinocerebellar systems in three classes of poikilothermic vertebrates. *J. Comp. Neurol.,* 1973, *149,* 477–495.

Heffner, R., and Masterton, B. Variation in form of the pyramidal tract and its relationship to digital dexterity. *Brain Behav. Evol.,* 1975, *12,* 161–200.

Heimer, L. Synaptic distribution of centripetal and centrifugal nerve fibers in the olfactory system of the rat. *J. Anat.,* 1968, *103,* 413–432.

Heimer, L. The secondary olfactory connections in mammals, reptiles and sharks. *Ann. N.Y. Acad. Sci.,* 1969, *167,* 129–147.

Heimer, L. The olfactory connections of the diencephalon in the rat. *Brain Behavo. Evol.,* 1972, *6,* 484–523.

Herrick, C. J. The fasciculus solitarius and its connections in amphibians and fishes. *J. Comp. Neurol.,* 1944, *81,* 307–331.

Herrick, C. J. *The Brain of the Tiger Salamander, Ambystoma tigrinum.* The University of Chicago Press, Chicago, 1948.

Hodos, W., and Karten, H. J. Visual intensity and pattern discrimination deficits after lesions of ectostriatum in pigeons. *J. Comp. Neurol.,* 1970, *140,* 53–68.

Hodos, W., Karten, H. J., and Bonbright, J. C., Jr. Visual intensity and pattern discrimination after lesions of the thalamofugal visual pathway in pigeons. *J. Comp. Neurol.,* 1973, *148,* 447–468.

Hopkins, D. A., and Holstege, G. Central amygdaloid nucleus projections to the lower brainstem in the cat: A horseradish peroxidase and autoradiographic study. *Anat. Rec.,* 1976, *184,* 432.

Ingle, D. Behavioral correlates of central visual function in anurans. In R. Llinás and W. Precht (eds.), *Frog Neurobiology.* Springer-Verlag, New York, 1976, pp. 435–451.

Joseph, B. S., and Whitlock, D. G. Central projections of selected spinal dorsal roots in anuran amphibians. *Anat. Rec.,* 1968a, *160,* 279–288.

Joseph, B. S., and Whitlock, D. G. The morphology of spinal afferent-efferent relationships in vertebrates. *Brain Behav. Evol.,* 1968b, *1,* 2–18.

Kaas, J., Hall, W. C., Killackey, H., and Diamond, I. T. Visual cortex of the tree shrew *(Tupaia glis).* Architectonic subdivisions and representations of the visual field. *Brain Res.,* 1972, *42,* 491–496.

Kare, M. Comparative study of taste. *Handbook of Sensory Physiology,* Vol. IV, No. 2. 1971, pp. 270–290.

Karten, H. J. The organization of the ascending auditory pathway in the pigeon *(Columba livia).* I. Diencephalic projections of the inferior colliculus (nucleus mesencephali lateralis, pars dorsalis). *Brain Res.,* 1967, *6,* 409–427.

Karten, H. J. The ascending auditory pathway in the pigeon *(Columba livia).* II. Telencephalic projections of the nucleus ovoidalis thalami. *Brain Res.,* 1968, *11,* 134–153.

Karten, H. J., and Nauta, W. J. H. Organization of retinothalamic projections in the pigeon and owl. *Anat. Rec.,* 1968, *160,* 373.

Karten, H. J., Hodos, W., Nauta, W. J. H., and Revzin, A. M. Neural connections of the "visual wulst" of the avian telencephalon: Experimental studies in the pigeon *(Columba livia)* and owl *(Speotyto cunicularia). J. Comp. Neurol.,* 1973, *150,* 253–278.

Krettek, J. E., and Price, J. L. A direct input from the amygdala to the thalamus and the cerebral cortex. *Brain Res.,* 1974, *67,* 169–174.

Kruger, L., and Berkowitz, E. C. The main afferent connections of the reptilian telencephalon as determined by degeneration and electrophysiological methods. *J. Comp. Neurol.,* 1960, *115,* 125–141.

Larsell, O. *The Comparative Anatomy and Histology of the Cerebellum from Myxinoids through Birds.* University Minnesota Press, Minneapolis, 1967.

La Vail, J. H., Winston, K. R., and Tish, A. A method based on retrograde axonal transport of protein for identification of cell bodies of origin of axons terminating within the C.N.S. *Brain Res.,* 1973, *58,* 470–477.

Lawrence, D. G., and Kuypers, H. G. J. M. Functional organization of the motor system in the monkey. II. The effect of lesions of the descending brainstem pathways. *Brain,* 1968, *91,* 15–36.

Leake, P. A. Central projections of the statoacoustic nerve in *Caiman crocodilus. Brain Behav. Evol.,* 1974, *10,* 170–196.

Le Gros Clark, W. E. *The Antecedents of Man.* Edinburgh University Press, Edinburgh, 1959.

Lettvin, J. Y., Maturana, H. R., McCullock, W. S., and Pitts, W. H. What the frog's eye tells the frog's brain. *Proc. Inst. Radio Engineers,* 1959, *47,* 1940–1951.

Liu, C. N., and Chambers, W. W. Experimental study of anatomical organization of frog's spinal cord. *Anat. Rec.,* 1957, *127,* 326.

Manley, G. A. A review of some current concepts of the functional evolution of the ear in terrestrial vertebrates. *Evolution,* 1972, *26,* 608–621.

Marler, P. Specific distinctiveness in the communication signals of birds. *Behaviour,* 1957, *11,* 13–39.

Marquis, D. G. Phylogenetic interpretation of the functions of the visual cortex. *Arch. Neurol. Psychiat.,* 1935, *33,* 807–815.

Masterton, R. B., and Diamond, I. T. Hearing: Central neural mechanisms. *Handbook of Perception,* Vol. III, 1973, pp. 409–448.

Masterton, R. B., Heffner, H., and Ravizza, R. The evolution of human hearing. *J. Acoust. Soc. Am.,* 1969, *45,* 966–985.

Masterton, R. B., Skeen, L. C., and RoBards, M. J. Origins of anthropoid intelligence. *Brain Behav. Evol.,* 1974, *10,* 322–353.

Masterton, R. B., Thompson, G. C., Bechtold, J. K., and RoBards, M. J. Neuroanatomical basis of binaural phase-difference analysis for sound localization: A comparative study. *J. Comp. Physiol. Psychol.,* 1975, *89,* 379–386.

Masterton, R. B., Bitterman, M. E., Campbell, C. B. G. and Hotten, N. (eds.). *Evolution of Brain and Behavior in Vertebrates.* Wiley, New York, 1976*a.*

Masterton, R. B., Hodos, W., and Jerison, H. (eds.). *Evolution, Brain and Behavior, Persistent Problems.* Wiley, New York, 1976*b.*

Mehler, W. R. Some observations on secondary ascending afferent systems in the central nervous system. In R. S. Knighton and P. R. Dumke (eds.), *Pain.* Little, Brown, Boston, 1966, pp. 11–32.

Mehler, W. R. Comparative anatomy of the vestibular nuclear complex in submammalian vertebrates. *Brain Res.,* 1972, *37,* 55–67.

Mehler, W. R., Feferman, M. E., and Nauta, W. J. H. Ascending axon degeneration following anterolateral cordotomy: An experimental study in the monkey. *Brain,* 1960, *83,* 718–750.

Miles, F. A. Centrifugal control of the avian retina. I. Receptive field properties of retinal ganglion cells. *Brain Res.,* 1972, *48,* 65–92.

Mishkin, M. Visual mechanisms beyond the striate cortex. In R. Russell (ed.), *Frontiers in Physiological Psychology,* Academic Press, New York, 1966.

Morest, D. K. The laminar structure of the medial geniculate body of the cat. *J. Anat. (London)*, 1965, *99*, 143–160.

Morest, D. K. The non-cortical neuronal architecture of the inferior colliculus of the cat. *Anat. Rec.*, 1966, *154*, 477.

Nachman, M., and Ashe, J. H. Effects of basolateral amygdala lesions on neophobia, learned taste aversions, and sodium appetite in rats. *J. Comp. Physiol. Psychol.*, 1974, *87*, 622–643.

Nauta, W. J. H., and Gygax, P. A. Silver impregnation of degenerating axons in the central nervous system: A modified technique. *Stain Tech.*, 1954, *29*, 91–93.

Nauta, W. J. H., and Karten, H. J. A general profile of the vertebrate brain, with sidelights on the ancestry of cerebral cortex. In F. O. Schmitt (ed.), *The Neurosciences: Second Study Program*. Rockefeller University Press, New York, 1970, pp. 7–26.

Negus, U. *Comparative Anatomy of the Nose and Paranasal Sinuses*. E & S Livingstone, London, 1958.

Nieuwenhuys, R. Topological analysis of the brainstem of the lamprey *Lampetra fluviatilis*. *J. Comp. Neurol.*, 1972, *145*, 165–178.

Noback, C. R. The heritage of the human brain. American Museum of Natural History, James Arthur Lecture, 1959.

Norgren, R. Taste pathways to hypothalamus and amygdala. *J. Comp. Neurol.*, 1976, *166*, 17–30.

Norgren, R., and Leonard, C. M. Ascending central gustatory pathways. *J. Comp. Neurol.*, 1973, *150*, 217–238.

Northcutt, R. G. Pallial projections of sciatic, ulnar and trigeminal afferents in a frog *(R. catesbeiana)*. *Anat. Rec.*, 1970, *166*, 356.

Norton, A. C., and Kruger, L. The dorsal column system of the spinal cord. Its anatomy, physiology, phylogeny and sensory function. An updated review. *Brain Inform. Ser.*, 1973.

Papez, J. W. Central acoustic tract in cat and man. *Anat. Rec.*, 1929, *42*, 60.

Parks, T. N., and Rubel, E. W. Organization and development of brainstem auditory nuclei of the chicken: Organization of projections from n. magnocellularis to n. laminaris. *J. Comp. Neurol.*, 1975, *164*, 435–448.

Parsons, T. S. Evolution of the nasal structure in the lower tetrapods. *Am. Zool.*, 1967, *7*, 397–413.

Parsons, T. S. The origin of Jacobson's organ. *Forma Functio*, 1970, *3*, 105–111.

Polyak, S. M. *The Vertebrate Visual System*. University of Chicago Press, Chicago, 1957.

Potter, D. H. Mesencephalic auditory region of the bullfrog. *J. Neurol.*, 1965, *28*, 1132–1154.

Price, J. L., and Powell, T. P. S. Certain observations on the olfactory pathway. *J. Anat.*, 1971, *110*, 105–126.

Pumphrey, R. J. Hearing. *Symp. Soc. Exp. Biol.*, *1950, 4*, 19–34.

Raczkowski, D., Diamond, I. T., and Winer, J. Organization of thalamo-cortical auditory system in the cat studied with horseradish peroxidase. *Brain Res.*, 1976, *101*, 345–354.

Raisman, G. An experimental study of the projection of the amygdala to the accessory olfactory bulb and its relationship to the concept of a dual olfactory system. *Exp. Brain. Res.*, 1972, *14*, 395–408.

Rexed, B., and Brodal, A. The nucleus cervicalis lateralis: A spinocerebellar relay nucleus. *J. Neurophysiol.*, 1951, *14*, 399–407.

RoBards, M. J., Watkins, D. W. III, and Masterton, R. B. An anatomical study of some somesthetic afferents to the intercollicular terminal zone of the midbrain of the opossum. *J. Comp. Neurol.*, 1976, *170*, 499–524.

Rockel, A. J., and Jones, E. G. The neuronal organization of the inferior colliculus of the adult cat. I. The central nucleus. *J. Comp. Neurol.*, 1973a, *147*, 11–60.

Rockel, A. J., and Jones, E. G. The neuronal organization of the inferior colliculus of the adult cat. II. The pericentral nucleus. *J. Comp. Neurol.*, 1973b, *149*, 301–334.

Rodieck, R. W. *The Vertebrate Retina*. Freeman, San Francisco, 1973.

Rubinson, K. The central distribution of VIII nerve afferents in larval petromyzon marinus. *Brain Behav. Evol.*, 1974, *10*, 121–129.

Rushton, W. A. H. A theory on the effects of fiber size in medullated nerve. *J. Physiol. (London)*, 1951, *115*, 101–122.

Sarnat, H. B., and Netsky, M. G. *Evolution of the Nervous System*. Oxford University Press, New York, 1974.

Scalia, F., and Winans, S. S. The differential projections of the olfactory bulb and accessory olfactory bulb in mammals. *J. Comp. Neurol.*, 1975, *161*, 31–56.

Scalia F., and Winans, S. S. New perspectives on the morphology of the olfactory system: Olfactory and vomeronasal pathways in mammals. In R. L. Doty (ed.), *Mammalian Olfaction, Reproductive Processes, and Behavior*. Academic Press, New York, 1976.

Schlaer, R. An eagle's eye: Quality of the retinal image. *Science,* 1972, *176*, 920–922.

Schneider, G. E. Two visual systems; brain mechanisms for localization and discrimination are dissociated by tectal and cortical lesions. *Science,* 1969, *163*, 895–902.

Schroeder, D. M., and Jane, J. A. The intercollicular area of the inferior colliculus. *Brain Behav. Evol.,* 1976, *13*, 125–141.

Scott, J. W., and Leonard, C. M. The olfactory connections of the lateral hypothalamus in the rat, mouse, and hamster. *J. Comp. Neurol.,* 1971, *141*, 331–344.

Shepherd, G. M. Synaptic organization of the mammalian olfactory bulb. *Physiol. Rev.,* 1972, *52*, 864–917.

Shorey, H. H. *Animal Communication by Pheromones.* Academic Press, New York, 1976.

Skeen, L. C., and Hall, W. C. Efferent projections on the main and the accessory olfactory bulb in the tree shrew *(Tupaia glis). J. Comp. Neurol.,* 1977, *172*, 1–36.

Sprague, J., and Meikle, T. The role of the superior colliculus in visually guided behavior. *Exp. Neurol.,* 1965, *11*, 115–146.

Sprague, J., Berlucchi, G., and DiBerardino, A. C. The superior colliculus and pretectum in visually guided behavior and visual discrimination in the cat. *Brain Behav. Evol.,* 1970, *3*, 285.

Stebbins. W. C. (ed.). *Animal Psychophysics: The Design and Conduct of Sensory Experiments.* Appleton-Century-Crofts, New York, 1970.

Stephan, F. K., and Nunez, A. A. Elimination of circadian rhythms in drinking, activity, sleep and temperature by isolation of the suprachiasmatic nuclei. *Behav. Biol.,* 1977, *20*, 1–16.

Stewart, W. A., and King, R. B. Fiber projections from the nucleus caudalis of the spinal trigeminal nucleus. *J. Comp. Neurol.,* 1963, *121*, 271–286.

Strominger, N. L., Nelson, R., and Dougherty, W. J. Second order auditory pathways in the chimpanzee. *J. Comp. Neurol.,* 1977, *172*, 349–366.

Suzuki, N., and Tucker, D. Amino acids as olfactory stimuli in freshwater catfish, *Ictalurus catus* (Linn.). *Comp. Biochem. Physiol.,* 1971, *40*, 399–404.

Swanson, L. W., Cowan, W. M., and Jones, E. G. An autoradiographic study of the efferent connections of the ventral lateral geniculate nucleus in the albino rat and the cat. *J. Comp. Neurol.,* 1974, *156*, 143–164.

Tansley, K. Vision. *Symp. Soc. Exp. Biol.,* 1950, *4*, 19–34.

Tansley, K. *Vision in Vertebrates.* Chapman and Hall, London, 1965.

Tigges, J. Untersuchungen über den Farbensinn von *Tupaia glis.* (Diard 1820). *Z. Morphol. Anthropol.,* 1963, *53*, 109–123.

Todd, J. H., Atema, J., and Bardach, J. E. Chemical communication in social behavior of a fish, the yellow bullhead *Ictalurus natalis. Science,* 1967, *158*, 672–673.

Truex, R. C., Taylor, M. J., Smythe, M. O., and Gildenberg, P. L. The lateral cervical nucleus of cat, dog and man. *J. Comp. Neurol.,* 1970, *139*, 93–104.

Tucker, D. Nonolfactory responses from the nasal cavity: Jacobson's organ and the trigeminal system. In L. M. Beidler (ed.), *Handbook of Sensory Physiology,* Vol. IV, Part I. Springer-Verlag, New York, 1971, pp. 151–181.

Tucker, D., and Smith, J. C. Vertebrate olfaction. In Masterton *et al.* (eds.), *Evolution of Brain and Behavior in Vertebrates,* Wiley, New York, 1976, pp. 25–52.

Tucker, D., and Suzuki, N. Olfactory responses to schreckstoff of catfish. In D. Schneider, (ed.), *Olfaction and Taste IV.* Wissenschaftliche Verlagesellschaft MBH, Stuttgart, 1972, pp. 121–127.

van Noort, J. *The Structure and Connections of the Inferior Colliculus: An Investigation of the Lower Auditory System.* Van Gorcum, Assen, 1969.

Vesselkin, N. P., Agayan, A. L., and Nomokonova, L. M. A study of thalamo-telencephalic afferent systems in frogs. *Brain Behav. Evol.,* 1971, *4*, 295–306.

Walls, G. L. Origin of the vertebrate eye. *Arch. Ophthalmol.,* 1939, *22*, 452.

Walls, G. *The Vertebrate Eye and Its Adaptive Radiation.* Cranbrook Institute, Bloomfield Hills, Mich., 1942, pp. 207–209.

Ward, J. P., and Masterton, B. Encephalization and visual cortex in the tree shrew. *Brain Behav. Evol.,* 1970, *3*, 421–469.

Warkentin, J. The visual acuity of some vertebrates. *Psychol. Bull.* 1937, *34*, 793.

Welker, W. I., and Seidenstein, S. Somatic sensory representation in the cerebral cortex of the raccoon *(Procyon lotor). J. Comp. Neurol.,* 1959, *111*, 469–501.

Wever, E. G. Origin and evolution of the ear in vertebrates. In R B. Masterton, M. E. Bitterman, C. B. G. Campbell, and N. Notten (eds.), *Evolution of Brain and Behavior in Vertebrates.* Wiley, New York, 1976, pp. 89–106.

Wever, E. G., and Werner, Y. L. The functions of the middle ear in lizards: *Crotophytus collaris* (Iguanidae). *J. Exp. Zool.,* 1970, *175*, 327–342.

Woolsey, C. N. Organization of cortical auditory system: A review and a synthesis. In G. L. Rasmussen and W. F. Windle (eds.), *Neural Mechanisms of the Auditory and Vestibular Systems.* Thomas, Springfield, Ill., 1960.

Woolsey, C. N., and Fairman, D. Contralateral, ipsilateral and bilateral representation of cutaneous receptors in somatic area I and II of the cerebral cortex of pig, sheep and other mammals. *Surgery,* 1946, *19*, 684–702.

Woolsey, T. A., Welker, C., and Schwartz, R. H. Comparative natomical studies of the sml face cortex with special reference to the occurrence of "barrels" in layer IV. *J. Comp. Neurol.,* 1975, *164*, 79–94.

Zeki, S. M. Representation of central visual fields in prestriate cortex of monkey. *Brain Res.,* 1969, *14*, 271–291.

2

Ontogeny of Sensory Systems

Timothy J. Cunningham and E. Hazel Murphy

Anatomical Development of Sensory Systems

The branch of neuroscience seeking relationships between the structural development of the sensory systems and the emergence of their function is still in its infancy. Although such relationships have been found, current knowledge is restricted to simple generalizations about functional capacities, such as the onset of vision or the onset of audition, and the most obvious of structural changes, such as the formation of synaptic connections between the eye or the ear and the brain. The inability to show more complicated relationships is due in part to difficulties in testing a wide variety of sensory functions in immature animals and in part to the subtlety of many of the developmental changes in the structure of neurons. Accordingly, this chapter is divided into two sections, the first focusing on anatomical structure and the second on function, both physiological and perceptual.

The emphasis of the chapter will be on interdependencies which exist during the ontogeny of sensory systems. These include the developmental dependence of one sensory structure on another and the relationship of sensory experience to both structural and functional development. With regard to the role of experience during development, three issues are of particular importance: (1) Are specific structures and functions genetically predetermined and manifested early in development, prior to sensory experience? (2) Are critical environmental and experiential features needed to maintain such structures and functions? (3) Are there examples of structures or functions which are not predetermined, i.e., which depend on critical environmental and experiential factors for normal maturation? These are the issues which will be emphasized in the following pages.

Timothy J. Cunningham and E. Hazel Murphy   Department of Anatomy, Medical College of Pennsylvania, Philadelphia, Pennsylvania 19129.

TIMOTHY J.
CUNNINGHAM AND
E. HAZEL MURPHY

The central nervous system gains access to the external environment via the sensory receptors. In general, there are three broad classes of receptors which can be defined according to their morphology and mode of innervation.

The first class consists of specialized ectodermal or mesodermal cells which are innervated by a neuron with one of its processes directed to the receptor and the other process directed to the central nervous system. The second class of receptors exists as a specialization of the neuron's peripheral process which itself is modified for sensory transduction. The third class, including, for example, encapsulated endings in the skin, fits into both categories because the peripheral nerve process is modified for sensory transduction and is associated with nonneural cells which can affect the quality of the stimulus.

Although considerable attention has been devoted to descriptions of receptor development (see Bradley and Mistretta, 1975, for review), much less is known about the factors which control this development. Obviously, receptors of a particular type must be formed in the correct position at an appropriate time. Receptor development is completed *in utero* in many mammals, and since the uterine environment seems to have little demand for sensory function it has been concluded that much of receptor development occurs independently of function.

However, the formation of receptors is not a completely autonomous process. The formation of some types of receptors is very likely dependent on the development of their innervating axons. For example, the taste buds of rats and rabbits degenerate rapidly after removal of their innervating axons (Guth, 1971; Oakley and Benjamin, 1966; Zelena, 1964). They then re-form after the axons regenerate. This morphogenetic dependence of the taste buds on their nerve supply is specific; i.e., only gustatory nerve fibers can induce the formation of taste receptors (Oakley, 1974). Experimentally rerouted axons from another system do not induce functional taste buds. Therefore, the peripheral nerve can be responsible for both the timing of receptor formation and the type of receptor which is produced.

Although direct experimental evidence of a similar relationship during the original development of taste receptors is not available, the normal morphogenesis of taste buds occurs at the time the gustatory epithelium is first invaded by taste fibers (Farbman, 1971).

The same temporal coincidence of nerve invasion and receptor information has been noted for skin receptors (Ramon y Cajal, 1929) and auditory hair cells (Sher, 1971). The relationship between retinal bipolar cell processes and the development of photoreceptors is not so clearly defined.

More direct evidence for the dependency of receptor development on the innervating axons has been derived from experiments on rat muscle receptors (Zelena, 1964). The muscle spindle begins to differentiate at 3 days before birth and is fully developed by postnatal day 10. At the onset of spindle formation the sensory axons are already present while the motor axons to intrafusal muscle fibers develop around birth. Denervation of the spindle 3 days before birth results in a failure of spindle development. The receptor does not show a similar dependency on the motor axons in that sectioning the ventral roots of newborn rats produces some atrophy of intrafusal muscle fibers but does not affect the progress of spindle differentiation. This experiment strongly indicates a dependency between receptor development and the development of innervating sensory axons.

In 1920, Olmstead attempted to explain the morphogenetic dependency of receptors on their nerve fibers by suggesting that receptor development was triggered by trophic substances secreted from the nerve axon. Although experimental evidence for this hypothesis is still technically impossible to obtain, it is accepted by most developmental neurobiologists. However, as Zelena (1964) points out, the concept of induction has been prominent in developmental biology for several years but no inductive agents have ever been isolated.

Another developmental event which may control the timing of receptor development is the growth of central axons and their contact with the central nervous system. This contact is made either by the central process of neurons whose peripheral process forms the receptor or by the central axons of ganglion cells whose peripheral axons innervate specialized receptor cells. For example, in the olfactory system, the peripheral process of the first-order bipolar cells is specialized for chemical reception and the central processes form connections with the olfactory bulb. An analysis of the development of olfactory receptors in the rat shows that the specialized "dendrites," or peripheral processes, appear in the olfactory epithelium at the same time the central processes make contact with the olfactory bulb (Cuschieri and Bannister, 1975; Hinds, 1972a,b). It has been previously suggested that receptor differentiation depends on this central contact with the bulb (Vinnikov and Titova, 1956).

In summary, receptor differentiation appears to occur independently of the development of sensory function but seems to be dependent on other morphogenetic events. For specialized receptor cells or receptor complexes, one of these events is the invasion of innervating axons; another may be the contact of the neuron's axon with its central target.

DIFFERENTIATION OF CENTRAL SENSORY NEURONS

CELL GENERATION. The neurons which form the sensory centers of the brain arise near the wall of the primitive neural tube. As the brain and spinal cord develop, the migration and further mitotic patterns of these neuroblasts ultimately produce the cell groups of the sensory receiving zones. The neurons which receive a projection from the receptors or their ganglia are found at all levels of the neuraxis and include cells which can be considered as primarily sensory in nature (such as neurons of the dorsal lateral geniculate nucleus) or primarily motor in nature (such as the motoneurons of the spinal cord). Thus it is inappropriate to consider the generation of neurons which receive sensory projections as a separate or special event from the generation of any other central neurons.

The understanding of cell generation in the central nervous system has recently been enhanced greatly by the technique of thymidine autoradiography. This technique depends on the fact that, before a cell divides, it synthesizes DNA.

TIMOTHY J.
CUNNINGHAM AND
E. HAZEL MURPHY

By labeling of a DNA precusor ([³H]thymidine), the "birthdate" of daughter cells can be determined (Sidman, 1970). Using this technique in mammals, it has been found that the majority of neurons in the central nervous system are produced by birth or shortly after birth. In addition, neurons forming specific nuclear groups (such as thalamic nuclei) or specific layers (such as the laminae of the cerebral cortex) are produced at a similar time and over a relatively short period. For example, the neurons of the neocortex are generated near the ependymal lining of the primitive forebrain and then migrate toward the surface of the developing cerebrum. The pattern of cell generation is such that the neurons forming the innermost lamina are produced first while those forming the outermost lamina are produced last. In rodents, most cells in a specific lamina of the cortex are generated within a period of about 24 hr during the final days of gestation. These newly formed neurons must migrate through other previously formed neurons to reach their appropriate laminar location (Angevine, 1965, 1970; Barry and Rogers, 1965; Brückner *et al.*, 1976; Caviness and Sidman, 1973; Hicks and D'Amato, 1968; Shimada and Langman, 1970). In the thalamus of the mouse, neurons forming the ventrocaudolateral nuclear groups are the first to be produced while those forming the dorsorostromedial groups are produced last (Angevine, 1970).

Although the functional significance of these temporal gradients of cell generation and patterns of cell migration is not clear, there is a great deal of experimental work which shows that these processes occur independently of afferent input or of sensory function. One of the clearest examples of this independence comes from studies of the development of the retinotectal system of chicks. Removal of one eye from the chick embryo has no effect on the production of tectal neurons or on their initial patterns of migration. It is only after this migratory phase of development that the neurons die if they fail to receive afferent connections (Cowan *et al.*, 1968; Kelly and Cowan, 1972). Likewise, visual function, which depends on afferent connections from the retina, must also have no effect on the generation of central neurons.

The fact that sensory axons have no effect on cell generation in the central nervous system does not mean that the incoming axons exert no influence whatever over the central cells. On the contrary, they exert a life-and-death control—so-called developmental neuron death. The importance of cell death during development has now been recognized for many embryonic systems (Cowan, 1973; Glucksmann, 1951; Jacobson, 1970; Lockshin and Beaulation, 1975; Saunders, 1966). In the nervous system, there seems to be a general overproduction of neurons initially, and then later a regulated death of the excess cells. Whether a neuron lives or dies appears to depend on its ability to make appropriate efferent connections and to receive appropriate afferent connections. For a homogeneous population of neurons, neuron death seems to be probabilistic or stochastic, because each cell has the same chance to make or receive an appropriate complement of terminal axons. However, the current ideas about neuron death during development are completely based on studies of nonmammals. Whether or not this scheme applies to the mammalian nervous system is not clear (Cowan, 1973).

CELL MATURATION. The generation, migration, and selective death and degeneration of central sensory neurons are only part of their total maturation. In addition to these developmental processes, each cell must develop a dendritic tree which will accommodate the terminals of innervating afferent fibers, and, still further, each cell must generate an axon which will form connections on still other central neurons. Unlike cell generation and migration, there is considerable evidence that these maturational processes are dependent on afferent innervation and some indication that they may be dependent on sensory experience.

Several studies have dealt with the maturation of neurons in sensory centers of the mammalian nervous system by application of the Golgi technique, for visualizing the entirety of a neuron, to embryonic and early postnatal animals. The kind of formation which can be obtained from applying the Golgi technique to young animals of various ages includes the day-to-day progress of maturation of a cell's dendritic tree or its axon. This technique has been employed in studies of the sensory receiving zones of the thalamus and brain stem (Morest, 1969a,b), cerebral cortex (Marin-Padilla, 1971; Morest, 1969a), and olfactory bulb (Hinds, 1972a) and spinal cord (Smith, 1969). In general, these studies have shown that the development of morphologically similar cells follows the same sequential pattern of dendritic maturation but not necessarily the same time.

In the olfactory bulb of the mouse (Hinds, 1972a,b) there is circumstantial evidence that the ingrowth of first-order afferent axons affects the maturation of the dendritic tree of the second-order mitral cells. The initial stage of maturation of the mitral cell's dendritic tree is characterized by the growth of processes which are tangential to the surface of the olfactory bulb. After the development of the terminal glomeruli of olfactory nerve axons at the surface of the bulb, the mitral dendrites change their orientation from tangential to radial. The subsequent differentiation of the dendritic tree occurs in close association with the primary olfactory axons. Morest (1969b) has noted the same spatial and temporal coincidence of axonal ingrowth and central differentiation in central sensory receiving zones of the auditory and visual systems and in the cerebral cortex. He has suggested that the growing tips of the afferent axons induce dendritic differentiation in their target cells, including the induction of the direction of growth of the cell's dendrites.

Experimental studies also indicate the same close relationship between dendritic orientation and afferent innervation. For example, section of dorsal roots on one side of the spinal cord in neonatal cats disrupts the usual orientation of the dendrites of neurons in Clark's nucleus (Smith, 1974). This disruption includes an abnormal redirection of the dendrites away from the denervated side of the spinal cord toward the normally innervated side.

Finally, the dependency of dendritic orientation on afferent axons appears to be a transneuronal phenomenon. For example, removal of an eye denervates the lateral geniculate nucleus, whose cells send a projection to the visual cortex. If one eye is removed from newborn rodents, there is abnormal development of the cortical cells which receive the geniculate projection (Valverde, 1968). The dendrites of these cells normally ramify freely in cortical layer IV (where the majority of geniculate axons terminate), but in newborn enucleates the dendrites tend to avoid this lamina. Another result of eye removal at birth in rats and rabbits is a drop in the number of dendritic spines on the apical dendrites of the pyramidal cells in the visual cortex (Globus and Schneibel, 1967a; Valverde, 1968). This spine loss occurs only in one population of pyramidal cells and is restricted to that portion of the dendrite which receives thalamocortical projections (Ryuga et al., 1975b). Similar changes in spinal density have also been reported for pyramidal cells in somatosensory cortex of rats after removal of their whiskers at birth (Ryugo et al., 1975a). Thus the available evidence indicates that developing afferent axons have effects on the ultimate form of the dendritic tree of sensory neurons—even those two or three synapses away.

Perhaps more significant, because of its far-reaching implications, is that alterations in the sensory environment can have the same effect on cortical dendrites as does loss of their sensory input. For example, loss and deformation of pyramidal cell spines have been demonstrated in the visual cortex of animals reared in the dark (Globus and Scheibel, 1967b; Valverde, 1967). One of the more reasonable explanations for this phenomenon is that the functional deprivation has modified the development of synaptic input to the cortical cells (see below).

In addition, the effects of visual deprivation are not limited to alterations in neurons of the visual cortex, but also interfere with the growth of cells in the lateral geniculate nucleus. For example, in a series of experiments on kittens (Guillery, 1972, 1973; Guillery and Stelzner, 1970; Sherman et al., 1974), there is evidence that unilateral eyelid suture arrests the growth of neurons which receive connections from the deprived eye. This effect apparently results from the inability of these neurons to compete with nondeprived neurons for synaptic space on the cells of the visual cortex. The functional consequences of these alterations are discussed in the second part of this chapter. In the present context, however, the structural alterations in lateral geniculate neurons are significant because visual deprivation produces minor changes in the cells of the retina and their axons in the optic nerve (Rasch et al., 1961; Sosula and Glow, 1971; Weiskrantz, 1958; Wiesel and Hubel, 1963a). Therefore, these results are another indication that receptor organs develop independently of function, but a reduction in the quality or quantity of the stimulation which they convey can affect the growth of central neurons.

Since environmental deprivation can affect the structure of dendrites, it might be expected that environmental enrichment might increase the number of dendritic spines. Although there are reports of such increases in spine counts on the pyramidal cells of rats raised in "enriched" environments (Globus et al., 1973; Schapiro and Vukovich, 1970), it seems a bit discomforting for humans to define "enriched" for rats. Furthermore, until more is known about the functional significance of dendritic spines, such results must be interpreted with caution. However, these experiments do show that some relatively small changes in the environment, whether enriching or not, result in changes in the structure of neurons and that these structural changes seem to include an increase in neuronal surface area.

So far, we have considered the development of receptors and the generation and maturation of central sensory neurons. For the proper function of the nervous system, however, these two sets of sensory structures must develop appropriate connections. In this section we consider some of the current ideas about the way sensory connections are formed and then the relationship of this synaptic development to the sensory experience of the animal.

The question of how developing neurons connect appropriately with each other is called the problem of *neuronal specificity.* Currently, there are several competing theories attempting to explain it. Sperry first recognized the importance of specificity in the nervous system and offered the suggestion that individual neurons or groups of neurons possess chemical affinities for each other. These affinities would allow one nerve cell to recognize the locus of other nerve cells with which it was to connect (Attardi and Sperry, 1963; Sperry, 1963). For the most part, Sperry's ideas were derived from observations on the orderly regeneration of retinotectal pathways in fish and amphibians. For example, he found that after section or crush of one optic tract the ganglion cell axons forming the tract always grew back to the proper part of the tectum, even if the eye had been rotated. That is, regeneration was always retinotopic and not dependent either on the visual field or on mechanical guidance of the axon. This point-to-point reconnection is easiest to explain on the basis of cell-to-cell recognition.

Since Sperry's original work, several investigators have amplified or modified this original hypothesis in order to explain the results of, now, hundreds of experiments concerned with regeneration and development of retinotectal connections. For the most part, these experiments deal with the nervous system of nonmammalian vertebrates (for reviews, see Gaze, 1970; Jacobson, 1970; Keating, 1976; Myer and Sperry, 1976).

A second view of the mechanism for the establishment of appropriate connections has been offered by Gaze and Keating (1972). They have proposed that, instead of point-to-point, or cell-to-cell affinities between neurons, there are somewhat less specific gradients in both the receptor organs and their central targets. These gradients, presumably chemical, are organized such that points along the receptor gradient will match up with corresponding points along the central gradients. They have termed this hypothesis "systems matching."

The results from still other experiments (Jacobson, 1970; Levine and Jacobson, 1974) suggest that in some cases axons may have intrinsic organizational properties (i.e., they have intrinsic affinities and know where to go without outside help), which determine their pattern of termination in spite of appropriate postsynaptic loci.

Thus the problem of neuronal specificity remains unsettled. Of course, it is not impossible that any or all of the specificity hypotheses are true and that the various factors such as point-to-point affinities, gradient systems, and intrinsic axonal affinities all act together to produce ordered connections during development. Under a given experimental situation, or with a given animal model, one of these factors may be expressed more than another. In this respect, it may be unwise to compare results from regeneration experiments with those from true developmental studies, or results using nonmammalian models (where there is regeneration of central pathways) with those using mammals (where there is little or no regeneration).

Whatever the mechanism of neuronal specification in the sensory systems, it is clear that this process occurs independently of sensory function. For example, several studies have shown that if the sensory map for a particular modality is modified experimentally, behavioral responses in that modality are also modified. In amphibians, if the optic nerve is sectioned and the eye is rotated about its axis, there is an inversion of visuomotor responses following regeneration of the retinal projection. The degree of this inversion of response corresponds to the degree of axial rotation of the eye. Furthermore, the abnormal reflexes persist. They are not corrected by experience (Sperry, 1944, 1951; Stone, 1944, 1953). This behavioral inversion (and, more recently, electrophysiological mapping studies, Jacobson, 1968) shows that the axons from the displaced ganglion cells regenerate as if they were in their normal position. The axons grow back to their original loci in the optic tectum. As another example, frogs with translocated skin show misdirected responses when the displaced skin is stimulated (Jacobson and Baker, 1969; Miner, 1956). This inappropriate behavior also never recovers; the sensory nerves selectively seek out the appropriate skin even when it has been reloacted (Bloom and Tompkins, 1976). In general, results such as these indicate that the topographic maps of the sensory systems, and the orderliness of axonal projections underlying them, are *not* affected by the experience of maladaptive behavioral responses.

Nevertheless, as a result of abnormal experience, there seems to be a quantitative effect on certain types of synaptic connections. As has already been described, lateral geniculate neurons of the kitten, which receive connections from an eye whose lid has been sutured, show atrophic changes. These changes have suggested an arrest in development due to a failure of competition by the neurons for terminal space (Sherman *et al.*, 1974). As also noted above, changes in the number of dendritic spines suggest either that visually deprived neurons projecting to cortical cells have failed to establish their full complement of connections or that there has been some dropout of early-forming synapses. This general idea is further supported by electron microscopic experiments which show changes in the size and density of synaptic profiles in the visual cortex after eyelid suture in young rats (Fifkova, 1970, 1971). Therefore, abnormal sensory experience does affect central connections quantitatively, although it does not affect their orderliness.

MECHANISMS OF STRUCTURAL CHANGES

A major concern in these studies on sensory deprivation is the mechanism of the observed structural changes. At present, it is not entirely clear whether changes in spine counts reflect a failure of spine maturation, failure of development of the axons which terminate on spines, or a dropout of the preformed spines and/or terminals via transneuronal degeneration. Similar interpretational difficulties arise when interpreting the studies which show changes in the quality and appearance of synaptic terminals after sensory deprivation. One study on the superior colliculus of the rat shows that eyelid suture results in the *failure* of a certain population of interneuronal terminals to develop (Lund and Lund, 1972), but the same systematic approach has not been applied to other sensory centers under conditions of deprivation.

PHYSIOLOGICAL DEVELOPMENT OF THE VISUAL SYSTEM

The preceding review of the role of the sensory environment in the structural development of sensory systems leads us to a consideration of parallel developmental processes in the functioning of these sensory systems. Since we have extensive knowledge of the development of the visual system and a relative paucity of information on the other sensory systems, this section of the chapter will be restricted largely to the visual system. In all mammals studied, the physiology of the visual system develops later in ontogeny than the physiology of tactile, olfactory or auditory systems (Rose and Ellingson, 1970). Thus ontogenetic sequences can be more easily studied in the visual system. In addition, experiential deprivation and its effects can be more easily studied in the visual system, by means of dark rearing or eyelid suturing, than in other systems. Since the visual system of the cat has been most extensively studied, this system will first be considered in detail. The visual system of other mammals will be considered later.

VISUAL PHYSIOLOGY OF THE MATURE CAT

In order to determine the extent to which the visual system of the neonate is prewired prior to sensory experience, a comparison of its function in the neonatal and adult cat must be made. On the one hand, if functions characteristic of the mature system are observed in the neonate, then these functions must not be dependent on visual experience. On the other hand, functions which are characteristic of the mature system but which are *not* observed in the neonate must be dependent on neural maturation, visual experience, or both. In order to make this comparison between the visual systems of the neonatal and adult cat, it is first necessary to review briefly the anatomy and physiology of the visual system of the cat. Details of any point in this brief review can be found in Chapters 5, 6, and 7.

MAJOR VISUAL PATHWAYS. The major visual pathway of the cat consists of the retinogeniculocortical pathway. The axons of retinal ganglion cells leave the eye in the optic nerve. At the optic chiasm, axons from the nasal retina decussate and project to lamina A of the contralateral dorsal lateral geniculate nucleus, while axons from the temporal retina project to lamina A1 of the ipsilateral dorsal lateral geniculate nucleus. Topographic organization is maintained such that neurons from adjacent sectors of laminae A and A1 are stimulated by the same points in the visual field, and their output, in turn, converges on neurons in the visual cortex. The second major pathway in the cat is the retinotectal pathway. Axons of retinal ganglion cells project to the dorsal layers of the superior colliculus and most of this projection is contralateral.

RECEPTIVE FIELD CHARACTERISTICS OF NEURONS OF THE CAT VISUAL SYSTEM. *Retina and Dorsal Lateral Geniculate Nucleus.* In the cat's retina, most ganglion cells have concentric receptive fields, having a center which responds to the onset or offset of light and an antagonistic surround. Three types of ganglion cells have been distinguished on the basis of their receptive field characteristics and the conduction rate of their axons. These are called X, Y, and W cells, and they maintain separate projections to central visual centers (Fukuda and Stone, 1974; Hoffman and Stone, 1973; Hoffman *et al.*, 1972; Stone and Fukuda, 1974; Wilson *et al.*, 1976). Neurons in the lateral geniculate nucleus also have concentric fields and can again be characterized as X, Y, and W cells (Hoffman *et al.*, 1972; Stone and Fukuda, 1974) (see Chapter 6).

Visual Cortex. At the cortical level, neurons have receptive fields which are orientation selective and have been classified as simple, complex, or hypercomplex (Hubel and Wiesel, 1962, 1965*a*). There is some evidence that X and Y cells may maintain separate and parallel pathways from the lateral geniculate nucleus to the simple and complex cells in the visual cortex, although the separation at the cortical level is not yet fully established (Denney *et al.*, 1968; Hoffman and Stone, 1971; Hoffman *et al.*, 1972; LeVay and Ferster, 1977; LeVay and Gilbert, 1976; Singer *et al.*, 1975; Stone, 1972; Stone and Dreher, 1973; Van Essen and Kelly, 1974). Three important response characteristics of neurons in the visual cortex should be noted. First, the neurons are binocularly activated (Hubel and Wiesel, 1962, 1965*a*). In the cat, about 85% of the neurons in striate cortex are driven by both eyes, although the response to each eye may not be equally strong. Many of these neurons are extremely sensitive to small disparities, giving a maximum response if the stimuli presented to each eye are perfectly aligned at their optimal disparity and showing considerable inhibition if the stimuli are misaligned. These neurons may play a critical role in binocular depth perception (Barlow *et al.*, 1967; Nikara *et al.*, 1968; Pettigrew *et al.*, 1968) (see Chapter 6).

The second characteristic to be noted is that each neuron has a preferred orientation and a slight misalignment from the optimal orientation of a stimulus will decrease the response of a neuron considerably. All orientations are represented at the cortical level, and radially organized cortical columns contain cells which have similar preferred orientations. The third characteristic is that most cortical cells also have a preferred direction, but this characteristic is not arranged in columns (see Chapter 6).

Finally, some cells in the visual cortex project to the superior colliculus.

Superior Colliculus. Most neurons in the dorsal layers of the superior colliculus have directionally selective receptive fields and most are binocularly driven. These receptive field characteristics appear to be functionally dependent on the corticotectal pathway, since ablation of visual cortex abolishes these response characteristics (Mize and Murphy, 1976; Rosenquist and Palmer, 1971; Sterling and Wickelgren, 1969; Wickelgren and Sterling, 1969) (see Chapter 5).

We can now compare the functioning of the visual system of the newborn kitten with that of the mature cat, as outlined above. The kitten opens its eye and receives its first patterned visual experience at approximately 6–9 days after birth, and this experience can be delayed by suturing the eyelids closed.

VISUAL CORTEX. The response characteristics of single neurons in the visual cortex of the neonatal cat were first described by Hubel and Wiesel (1963). They reported that, although many cells were sluggish and fast adapting, orientation selectivity of cortical neurons was present and "much of the richness of visual physiology in the cortex of the adult cat . . . was present in very young kittens without visual experience." Although this conclusion has been challenged (Barlow and Pettigrew, 1971; Pettigrew, 1974), an increasing body of evidence indicates that at least some percentage of cells in kitten visual cortex do show orientation selectivity in the absence of visual experience (Blakemore and Van Sluyters, 1975; Buisseret and Imbert, 1974, 1976; Imbert and Buisseret, 1975; Wiesel and Hubel, 1974), and radially organized orientation columns have also been observed (Blakemore and Van Sluyters, 1975; Hubel and Wiesel, 1963). Thus the evidence indicates that orientation selectivity is genetically specified, at least for some cortical neurons, and that visual experience is not essential for its appearance.

The percentage and distribution of binocularly driven cortical cells typical of the mature visual system are also seen in neurons of the cortex of the visually naive kitten (Hubel and Wiesel, 1963; Imbert and Buisseret, 1975; Schechter and Murphy, 1976). Thus this ocular dominance organization is also genetically specified and is not dependent on visual experience. However, the fine disparity tuning typical of the mature visual system is apparently not present in neurons in the visual cortex of the naive kitten (Barlow and Pettigrew, 1971; Pettigrew, 1974). As will be seen below, this is a crucial finding for theoretical interpretations of the developmental processes in the visual system.

The decrease in fatigability and increase in the percentage of orientation-selective cells and in disparity tuning occur rapidly in the early postnatal period, and the functioning of the kitten visual cortex appears to be essentially mature by the age of 4 weeks.

DORSAL LATERAL GENICULATE NUCLEUS. In the lateral geniculate nucleus, small and precisely defined receptive fields can be recorded at the time of eye opening (Norman *et al.*, 1975). However, the receptive fields differ from the concentrically organized fields of the adult in that the responses of the antagonistic surround are not fully developed. These responses, characteristic of the antagonistic surround, appear in most cells by the end of the third postnatal week. Thus the age of 4 weeks for the appearance of relatively adult characteristics in the visual cortex coincides with the development of surround inhibition in the lateral geniculate nucleus. This suggests that the functional immaturity of some cortical cells during the first 3–4 weeks may depend, at least in part, on the immaturity of geniculate cells.

SUPERIOR COLLICULUS. In the superior colliculus of the young kitten, single neurons have characteristics similar to those found in the adult cat following visual cortical ablation; that is, most of the cells are responsive to the onset or offset of light or to movement. Adult characteristics of direction selectivity and binocular activation develop between 15 and 35 days postnatally, indicating that the development and maturing of the corticotectal pathway are occurring during this period (Norton, 1974; Stein *et al.,* 1973).

SUMMARY. Of the various aspects of functional organization seen in the visual cortex of the adult cat, columnar organization and ocular dominance distribution are apparently present as soon as the eyes open. Some but probably not all cells show direction selectivity, but fine disparity tuning is not present. The maturation of those response characteristics which are not fully developed in the neonate occurs very rapidly during the first 4 weeks: the percentage of orientation-selective cells increases, the responsivity and narrowness of orientation tuning increase, and disparity-sensitive neurons appear. During this same period, lateral geniculate cells develop surround inhibition and the corticotectal pathway matures. However, as will be seen, this rapid maturation during the first 4 postnatal weeks is dependent, at least in part, on normal visual experience.

EFFECTS OF VISUAL DEPRIVATION ON DEVELOPMENT OF THE CAT VISUAL SYSTEM

VISUAL CORTEX. *Binocular Deprivation.* Binocular visual deprivation can be achieved by suturing both eyelids closed—which prevents the kitten from experiencing visual patterned stimulation—or by dark rearing—which deprives the kitten not only of patterned stimulation but also of all light stimulation. The fact that the physiological consequences of these two forms of deprivation do not seem to differ to any great extent suggests that the experience of visual patterns is the most critical element of early visual stimulation.

The most dramatic consequences of visual deprivation occur at the level of the visual cortex, following either dark rearing or lid suture. Following binocular suture for the first 3–6 months of life, many neurons in the visual cortex are found to be unresponsive to light stimulation. Of those neurons which retain visual responsivity, many do not have normal receptive field characteristics. In contrast to the previously cited reports of orientation selectivity in cortical neurons of the young visually naive kitten, several investigators report a decrease or complete absence of orientation selectivity in cortical neurons following weeks or months of dark rearing or binocular lid suture. A decrease in the overall level of responsivity of visual cortical neurons occurs in visually deprived kittens as young as 19 days, compared with normally reared 19 day-old-kittens (Baxter, 1966; Blakemore and Van Sluyters, 1975; Buisseret and Imbert, 1974, 1976; Cynader *et al.,* 1976; Sherk and Stryker, 1976).

These results suggest that deprivation has two effects on receptive field properties of visual cortical neurons. First, it prevents the maturation which normally occurs rapidly during the first 4 postnatal weeks. Second, it causes a breakdown of preexisting organization in that percentage of cells which show orientation selectivity at the time of eye opening, prior to visual experience.

The normal ocular dominance distribution observed in 8-day-old visually naive kittens is also seen in dark-reared kittens and in kittens reared with binocular lid suture (Blakemore and Van Sluyters, 1975; Buisseret and Imbert, 1974, 1976; Imbert and Buisseret, 1975; Sherk and Stryker, 1976; Wiesel and Hubel, 1965a). Thus visual experience is not necessary either for the maturation or for the maintenance of this organization. Disparity-sensitive neurons, however, are not found in visually deprived cats and apparently their development is dependent on visual experience (Barlow and Pettigrew, 1971; Pettigrew, 1974).

Monocular Deprivation. The effects of depriving a kitten of visual experience in one eye, by monocular suture, differ from the effects of binocular deprivation. Monocular suture results in an imbalance in the converging inputs from the two eyes onto cortical neurons. Following monocular lid suture, most neurons in visual cortex can be driven only by the open, experienced eye, and are not responsive to stimulation of the sutured eye (Wiesel and Hubel, 1963b). It has been suggested that inputs from each eye compete for synaptic space on cortical neurons and that the imbalance results in a tendency for the input from the experienced eye to win space at the expense of input from the deprived eye. Receptive field properties are quite normal except for their abnormal ocular dominance distribution (Blakemore and Van Sluyters, 1975; Pettigrew, 1974; Schechter and Murphy, 1976; Wiesel and Hubel, 1965a). Thus, although binocular activation of cortical neurons is present in the visually naive kitten and is not dependent on visual experience for its maintenance, it can be disrupted by this form of abnormal visual experience.

Discrepant Visual Stimulation. In conditions of monocular suture, two processes are thus involved: (1) deprivation of one eye, resulting in a bias toward the experienced eye; and (2) differential input to the two eyes. Differential input to the two eyes is, alone, sufficient to disrupt the normal binocular activation of cortical neurons. If an occluder is placed on one or the other eye on alternate days, or if kittens are reared with artificially induced ocular strabismus, with eye rotation, or with goggles which present different visual stimulation to each eye, then the same points on each retina never experience identical simultaneous visual stimulation. Under these conditions, there is no deprivation and no loss of visual responsivity in visual cortical cells, but almost total loss of binocularity, i.e., all cells have receptive fields and are responsive to one or the other eye (Blake *et al.,* 1974; Blakemore, 1976; Hirsch and Spinelli, 1970; Hubel and Wiesel, 1965b). Asynchrony of eye movements may also disrupt binocularity (Maffei and Bisti, 1976).

SUBCORTICAL VISUAL AREAS. These results lead us to a consideration of the extent to which the dramatic changes in visual cortex physiology resulting from visual deprivation are secondary to changes at subcortical sites. At the lateral geniculate nucleus, the predominant effect of deprivation is a selective loss of Y cells. It has been shown that in monocularly and binocularly deprived cats, Y cells can be recorded only rarely, but X cells appear in normal frequency (Sherman *et al.,* 1972). In monocularly deprived cats, the Y cell loss is very severe in the binocular segment of the lateral geniculate nucleus but is not apparent in the monocular segment. In binocularly deprived cats, Y cell loss is less severe, but occurs throughout the monocular and binocular segments of the nucleus. These effects occur postretinally, since the retinal ganglion cell populations and their axons are normal (Sherman and Stone, 1973).

In the superior colliculus, the effects of monocular and binocular deprivation differ, as they do in the lateral geniculate nucleus. Following binocular deprivation, a severe loss occurs in the Y direct input from the retina to the superior colliculus, and also in the Y indirect pathway from the cortex to the superior colliculus. In contrast, following monocular deprivation, the Y direct pathway appears normal, but the Y indirect pathway from the deprived eye via the cortex is essentially lost (Berman and Sterling, 1976; Hoffman and Sherman, 1974, 1975).

These data on the effects of deprivation on subcortical visual areas are of interest for several reasons. They suggest that the effects of visual deprivation on cortical physiology may be occurring, at least in part, as a consequence of changes at the lateral geniculate nucleus, and there is other evidence of abnormalities in receptive field properties of lateral geniculate neurons following visual deprivation (Hamasaki and Winters, 1973; Hamasaki *et al.,* 1972; Sherman and Sanderson, 1972). The effects both in lateral geniculate nucleus and in superior colliculus also reflect a difference in the severity of consequences of monocular and binocular deprivation which is paralleled in the physiology of cortical consequences of deprivation, described above. However, an indication that subcortical changes are not the sole determinants of cortical abnormalities is found in a recent study showing that cortical function in the monocular segment of visual cortical neurons in monocularly deprived cats is abnormal, unlike the monocular segment of the lateral geniculate nucleus in these cats (Watkins and Sherman, 1975; Wilson and Sherman, 1977). In addition, since Y cell loss predominates in the lateral geniculate nucleus, and since Y cells are believed to project predominantly to complex cells in the visual cortex, one might expect a selective loss of complex cells in visual cortex. This has not been reported, in binocular areas of striate cortex, again indicating that subcortical changes cannot be the sole determinant of functional changes at the cortical level. Much more research is needed to elucidate the significance of the selective Y cell loss in subcortical sites and the functional significance of the X and Y cell input to visual cortex. However, the data reported to date suggest that much of the physiological change occurring in the visual cortex as a consequence of visual deprivation cannot be attributed solely to subcortical abnormalities.

The lid suture technique which results in these changes in visual cortical function has traditionally been regarded as a technique for depriving an animal of patterned stimulation but not of light stimulation. However, it is apparent that lid suture results in deprivation not only of patterns but also of movement of stimuli in the visual environment. Recent evidence indicates that experience of moving stimuli during the early postnatal period is a critical factor in the ontogeny and maintenance of normal function of the visual cortex. Rearing kittens in an environment in which all perceived motion is undirectional or in an environment which is stroboscopically illuminated and which therefore prevents experience of movement but not of patterns results in significant loss of direction selectivity in visual cortical neurons (Berman and Daw, 1977; Cynader *et al.*, 1973, 1975; Cynader and Chernenko, 1976; Daw and Wyatt, 1976; Olson and Pettigrew, 1974; Singer, 1976; Tretter *et al.*, 1975). Thus lid suture should be regarded as a technique for depriving an animal of experience of both patterned and moving stimuli. Since visual cortical neurons of newborn visually naive kittens have the property of direction selectivity, it is clear that deprivation of experience of moving stimuli results in a breakdown or rearrangement of genetically specified functional organization.

The problem of accounting for the adaptive significance of a sensory system which is so plastic, and is so easily disrupted by abnormal sensory input, is considerable. However, before addressing this central issue, the time period of susceptibility to deprivation and the extent to which these changes are reversible will be considered.

CRITICAL PERIODS AND REVERSIBILITY OF DEPRIVATION EFFECTS. Reports of neural plasticity in the adult are sparse (Brown and Salinger, 1975; Creutzfeld and Heggelund, 1975), and most investigators report that the period of susceptibility to deprivation is limited to the early postnatal period. In the cat, lid suture during the fourth and fifth postnatal weeks has the most deleterious effects. The critical period for these effects is essentially complete by the end of the third month, and lid suture in the adult has minimal effects (Hubel and Wiesel, 1970). It is of interest to note that the critical period for these effects of visual deprivation extends considerably beyond the period (4 weeks) at which the cortical physiology of the kitten visual system has developed essentially adult characteristics. The binocularity of cortical neurons seems particularly fragile, and recent studies have shown that, during the fourth postnatal week, as little as a few hours of monocular lid suture is sufficient to cause significant loss of binocularity and significant bias toward the experienced eye (Olson and Freeman, 1975; Peck and Blakemore, 1975; Pettigrew *et al.*, 1973*a*; Schechter and Murphy, 1976). It seems unlikely that such short periods of binocular deprivation would cause similarly rapid effects of receptive field characteristics, but this has not yet been investigated. The critical period for deprivation of movement overlaps with but is not identical to the critical period for lid suture.

A question of central importance is the extent to which these cortical abnormalities are reversible. The evidence indicates that they are remarkably persistent. Even if the deprived eye is opened for 12 months following the early brief period of monocular lid suture, the percentage of cortical cells which can subsequently be driven by the deprived eye remains very small (Wiesel and Hubel, 1965*b*). This is true even if the "cross-suture" technique is used, which involves suturing the originally experienced eye when the deprived eye is opened, thus forcing usage of the originally deprived eye (Chow and Stewart, 1972).

Nevertheless, reversibility of the effects of early deprivation can be demonstrated during a critical period (Berman and Daw, 1977; Blakemore and Van Sluyters, 1974; Movshon, 1976). It has been shown that the period between the fourth week and the fourth month, when kittens are most susceptible to the effects of deprivation, coincides with the period when they also demonstrate a potential for recovery, if the cross-suture technique is used. Thus cross-suturing at 5 weeks caused a complete reversal in ocular dominance of cortical cells, i.e., cells respond only to the eye which was closed for the first 5 weeks and then opened.

FUNCTIONAL SIGNIFICANCE OF CORTICAL PLASTICITY

The experimental data reviewed above indicate that at least three aspects of visual cortical function are affected by deprivation: binocular interaction, orientation specificity, and direction selectivity. The data also indicate that many components of these functional characteristics are present prior to visual experience and are then disrupted by abnormal visual experience. The adaptiveness of a largely prewired system which is so sensitive to disruption by abnormal visual experience is hard to explain. Ideally, a genetically determined prewired system would be quite resistant to idiosyncratic variants of environmental experiences. To account for this susceptibility to disruption of functional organization during development, many investigators have hypothesized that there must be some critical aspects of visual function which cannot be totally prespecified and for which visual experience must be an essential component. This idea has been convincingly argued, by several investigators, with reference to the functional organization of binocular activation of cortical neurons (Barlow, 1975; Blakemore and Van Sluyters, 1975; Grobstein and Chow, 1975; Pettigrew, 1974). For example, the size, optics, and position of the two eyes develop independently, and, in order to achieve the precise interocular interactions seen in disparity-sensitive cortical cells, visual experience would have to produce changes in cortical organization at some point during normal development. Such changes in disparity tuning of cortical neurons do occur if the discrepancy in input to the two eyes is limited to a range that can be accommodated physiologically (Shlaer, 1971), and this evidence supports this interpretation of the functional significance of neonatal plasticity in interocular interactions.

The functional adaptiveness of plasticity of orientation selectivity and direction selectivity of cortical neurons is much harder to explain since, unlike disparity sensitivity, these characteristics are largely specified prior to visual experience. Two arguments have been put forward to account for this plasticity of orientation selectivity: one argues that visual experience serves to enhance physiological and perceptual resolution of orientations and contours most frequently encountered in the individual environment of the animal; the other argument suggests that experience may serve to enhance matching of orientation selectivity for each eye in binocularly driven neurons; interocular matching of orientation sensitivity is closely related to the phenomenon of interocular alignment and disparity tuning, and so this argument could explain both forms of plasticity of neurons of the kitten visual cortex. The hypothesis is both plausible and parsimonious, but awaits experimental verification. The first hypothesis seems somewhat less plausible, since most environments probably include a richly variegated offering of orientations and contours. However, it is susceptible to experimental testing and has provoked extensive research involving selective deprivation of specific orientations in the visual environment (Blakemore, 1974*a,b;* Blakemore and Cooper, 1970;

Blasdel *et al.*, 1977; Freeman and Pettigrew, 1973; Hirsch and Spinelli, 1970; Pettigrew and Freeman, 1973; Pettigrew and Garey, 1974; Pettigrew *et al.*, 1973*b;* Van Sluyters and Blakemore, 1973).

55

ONTOGENY OF
SENSORY SYSTEMS

EFFECTS OF SELECTIVE DEPRIVATION ON DEVELOPMENT OF THE CAT VISUAL SYSTEM

If kittens are reared in special striped environments, or with goggles over their eyes, thus restricting their early visual experience to horizontal or vertical lines, then an increased percentage of visual cortical neurons are found to respond to orientations similar to those experienced in the restricted environment (Blakemore, 1974*a,b;* Blakemore and Cooper, 1970; Blasdel *et al.*, 1977; Hirsch and Spinelli, 1970; Pettigrew *et al.*, 1973*b*). A recent failure to replicate this effect suggests that some specific aspects of the rearing environment may be critical in producing this effect (Stryker and Sherk, 1975), but the weight of the evidence suggests that visual experience can modify the physiological organization of visual cortex in such a way that it reflects the visual environment. However, the way in which such changes are achieved is not clear. Two hypotheses can be put forward: the absence of stimulation of specific orientations might cause cells which were prespecified to respond to such orientation to become nonfunctional, and thus activity would be recorded only from those cells prespecified to respond to the experienced orientation; alternatively, cells might change their prespecified orientation preferences in response to such stimulation. The data obtained from kittens reared with goggles suggest the first alternative, since large "silent" areas of cortex occurred in which no responsive cells could be isolated. However, if instead of wearing goggles kittens are reared in a striped environment, then no such silent areas are found. Thus, although the issue of whether restricted visual experience results in loss of function of nonstimulated cells or in an active change in response properties is of critical theoretical importance, conflicting data and methodological problems confound resolution of the issue. An alternative approach to this issue is to attempt to alter receptive field properties of a neuron by stimulating its receptive field while recording its activity. However, such attempts have resulted in rather temporary and unconvincing changes (Pettigrew *et al.*, 1973*a*). Again the data are hard to interpret. The failure to observe changes in receptive field properties could be a function of the fact that the experience is occurring in a paralyzed, anesthetized animal, or of the need for a consolidation period, or it could be considered evidence in favor of the hypothesis that cells do *not* change their properties but merely become nonfunctional if they do not receive adequate stimulation. Thus, although there is now ample evidence that aberrant early visual experience does result in abnormalities of receptive field properties, the central issue of interpreting the mechanisms by which these changes are achieved awaits resolution.

SUMMARY

Several features of the organization of the cat visual system are genetically specified and are present in the visually naive kitten. Other features develop rapidly during the first 4 postnatal weeks. Deprivation during a critical period appears to result both in a failure of this rapid maturation and in a breakdown of preexisting organization. The most dramatic changes occur at the cortical level and cannot be wholly attributed to changes at subcortical sites, and these cortical changes in response to deprivation appear to be largely irreversible after the third month of life. The functional significance of this plasticity, utilizing visual experience to achieve the precise interocular integration of both disparity sensitivity and orientation and direction selectivity of the mature visual system, is hypothesized but awaits experimental verification.

Visual System Development in Other Mammals

A major problem in the analysis of sensory development is that, although most physiological and anatomical data derive from cats, most behavioral studies of the ontogeny of perception have used human infants as subjects. If we are to draw conclusions from such disparate sets of data, we must consider to what extent the visual system of the cat can be considered to provide an adequate model for other mammals, including humans. Ontogenetic development of visual system function has been studied in a variety of mammals, which differ considerably in the state of maturity of the central nervous system at birth. In the rabbit, in which only about 25% of visual cortical neurons are orientation selective in the mature animal, no orientation-selective cells are present prior to eye opening at 10–11 days of age (Chow *et al.*, 1971; Mathers *et al.*, 1974). In contrast, the monkey, which is born with its eyes open, apparently has the full complement of finely tuned orientation selectivity, columnar organization, and binocular integration in visual cortical cells at the time of birth (Wiesel and Hubel, 1974). Thus the cat appears to be intermediate between the rabbit and the monkey, in terms of the presence of orientation selectivity of visual cortical cells prior to visual experience.

In the monkey, as in the cat, monocular lid suture during the early postnatal period results in a significant loss of cortical cells driven by the deprived eye (Baker *et al.*, 1974). Binocular suture results in the loss of normal receptive field characteristics and the appearance of visually unresponsive cells (Wiesel and Hubel, 1974). Clearly, in the monkey, the effect of deprivation is one of a breakdown of prespecified organization in a system which is physiologically quite mature at birth. However, it is not known whether disparity-sensitive neurons, which are found in cortical area 18 but not in area 17 in the monkey (Baker *et al.*, 1974), are present at birth or are dependent on visual experience, as appears to be the case for the cat.

In contrast to the cat and the monkey, the rabbit appears to be quite resistant to the effects of monocular and binocular lid suture. Binocular activation of cortical cells is not disrupted by monocular lid suture (Van Sluyters and Stewart, 1974) and orientation selectivity appears normal following extended lid suture, although the appearance of this receptive field characteristic is delayed by deprivation (Chow and Spear, 1972; Grobstein *et al.*, 1975). Rabbits also show no change in the distribution of orientation preferences following rearing in a restricted environment of vertical or horizontal lines (Mize and Murphy, 1973). In attempting to account for this relative insensitivity of the rabbit visual system to the effects of early deprivation, it seems plausible that retinal organization may be a critical factor in determining plasticity of cortical function in the visual system. The complex anatomical and physiological features of retinal organization in the rabbit may permit less capacity for reorganization at more central levels (Barlow and Hill, 1963; Dowling, 1970). In rats, cats, and monkeys, in which anatomical and physiological organization of the retina is similar and in which concentric receptive fields predominate in retinal ganglion cells, early deprivation results in disruption of visual cortical function. Thus it can be hoped that physiological data from these species will prove appropriate models for the similarly organized human system.

Ontogeny of Visual Perception

Visual Discrimination in the Neonate

Investigations of sensory and perceptual capacities present at birth, and of their development during the early postnatal period, are made difficult by the immaturity of the motor system of most neonatal mammals. Over the past few years, a variety of ingenious and highly sensitive techniques for the study of visual capacities in human infants have been developed (Fantz, 1961, 1965, 1966). One method frequently used involves observing an infant's visual fixation of two simultaneously presented stimuli. If the infant spends more time looking at one stimulus than the other, then a discrimination between the two stimuli can be assumed. This "visual preference" method offers a highly sensitive means of examining discrimination of various visual dimensions. However, it should be noted that a failure to obtain differences in fixation time for two stimuli may indicate a lack of preference for either stimulus rather than a failure to discriminate between them.

Through the use of such techniques, it has emerged that the visual capacities of the human neonate are much more highly developed than had been previously recognized. Unfortunately, these methods have rarely been adapted by psychologists studying nonhuman mammals, and there is a dearth of information on those species which have been studied most extensively by neurophysiologists and anatomists. Thus much of the following section will be devoted to the development of visual capacities in the human infant. Three types of visual behaviors will be considered: (1) visuomotor coordination and spatial localization, (2) acuity and visual resolution, and (3) pattern and object discrimination. As was done in the previous section on the physiological development of the visual system, these visual behaviors will be considered in relation to (1) visual capacities which are present in the neonate and therefore not dependent on visual experience, (2) maturation of visual capacities during the early postnatal period, and (3) the effects of sensory deprivation on these visual behaviors.

VISUOMOTOR COORDINATION AND SPATIAL LOCALIZATION. *Eye Movements.* If the human infant is presented with a display of moving stripes, an ocular following response called optokinetic nystagmus is elicited. This response appears within the

TIMOTHY J.
CUNNINGHAM AND
E. HAZEL MURPHY

first 12 hr of life and has also been observed in premature infants (McGinnis, 1930). Ocular pursuit movements, which involve fixation and visual following of objects through space, also occur within the first few hours of life (Dayton *et al.*, 1964*b*). Conjugate eye movements toward a stationary object are less easily elicited in the infant, but probably do occur (Hershenson, 1964, 1967). Visual scanning of geometric forms also appears shortly after birth (Salapatek, 1968; Salapatek and Kessen, 1966). Infants show ocular orientation toward a triangle and scanning movements around its vertices. Similar scanning movements are made by adult subjects during observation of geometric forms (Noton and Stark, 1971) and may be an essential component of object recognition.

Discrimination of Distance and Radial Movement. A variety of monocular and binocular cues can be used to estimate distance and radial movement. For binocular cues, the convergence angle of the eyes and binocular disparity are a joint function of distance and interocular separation. However, since the interocular separation changes considerably from 3 cm in the human infant to 6 cm in the adult (Bower, 1974), the use of this cue would have to be constantly tuned with experience. Nevertheless, young infants can use binocular parallax cues to specify an object in depth, even though depth estimation may not be precise (Bower *et al.*, 1970*a,b*).

Alternatively, infants can use monocular cues, such as motion parallax or optical expansion patterns, to discriminate distance and radial movement. Cues of optical expansion (increase in size of the image on the retina as an object moves toward the infant) are used by very young infants, who show a coordinated defensive response to an object approaching from straight ahead (Bower, 1974).

Depth perception is a particular case of this distance perception and has been studied in a variety of species, using the visual cliff apparatus (Hinds, 1972*a*). Human infants aged 6 months show a clear preference for the shallow or "safe" side of the visual cliff. Because the visual cliff requires some level of motor ability for testing to be carried out, it cannot be used with newborn infants. However, evidence from other species clearly indicates that depth perception is not dependent on experience. In chicks and in ungulates, which are motorically precocial, virtually perfect performance is demonstrated on the visual cliff within hours of birth (Gibson and Walk, 1960). Other animals, such as the cat and rabbit, show a preference for the shallow side of the visual cliff coincidentally with the development of a level of visual acuity adequate to make the depth discrimination (Karmel *et al.*, 1970; Stewart and Riesen, 1972; Warkentin, 1937; Warkentin and Smith, 1937).

Perception of distance of objects occurs in 2-week-old infants, but accurate estimation of distance develops somewhat later (Bower, 1974; Bower *et al.*, 1970*b*; White *et al.*, 1964).

Localization of an object in space is often specified by cues in more than one sensory modality, and the ability to integrate information from different sensory modalities is present at birth. Thus human infants, immediately after birth, will orient visually toward the source of an auditory stimulus (Wertheimer, 1961), and will turn their heads away from unpleasant odors (Aronson and Rosenblum, 1971; Engen *et al.*, 1963).

VISUAL ACUITY. Visual accommodation in human infants is quite poor at birth. The newborn can focus its eyes only at a particular distance (median 19 cm) but the range of accommodation increases rapidly and reaches adult levels by about the fourth month of life (Haynes *et al.*, 1965). Despite this poor level of accommodation in the newborn infant, visual acuity is reasonably good and estimates indicate that it is at least 20/150 with the Snellen scale (Dayton *et al.*, 1964a; Fantz, 1966; Gorman *et al.*, 1957; Marg *et al.*, 1976). Acuity improves rapidly during the early postnatal months, and an adult level of acuity (Snellen 20/20) is achieved by the fifth or sixth month of life (Atkinson *et al.*, 1974; Fantz, 1966). Rapid postnatal improvement in visual acuity occurs in other mammals, and appears to be a function of maturation, not of visual experience, since there is no correlation between time of eye opening and development of visual acuity (Freeman and Marg, 1975; Vestal and King, 1968, 1971; Warkentin and Smith, 1937).

Thus, in all mammals tested, optokinetic nystagmus can be elicited at birth or at the time of eye opening, and a rapid increase in visual acuity occurs during the early postnatal months. Brightness and color discrimination also improve rapidly during this period, and, in human infants, reach essentially adult levels within a few months (Bernstein *et al.*, 1976; Dobson, 1976; Dorsi and Cooper, 1966; Mitchell *et al.*, 1976; Ordy *et al.*, 1964; Peeples and Teller, 1975).

PATTERN PERCEPTION. Studies of visual fixation of patterned vs. unpatterned stimuli indicate that infants do discriminate patterns and show preferences for complex patterns within the first week of life (Fantz, 1966, 1967). Fantz suggests that this innate interest in form and pattern is highly adaptive in that it plays an important role in focusing attention on stimulus characteristics which will later have significance for the recognition and discrimination of objects. Color and brightness would then be less potent stimuli because these features are not crucial in object recognition.

The evidence reviewed above clearly indicates that, at least for the human infant, discrimination of brightness, color, pattern, spatial localization, distance, and movement is present at or near the time of birth, along with the capacity to fixate, follow, and orient toward visual stimuli. During the early postnatal months, rapid increases in brightness sensitivity, acuity, and accuracy of visual following occur. Thus, despite the immaturity of the motor systems, the human infant is well able to passively explore his visual world.

EFFECTS OF DEPRIVATION ON VISUAL DISCRIMINATION

The effects of depriving an animal of pattern experience during the early postnatal period have been studied in a variety of animals. In most cases, the effects of dark rearing and of binocular lid suture do not differ significantly. The effects of monocular lid suture, however, tend to be more severe. When animals are first exposed to a patterned environment after a period of dark rearing or lid suture, they appear behaviorally blind, but many visual behaviors return. The time course of the return of visually guided behaviors depends on the amount of time of prior deprivation and on the visual behavior being tested.

VISUOMOTOR COORDINATION AND SPATIAL LOCALIZATION. *Eye Movements.* Optokinetic nystagmus is only partially suppressed by visual deprivation. Immediately after the deprivation period, it is elicited less easily than in the normally reared animal, but recovers with normal visual experience (Fitch, 1971; Riesen, 1947; Van Hof-Van Duin, 1976). Visual tracking is more severely suppressed by early deprivation but still recovers in all species tested (Fantz, 1965; Ganz and Fitch, 1968; Riesen, 1947; Van Hof-Van Duin, 1976). Both patterned visual stimulation and experience of moving objects are important in maintaining this visual following. Monkeys reared in a stroboscopically illuminated environment (thus eliminating experience of moving objects) are unable to track moving objects smoothly, but also improve with experience (Orbach and Miller, 1969). Thus visual following of moving objects and optokinetic nystagmus, both of which are seen in most animals at birth or soon after, are suppressed by deprivation but recover with experience in a normal visual environment.

Discrimination of Distance and Radial Movement. Cats and monkeys reared with binocular deprivation do not show a blink response to rapidly approaching objects, but the response appears after experience with a normal visual environment (Peck and Blakemore, 1975; Walk and Gibson, 1961; Wilson and Riesen, 1966). Depth discrimination, measured by the visual cliff apparatus, is also lost after a period of deprivation, but reappears with visual experience (Fantz, 1965; Held and Hein, 1963; Nealy and Riley, 1963; Walk and Gibson, 1961; Walk *et al.*, 1957; Wilson and Riesen, 1966). The data indicate that an unlearned aversion to depth is suppressed by visual deprivation but that this suppression is reversible. Similar results are reported for visual placing and visually guided reaching (Fantz, 1965; Foley, 1935; Ganz, 1975; Ganz and Fitch, 1968; Hein, 1970; Hines, 1942; Norton, 1974; Riesen, 1961; Tinklepaugh and Hartman, 1932; Wilson and Riesen, 1966). For many aspects of visuomotor coordination, patterned visual experience is not sufficient, but correlated visual and motor experience is needed. This literature has been reviewed elsewhere (Ganz, 1975) and will not be discussed further here.

VISUAL ACUITY. When acuity is measured by eliciting optokinetic nystagmus, there appear to be only minimal long-lasting effects of visual deprivation, although there is often a temporary loss of acuity immediately after the deprivation period (Ganz and Fitch, 1968; Ordy *et al.*, 1962; Riesen, 1958). However, optokinetic nystagmus survives cortical ablation and is probably subserved by subcortical structures. If other measures of acuity are used, which depend on cortical integrity, such as discrimination of stripes or of gaps in a line or circle, then acuity deficits may be permanent (Dews and Wiesel, 1970; Van Hof, 1971; Van Hof and Kobayashi, 1972;), especially if monocular lid suture is used. In both humans and monkeys, very brief periods of monocular occlusion during an early critical period appear to result in severe and permanent amblyopia of the occluded eye and in deficits in binocular vision (Banks *et al.*, 1975; Von Noorden, 1973; Von Noorden *et al.*, 1970).

PATTERN PERCEPTION. Pattern discrimination and object recognition are severely disrupted by deprivation, and the deficits are often permanent. These discriminations are dependent on visual cortical function in most mammals and are lost following ablation of visual cortex. These data have been reviewed recently in detail (Riesen and Zilbert, 1975) and will be only briefly summarized here. Von Senden (1960) provides vivid descriptions of the limited visual capacities of humans who, in early life, developed cataracts which were surgically removed in later life. These patients had severe difficulties in learning to discriminate such simple forms as square and triangle, and in recognizing simple objects presented in different aspects. Generalization of objects, such as boxes or rings, was extremely difficult. More recent case studies (Ackroyd *et al.,* 1974; Sherman *et al.,* 1974) present some conflicting evidence, but, in at least one case, pattern and object recognition were never achieved by the patient, despite quite good discrimination of brightness and movement. Nonhuman subjects experience similar difficulties. Monkeys reared in the dark until the age of 16 months are very slow to learn to recognize objects (Jacobson, 1970). Cats and rats also show difficulties in learning complex pattern discriminations following deprivation (Ganz *et al.,* 1972; Resen *et al.,* 1953; Tees, 1968), although rabbits seem more resistant to such deprivation (Van Hof, 1971). Thus pattern discrimination and object recognition appear to differ from those other visual capacities reviewed above, in that visual deprivation results in severe and long-lasting deficits. Since human and monkey newborn infants show pattern discrimination and pattern preferences shortly after birth, this effect appears to signify a loss of innate ability to discriminate patterns. Visual fixation preferences for patterned stimuli are also lost, and color and brightness become the preferred stimulus attributes.

The physiological abnormalities of visual cortex which result from deprivation, reviewed earlier, are largely irreversible, so it is not surprising that those visual capacities which are strongly dependent on the integrity of visual cortical function should also show long-lasting deficits. However, most of the visual abilities reviewed above, other than pattern and object discrimination, show rather temporary deficits following deprivation. If these capacities are subserved by subcortical sites, then one might expect that the physiological changes which occur in subcortical visual areas following deprivation should also show recovery following exposure to a normal visual environment. This appears to be the case, at least for neurons of the lateral geniculate nucleus (Hoffman and Cynader, 1975).

EFFECTS OF SELECTIVE VISUAL EXPERIENCE ON VISUAL PERCEPTION

Selective restriction of visual experience to selected orientations, during development, affects visual discrimination, although the effects are more subtle than those resulting from total deprivation. If cats are reared with their visual experience restricted to vertical or horizontal lines, then, on their first exposure to a normal environment, they appear blind to lines of an orientation orthogonal to those experienced (Blakemore and Cooper, 1970). However, this apparent blindness is only temporary, and the only permanent effect appears to be a reduction in sensitivity of resolution of gratings of the nonexperienced orientation (Muir and Mitchell, 1973). In human infants, astigmatism, which can deprive the infants of experience of sharp images of specific orientations, can also result in a reduced acuity for those orientations (Freeman *et al.,* 1972; Mitchell *et al.,* 1973; Mitchell

TIMOTHY J.
CUNNINGHAM AND
E. HAZEL MURPHY

and Wilkinson, 1974). Further, humans reared in an environment relatively free of vertical and horizontal contours do not show the enhanced resolution of vertical and horizontal orientations which is found in individuals in whose environment these orientations predominate (Annis and Frost, 1973). This seems to indicate that visual experience serves to enhance resolution of commonly experienced orientations. However, newborn infants have higher resolutions of vertical and horizontal orientations than of other orientations, and so the differential resolution of orientations may be genetically determined. Therefore, while experience might appear to enhance resolution of commonly viewed orientations, it might be more accurate to conclude that deprivation produces a decrease in resolution for nonexperienced orientations including those for which resolution is inherently optimal. Overall, the consequences of selective visual experience during development appear to have only a subtle influence on perceptual abilities, and these findings do not lend strong support to the hypothesis, discussed earlier, that plasticity of orientation selectivity of visual cortical neurons might serve to enhance visual discrimination of frequently encountered environmental events.

Conclusions

Many structural and functional features of adult mammalian sensory systems appear to develop independently of appropriate sensory experience. However, deprivation during critical periods early in life may produce profound and irreversible deficits in sensory functioning, primarily of those functions which depend on the integrity of the cerebral cortex. These functional deficits can be shown with both electrophysiological and behavioral testing methods. The structural changes which underlie these deficits are not clear, but they may include alterations in the morphology and quantity of synaptic terminals in the central sensory receiving zones.

On the other hand, certain sensory functions and possibly some aspects of the structure of sensory neurons depend on appropriate experience for normal development. At present, there are few examples of this experience-dependent development. However, it would be unwise to suggest that most sensory structures and functions are genetically predetermined. It is more likely that the experience-dependent properties of developing sensory systems are technically inaccessible to modern neurobiology. When anatomical and physiological techniques can detect the subtleties of sensory perception, we expect that such properties will be the rule rather than the exception.

In attempting to draw conclusions from such a vast set of data, in which methods, subjects, and philosophical biases are so diverse, we present a boldness which is pretended, not real. Clearly, there is no resolution to the nature-nurture issue; both nature and nurture interact to produce the final complex product of a perceiving individual. The central problem facing developmental neurobiologists today is to achieve an insight into the mechanisms by which these interactions occur.

Ackroyd, C., Humphrey, N. K., and Warrington, E. K. Lasting effects of early blindness: A case study. *Quart. J. Exp. Psychol.,* 1974, *26,* 114–124.

Angevine, J. B. Time of neuron origin in the hippocampal region: An autoradiographic study in the mouse. *Exp. Neurol. Suppl.,* 1965, *2,* 1–70.

Angevine, J. B. Time of neuron origin in the diencephalon of the mouse: An autoradiographic study. *J. Comp. Neurol.,* 1970, *139,* 129–188.

Angevine, J. B., and Sidman, R. L. Autoradiographic study of cell migration during histogenesis of cerebral cortex of the mouse. *Nature,* 1961, *192,* 766–768.

Annis, R. C., and Frost, B. Human visual ecology and orientation anisotropies in acuity. *Science,* 1973, *182,* 729.

Aronson, E., and Rosenblum, S. Space perception in early infancy: Perception within a common auditory-visual space. *Science,* 1971, *172,* 1161–1163.

Atkinson, J., Braddick, O., and Braddick, F. Acuity and contrast sensitivity of infant vision. *Nature,* 1974, *247,* 403.

Attardi, D. G., and Sperry, R. W. Preferential selection of central pathways by regenerating optic fibers. *Exp. Neurol.,* 1963, *7,* 46–64.

Baker, F. H., Grigg, P., and Von Noorden, G. K. Effects of visual deprivation and strabismus on the response of neurons in the visual cortex of the monkey, including studies on the striate and prestriate cortex in the normal animal. *Brain Res.,* 1974, *66,* 185–208.

Banks, M. S., Aslin, R. N., and Letson, R. D. Sensitive period for the development of human binocular vision. *Science,* 1975, *190,* 675–677.

Barlow, H. B. Visual experience and cortical development. *Nature,* 1975, *258,* 199–204.

Barlow, H. B., and Hill, R. M. Selective sensitivity to direction of movement in ganglion cells of the rabbit retina. *Science,* 1963, *193,* 421–422.

Barlow, H. B., and Pettigrew, J. D. Lack of specificity of neurons in the visual cortex of young kittens. *J. Physiol. (London),* 1971, *218,* 98–100.

Barlow, H. B., Blakemore, C., and Pettigrew, J. P. The neural mechanism of binocular depth discrimination. *J. Physiol. (London),* 1967, *193,* 327–342.

Baxter, B. L. Effect of visual deprivation during postnatal maturation on the electroencephalogram of the cat. *Exp. Neurol.,* 1966, *14,* 224–237.

Berman, N., and Daw, N. W. Comparison of the critical periods for monocular and directional deprivation in cats. *J. Physiol. (London),* 1977, *265,* 249–259.

Berman, N., and Sterling, P. Cortical suppression of the retino-collicular pathway in the monocularly deprived cat. *J. Physiol. (London),* 1976, *255,* 263–273.

Bernstein, M. H., Kessen, W., and Weiskopf, S. The categories of hue in infancy. *Science,* 1976, *191,* 201–202.

Berry, M., and Rogers, A. W. The migration of neuroblasts in the developing cerebral cortex. *J. Anat. (London),* 1965, *99,* 691–709.

Blake, R., Crawford, M. L. J., and Hirsch, H. V. B. Consequences of alternating monocular deprivation on eye alignment and convergence in cats. *Invest. Opthalmol.,* 1974, *13,* 121–126.

Blakemore, C. Developmental factors in the formation of feature extracting neurons. In F. O. Schmitt and F. G. Worden (eds.), *The Neurosciences: Third Study Program.* MIT Press, Cambridge, Mass., 1974*a*.

Blakemore, C. Development of the mammalian visual system. *Br. Med. Bull.,* 1974*b*, *30(2),* 152–157.

Blakemore, C. The conditions required for the maintenance of binocularity in the kitten's visual cortex. *J. Physiol. (London),* 1976, *261,* 423–444.

Blakemore, C., and Cooper, G. F. Development of the brain depends on the visual environment. *Nature,* 1970, *228,* 447–478.

Blakemore, C., and Van Sluyters, R. C. Reversal of the physiological effects of monocular deprivation in kittens: Further evidence for a sensitive period. *J. Physiol. (London),* 1974, *237,* 195–216.

Blakemore, C., and Van Sluyters, R. C. Innate and environmental factors in the development of the kitten's visual cortex. *J. Physiol. (London),* 1975, *248,* 663–716.

Blasdel, G. G., Mitchell, D. E., Muir, D. W., and Pettigrew, J. D. A physiological and behavioral study in cats of the effects of early visual experience with contours of a single orientation. *J. Physiol. (London),* 1977, *265,* 615–636.

Bloom, E. M., and Tompkins, R. Selective reinnervation in skin rotation grafts in *Rana pipiens, J. Exp. Zool.*, 1976, *195*, 237–246.

Bower, T. G. R. *Development in Infancy.* Freeman, San Francisco, 1974.

Bower, T. G. R., Broughton, J. M., and Moore, M. K. The co-ordination of vision and touch in infancy. *Percept. Psychophys.*, 1970a, *8*, 51–53.

Bower, T. G. R., Broughton, J. M., and Moore, M. K. Demonstration of intention in the reaching behavior of neonate humans. *Nature,* 1970b, *228*, 679–681.

Bradley, R. M., and Mistretta, C. M. Fetal sensory receptors. *Physiol. Rev.*, 1975, *55*, 352–382.

Brown, D. L., and Salinger, W. L. Loss of X-cells in lateral geniculate nucleus with monocular paralysis: Neural plasticity in the adult cat. *Science,* 1975, *189*, 1011–1012.

Brückner, G., Vladislav, M., and Biesold, D. Neurogenesis in the visual system of the rat: An autoradiographic investigation. *J. Comp. Neurol.*, 1976, *166*, 245–256.

Buisseret, P., and Imbert, M. Responses of neurons in the striate cortex observed in normal and dark-reared kittens during post-natal life. *J. Physiol. (London)*, 1974, *246*, 98–99P.

Buisseret, D., and Imbert, M. Visual cortical cells: Their developmental properties in normal and dark-reared kittens. *J. Physiol. (London)*, 1976, *255*, 511–525.

Caviness, V. S., and Sidman, R. L. Time of origin of corresponding cell classes in the cerebral cortex of normal and reeler mutant mice. *J. Comp. Neurol.*, 1973, *148*, 141–151.

Chow, K. L., and Spear, P. D. Morphological and functional effects of visual deprivation on the rabbit visual system. *Exp. Neurol.*, 1972, *34*, 409–433.

Chow, K. L., and Stewart, D. L. Reversal of structural and functional effects of long-term visual deprivation in cats. *Exp. Neurol.*, 1972, *34*, 409–433.

Chow, K. L., Masland, R. H., and Stewart, D. L. Receptive field characteristics of striate cortical neurons in the rabbit. *Brain Res.*, 1971, *33*, 337–352.

Cowan, W. M. Neuronal death as a regulative mechanism in the control of cell numbers in the nervous system. In M. Rockstein (ed.), *Development and Aging in the Nervous System.* Academic Press, New York, 1973, pp. 19–34.

Cowan, W. M., Martin, A. H., and Wenger, E. Mitotic patterns in the optic tectum of the chick during normal development and after early removal of the optic vesicle. *J. Exp. Zool.*, 1968, *169*, 71–92.

Creutzfeld, O. D., and Heggelund, P. Neural plasticity in visual cortex of adult cats after exposure to visual patterns. *Science,* 1975, *188*, 1025–1027.

Cuschieri, A., and Bannister, L. H. The development of the olfactory mucosa in the mouse: Light microscopy. *J. Anat. (London)*, 1975, *119*, 277–284.

Cynader, M., and Chernenko, G. Abolition of direction selectivity in the visual cortex of the cat. *Science,* 1976, *193*, 504–505.

Cynader, M., Berman, N., and Hein, A. Cats reared in stroboscopic illumination: Effects on receptive fields in visual cortex. *Proc. Natl. Acad. Sci. (USA)*, 1973, *70*, 1353–1354.

Cynader, M., Berman, N., and Hein, A. Cats raised in a one-directional world: Effects on receptive fields in visual cortex and superior colliculus. *Exp. Brain Res.*, 1975, *22*, 267–280.

Cynader, M., Berman N., and Hein, A. Recovery of function in cat visual cortex following prolonged deprivation. *Exp. Brain. Res.*, 1976, *25*, 139–156.

Daw, N. W., and Wyatt, H. J. Kittens reared in a unidirectional environment: Evidence for a critical period. *J. Physiol. (London)*, 1976, *257*, 155–170.

Dayton, G. O., Jones, M. H., Aiu, P., Rawson, R. A., Steele, B., and Rose, M. Developmental study of co-ordinated eye movements in the human infant. I. Visual acuity in the newborn human: a study based on induced optokinetic nystagmus recorded by electro-oculography. *Arch. Ophthalmol.*, 1964a, *71*, 865–870.

Dayton, G. O., Jones, M. H., Steele, B., and Rose, M. Developmental study of co-ordinated eye movements in the human infant. II. An electro-oculographic study of the fixation reflex in the newborn. *Arch. Ophthalmol.*, 1964b, *71*, 871–875.

Denney, D., Baumgartner, G., and Adoriani, C. Responses of cortical neurons to stimulation of the visual afferent radiations. *Exp. Brain Res.*, 1968, *6*, 265–272.

Dews, P. B., and Wiesel, T. N. Consequences of monocular deprivation on visual behavior in kittens. *J. Physiol. (London)*, 1970, *206*, 437–455.

Dobson, V. Spectral sensitivity of the 2-month infant as measured by the visually evoked cortical potential. *Vision Res.*, 1976, *16*, 367–374.

Doris, J., and Cooper, L. Brightness discrimination in infancy. *J. Exp. Child Psychol.*, 1966, *3*, 31–39.

Dowling, J. E. Organization of vertebrate retinas. *Invest. Ophthalmol.*, 1970, *9*, 655–680.

Engen, T., Lipsitt, L. P., and Kaye, H. Olfactory responses and adaptation in the human neonate. *J. Comp. Physiol. Psychol.*, 1963, *56*, 73–77.

Fantz, R. L. The origin of form perception. *Sci. Am.*, 1961, *204*, 66–72.

Fantz, R. L. Ontogeny of perception. In A. M. Schrier and H. F. Harlow (eds.), *Behavior of Nonhuman Primates: Modern Research Trends*, Vol. 2. Academic Press, New York, 1965, pp. 365–403.

Fantz, R. L. Pattern discrimination and selective attention as determinants of perceptual development from birth. In A. H. Kidd and J. L. Rivoire (eds.), *Perceptual Development of Children.* 1966, International Universities Press, New York, pp. 143–173.

Fantz, R. L. Visual perception and experience in early infancy: A look at the hidden side of behavior development. In (H. W. Stevenson *et al.,* eds.), *Early Behavior: Comparitive and Developmental Approaches.* Wiley, New York, 1967, pp. 181–224.

Farbman, A. I. Development of the taste bud. In L. M. Biedler (ed.), *Handbook of Sensory Physiology,* Vol. IV: *Chemical Senses,* Part 2. Springer, New York, 1971, pp. 51–62.

Fifkova, E. The effect of monocular deprivation on the synaptic contacts of the visual cortex. *J. Neurobiol.,* 1970, *1*, 285–295.

Fifkova, E. Changes of axosomatic synapses in the visual cortex of monocularly deprived rats. *J. Neurobiol.,* 1971, *2*, 61–71.

Fitch, M. H. Development of visuomotor behaviors following monocular and binocular patterned visual deprivation in the cat. Thesis, University of California at Riverside, 1971.

Foley, J. P., Jr. Two year development of a rhesus monkey *(Macaca mulatta)* reared in isolation. *J. Genet. Psychol.,* 1935, *47*, 73–97.

Freeman, D. N., and Marg, E. Visual acuity development coincides with the sensitive period in kittens. *Nature,* 1975, *254*, 614–615.

Freeman, R. D., and Pettigrew, J. D. Alteration of visual cortex from environmental asymmetries. *Nature,* 1973, *246*, 359–360.

Freeman, R. D., Mitchell, D. E., and Millodot, M. A neural effect of partial visual deprivation in humans. *Science,* 1972, *175*, 1384–1386.

Fukuda, Y., and Stone, J. Retinal distribution and central projections of Y-, X- and W-cells of the cat's retina. *J. Neurophysiol.,* 1974, *37*, 749–772.

Ganz, L. Orientation in visual space by neonates and its modification by visual deprivation. In A. H. Riesen (ed.), *The Developmental Neuropsychology of Sensory Deprivation.* Academic Press, New York, 1975, pp. 169–210.

Ganz, L., and Fitch, M. The effect of visual deprivation on perceptual behavior. *Exp. Neurol.,* 1968, *22*, 638–660.

Ganz, L., Hirsch, H. V. B., and Tieman, S. B. The nature of perceptual deficits in visually deprived cats. *Brain Res.,* 1972, *44*, 547–568.

Gaze, R. M. *The Formation of Nerve Connections.* Academic Press, New York, 1970.

Gaze, R. M., and Keating, M. J. The visual system and neuronal specificity. *Nature (London),* 1972, *237*, 375–378.

Gibson, E. J., and Walk, R. D. The "visual cliff." *Sci. Am.,* 1960, *202*, 64–71.

Globus, A., and Scheibel, A. Synaptic loci on visual cortical neurons of the rabbit: The specific afferent radiation. *Exp. Neurol.,* 1967a, *18*, 116–131.

Globus, A., and Scheibel, A. The effect of visual deprivation on cortical neurons: A Golgi study. *Exp. Neurol.,* 1967b, *19*, 331–345.

Globus, A., Rosenzweig, M. R., Bennet, E. L., and Diamond, M. C. Effects of differential experience on dendritic spine counts in rat cerebral cortex. *J. Comp. Physiol. Psychol.,* 1973, *82*, 175–181.

Glucksmann, A. Cell death in normal vertebrate ontogeny. *Biol. Rev.,* 1951, *26*, 59–86.

Goodman, L. Effect of total absence of function on the optic system of rabbit. *Am. J. Physiol.,* 1932, *100*, 46–63.

Gorman, J. J., Cogan, D. G., and Gellis, S. S. Apparatus for grading visual acuity of infants on basis of optokinetic nystagmus. *Pediatrics,* 1957, *19*, 1088–1092.

Gregory, R. L., and Wallace, J. G. Recovery from early blindness: A case study. *Exp. Psychol. Soc. Monogr.,* 1963, No. 2.

Grobstein, P., and Chow, K. L. Receptive field development and individual experience. *Science,* 1975, *190*, 352–358.

Grobstein, P., Chow, K. L., and Fox, P. C. Development of receptive fields in rabbit visual cortex: Changes in time course due to delayed eye-opening. *Proc. Natl. Acad. Sci. (USA),* 1975, *72*, 1543–1545.

Guillery, R. W. Binocular competition in control of geniculate cell growth. *J. Comp. Neurol.*, 1972, *144*, 117–127.

Guillery, R. W. The effect of lid suture on the growth of cells in the dorsal lateral geniculate nucleus of kittens. *J. Comp. Neurol.*, 1973, *148*, 417–422.

Guillery, R. W., and Stelzner, D. J. The differential effects of unilateral lid closure upon the monocular and binocular segments of the dorsal lateral geniculate nucleus in the cat. *J. Comp. Neurol.*, 1970, *139*, 413–422.

Guth, L. Degeneration and regeneration of taste buds. In L. M. Biedler (ed.), *Handbook of Sensory Physiology,* Vol. IV: *Chemical Senses,* Part 2. Springer, New York, 1971, pp. 63–74.

Hamasaki, D. I., and Winters, R. W. Intensity-response functions of visually deprived LGN neurons in cats. *Vision Res.,* 1973, *13*, 925–936.

Hamasaki, D. I., Rackensperger, W., and Vesper, J. Spatial organization of normal and visually deprived units in the lateral geniculate nucleus of the cat. *Vision Res.,* 1972, *12*, 843–854.

Haynes, H., White, B. L., and Held, R. Visual accommodation in human infants. *Science,* 1965, *148*, 528–530.

Hein, A. Recovering spatial motor co-ordination after visual cortex lesions. In D. Hamburg (ed.), *Perception and Its Disorders.* Research Publications of the Association for Research in Nervous Mental Disease, Vol. 48. Williams and Wilkins, Baltimore, 1970.

Held, R., and Hein, A. Movement-produced stimulation in the development of visually guided behavior. *J. Comp. Physiol. Psychol.,* 1963, *56*, 872–876.

Hershenson, M. Visual discrimination in the human newborn. *J. Comp. Physiol. Psychol.,* 1964, *58*, 270–276.

Hershenson, M. Development of the perception of form. *Psychol. Bull.,* 1967, *67*, 326–336.

Hicks, S. P., and D'Amato, C. J. Cell migrations to the isocortex in the rat. *Anat. Rec.,* 1968, *160*, 619–634.

Hinds, J. W. Early neuron differentiation in the mouse olfactory bulb. I. Light microscopy. *J. Comp. Neurol.,* 1972*a*, *146*, 233–252.

Hinds, J. W. Early neuron differentiation in the mouse olfactory bulb. II. Electron microscopy. *J. Comp. Neurol.,* 1972*b*, *146*, 253–276.

Hines, M. The development and regression of reflexes, postures and progression in the young macaque. *Contrib. Embryol. Carnegie Inst. (Washington, D.C.),* 1942, *30*, 153–209.

Hirsch, H. V. B., and Spinelli, D. N. Visual experience modifies distribution of horizontally oriented receptive fields in cats. *Science,* 1970, *168*, 869–871.

Hoffman, K. P., and Cynader, M. Recovery in the LGN of the cat after early visual deprivation. *Brain Res.,* 1975, 85–179.

Hoffman, K. P., and Sherman, S. M. Effects of early monocular deprivation on visual input to cat superior colliculus. *J. Neurophysiol.,* 1974, *37*, 1276–1286.

Hoffman, K. P., and Sherman, S. M. Effects of early binocular deprivation on visual input to cat superior colliculus. *J. Neurophysiol.,* 1975, *38*, 1049–1059.

Hoffman, K. P., and Stone, J. Conduction velocity of afferents to cat visual cortex: A correlation with cortical receptive field properties. *Brain Res.,* 1971, *32*, 460–466.

Hoffman, K. P., and Stone, J. Central terminations of W-, X- and Y-type ganglion cells from cat retina. *Brain Res.,* 1973, *49*, 500–501.

Hoffman, K. P., Stone, J., and Sherman, S. M. Relay of receptive field properties in dorsal lateral geniculate nucleus of the cat. *J. Neurophysiol.,* 1972, *35*, 518–531.

Hubel, D. H., and Wiesel, T. N. Receptive fields, binocular interaction and functional architecture in the cat's visual cortex. *J. Physiol. (London),* 1962, *160*, 106–154.

Hubel, D. H., and Wiesel, T. N. Receptive fields of cells in striate cortex of very young, visually inexperienced kittens. *J. Neurophysiol.,* 1963, *26*, 944–1002.

Hubel, D. H., and Wiesel, T. N. Receptive fields and functional architecture in two nonstriate visual areas (18 and 19) of the cat. *J. Neurophysiol.,* 1965*a*, *28*, 229–289.

Hubel, D. H., and Wiesel, T. N. Binocular interaction in striate cortex of kittens reared with artificial squint. *J. Neurophysiol.,* 1965*b*, *28*, 1041–1059.

Hubel, D. H., and Wiesel, T. N. The period of susceptibility to the physiological effects of unilateral eye closure in kittens. *J. Physiol. (London),* 1970, *206*, 419–436.

Imbert, M., and Buisseret, P. Receptive field characteristics and plastic properties of visual cortical cells in kittens reared with or without visual experience. *Exp. Brain Res.,* 1975, *22*, 25–36.

Jacobson, M. Development of neuronal specificity in retinal ganglion cells of *Xenopus. Dev. Biol.,* 1968, *17*, 202–218.

Jacobson, M. *Developmental Neurobiology.* Holt, Rinehart and Winston, New York, 1970.

Jacobson, M., and Baker, R. E. Development of neuronal connections with skin grafts in frogs: Behavioral and electrophysiological studies. *J. Comp. Neurol.*, 1969, *137*, 121–142.

Karmel, B. Z., Miller, P. N., Dettweiler, L., and Anderson, G. Texture density and normal development of visual depth avoidance. *Dev. Psychobiol.*, 1970, *3*, 73–90.

Keating, M. J. The formation of visual neuronal connections: An appraisal of the present status of the theory of neuronal specificity. In G. Gottlieb (ed.), *Studies on the Development of Behavior and the Nervous System,* Vol. 3: *Neural and Behavioral Specificity.* Academic Press, New York, 1976, pp. 59–110.

Kelly, J. P., and Cowan, W. M. Studies on the development of the chick optic tectum. III. Effects of early eye removal. *Brain Res.*, 1972, *42*, 263–288.

Leehey, S. C., Moskowitz-Cook, A., Brill, S., and Held, R. Orientational anisotrophy in infant vision. *Science*, 1975, *190*, 900–901.

LeVay, S., and Ferster, D. Relay cell classes in the lateral geniculate nucleus of the cat and the effects of visual deprivation. *J. Comp. Neurol.*, 1977, *172*, 563–584.

LeVay, S., and Gilbert, C. D. Laminar patterns of geniculocortical projection in the cat. *Brain Res.*, 1976, *113*, 1–19.

Levine, R. L., and Jacobson, M. Deployment of optic nerve fibers is determined by positional markers in the frog's tectum. *Exp. Neurol.*, 1974, *43*, 527–538.

Lockshin, R. A., and Beaulation, J. Programmed cell death. *Life Sci.*, 1975, *15*, 1549–1565.

Lund, J. S., and Lund, R. D. The effects of varying periods of visual deprivation on synaptogenesis in the superior colliculus of the rat. *Brain Res.*, 1972, *42*, 21–32.

Maffei, L., and Bisti, S. Binocular interaction in strabismic kittens deprived of vision. *Science*, 1976, *191*, 579–580.

Marg, E., Freeman, D. N., Peltzman, P., and Goldstein, P. J. Visual acuity development in human infants: Evoked potential measurements. *Invest. Ophthalmol.*, 1976, *15*, 150–153.

Marin-Padilla, M. Early postnatal ontogenesis of the cerebral cortex (neocortex) of the cat *(Felis domestica).* A Golgi study. I. The primordial neocortical organization. *Z. Anat. Entwickl.-Gesch.*, 1971, *134*, 117–145.

Mathers, L. H., Chow, K. L., Spear, P. D., and Grobstein, P. Ontogenesis of receptive fields in the rabbit striate cortex. *Exp. Brain Res.*, 1974, *19*, 20–35.

McGinnis, J. M. Eye movements and optic nystagmus in early infancy. *Genet. Psychol. Monogr.*, 1930, *8*, 321–430.

Miner, N. Integumental specification of sensory fibers in the development of cutaneous local sign. *J. Comp. Neurol.*, 1956, *105*, 161–170.

Mitchell, D. E., and Wilkinson, F. The effect of early astigmatism on the visual resolution of gratings. *J. Physiol. (London)*, 1974, *243*, 729–756.

Mitchell, D. E., Freeman, R. D., Millodot, M., and Haegerstrom, G. Meridional amblyopia: Evidence for modification of the human visual system by early visual experience. *Vision Res.*, 1973, *13*, 535–558.

Mitchell, D. E., Giffin, F., Wilkinson, F., Anderson, P., and Smith, M. L. Visual resolution in young kittens. *Vision Res.*, 1976, *16*, 363–366.

Mize, R. R., and Murphy, E. H. Selective visual experience fails to modify receptive field properties of rabbit cortex neurons. *Science*, 1973, *180*, 320–323.

Mize, R. R., and Murphy, E. H. Alterations in receptive field properties of superior colliculus cells by visual cortex ablation in infant and adult cats. *J. Comp. Neurol.*, 1976, *168*, 393–424.

Morest, D. K. The differentiation of cerebral dendrites: A study of the post migratory neuroblast in the medical trapezoid body. *Z. Entwickl.-Gesch.*, 1969a, *128*, 271–289.

Morest, D. R. The growth of dendrites in the mammalian brain. *Z. Entwickl.-Gesch.*, 1969b, *128*, 290–317.

Movshon, A. J. Reversal of the physiological effects of monocular deprivation in the kitten's visual cortex. *J. Physiol. (London)*, 1976, *261*, 125–174.

Muir, D. W., and Mitchell, D. E. Visual resolution and experience: Acuity deficits in cats following early selective visual deprivation. *Science*, 1973, *180*, 420–422.

Myer, R. L., and Sperry, R. W. Retinotectal specificity: Chemoaffinity theory. In G. Gottlieb (ed.), *Studies on the Development of Behavior and the Nervous System,* Vol. 3: *Neural and Behavioral Specificity.* Academic Press, New York, 1976, pp. 111–149.

Nealy, S. M., and Riley, D. A. Loss and recovery of visual depth in dark reared rat. *Am. J. Psychol.*, 1963, *76*, 329–333.

TIMOTHY J.
CUNNINGHAM AND
E. HAZEL MURPHY

Nikara, T., Bishop, P. O., and Pettigrew, J. D. Analysis of retinal correspondence by studying receptive fields of binocular single units in cat striate cortex. *Exp. Brain Res.*, 1968, *6*, 353–372.

Norman, J. L., Daniels, J. D., and Pettigrew, J. D. Absence of surround antagonism in unit responses of the LGN in young kittens. *Neurosci. Abstr.*, 1975, *1*, 88.

Norton, T. T. Receptive-field properties of superior colliculus cells and development of visual behavior in kittens. *J. Neurophysiol.*, 1974, *37*, 674–690.

Noton, D., and Stark, L. Eye movements and visual perception. *Sci. Am.*, 1971, *224*, 34–43.

Oakley, B. On the specification of neurons in the rat tongue. *Brain Res.*, 1974, *75*, 85–96.

Oakley, B., and Benjamin, R. M. Neural mechanisms of taste. *Physiol. Rev.*, 1966, *46*, 173–211.

Olmstead, J. M. D. The result of cutting the seventh cranial nerve in *Ameiurus nebulosus* (Lesueur). *J. Exp. Zool.*, 1920, *31*, 369–401.

Olson, C. R., and Freeman, R. D. Progressive changes in kitten striate cortex during monocular vision. *J. Neurophysiol.*, 1975, *38*, 26–32.

Olson, C. R., and Pettigrew, J. D. Single units in visual cortex of kittens reared in stroboscopic illumination. *Brain Res.*, 1974, *70*, 109–204.

Orbach, J., and Miller, M. H. Visual performance of infrahuman primates reared in an intermittently illuminated room. *Vision Res.*, 1969, *9*, 713–716.

Ordy, J. M., Massopust, L. C., and Wolin, L. R. Postnatal development of the retina, ERG and acuity in the rhesus monkey. *Exp. Neurol.*, 1962, *5*, 364–382.

Ordy, J. M., Latanick, A., Samorajski, T., and Massopust, L. C. Visual acuity in newborn primate infants. *Proc. Soc. Exp. Biol. Med.*, 1964, *115*, 677–680.

Palmer, L. A., and Rosenquist, A. C. Visual receptive fields of single striate cortical units projecting to the superior colliculus in the cat. *Brain Res.*, 1974, *67*, 27–42.

Peck, C. K., and Blakemore, C. Modification of single neurons in the kitten's visual cortex after brief periods of monocular vision experience. *Exp. Brain Res.*, 1975, *22*, 57–68.

Peeples, D. P., and Teller, D. Y. Color vision and brightness discrimination in two-month-old human infants. *Science*, 1975, *189*, 1102–1103.

Pettigrew, J. D. The effect of visual experience on the development of stimulus specificity by kitten cortical neurons. *J. Physiol. (London)*, 1974, *237*, 49–74.

Pettigrew, J. D., and Freeman, R. D. Visual experience without lines: Effect on developing cortical neurons. *Science*, 1973, *182*, 599–601.

Pettigrew, J. D., and Garey, L. J. Selective modification of single neuron properties in the visual cortex of kittens. *Brain Res.*, 1974, *66*, 160–164.

Pettigrew, J. D., Nikara, T., and Bishop, P. O. Responses to moving slits by single units in cat striate cortex. *Exp. Brain Res.*, 1968, *6*, 373–390.

Pettigrew, J. D., Olson, C., and Barlow, H. B. Kitten visual cortex: Short-term stimulus-induced changes in connectivity. *Science*, 1973a, *180*, 1202–1203.

Pettigrew, J. D., Olson, C., and Hirsch, H. V. B. Cortical effect of selective visual experience: Degeneration or re-organization? *Brain Res.*, 1973b, *51*, 345–351.

Ramon y Cajal, S. *The Mechanism of Development of Intraepithelial Sensory and Special Sense Nerve Terminations. Studies on Vertebrate Neurogenesis.* Thomas, Springfield, Ill., 1929.

Rasch, E., Swift, H., and Riesen, A. H. Altered structure and composition of retinal cells in dark reared mammals. *Exp. Cell Res.*, 1961, *25*, 348–363.

Riesen, A. H. The development of visual perception in man and chimpanzee. *Science*, 1947, *106*, 107–108.

Riesen, A. H. Plasticity of behavior: Psychological aspects. In H. F. Harlow and C. N. Woolsey (eds.), *Biological and Biochemical Bases of Behavior.* University of Wisconsin Press, Madison, Wis., 1958.

Riesen, A. H. Studying perceptual development using the technique of sensory deprivation. *J. Nerv. Ment. Dis.*, 1961, *132*, 21–25.

Riesen, A. H. Sensory deprivation. In Stellar and J. M. Sprague (eds.), *Progress in Physiological Psychology*, Vol. 1. Academic Press, New York, 1966, pp. 117–147.

Riesen, A. H., Kurke, M. I., and Mellinger, J. C. Interocular transfer of habits learned monocularly in visually naive and visually experienced cats. *J. Comp. Physiol. Psychol.*, 1953, *46*, 166–172.

Riesen, A. H., and Zilbert, D. E. Behavioral consequences of variations in early sensory environments. In A. H. Riesen (ed.), *The Developmental Neuropsychology of Sensory Deprivation.* Academic Press, New York, 1975, pp. 211–252.

Rose, G. H., and Ellingson, R. J. Ontogenesis of evoked responses. In W. A. Himwich (ed.), *Developmental Neurobiology.* Thomas, Springfield, Ill., 1970, pp. 393–440.

Rosenquist, A. C., and Palmer, L. A. Visual receptive field properties of cells of the superior colliculus after cortical lesions in the cat. *Exp. Neurol.,* 1971, *33*, 629–652.

Ryugo, D. K., Ryugo, R., and Killackey, H. P. Changes in pyramidal cell spine density consequent to vibrissae removal in the newborn rat. *Brain Res.,* 1975a, *96*, 82–87.

Ryugo, R., Ryugo, D. K., and Killackey, H. P. Differential effect of enucleation on two populations of layer V pyramidal cells. *Brain Res.,* 1975b, *88*, 554–559.

Salapatek, P. Visual scanning of geometric figures by the human newborn. *J. Comp. Physiol. Psychol.,* 1968, *66*, 247–258.

Salapatek, P., and Kessen, W. Visual scanning of triangles by the human newborn. *J. Exp. Child Psychol.,* 1966, *3*, 155–167.

Saunders, J. W. Death in embryonic systems. *Science,* 1966, *154*, 604–612.

Schapiro, S., and Vukovich, V. R. Early experience effects on cortical dendrites: A proposed model for development. *Science,* 1970, *167*, 292–294.

Schechter, P. B., and Murphy, E. H. Brief monocular visual experience and kitten cortical binocularity. *Brain Res.,* 1976, *109*, 165–168.

Shaw, C., Yinon, U., and Auerbach, E. Diminution of evoked neuronal activity in the visual cortex of pattern deprived rats. *Exp. Neurol.,* 1974, *45*, 42–50.

Sher, A. E. The embryonic and postnatal development of the inner ear of the mouse. *Acta Oto-Laryngol. Suppl.,* 1971, *285*, 1–77.

Sherk, H., and Stryker, M. P. Quantitative study of cortical orientation selectivity in visually inexperienced kitten. *J. Neurophysiol.,* 1976, *39*, 63–70.

Sherman, S. M., and Sanderson, K. J. Binocular interaction of cells of the dorsal lateral geniculate nucleus of visually deprived cats. *Brain Res.,* 1972, *37*, 126–131.

Sherman, S. M., and Stone, J. Physiological normality of the retina in visually deprived cats. *Brain Res.,* 1973, *60*, 224–230.

Sherman, S. M., Hoffman, K. P., and Stone, J. Loss of specific cell type from dorsal lateral geniculate nucleus in visually deprived cats. *J. Neurophysiol.,* 1972, *35*, 532–541.

Sherman, S. M., Guillery, R. W., Kaas, J. H. and Sanderson, K. J. Behavioral, electrophysiological, and morphological studies of binocular competition in the development of geniculo-cortical pathways of cats. *J. Comp. Neurol.,* 1974, *158*, 1–18.

Shimada, M., and Langman, J. Cell proliferation migration, and differentiation in the cerebral cortex of the golden hamster. *J. Comp. Neurol.,* 1970, *139*, 227–244.

Shlaer, R. Shift in binocular disparity causes compensatory changes in the cortical structure of kittens. *Science,* 1971, *173*, 638–641.

Sidman, R. L. Autoradiographic methods and principles for study of the nervous system with thymidine-³H. In W. J. H. Nauta and S. O. E. Ebbesson (eds.), *Contemporary Research Methods in Neuroanatomy.* Springer, New York, 1970, pp. 252–274.

Singer, W. Modification of orientation and direction selectivity of cortical cells in kittens with monocular vision. *Brain Res.,* 1976, *118*, 460–468.

Singer, W., Tretter, F., and Cynader, M. Organization of cat striate cortex: A correlation of receptive field properties with afferent and efferent connections. *J. Neurophysiol.,* 1975, *38*, 1080–1098.

Smith, D. E. Observations on the postnatal development of Clarke's column in the kitten. *J. Comp. Neurol.,* 1969, *135*, 263–274.

Smith, D. E. The effect of deafferentation on the postnatal development of Clark's nucleus in the kitten: A Golgi study. *Brain Res.,* 1974, *74*, 119–130.

Sosula, L., and Glow, P. H. Increase in the number of synapses in the inner plexiform layer of light deprived rat retinae: Quantitative electron microscopy. *J. Comp. Neurol.,* 1971, *141*, 427–452.

Sperry, R. W. Optic nerve regeneration with return of vision in anurans. *J. Neurophysiol.,* 1944, *7*, 57–69.

Sperry, R. W. Mechanisms of neural maturation. In S. S. Stevens (ed.), *Handbook of Experimental Psychology.* Wiley, New York, 1951, pp. 236–280.

Sperry, R. W. Chemoaffinity in the orderly growth of nerve fiber patterns and connections. *Proc. Natl. Acad. Sci. (USA),* 1963, *50*, 703–710.

Stein, B. E., Labos, E., and Kruger, L. Sequence of changes in the properties of neurons of superior colliculus of the kitten during maturation. *J. Neurophysiol.,* 1973, *36*, 667–679.

Sterling, P., and Wickelgren, B. G. Visual receptive fields in the superior colliculus of the cat. *J. Neurophysiol.,* 1969, *32*, 1–15.

Stewart, D. L., and Riesen, A. H. Adult versus infant brain damage: Behavioral and electrophysiological

TIMOTHY J.
CUNNINGHAM AND
E. HAZEL MURPHY

effects of striatectomy in adult and neonatal rabbits. In G. Newton and A. H. Riesen (eds.), *Advances in Psychobiology*, Vol. 1. Wiley, New York, 1972, pp. 171–211.

Stone, J. Morphology and physiology of the geniculocortical synapse in the cat: The question of parallel input to the striate cortex. *Invest. Ophthalmol.*, 1972, *11*, 338–344.

Stone, J., and Dreher, B. Projection of X- and Y-cells of the cat's lateral geniculate nucleus to areas 17 and 18 of visual cortex. *J. Neurophysiol.*, 1973, *36*, 551–567.

Stone, J., and Fukuda, Y. Properties of cat retinal ganglion cells: A comparison of W-cells with X- and Y-cells. *J. Neurophysiol.*, 1974, *37*, 722–748.

Stone, L. S. Functional polarization in retinal development and its re-establishment in regenerated retinae of rotated eyes. *Proc. Soc. Exp. Biol. Med.*, 1944, *57*, 13–14.

Stone, L. S. Normal and reversed vision in transplanted eyes. *Arch. Ophthalmol. (Chicago)*, 1953, *49*, 28–35.

Stryker, M. P., and Sherk, H. Modification of cortical orientation selectivity in the cat by restricted visual experience: A re-evaluation. *Science*, 1975, *190*, 904–906.

Tees, R. C. Effect of early visual restriction on later form discrimination in the rat. *Can. J. Psychol.*, 1968, *22*, 294–301.

Tinklepaugh, O. L., and Hartman, C. G. Behavior and maternal care of the newborn monkey *(Macaca mulatta)*. *J. Genet. Psychol.*, 1932, *40*, 257–286.

Tretter, F., Cynader, M., and Singer, W. Modification of direction selectivity of neurons in the visual cortex of kittens. *Brain Res.*, 1975, *84*, 143–149.

Valverde, F. Apical dendritic spines of the visual cortex and light deprivation in the mouse. *Exp. Brain Res.*, 1967, *3*, 337–352.

Valverde, F. Structural changes in the area striata of the mouse after enucleation. *Exp. Brain Res.*, 1968, *5*, 274–292.

Van Essen, D. C., and Kelly, J. P. Cell structure and function in the visual cortex of the cat. *J. Physiol. (London)*, 1974, *238*, 515–547.

Van Hof, M. W. Orientation discrimination in normal and light-deprived rabbits. *Docum. Ophthalmol.*, 1971, *30*, 299–311.

Van Hof, M. W., and Kobayashi, K. Pattern discrimination in rabbits deprived of light for 7 months after birth. *Exp. Neurol.*, 1972, *35*, 551–557.

Van Hof-Van Duin, J. Development of visuomotor behavior in normal and dark-reared cats. *Brain Res.*, 1976, *104*, 233–241.

Van Sluyters, R. C., and Blakemore, C. Experimental creation of unusual neuronal properties in visual cortex of kitten. *Nature*, 1973, *246*, 506–508.

Van Sluyters, R. C., and Stewart, D. L. Binocular neurons of the rabbit's visual cortex: Effects of monocular sensory deprivation. *Exp. Brain Res.*, 1974, *19*, 196–204.

Vestal, B. M., and King, J. A. Relationship of age at eye opening to the first optokinetic response in deermice. *Dev. Psychobiol.*, 1968, *1*, 30–34.

Vestal, B. M., and King, J. A. Effect of repeated testing on development of visual acuity in prairie deermice. *Psychon. Sci.*, 1971, *25*, 297–298.

Vinnikov, Y. A., and Titova, L. A. The development of vertebrate sense organs. *Prabl. Sorr. Embriol. (Leningrad)*, 1956, *89*, 96.

Vital-Durand, F., and Jeannerod, M. Maturation of the optokinetic response: Genetic and environmental factors. *Brain Res.*, 1974, *71*, 237–249.

Von Noorden, G. K. Experimental amblyopia in monkeys: Further behavioral observations and clinical correlations. *Invest. Ophthalmol.*, 1973, *12*, 721–726.

Von Noorden, G. K., Dowling, J. E., and Ferguson, D. C. Experimental amblyopia in monkeys: Behavioral studies of stimulus deprivation amblyopia. *Arch. Ophthalmol.*, 1970, *84*, 206–214.

Von Senden, M. *Space and Sight.* Methuen, London, 1960.

Walk, R. D., and Gibson, E. J. A comparative and analytic study of depth perception. *Psychol. Monogr.*, 1961, *75*, 44.

Walk, R. D., Gibson, E. J., and Tighe, T. J. Behavior of light and dark reared rats on the visual cliff. *Science*, 1957, *126*, 80–81.

Warkentin, J. An experimental study of the ontogeny of vision in the rabbit. *Psychol. Bull.*, 1937, *50*, 542–543.

Warkentin, J., and Smith, J. U. The development of visual acuity in the cat. *J. Genet. Psychol.*, 1937, *50*, 371–399.

Watkins, D. W., and Sherman, S. M. Effects of binocular deprivation on cat striate cortex. *Neurosci. Abstr.*, 1975, *1*, 86.

Weiskrantz, L. Sensory deprivation and the cat's optic nervous system. *Nature,* 1958, *181*, 1047–1050.

Wertheimer, M. Psychomotor co-ordination of auditory-visual space at birth. *Science* 1961, *134*, 1692.

White, B. L., Castle, P., and Held, R. Observations on the development of visually directed reaching. *Child Dev.,* 1964, *35*, 349–364.

Wickelgren, B. G., and Sterling, P. Influence of visual cortex on receptive field properties in the superior colliculus of the cat. *J. Neurophysiol.,* 1969, *32*, 16–23.

Wiesel, T. N., and Hubel, D. H. Effects of visual deprivation on morphology and physiology of cells in the cat's lateral geniculate body. *J. Neurophysiol.,* 1963*a*, *26*, 978–993.

Wiesel, T. N., and Hubel, D. H. Single cell responses in striate cortex of kittens deprived of vision in one eye. *J. Neurophysiol.,* 1963*b*, *26*, 1003–1017.

Wiesel, T. N., and Hubel, D. H. Comparison of the effects of unilateral and bilateral eye closure on cortical unit responses in kittens. *J. Neurophysiol.,* 1965*a*, *28*, 1029–1040.

Wiesel, T. N., and Hubel, D. H. Extent of recovery from the effects of visual deprivation in kittens. *J. Neurophysiol.,* 1965*b*, *28*, 1060–1072.

Wiesel, T. N., and Hubel, D. H. Ordered arrangement of orientation columns in monkeys lacking visual experience. *J. Comp. Neurol.,* 1974, *158*, 307–318.

Wilson, J. R., and Sherman, S. M. Differential effects of early monocular deprivation on binocular and monocular segments of cat striate cortex. *J. Neurophysiol.,* 1977, *40*, 891–903.

Wilson, P. D., and Riesen, A. H. Visual development in rhesus monkeys neonatally deprived of patterned light. *J. Comp. Physiol. Psychol.,* 1966, *61*, 87–95.

Wilson, P. D., Rowe, M. H., and Stone, J. Properties of relay cells in cat's lateral geniculate nucleus: A comparison of W-cells with X- and Y-cells. *J. Neurophysiol.,* 1976, *39*, 1193–1209.

Zelena, J. Development, degeneration and regeneration of receptor organs. In M. Singer and J. P. Schade (eds.), *Mechanisms of Neural Recognition, Progress in Brain Research,* Vol. 13. Elsevier, Amsterdam, 1964, pp. 175–213.

3

Common Properties of Sensory Systems

ROBERT P. ERICKSON

> Science is built up with facts, as a house is with
> stones. But a collection of facts is no more a science
> than a heap of stones is a house.
> —Poincaré

INTRODUCTION

On the surface, vision appears to have little in common with pain, and neither vision nor pain reminds us of taste; why, then, a discussion of their common properties? These systems do have the common tasks of conveying sensory information to the brain, which must integrate all messages from both within and across sensory systems. To the extent that the similarities of these sensory coding and integration processes require common underlying principles,[1] our knowledge of sensory processes will be constrained if we resist seeing beyond the idiosyncracies of each system. The eventual value of any scientific statement is in direct proportion to its generality.

It may seem that our science is still too young to support such general principles. But we are in an age of technological excellence in neurophysiology in

[1] These principles may be broader still, extending beyond sensory functions, to memory, movement, emotion, and motivation. As discussed elsewhere (Erickson, 1973), these functions share the basic problems and neural resources of sensory systems, and must be compatible (interface) with each other.

ROBERT P. ERICKSON Departments of Psychology and Physiology, Duke University, Durham, North Carolina 27706. Research supported in part by grants from the National Science Foundation and the U.S. Army.

which the rate of increase in the production of data is explosive. This advance has had two simultaneous effects which are now in partial, but unnecessary, conflict. First, it has provided a sufficient data base for forming general principles of sensory function; and data are certainly a necessary, although not a sufficient, aspect of science. However, this data explosion seems to have generated a preoccupation with data themselves at the expense of the second major aspect of science, a search for the systematizing principles called theories.

An example of the interaction of data and theory may be drawn from current neurophysiological studies. The fact that a visual cortical neuron may respond best to a vertical straight line is quite uninteresting when considered alone. But, of course, to most of us this finding is extremely exciting, because it suggests that we are somehow closer to an understanding of how animals, and perhaps even man, perceive the visual world; or that we are on the threshold of understanding something important about how the nervous system is wired. In this way, it is their usefulness in relating events (rather than standing "alone") or in showing the way toward new knowledge that makes some facts interesting, and others not. And with these "interesting" facts, the slip from data to new and exciting knowledge seems as easy as it is fascinating.

But the smooth movement from facts to insights or understanding is provided only by the vehicle of theory. Each scientist who makes the connection between the cat's cortical visual neurons and human percepts is doing so only on the basis of an implicit mini-theory—perhaps that the activity of these neurons provides the substrate for, or is equivalent to, the perception of a vertical straight line—an unexplained and undefended theory that the neural basis for percepts is to be found in the activity of individual neurons. Such theories, of course, are the "formers" upon which Poincaré (1952) suggested that the facts may take meaningful shape (prefatory quote).

In some areas of science the theories are broad and detailed, but in the neural sciences we are faced with an abundance of facts of uncertain relationships, connected with only limited and tentative sets of unifying rules. However, although vision and taste are by definition very different, they may differ in the way that, by crude analogy, sodium and chlorine differ in chemistry. These very different chemical elements fit tightly into the general, but simple, scheme of atomic structure which uses the same few rules, and particles, for all matter. It was Mendeleev's systematization of the similarities and differences among the various chemical elements which led to this extremely useful and general theory. In turn, this theory put order and understanding into the idiosyncratic behavior of each element, and helped bring into mutual relationship under one set of rules practically all knowledge of chemistry.

A systematic treatment of sensory neural function should point out the similarities among systems and include the differences as instances from which the general rules are derived; for example, differences in fiber diameter and related differences in conduction velocity provide the basis for a general principle of nerve conduction—that conduction velocity is directly proportional to fiber diameter. Similarly, in chemistry, the systematic nature of the differences among the elements provides the common general laws of atomic theory. The discussion to

follow will center on similarities and differences among sensory systems which 75
may be relevant to the formation of general rules of sensory neural function.

COMMON PROPERTIES
OF SENSORY SYSTEMS

Neural Mechanisms Available for Coding

Let us imagine ourselves within the nervous system, observing the activity at some point in a sensory pathway. We should find it very difficult to distinguish one sensory system from another on the basis of the characteristics of the neural activity or the nature of the connections seen. (The experimenter is relieved of this problem since he has the extra information of what the stimulus is and where the electrode is placed.) These similarities suggest at the outset that coding mechanisms are extensively similar across systems, rather than being unique to each. The neurons composing one sense are largely similar in structure and function to those composing another; each set has basically the same ionic mechanisms of function, from the electrically inexcitable dendritic systems and the excitable axonic systems to neurohumoral secretory synaptic action. Also, each uses the same general types of excitations and inhibitions, divergences and convergences, interneuronal pools providing inhibitory networks for lateral inhibition, and feedback systems. And, although an olfactory mitral cell, for example, is at least as different from an alpha motoneuron (Shepherd, 1975) as sight is from sound, the similarities in both cases are great, and must be understood before the meaning of their differences may be clearly appreciated.

The general CNS pathways of the various sensory systems may be most clearly and concisely understood in terms of their general common plan of ascending projections. There is a remarkable and instructive similarity in the course of most sensory systems from periphery to cortex. The olfactory input descending from the anterior end of the nervous system is a notable exception; but to view olfaction in the context of the general rules for afferent pathways (Bishop, 1959; Herrick, 1948) sheds light on its special functions, as well as on the contrasting functions of the other systems. That is, why should the other systems share a common plan in which olfaction does not partake? Why do certain variations on this plan exist among the nonolfactory systems? The complexities of these similarities and differences will become simple when the rationale of sensory systems in general is understood.

Some aspects of sensory systems seem so unique that they could hardly be instances of general principles; for example, the receptor transducers must be unique to sort out the proper stimulus energies. Only in these cases does it seem clear that the organism has resorted to categorically dissimilar mechanisms in its search to distinguish among the various relevant stimulus energies.

The binocular comparison process in depth vision and the fine interaural time sensitivities of the auditory system seem unique to those systems, but the neural mechanisms for these and other afferent idiosyncracies may not involve entirely different principles of synaptic organization. These systems probably gain their "uniqueness" through unusual combinations of common principles, transforming these special coding problems into a common neural currency. Thus the mechanisms for binocular fusion and depth perception may simply be those of convergence, but in unique anatomical arrangements with the two sources. This raises the problem treated further in the next section, of whether certain sensory systems have truly distinct stimulus parameters that are categorically distinct from those of other systems, in addition to the analogous parameters.

ISSUES IN SENSORY NEURAL CODING

REQUIREMENTS OF SENSORY SYSTEMS

RANGE OF CODING PARAMETERS. In addition to their evident structural and physiological similarities, the sensory systems share many coding problems as well as solutions to these problems. All sensory systems have certain similar general coding problems. The broadest, most general statement of this problem is the same for each system: that the discriminable aspects of the stimulus world must be represented. The stimulus world, both historically and for experimental expediency (which does not assure the correctness of this procedure), is fractionated into "stimulus attributes," including at least the following: stimulus quality ("what" is perceived), location or position, intensity, and duration. The classic defining criterion of an attribute is that if it is reduced to zero, the sensation does not exist (Wundt, 1907). If this criterion is ignored, an enormous increase in the range of aspects of the sensory world to be encoded results, with a corresponding reduction in the possibilities of systematization. In vision, for example, not only may stimulus movement be added to the issues of color, form, and position, but also a limitless range of other stimulus parameters such as acceleration of movement and change in rate of acceleration, visual depth and extent of depth, curvature, changes in intensity or color, spatial frequencies, and various levels of complex form perception, etc.: the potential list is limitless! Can these all be separate topics for the nervous system with different sets of specialized neurons for each? It is to be hoped that, on closer inspection, they will be seen to be aspects of a few general neural problems, and thus amenable to systematization.

This possibility, that the general coding issues are few, and similar across systems, is the thesis of at least one approach to neural function (Erickson, 1968, 1973), in which all aspects of the stimulus world are reduced to the attributes of quality, intensity, and duration—any other aspects of the stimuli being treated by the nervous system as subdivisions of these.

LIMITED NEURAL RESOURCES. In each sensory system, there is the very real problem of accomplishing a great deal of coding with a very limited number of neurons. For example, in terms of the commonplace understanding of the magnitudes of numbers, when one counts the number of neurons available to the visual system to carry out its functions, the number seems very large; however, the number of neurons available does not seem so abundant if one thinks seriously about the load put on these neurons by the even more enormous complexity of the visual world, the fantastic array of colors and complicated forms, and the relations between forms and movements which make up the visual stimuli to which we respond. If one is to relate in any straightforward way the amount of visual information processed by the nervous system to the number of neurons available, this process would quickly overwhelm the total visual system, and the whole brain. This issue of maximum capacity is a major problem for all sensory systems and should be included as a basic provision in any theory of sensory neural function.

READOUT. Each sensory system also has the problem of being accessible to the "response" side of the nervous system, whether the responses be considered as percepts, thoughts, memories, or movements. In this regard, the various systems share at some central level the common coding problem of being accessible to "readout." "Pontifical" neurons, "command" cells, and "grandmother" neurons of various types are almost always invoked for this function, although usually only by implication rather than explicitly. All of these readout neurons require the "funneling" of neural activity representing either a feature or the whole of a complex stimulus onto a single neuron or small group of neurons.

These approaches may be contrasted with the "across-fiber pattern" theory, in which it is held that such "readout" cells are not only unnecessary but also untenable as ultimate stages of neural processing (Erickson, 1973). All the same, each system does seem to proceed through certain levels of "feature extraction," the construction of sensitivities to complex pieces of stimuli which are undoubtedly important in meeting the response requirements of the nervous system. As this idea is carried to extreme levels (Kuffler, 1973) of individual neurons as "object detectors," the range of responsiveness of the nervous system to a variety of stimuli is progressively reduced (Erickson, 1973). We do not yet have a good, quantitative understanding of how this refining process, carried to a particular level and no further, economically meets the requirements of response or output from the nervous system; until this is clear, we do not understand either of the related problems of feature extraction and readout.

It should be noted that contemporary approaches to these requirements for sensory systems have been quite unsystematic. For example, does temperature have both intensive and qualitative attributes? Do the kinesthetic or vestibular senses have either? Do the various sensory systems require different degrees of extraction or detection?

OTHER ISSUES

Several other issues are in similar need of systematization in that it is not clear how general they are or should be; examples are the issues of primaries, classes of neurons, specificity, and the complementary processes of analysis and synthesis.

SENSORY PRIMARIES. The idea of primaries[2] seems to apply to color vision, taste, and somesthesis. But why is this concept relevant to these senses and not others? The definitions of the term itself is often unclear, in that it may apply in unrelated, or related, fashion to primary sensations, primary stimuli, primary types of neurons, or other primary subdivisions of a sensory system (cold vs. touch, etc.). The idea of neural primaries is closely related to that of neuron classes, such as edge detectors, simple cortical visual cells, frequency analysis neurons, and the various classes of somesthetic neurons (touch, pressure, cold and warm, etc.). Such

[2]See the glossary at the end of this chapter.

classes are of obvious usefulness in the investigation of the various selective receptor processes and in determining how the nervous system sorts out and classifies the input.

It is not clear, however, that these classes (primary, etc.) may be directly related to classes of behaviors or perceptions. It is yet to be demonstrated that the nervous system uses such classifications as tools (such as basic mechanisms in perception or behavior) beyond the methods of simplest transduction and neural connectivism. Clearly, neural classes are not equivalent to neural codes. The only safe assumption is that such "classes" give the response characteristics of a particular group of neurons, which leaves us with the same problem as with other neurons—what is the role, if any, of activity in these (classified) neurons in neural codes?

ANALYSIS AND SYNTHESIS. In some cases, sensory systems appear to fuse stimuli, and in others the nervous system seems to be designed to keep stimuli separate; these two processes may be termed "synthesis" and "analysis." The most apparent example of synthesis is that in which colors lose their individual identity when mixing to form another perceived color; similar events seem to operate in the temperature sense and the chemical senses, although it is not yet clear to what extent the latter are synthetic. The auditory sense is analytic with respect to the separation of tones, and the somesthetic and visual senses are analytic with respect to position. Why and how is analysis accomplished in some cases and synthesis in others? Are these processes omitted or irrelevant for kinesthesis and the vestibular senses? Again, systematic treatment of these problems is lacking.

SPECIFICITY. Specificity is another general topic with poor systematic consideration which crosses the lines of sensory domains; it is probably the most overworked and underdefined term in sensory neurophysiology. This term has at least four common usages: (1) narrowness of neural tuning (e.g., narrow auditory response areas); (2) complexity of sensitivity ("grandmother" cells); (3) range of excitatory stimuli (some "unspecific" somesthetic neurons respond to temperature as well as touch); and (4) perceptual specificity (yellow is perceived as a "specific" color). The result is that workers in various areas may seem to be agreeing or disagreeing on the presence or absence of "specificity," when the term may simply have been left undefined.[3]

---

[3]This problem of definition of the terms used in our scientific language is a very serious one: thus the glossary that appears at the end of this chapter containing a list of a few common terms used in the study of sensory processes which have particularly vague or multiple definitions. The function of this list could not possibly be to provide the best or proper definitions of these terms, but only to point out the importance of making clear definitions when they, or similarly vague terms, are used. As Humpty Dumpty put the problem in *Through the Looking Glass*, "'When *I* use a word, . . . it means just what I choose it to mean—neither more nor less.' 'The question is,' said Alice, 'whether you *can* make words mean so many different things.' 'The question is,' said Humpty Dumpty, 'which is to be master—that's all.'" Humpty Dumpty is probably right. Words will be our masters if we search to find their meaning; or, on the other hand, we may require them to express the meanings dictated by our data. With due homage to common usage (there is no sense in using "white" to mean black), the words we use may take any meaning we need as long as the meaning is made clear. It would be better to use terms, as in Carroll's *Jabberwocky,* that have so little intrinsic meaning that their total meaning comes from the author's definition. For example, compare the confusion of ideas evoked by the terms "inhibition" or "specificity" (see glossary), with "brillig"; "brillig" has no immediately intuitive and thus no unintended surplus meaning, gaining its complete definition from Humpty Dumpty, "four o'clock in the afternoon."

There have been nearly as many neural codes nominated as there have been experimenters in this area! Perkel and Bullock (1969) have listed a large number of these candidate codes. Of course, the nervous system might be using any one or any combination of them, but then again its function may be only vaguely related to this set of codes. Concerning the validity of any candidate code, whether it qualifies as a neural variation used by the nervous system in coding or simply as a "sign" (Uttal, 1973) to the experimenter that a stimulus has occurred can be determined only if it is described in enough detail that crucial and testable predictions can be made from it. We seldom provide for such tests; when left untested, the experimenter's codes may not be the nervous system's codes. It is a most instructive maneuver to imagine oneself decoding neural activity without the knowledge of what the stimulus is (which knowledge, as mentioned above, is one of the "reliefs" afforded the experimenter). If one can know what the stimulus was on the basis of the evoked neural activity, then and only then can it be said that the neural code is understood, and this usually is not done (see Erickson, 1973).

The *sine qua non* of coding is only that the nervous system responds differentially to discriminably different stimuli. Within this broad requirement, any neural differences may be the candidates as codes; the question is, which are the valid differences? In large measure, we have accepted the idea that these valid differences have to do with the tuning of neurons to particular realms of stimuli such that the identity of the neuron activated gives the identity of the stimulus, discussed as "labeled-lines" in "Spatial Codes" below. The other main coding possibility, that the temporal aspects of neural activity are responsible for the identification of the stimulus, is discussed in "Temporal Codes" to follow.

It is possible, of course, that the coding process changes from one level of the nervous system to the next, and across sensory systems; but one should expect a certain parsimony throughout.

SPATIAL CODES. In general, spatial codes include mechanisms that use as their basic mechanism the parameter of "which" neurons are responding. They include the most ancient and respected of all coding theories (Mueller, 1833; see Boring, 1942), the doctrine of specific nerve energies. This line of theorizing predates, by about a century, the advent of electrophysiological recording methods, originating in the work of Bell and Magendie in the second decade of the nineteenth century. These men pointed out in terms of some very simple and decisive experiments that the dorsal roots of the spinal cord are sensory in function, and the ventral roots are motor. Theirs was probably the first statement of the idea that certain neurons have specific functions, even though the functions were rather general; our basic ideas of neural function have not changed significantly since then. The most famous articulation of this principle was achieved by Johannes Müller, who in 1838 formulated the doctrine of specific nerve energies. He stated that, however stimulated, activity in the visual nerve will evoke only visual sensations, the auditory nerve only auditory sensations, and so forth. Thus the very important biological principle that certain structures have certain definite functions was given embodiment in the nervous system.

Brain Centers. The idea that particular neural structures are responsible for particular functions is very nearly the only important neural coding doctrine now in use. It has been used more extensively than is commonly recognized; in some cases it clearly has been overextended. For example, it has given rise to the search for isolated groups of CNS neurons, or neural "centers," which mediate a particular behavior, such as hunger, sleep, happiness, or memory. This approach suits our intuitions as well as our methods, and obviously must be correct to a certain degree; but it contains two difficult problems. First, the range of different behaviors to be mediated seems endless; it is difficult at this time to form a clear image of how far the search for more elaborate functions in isolated centers may proceed, or, on the other hand, to what extent the list is limited. As with the question of the range of stimulus attributes to be encoded discussed above, it is of basic importance here to gain some perspective on the limits of the vocabulary of the nervous system, which is undoubtedly more restrained and differently organized than our verbal behavior in naming functions which should have structures. Second, there is a growing awareness of the problems of the "center" approach, which in its extreme form is reminiscent of the phrenology of Gall. Clearly, the brain is heterogeneous in function and structure, but it functions as a coordinated whole. An understanding has developed (e.g., Morgane, 1975) that, although we do not have the tools to study it in this way, the nervous system probably works *en masse* as a complex of interconnected circuits through which functions are distributed, rather than in terms of easily studied centers. Still, the exigencies of our methods force the experimental results into the mold of "centers."

Labeled-Line Codes. Well before the idea of specific nerves, or of specific nerve centers, impetus for the idea that individual nerve cells might have particular functions originated in the work of Young; in 1802, he hypothesized that individual visual elements might carry the code for different colors. Young's approach was elaborated and given clear form by Helmholtz in 1858 in his statement of the trichromatic theory of color vision. Helmholtz stated as one aspect of this theory that activity in a particular neuron gives the sensation appropriate to that neuron; for example, activity in a "red" neuron is equivalent to the sensation of red. Helmholtz carried this type of coding forward in his resonance theory of hearing in which the representation of particular tones is given to the activity of individual auditory neurons.

The major modern statement of the idea that particular neurons may have particular functions, such that activity in any particular neuron is interpretable as a code, has been termed "labeled-line" theory (Mountcastle, 1968; Perkel and Bullock, 1969). In this theory, largely developed from studies in somesthesis, the meaning for the nervous system of the activity of a particular neuron is identical to the singular stimulus to which it is most sensitive; thus individual neurons presumably signal precise skin locations, temperatures, tones, etc. The hypothesis is not expressed in enough detail to indicate whether labeling of lines is to be expected in all sensory neurons, with "salty" or "red" neurons, or whether it is appropriate only for certain somesthetic neurons. An hypothesis that is applicable to all sensory systems is, of course, preferable to a situation in which many hypotheses are required.

Population Codes. Although it need not be, trichromatic theory as seen by Helmholtz is a labeled-line theory, in that individual neurons give sensations of red or green or blue; the code for any color is given in the relative amounts of activity in several parallel neural channels. The synthesis of the neural activity representing these primary sensations into the other colors is unresolved in this theory, evidently being left for higher centers. But the problem of the synthesis of the color sensations need not be left unsolved since the sufficient neural differences for any particular color are given in the relative amounts of activity in a few types of neurons. Inherent in the theory of Young and Helmholtz is the idea that the coding process may therein be complete, with no further decoding necessary of the three separate primary sensations by an "inner man" at a higher center. The view that the code for simple or complex stimuli is entirely given in the simultaneous relative activities of a population of neurons forms the basis for one variation on spatial approaches to neural coding, the "across-fiber pattern" theory (Erickson, 1968, 1973). This variation on the spatial codes accepts the fact of the precise stimulus selectivity of afferent neurons, and thus that it is important "which" neurons are active, but in addition recognizes the importance of the precise relative amounts of activity in each of a population of these neurons for stimulus quality coding. Since it takes its origin in the work of Young and Helmholtz, this view of neural organization dates from 1802. Its more immediate roots are to be found in the works of Pfaffmann (1955) in gustation.

Illustrations of the Codes. The across-fiber and labeled-line points of view may be elucidated and compared in reference to Fig. 1. In part A of this figure is schematized the typical responsiveness of sensory neurons. The abscissa represents any stimulus dimension; the ordinate, neural responsiveness (amount of response, 1/threshold, etc.). The curves, here termed "neural response functions" (NRFs), represent the responsiveness of receptors or neurons along this dimension. The NRFs are always simple and smooth in form, and are usually bell-shaped as shown, but variations in form exist (as the monotonic kinesthetic or S-shaped opponent-process color-coded neurons) which do not change the logic of the coding theories described below. In all sensory systems, NRFs typically overlap extensively as shown, and are broadly tuned (color, taste, olfaction, line orientation, temperature, vestibular, and others); these are the nontopographic modalities (Erickson, 1968). In topographic modalities (skin or visual position, auditory tones), the illustrated section of the stimulus dimension is only a small part of the total dimension, and the neurons are thus "narrowly tuned."

Labeled-Lines. Figure 1B shows the specific neuron or labeled-line neural code (parts B and C derive from part A). In this view, the meaning of the activity of each neuron is unique, and corresponds to the stimulus to which it is most responsive, at the "peak" of its NRF. Thus the meaning for the organism of activity in a color-coded neuron which peaks in the blue, a "blue" neuron, is blueness. However, each neuron responds in various degrees to a range of stimuli. Consider that neuron 1 is a "blue" neuron; it responds equivalently to stimuli P and Q, and thus within this neuron the messages for these two stimuli are confounded. Intensity messages are also confounded within this neuron, since the small response to stimulus R is interpretable as a less intense P or Q.

Population Codes. Figure 1C shows the across-fiber-pattern view, a population code. In this view, the meaning of the activity of each neuron is given only in the context of the activity of other neurons responding to the stimulus. The nervous system does not attach special meaning to the peaks of the NRFs, as in B; however,

ROBERT P. ERICKSON

these peaks serve as useful label points for the experimenter ("blue" neurons, etc.). The concern of this theory is in the representation of a stimulus rather than in the responsiveness of individual neurons; to suppose that these are the same issue assumes that the doctrine of specific nerve energies is valid in a very strict sense at the level of the individual neuron. Thus the data are arranged by stimuli rather than in the customary method by neuron (B). The quality of the

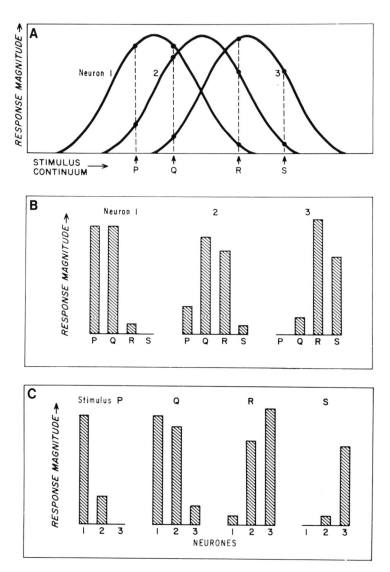

Fig. 1. Illustrations of spatial codes. A: Responsiveness of three neurons along a stimulus dimension. The responses of these neurons to four stimuli (*P, Q, R,* and *S*) along this dimension provide the data for the rest of this figure. B: The labeled-line scheme. Since the emphasis in this approach is on the sensitivity of the individual neuron, the data are arranged by neurons. The responses of each neuron to the four stimuli are illustrated. C: The across-fiber-pattern scheme. Since the emphasis in this approach is on the neural representation of a stimulus, the data are arranged by stimuli. The responses to each stimulus of all neurons are illustrated (after Erickson, 1968).

stimulus is given in the pattern (ratios) shown of amounts of response across the neural population, rather than being seen in the responses of individual neurons.

The following points may be noted about this population coding scheme: (1) each stimulus evokes a unique response in that no two stimuli may evoke the same across-fiber pattern; (2) the number of stimuli encodable (i.e., the number of across-fiber patterns) is greater than the number of neurons—indeed, a continuum of stimuli may be supported across a small population; and (3) intensity changes do not confound the message, changing the height of the response but not the pattern.

But, primarily, the across-fiber-pattern theory has the advantage of providing for the encoding of many stimuli with few neurons. This advantage was a major consideration for the color theory of Young and Helmholtz; they realized that at each point in the retina only a very few neurons were available to encode the visible spectrum. Certainly there could not be a receptor for each discriminable wavelength at each point in the retina and, even if there were, the problem would not be solved inasmuch as we see a continuum of colors, not discrete color steps. Helmholtz saw the solution to this problem in stimulus specification by unique patterns of activity in three broadly tuned receptor types. The across-fiber-pattern theory extends Helmholtz's idea to deal with the fact that all sensory neurons are much more broadly tuned across their parameters than the facts of discriminability would immediately lead us to expect; the discrepancy between the broad range of stimuli to which a neuron typically responds and the singular sensation hypothesized is a major difficulty for labeled-line theory.

The across-fiber-pattern theory provides other advantages in the coding process, which are less obvious in Fig. 1 and are discussed elsewhere (Erickson, 1968, 1973); these are (4) that it has potential for redundancy and resulting stability of the neural messages in the face of the variability of response of each neuron, or neuron loss or damage, and (5) that both the presence of fiber "types" and the nature of the stimulus dimensions may be derived from analysis of the across-fiber patterns to many stimuli (e.g., in taste and olfaction, there appear to be no fiber types, and the stimulus spaces are three-dimensional; Erickson and Schiffman, 1975).

General Comments on Spatial Codes. Thus far, the spatial codes have been discussed as if each neuron were selectively tuned along only one parameter. Obviously each is tuned along many parameters (a visual neuron tuned along the wavelength dimension may also be critically tuned for position, movement, object orientation, etc.), a process which reduces the generality of its responsiveness. As this process becomes more refined, it becomes the process of "feature extraction" and finally "object detection."

All spatial theories are related to the observable fact of topographic organization, in which a stimulus parameter such as visual (retinal) location, somesthetic space, or auditory frequency is laid out in an orderly fashion across neural areas. The two basic requirements for topographic organization are (1) that the individual neurons are differentially responsive to different portions of that particular stimulus dimension and (2) that they are laid out in an orderly sequence across neural tissue. The fact of topographic relationships between neural projections and stimulus dimensions is, of course, not in itself a code, but merely a statement that the neurons are differentially tuned and laid out in order. The function of topographic organization remains an interesting puzzle, perhaps providing a convenient ballpark in which neural effects based on spatial proximity, such as lateral inhibition, may be conveniently organized; or it may be just ontogenetically simpler to lay out the nervous system this way.

TEMPORAL CODES. For spatial codes, the main parameter of concern for sensory quality is "which" neurons are active and also, in across-fiber patterning, to what extent they are active. The second major class of neural code is concerned with the relationships between the rates of neural activity at several points in time, e.g., in some subtle variations in the intervals (rates) between successive impulses or in rate of change of frequency (Parkel, 1970; Segundo, 1970; Terzuolo, 1970). Interesting interspike interval variations are obvious in almost all sensory systems; the few systems in which such variations are not prominent are those of the simplest and most information-poor systems, such as the crustacean stretch receptor. Certainly, such variations hold the potential for considerable neural coding.

Definitions of Temporal Codes. In its purest form, in which it is absolutely distinguished from spatial codes, a temporal code is exemplified in a frequency theory of auditory tone perception. In this theory, the message for any particular tone is given only in the frequency of impulses in the auditory system, with no concern for which auditory neurons are responding. Of course, it would take an extreme position on homogeneity of brain function to support a pure temporal coding point of view, because even in the example given for audition it must be understood that only the auditory neurons, and none other, could be concerned for the coding of tones; i.e., it does matter "which" neurons are responding. Therefore, in practice, temporal coding points of view have always been a combination of spatial codes (specific neurons) and temporal codes.

Conversely, it will be recalled that the specific neuron points of view usually employ some analysis of the temporal aspects of the neural activity, even if it is simply an accounting of the rate of neural impulses at one point in time. Relative rates of firing across a population constitute the code for quality in the across-fiber-pattern view; thus it is truly a spatial and temporal theory of coding. In the pure labeled-line neuron, however, rate is strictly related to intensity and does not influence quality.

With a thoughtful consideration of the temporal aspects of neural activity, it is clear that there is a vast array possible, ranging from the microfluctuations in impulse rate from one interspike interval to the next, and all the combinations of temporally adjacent interspike intervals, through the analysis of longer and longer macrofluctuations in impulse frequency, to hours, days, or longer. The shorter periods may correspond with fleeting sensory impressions, and the longer periods may be related to backgrounds for sensory activity or to more permanent conditions of memory.

Problems in Temporal Coding. A major problem for temporal codes is posed by the limited ability of a synapse to "see" and respond to these variations, especially those at the extremes either of a finer, more rapid grain or of a very long period. Compounding this problem, the postsynaptic membrane is receiving many inputs at once, and the temporal pacing of one input is not apt to be in synchrony with the others; thus the timing of any presynaptic spike train may easily be lost. Since the synapse is looking at many temporal trains at once, it has a different order of problem than the single-neuron physiologist who has the luxury of looking at only one train at a time. Also, the postsynaptic membrane is quite sluggish in comparison to the ability of the experimenter to measure subtle variations in the timing of neuron spikes; thus the membrane may respond only to the temporally grosser measures, such as mean frequency over short periods (tens of milliseconds), rather than more fine-grained aspects, such as variations in length of successive interspike intervals (e.g., standard deviations). At least we should not assume that the nervous system can make all the fine temporal measurements that our instruments can, just as we also should not assume that it is limited to our methods of analysis.

Temporal Coding and Intensity. Certain aspects of temporal signs in neural trains usually associated with intensity have not yet found clear relationships within the larger body of thinking concerning neural coding. For example, although rate of activity is typically related to sensory intensity, Hyvärinen *et al.* (1968) have related impulse frequency in certain somatosensory neurons with the sensations of various rates of vibration. On the other hand, Mountcastle *et al.* (1965) found that rate of discharge in kinesthetic neurons follows the intensity power law as the limb's position is changed. And temperature neurons show bell-shaped neural response functions across temperatures, with frequency of discharge decreasing as the "intensity" increases (Poulos and Lende, 1970; Zotterman, 1959). What is the relation in these cases between rate of discharge and "intensity"? Should we expect rate of firing to be a positive function of intensity in the "typical" case, a negative function in others (e.g., temperature), and unrelated to intensity in still others (rate of vibration, kinesthetic position)? Probably, the nervous system is using a more internally consistent code.

COMPARISONS OF THE CODES

In conclusion, it should be pointed out that spatial codes have one advantage over the temporal codes in their congruence with the motor outflow for which they are responsible; this is because differences in responses (arm vs. leg or extension vs. flexion, etc.) are largely differences in which neurons are responding.[4] On the other hand, the obvious temporal properties of movements are more in accord with the temporal codes. Here is an example where our chosen rubrics may have proven to be impediments. A concept of "spatiotemporal" might prove more appropriate for neural function than spatial or temporal concepts.

INFLUENCES OF TECHNIQUES AND LANGUAGE

Our concepts concerning sensory neural function have been dictated to a rather dismaying degree by factors which may be irrelevant or misleading. Some

---

[4]There is evidence that to some extent the temporal pattern of impulses may determine which postsynaptic elements are activated (Parnas, 1972).

of these factors remain unnoticed because of their extreme conspicuousness, being common to all workers in an area.

Experiment Techniques

The first factor concerns the techniques available for measurement of neural structure and function. Whether it is the microelectrode, the lesion-producing device, the staining method, or any of the other variety of tools in use, our ideas seem to be largely directed and constrained by these techniques. For example, the microelectrode seems to generate concepts of the nervous system confined to information carried in individual neurons; the stimulating electrode and lesion-producing device give us neural concepts of functionally unitary brain "pathways," "centers," or "levels." The various cell-staining methods give us views of limited neural pathways that largely omit the physiological problems of the kind and amount of influence exerted at the neuron terminals thus defined, as well as the precise identity of the neurons thus influenced; at best, they show a very limited section of a neural circuit.

The choice of stimuli for testing a sensory neural system in physiological or behavioral studies heavily influences the conceptual view of the nervous system generated by these studies. For example, the greatest recent strides in neural studies of visual organization have taught us that the choice of stimuli markedly influences our ideas of neural organization. Our understanding in this area was very constrained as long as very simple stimuli were used; with the use of complex stimuli our view of nervous system function has advanced dramatically. Studies of the auditory system have only recently begun to struggle beyond the limitations imposed by the use of very simple stimuli, such as pure tones; it is becoming evident that the language of the auditory system is in large degree couched in more complex terms. Studies of taste are still constrained within the limits of "sweet," "sour," "salty," and "bitter."

Language

Just as we are influenced by our techniques, we are also strongly guided by our language. The fact that we use the rubrics "color" vision, "form" vision, and "salty" and "sweet" tastes affects from its inception the direction of our research, and the conclusions derived. Color was long studied disregarding form, and *vice versa,* and intensity was studied disregarding both. These and other parameters have recently been studied simultaneously (e.g., Wagner *et al.,* 1960), and it is becoming clear that there are not separate codes or separate populations of neurons for each of the experimenter's separate topics so much as there is a general code encompassing all aspects of the stimulus within the same neurons. Of course, our use of these terms has come only with considerable labor, and their survival in our work attests to a certain success in their use; still, because they are of such powerful influence, largely determining the design of our experiments and our thoughts, they must remain under careful scrutiny. That the nervous system may not be working in terms of our chosen rubrics remains one of the primary impediments to our science.

Scientists are often accused of doing only expedient research (e.g., Daniel Bell, in Wade, 1975); it is the unusually thoughtful investigator who is aware of the influence of his techniques and language, the rare and creative investigator who can in a reasonable manner conceive of neural function beyond them. In short, each technically limited approach exerts heavy pressure toward the development of similarly limited views of neural functions. But problem-oriented research (e.g., how does the nervous system represent a stimulus?) is infinitely more useful than technique-centered research (e.g., what does the microelectrode see?) but almost always more difficult. Many workers in the area would probably agree that a definition of this problem toward which we should ultimately be oriented is, very simply, to show how the sensory systems provide for responses—the responses conceived broadly as movements or percepts, etc. A statement of the state of the art might be that there are only unclear and distant connections between this simple goal and the actual performance of our science in which technique-centered data can easily become a substitute for this goal.

CONCLUSION

It is suggested throughout this chapter that it would be useful to determine whether our data are getting us any closer to broad and general concepts of neural function, and some guidelines to this end are suggested. It is for the reader to judge in his excursions through the chapters to follow to what extent the materials are, or could be, related to a general view. A good, general theory of neural function would incorporate, and reduce to simple form, large amounts of data from as many sensory systems as possible; and "good" data, then, would be those which bear on such a theory. Poincaré (1952) expressed the issue very concisely: "What then is a good experiment? It is that which informs us of something besides an isolated fact; it is that which enables us to predict, and to generalize."

It is suggested here that the various sensory systems have a significant number of common principles amenable to systematization. The implementation of these principles may vary enough between systems to appear as differences, but those are differences of detail or amount rather than kind, and may be used to disclose the principles themselves. The sensory systems share the few coding topics of stimulus attributes (such as quality and intensity), and they share a common neural machinery for the encoding of these attributes, as well as common potential neural codes. None of the sensory systems is spared the difficulties imposed by our techniques, theoretical biases, and language. This situation makes it appear probable that the principles for which we search in sensory coding mechanisms are more extensively similar for all systems than would be immediately evident. This probability, coupled with the knowledge that it is just such common general principles which promote understanding, should encourage the sensory neurophysiologist to inspect closely the problems, definitions, theories, and findings in systems other than his own, and to search for the elusive relationships among systems which will lead to a larger and clearer view of neural function.

ROBERT P. ERICKSON

Listed below are a few terms commonly used in sensory neurophysiology, which are notable for inconsistent usage or vagueness of definition. That the reader may take exception to them can only serve to emphasize this point, and the further point that, whenever a term is used, its implied meaning should be made explicit. It would be an interesting exercise, for both reader and experimenter, for published papers to include a list of definitions of the terms used.

1. *Feature detector*. This term may refer to the complex stimulus selectivity shown by some central neurons. It may also imply a functional meaning: the role of such a neuron in sensory organization. In any case, these meanings should be held distinct from the synaptic mechanisms of attaining this organization, the process of "feature extraction."

2. *Inhibition*. This term often refers indiscriminately to synaptic interactions by which one input will reduce the effectiveness of another (excitatory) input. However, this term is usually considered to be inappropriate unless certain other criteria are met concerning the mechanisms involved. For example, if the mechanism of occlusion (refractory states) is responsible, then the reduction in responsiveness is not an example of inhibition. Even excluding occlusion, several quite dissimilar neurophysiological mechanisms are included under this rubric. Selective ionic (K^+, Cl^-) permeability changes (which may cause hyperpolarization—i.p.s.p.'s) produced by neurotransmitters and resulting in reduced excitability of the membrane account for one type of inhibition. However, the presynaptic neuron may inject hyperpolarizing current into the postsynaptic membrane, a second type of inhibition. A third type of inhibition is very dissimilar from these in mechanism, resulting from an excitatory (depolarizing) effect on the presynaptic terminals, leading to a diminished spike amplitude and consequent reduction of transmitter output. It should be obvious that none of these may serve as a direct explanation for Pavlovian, Skinnerian, or Freudian inhibition.

3. *Lateral inhibition*. This term is often used whenever lateral neural or psychophysical effects are seen. In a pure sense, as it derived from studies on *Limulus*, the effects between the two stimuli should be mutual; this criterion is often omitted. The neural machinery for these various effects differs from *Limulus* to mammal, and from spinal cord to olfactory bulb, and only in some cases involves cell hyperpolarization. The function may vary from a "sharpening" process to other re-encoding processes. The term is also used for psychophysical events which may or may not be related to the neural events described.

4. *Primaries*. This term is used to describe types of neurons, types of stimuli, or psychophysically pure sensations. In each definition, typical types are "yellow," "salty," etc. These levels of description are clearly different, and a pure salty taste does not necessarily indicate a salt neuron type, and neither pure taste nor neuron type requires a distinct category of salty receptors or stimuli. It would be clearer to give each a separate nonsense

name which carries little excess meaning ("neuraries," "stimaries," "psy-maries") than to include all under one term.

5. *Spatial frequency analyzers.* This term has several definitions which are often taken to be identical but which, in fact, may be unrelated. A frequency analyzer neuron may be sensitive to spatial frequencies; these frequencies could be visual, auditory, somesthetic, or other. The reference may be to a central neural process of unknown detail, defined by its sensitivity to psychophysical manipulations (adaptation). The characteristics of these psychophysical effects may be called frequency analysis without strict reference to neural processes.

6. *Specificity.* There is a variety of usage of this term, and the distinctions are seldom made clear. This term is used interchangeably to describe the following unrelated situations: the sensitivity of neurons to complex aspects of a stimulus, the narrowness of tuning of a neuron along some parameter, the selectivity of a neuron to only one stimulus species, and types of neurons and types of stimuli. The latter two uses also overlap with the definitions of "primaries."

REFERENCES

Bishop, G. H. The relation between nerve fiber size and sensory modality: Phylogenetic implications of the afferent innervation of cortex. *J. Nerv. Ment. Dis.,* 1959, *128,* 89–114.

Boring, E. G. *Sensation and Perception in the History of Experimental Psychology.* Appleton-Century-Crofts, New York, 1942.

Erickson, R. P. Stimulus coding in topographic and non-topographic afferent modalities: On the significance of the activity of individual sensory neurons. *Psychol. Rev.,* 1968, *75,* 447–465.

Erickson, R. P. Parallel "population" neural coding in feature extraction. In F. O. Schmitt *et al.* (eds.), *The Neurosciences: Third Study Program.* MIT Press, Cambridge, Mass., 1973, pp. 155–169.

Erickson, R. P., and Schiffman, S. S. The chemical senses: A systematic approach. In M. S. Gazzaniga and C. Blakemore (eds.), *Handbook of Psychobiology.* Academic Press, New York, 1975, pp. 393–426.

Herrick, C. J. *The Brain of the Tiger Salamander.* University of Chicago Press, Chicago, 1948.

Hyvärinen, J., Sakata, H., Talbot, W. H., and Mountcastle, V. B. Neural coding by cortical cells of the frequency of oscillating peripheral stimuli. *Science,* 1968, *162,* 1130–1132.

Kuffler, S. W. The single-cell approach in the visual system and the study of receptive fields. *Invest. Ophthalmol.,* 1973, *12,* 794–813.

Morgane, P. J. Anatomical and neurobiochemical bases of the central nervous control of physiological regulations and behavior. In G. Mogenson and F. Calarens (eds.), *Neural Integration of Physiological Mechanisms and Behavior,* University of Toronto Press, 1975.

Mountcastle, V. B. Physiology of sensory receptors: Introduction to sensory processes. In *Medical Physiology,* Vol. 2, 12th ed. Mosby, St. Louis, 1968.

Mountcastle, V. B., Poggio, G. F., and Werner, G. The relation of thalamic cell response to peripheral stimuli varied over an intensity continuum. *J. Neurophysiol.,* 1963, *26,* 807–834.

Mueller, J. *Handbuch der Physiologie des Menschen,* Vols. 1 and 2. Holscher, Coblenz, 1833/1834.

Parnas, I. Differential block at high frequency of branches of a single axon innervating two muscles. *J. Neurophysiol.,* 1972, *35,* 903–913.

Perkel, D. H. Spike trains as carriers of information, In F. O. Schmitt (ed.), *The Neurosciences: Second Study Program.* Rockefeller University Press, New York, 1970, pp. 587–596.

Perkel, D. H., and Bullock, T. H. Neural coding. In F. O. Schmitt, T. Melnechuk, G. C. Quarton, and G. Adelman (eds.), *Neurosciences Research Symposium Summaries,* Vol. 3. MIT Press, Cambridge, Mass., 1969.

Pfaffmann, C. Gustatory nerve impulses in rat, cat and rabbit. *J. Neurophysiol.,* 1955, *18,* 429–440.

Poincaré, H. Hypotheses in physics. In *Science and Hypothesis,* Chapter 9. Dover, New York, 1952.

Poulos, D. A., and Lende, R. A. Response of trigeminal ganglion neurons to thermal stimulation of oral-facial regions. I. Steady-state response *J. Neurophysiol.*, 1970, *33*, 508–517.

Segundo, J. P. Communication and coding by nerve cells. In F. O. Schmitt (ed.), *The Neurosciences: Second Study Program*. Rockefeller University Press, New York, 1970, pp. 569–586.

Shepherd, G. M. Axons, dendrites and synapses. *Fed. Proc.*, 1975, *34*, 1395–1397.

Terzuolo, C. A. Data transmission by spike trains. In F. O. Schmitt (ed.), *The Neurosciences: Second Study Program*. Rockefeller University Press, New York, 1970, pp. 661–671.

Uttal, W. *The Psychobiology of Sensory Coding*. Harper and Row, New York, 1973.

Wade, N. Daniel Bell: Science as the imago of the future society. *Science*, 1975, *188*, 35–37.

Wagner, H. G., MacNichol, E. F., Jr., and Wolbarsht, M. L. The response properties of single ganglion cells in the goldfish retina. *J. Gen. Physiol.*, 1960, *43*, 45–62.

Wundt, W. *Lectures on Human and Animal Psychology*. Macmillan, New York, 1907.

Zotterman, Y. Thermal sensations. In J. Field (ed.), *Handbook of Physiology*, Section I: *Neurophysiology*, Vol. I. American Physiological Society, Washington, D.C., 1959, pp. 431–458.

4

Olfaction

D. G. MOULTON

INTRODUCTION

The relative significance assigned to olfactory function has, in the past, been largely a matter of disciplinary approach. Thus, in contrast to its fluctuating fortunes in the hands of neuroanatomists assessing components of forebrain function, olfaction has long been accorded a major role by animal behaviorists in sexual and social behavior, trail following, feeding behavior, and identification of territory. Or consider the view that olfaction can directly influence certain physiological functions. Until about the middle of this century this suggestion would have had little support. Then came evidence that, in mice, the odors of a strange male can block the pregnancy of females, while isolation of nonpregnant mice in a large group away from males induces anestrus in a proportion of them (Parkes and Bruce, 1961; Bruce, 1970; Whitten, 1959). Since then, numerous studies have pointed to close functional links between olfaction and endocrine activity. Other reports claimed that olfactory input can influence growth, water balance, and temperature regulation, and that bulbectomy causes marked changes in norepinephrine content of several brain regions (Digiesi *et al.*, 1963; Nováková and Dlouhá, 1960; Edwards and Roberts, 1972; Pohorecky *et al.*, 1969; Eichelman *et al.*, 1972; King and Cairncross, 1974). Similarly, there was until recently limited evidence to support Herrick's (1933) contention that the olfactory system serves as a nonspecific activator for all cortical functions. It is now known that bulbectomized animals show a tendency toward increased aggression and hyperactivity and are slower to habituate. Indeed, the olfactory system appears to be implicated in many functions attributed to limbic and hypothalamic structures (see Wenzel, 1974).

D. G. MOULTON   Monell Chemical Senses Center and Department of Physiology, University of Pennsylvania, and Veterans Administration Hospital, Philadelphia, Pennsylvania 19104.

But while there has been a growing realization of the critical role of olfaction, particularly in controlling certain behavioral activities, the extent to which olfaction alone mediates the observed responses remains controversial. Recent emphasis on the existence of a dual olfactory system has quickened awareness and interest in one aspect of this problem, but, in fact, many vertebrates have three and sometimes four different chemosensitive regions in the nose. We know little about certain of these organs, but there is some indication that they influence distinct behavioral activities or physiological mechanisms. Thus it is pertinent to begin with a brief overview of their structure and functional properties. In the remainder of this chapter, we shall examine some basic aspects of the olfactory organ, bulb, and central projections as well as the problem of olfactory coding. Unless otherwise noted, these descriptions refer primarily to mammals.

NASOCHEMOSENSORY SYSTEMS

INTRODUCTION

The four nasochemosensory systems are the olfactory organ, the septal organ, the vomeronasal or Jacobson's organ, and the trigeminal supply to the nasal mucosa. It might be argued that—for the purposes of analyzing the role of odors in controlling behavior—the vomeronasal and septal organs, and even the nasotrigeminal system, can be considered simply as accessory olfactory organs. In the case of the septal organ this may be useful. But to do so in the remaining cases, at least, is to minimize the potential implications of their major differences: their location in the nasal region, the conditions governing access of odorous molecules to their receptors, the nature of their central projections, and evidence suggesting a particular role for the vomeronasal organ in the control of mating behavior in mammals.

Throughout the vertebrates there are such wide variations in nasal architecture, in the presence or absence of the vomeronasal organ (and, possibly, the septal organ), and in the location and extent of certain of these organs that few generalizations concerning their structure and function are possible. Of the four systems, the olfactory, septal, and vomeronasal organs are the most closely related in that their receptors are similar and their axonal connections are with the olfactory bulbs. Least is known about the septal organ. The nasotrigeminal sense is part of what was once known as the "common chemical sense"—which meant the ability, shared by all exposed mucous membranes, to detect primarily irritating chemicals.

The interrelations among these four systems and their relations to other chemosensory systems are outlined in Fig. 1 and have been discussed by Moulton (1967a). In addition, Tucker (1971) has reviewed in-depth knowledge of these systems and of the curious nervus terminalis—a nerve thought to be sensory but otherwise of unknown function—innervating the nasal region.

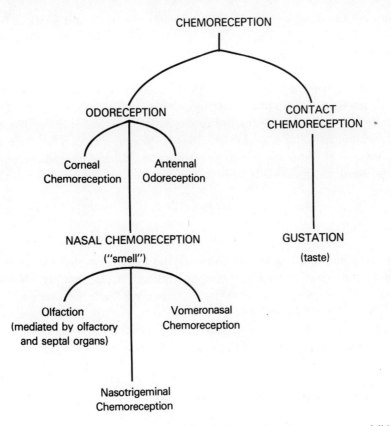

Fig. 1. Components of nasal chemoreception and its relation to other chemosensory modalities. For definitions, see text.

THE MAIN OLFACTORY ORGAN

An olfactory organ is present in almost all vertebrate groups (with the notable exception of certain aquatic mammals). In tetrapods the olfactory organ is generally situated dorsally in the main nasal cavity (or cavum nasi proprium). It contains Bowman's glands, and projects to the main olfactory bulb by way of the primary olfactory neurons. In addition, the receptors possess cilia in almost all species so far studied, and, in the rat at least, the organ is not innervated by branches of the trigeminal nerve (Bojsen-Møller, 1975). (For a fuller description, see "Olfactory Epithelium" below.)

THE SEPTAL ORGAN

The septal organ (or septal olfactory organ or organ of Rodolfo-Masera) has so far been studied only in certain rodents, rabbits, and one species of opossum (*Didelphys*). There is no available information about its presence or absence in other species (Broman, 1921; Rodolfo-Masera, 1943; Adams and McFarland, 1971; Bojsen-Møller, 1975). It lies like an island in the respiratory epithelium on both sides of the nasal septum and is positioned rostral to, and separate from, the olfactory epithelium. (In the rat, it is a 1×2 mm area at the junction of the nasopharynx and the nasal cavity; Bojsen-Møller, 1975.) The epithelium appears similar, if not identical, to that of the olfactory organ. It contains Bowman's glands and the receptors possess cilia. Although it also sends fibers to the main olfactory bulb, the nerve so differs in its histology, course, and termination from those of either the olfactory or vomeronasal organ as to justify considering it a separate organ (Adams and McFarland, 1971; Bojsen-Møller, 1975). There are speculations that it may be involved in monitoring air during quiet breathing or in assessing food palatability, but as yet there has been no specific study of its function.

The Vomeronasal Organ

In mammals and reptiles the vomeronasal or Jacobson's organ generally lies ventral to the nasal chamber in a blind-ending sac. Depending on species, it connects with the nasal or oral cavity or sometimes both. Entrance to the nasal cavity is by way of a duct that often opens in the base of the anterior section of the nasal septum or in the floor of the nasal cavity. (In the rat, it opens into the nasal chamber close to the opening of the sphenopalatine canal.) Entrance to the mouth is either by way of the sphenopalatine canal or by a direct opening anteriorly (Kratzing, 1971; Estes, 1972; Scalia and Winans, 1975). Where it opens into the mouth, the organ has the possibility of responding to taste compounds, and thus, in a sense, acting as an accessory contact chemoreceptor. The vomeronasal organ reaches its highest degree of development relative to the olfactory organ in snakes and lizards, where it plays an essential role in controlling a variety of behavior patterns (Burghardt, 1970). It is prominent in many mammals including marsupials, certain bats, rodents, ungulates, and carnivores, but is generally vestigial in adult man.

The receptors are similar, histologically, to olfactory receptors but possess microvilli rather than cilia. Their axons pass exclusively—by way of the vomeronasal nerve—to the accessory olfactory bulb. The epithelium lacks Bowman's glands but is apparently innervated by the nervus terminalis (Barber and Field, 1975; Bojsen-Møller, 1975). Since the organ lies remote from the main respiratory stream, special mechanisms exist—at least in some species—to convey odorants or increase their access to the receptors (Hamlin, 1929; Mann, 1961).

In a study of the accessory bulb in several species of bats, Mann (1961) found no relation between its volume and either that of the main bulb or that of the size of the animal as a whole (insofar as this was indicated by the volume of the myelencephalon). This might suggest that its function does not coincide with that of the olfactory organ.

The vomeronasal organ seemed to intrigue early investigators, who speculated widely on its possible function. For Broman (1920) it was a water-smelling organ ("ein Wassergeruchsorgan"), for Kölliker (1877) a self-smelling organ, and for Jacobson (1811) an organ providing lubrication for the nasal passageways.

More recently, Estes (1972) in a review of the literature concluded that in mammals it may function primarily as a specialized chemoreceptor of excreted sex hormones and their breakdown products, or both. Critical evidence, however, is still lacking in the case of mammals, and the problem remains controversial. For example, Powers and Winans (1975) claim that the vomeronasal organ plays a critical role in mediating sexual behavior in the male hamster, but Devor and Murphy (1973) found that the mating behavior in this species was not impaired by severing of the vomeronasal nerve. In view of its central connections (see "Tertiary Olfactory Connections" below), the possibility that it at least participates in the control of sexual behavior remains a very active one. On the other hand, recordings from bundles of primary vomeronasal neurons in tortoise and rabbit indicate a response spectrum and sensitivity to odors somewhat comparable to that of the olfactory organ (Tucker, 1963*a,b*) showing that it is equipped to transmit information on a diverse range of compounds. However, the possibility that it may be especially sensitive to specific sex (or food) odors has not been investigated electrophysiologically.

TRIGEMINAL SUPPLY TO THE NASAL MUCOSA

Nasotrigeminal chemoreception is mediated by "free nerve endings" in the respiratory part of the nasal cavity. These stem from branches of the ophthalmic and maxillary divisions of the trigeminal nerve. Details of anatomy and function are reviewed by Tucker (1971).

Autonomic responses are frequent concomitants of trigeminal nerve stimulation (e.g., the oculocardiac reflex of the ophthalmic branch). Responses elicited by stimulating the trigeminal supply to the nasal mucosa seem to be no exception to this general rule. For example, Tucker (1963*b*) found that the amount of sympathetic activity often followed, reflexively, the trigeminal responses to odorants. In the rabbit, sectioning of the cervical sympathetic and seventh cranial nerves abolished all of the efferent activity in the ethmoidal branch of the trigeminal supply to the nasal mucosa (Tucker and Beidler, 1956). Among other effects reported to be initiated by nasotrigeminal receptors is the reflex inhibition of spontaneous muscle action potentials associated with ether stimulation of the nose (Anderson, 1954).

It appears likely, from this and related evidence, that a major function of the nasotrigeminal system is to inhibit inhalation of harmful vapors. It may also form the afferent limb of a reflex that initiates sneezing and mucus secretion. These reflexes could in turn remove or reduce the concentration of any such vapor that enters the nasal airways. But is this the only function of the system? Is its sensitivity to odors such that it also extends and amplifies the functions of the olfactory organ? The classical view was that most odorants were pure olfactory stimuli while the nasotrigeminal receptors responded only to irritating or noxious vapors. Some support for this concept of a limited response range in the trigeminal system comes from the work of Doty (1975), who found that human subjects lacking olfactory function reported detecting only one-fourth of 31 commonly used laboratory odorants. When psychophysical thresholds were determined for two of these compounds, "anosmic" subjects were found to be less sensitive than normal subjects by about 2 log units. Similarly, bulbectomized pigeons have thresholds for amyl acetate, butyl acetate, and butyric acid ½–1 log unit higher than those of normal pigeons (Henton *et al.,* 1969).

But other evidence suggests that the trigeminal system is quite capable of mediating responses to odors comparable in threshold to those mediated by the olfactory system. Instead of using subjects rendered "anosmic" by disease or by injury, Cain (1974) used subjects who were normal except for unilateral destruction of the trigeminal nerve. He found no significant differences in odor threshold between the deficient and normal nostrils. (On the other hand, perceived magnitude was consistently lower on the deficient side, particularly at higher concentrations.) More striking is the electrophysiological evidence: Tucker (1963*a,b*) found no odors to which the tortoise trigeminal nerve would not show some response. Furthermore, in the rabbit, trigeminal thresholds for phenyl ethyl acetate and coffee were lower than the corresponding olfactory thresholds. The greatest difference seen between olfactory and trigeminal thresholds was for amyl acetate $(10^{-3}:10^{-1}$ of vapor saturation at 20°C).

Much of the existing data can be explained by assuming that the main function of the nasotrigeminal system is protective: for the initiation of inhibitory reflexes and avoidance behavior. Unless vapors are present in concentrations that are potentially harmful, the response of the trigeminal system does not usually reach the level of conscious perception and may contribute little if anything to the detection and discrimination of odors. However, the viability of this hypothesis has yet to be tested. In particular, systematic behavioral and electrophysiological investigations have not been made on the same species.

Other functions that have been ascribed to nasochemoreception include reduction in the magnitude of adaptation to stimuli of high and possibly moderate intensity, and localization of the source of an odor (Cain, 1974; von Skramlik, 1925; Schneider and Schmidt, 1967).

TERMINOLOGY

When a mammal responds behaviorally to an odor it is generally not clear whether the response is mediated by olfactory, septal, vomeronasal, or trigeminal chemoreceptors, or by some combination of them. Attempts to isolate one or more of these components or to produce "anosmia" have generally involved bulbectomy or application of agents or procedures which block or destroy olfactory receptors. The variety of techniques in use and the variety of combinations of sensory and nonsensory structures which they can damage or destroy greatly complicate the interpretation of much of the existing evidence (see Alberts, 1974; Sieck and Daumbach, 1974). For example, bulbectomy destroys the main bulb and either the vomeronasal nerve or accessory bulb or both, but may or may not leave intact either the ethmoidal branch of the trigeminal supply to the nasal mucosa or the nervus terminalis. In addition, bulbectomy may destroy portions of the anterior olfactory nucleus, and influence a variety of behavior patterns that depend on an intact bulb but not necessarily on intact olfactory receptors. For example, attempts to produce peripheral "anosmia" have frequently involved necrotic destruction of the olfactory epithelium by perfusion of the nasal chamber with a solution of zinc sulfate. However, unless special precautions are taken, this procedure may destroy or damage vomeronasal receptors as well. Conversely, it may not eliminate all olfactory receptors (e.g., Powers and Winans, 1975).

One consequence of these technical difficulties is that existing terminology is often misleading or insufficiently precise (e.g., "olfaction," "olfactory," "anosmia"). For this reason it is helpful to define *olfaction* as the form of nasal chemoreception that is initiated by olfactory receptors that send their axons to the main olfactory bulb. *Nasal chemoreception* ("smell") in turn refers to the responses mediated by all receptors within both the nasal cavity and the vomeronasal organ (despite the fact that in some species it may connect only to the oral cavity). *Odoreception* can then be used as a term covering nasal chemoreception as well as other forms of chemoreception in which the stimuli are chemicals delivered in the vapor phase (e.g., via antennal chemoreceptors). Although the use of "olfaction" in a much broader context is so firmly entrenched that confusion is likely to persist, it is these more limited definitions that will be used in the remainder of this chapter.

OLFACTORY EPITHELIUM: SOME STRUCTURAL AND FUNCTIONAL ASPECTS

The purpose of this section is to provide a brief overview of the anatomy and function of the peripheral olfactory systems. More detailed accounts and further references are given by Moulton and Beidler (1967), Graziadei (1971), and Altner and Kolnberger (1975). The most basic features are outlined schematically in Fig. 2.

It is sometimes assumed that the absolute area of the olfactory surface is a guide to the olfactory powers of an animal. If this is so, the relation is not a simple one since man—a so-called microsmatic mammal said to have poor olfactory powers—has a total olfactory area estimated to be 10 cm² (von Brunn, 1892), while the rabbit—a so-called macrosmatic animal assumed to have well-developed olfactory powers—has a surface area of 9.3 cm² (Allison and Warwick, 1949). Factors complicating such comparisons are the absence of pertinent behavioral data and the wide variation among species in the density of receptor cells per unit area of the olfactory surface (see Moulton and Beidler, 1967; Kolnberger, 1971) and in the number of cilia per receptor. (The dog, for example, has 100–150 cilia per receptor while the rabbit has only 9–16 per receptor; Okano *et al.,* 1967; Le Gros Clark, 1956.)

The olfactory epithelium is surprisingly uniform in structure throughout the vertebrates. The receptors themselves are bipolar neurons providing both a receptive surface that penetrates into the overlying mucous secretions and an axon connecting without branch or collateral directly to the olfactory bulb (Fig. 2).

There is no convincing evidence that receptors are electrically coupled by low-resistance junctions. Within the olfactory epithelium the receptors surround supporting cells thought to have a secretory function. Underlying the receptor and supporting cells is a layer composed of the third cell type of the olfactory epithelium: the basal cell. The continuous division of these cells provides daughter cells, some of which migrate peripherally to replace receptor cells. The entire epithelium has a turnover time of 28.6 ± 6.6 days in the mouse (see Moulton, 1974, 1975).

The possibility that the olfactory receptors regenerate in higher vertebrates has been questioned in the past (see Takagi, 1971; Moulton, 1974). This problem has been reexamined by Tucker *et al.* (1975) using the pigeon. They report not only that cut olfactory nerves regenerate after a month or more but also that odor quality discrimination is fully restored (as judged by conditioned suppression of key pecking during odor presentation).

When an odor is puffed onto the olfactory epithelium, a slow negative voltage shift can be recorded from the surface. This transient is the electroolfactogram (EOG) first studied extensively by Ottoson (1956). Intracellular recordings, and other evidence, indicate that at least a major component of the potential is derived from the receptor, but leave open the possibility that some contribution may also come from the supporting cell (Getchell, 1974*b*, 1975).

It is generally assumed that the receptor membrane contains specialized loci, or sites, with which odorous molecules interact. "Cross-adaptation" studies of single receptor responses (adapt to one odorant, test with a second) indicate that at least a proportion of the receptors may bear two or more types of receptor sites (Baylin and Moulton, 1975). The location, structure, and number of different types of receptor sites are unknown, but there is some indication that the sites themselves are proteins (Getchell and Gesteland, 1972; Getchell and Getchell, 1974).

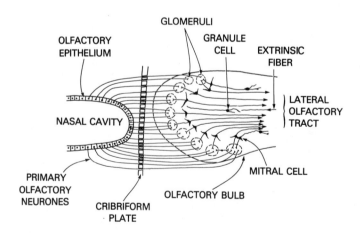

Fig. 2. Semischematic diagram of olfactory epithelium and bulb. The bulb and epithelium are normally separated only by the cribriform plate. The ratios of primary neurons, glomeruli, mitral cells, and granule cells are not accurate.

The poverty of our knowledge concerning the basic events in the odorant–receptor interaction has provided a fertile ground for odor theorists but no generally accepted account of the transduction process.

The unmyelinated axons of the olfactory receptors are among the smallest in the body: a selected sample in the cat had a mean diameter of $0.276 \pm 0.055\mu m$ (Freeman, 1972a; see also Willey, 1973). The slow conduction velocity associated with such fibers (about 0.2 m/sec) accounts for a significant fraction of the total reaction time to an odor: possibly 20 msec or more in species with relatively long fibers.

ODOR QUALITY CODING

Extracellular unit recordings from frogs, tortoises, and vultures show many receptors to be broadly tuned, responding to the majority of stimuli presented, although a few show more restricted response spectra. Some can discriminate among sterically related molecules eliciting similar odor sensations but no two receptors have identical response spectra, and, as yet, there is no basis for classifying receptors (Gesteland et al., 1963, 1965; Takagi and Omura, 1963; Shibuya and Shibuya, 1963; Altner and Boeckh, 1967; O'Connell and Mozell, 1969; Mathews, 1972; Getchell, 1974a; Duchamp et al., 1974; Blank, 1974).

While it would be possible to overlook a population of highly specific odor receptors among the several millions or tens of millions in the olfactory epithelium, there is no general support for the idea of a receptor subpopulation operating on the principle of labeled-line coding (see Chapter 3). More probably the identity of individual odors is signaled by an ensemble of neurons firing in concert to produce an odor-specific pattern. The central question, however, is the nature of the pattern and, in particular, whether it varies from one place to another across the epithelial surface (see Moulton, 1976).

The suggestion that different odors might elicit different patterns of excitation at different places on the receptor organ's surface was first proposed by Adrian (1950, 1956, 1959), who also made the first major contributions to an understanding of the electrophysiology of the olfactory bulb. He found that certain esters were more effective stimuli for single units located anteriorly in the rabbit olfactory bulb while hydrocarbons were more effective posteriorly. He ascribed these patterns to relative differences in the mode of dispersal of odorous molecules across the receptor sheet and later suggested that the principles governing their distribution may be analogous to those operating in chromatography; that is, their dispersal may depend on differences in their sorptive properties. Clearly, if this or any other hypothesis that implicates spatial patterning as a component of odor quality coding is valid, there must be some topographic projection to the bulb from the epithelium (in other words, the epithelium must be mapped onto the bulb).

Anatomical studies have borne out this general expectation: the dorsal surface of the epithelium projects to the dorsal surface of the bulb and the ventral epithelium projects to the ventral bulb. However, this map is not a precise point-to-point projection. It is, in fact, least precise in the direction most relevant to Adrian's studies: the anteroposterior plane. Its sharpest focus is on the dorsal surface of the bulb (Le Gros Clark, 1951, 1957; Land, 1973; Land and Shepherd, 1974). Nevertheless, the spatial correspondence between the epithelium and the bulb is such that any spatial patterning of receptors according to different odor specificities is likely to be reflected in the bulb.

Two electrophysiological studies, however, have picked out another layer of complexity. One of these involves responses of second-order neurons in the bullfrog bulb to electrical stimulation of primary olfactory nerves. Apparently two kinds of units exist: those receiving a widespread projection from the entire dorsal mucosa and those more selective in their response. Among the most selective are some that respond only to stimulation of corresponding regions in the mucosa (Costanzo and Mozell, 1974). Diffuseness of projection was also noted by Freeman (1974), who mapped evoked responses on the surface of the bulb to low-level electrical stimulation of primary olfactory neurons. He concluded that activity from every point stimulated experimentally in the primary neurons diverged over the entire bulb.

These results raise the possibility that there are two kinds of projection from receptor surface to bulb: one which preserves at least some features of the map and one which diffuses it. The main point, however, is that a map of the receptor surface (diffuse anteroposteriorly and sharper dorsally) does indeed exist in the bulb and the evidence is sufficient to justify pursuing further the question of a possible spatial component to odor quality coding.

In abstract this spatial patterning could be of two types: imposed or inherent. Imposed patterning is like the kind generated in the retina, responding directly to a pattern of graded light intensities in the external environment. In the nose, imposed patterning refers to a pattern set up by differential filtering and shunting of molecules as they pass through the nasal airways and over the olfactory surface. In contrast, inherent patterning is that which is determined by inherent differences in the properties of receptors and the way in which they are distributed on an organ according to these differences. In the nose, it refers to a pattern generated by receptors organized topographically according to their different odor specificities.

Evidence for imposed patterning has come chiefly from Mozell and his associates. They have shown that the sorptive properties of the bullfrog olfactory epithelium are sufficient to impose a marked concentration gradient in an antero-posterior direction on certain odorants as they pass through the olfactory sac. Anteroposterior patterning also appears in the relative responses of primary olfactory neurons innervating anterior and posterior regions of the mucosa to certain odorants. To account for these and related findings, Mozell has proposed a chromatographic theory of olfaction. This assumes, first, that when odorants cross the olfactory surface they are sorted out according to principles analogous to those operating in chromatography, and, second, that this sorting provides supplementary information that can be used by the organism in identifying odors (Mozell, 1964, 1966; Mozell and Jagodowicz, 1973; Hornung et al., 1975).

There can be little doubt that sorptive patterning could be effective in sorting odorants into, at least, a few general groups. But beyond this its potential contribution to odor discrimination is less clear. It appears that an odorant would be correctly recognized by this mechanism if it elicited one specific activity pattern among many thousands that could be generated. But odorants can be recognized in one sniff and under widely varying conditions (e.g., breathing normally, sniffing, and by the retronasal route) that should result in a considerable range of activity gradients for the same odor if the analogy with chromatography were to hold. Furthermore, the nose-to-bulb projection is particularly diffuse in the anteroposterior direction. In other words, the system is not constructed in a way that would favor fidelity of transfer of "chromatographic" patterning.

Evidence for the existence of inherent patterning has begun to accumulate more recently. Simultaneous recordings from several sites in the olfactory bulb responding to odor stimulation showed spatial patterning that could best be ascribed to a combination of inherent and imposed patterning, inherent patterning being dominant (Moulton, 1967*b*, 1969). At the epithelial level, Mustaparta (1973) found evidence of nonhomogeneity in the distribution of receptors as judged by electroolfactograms recorded from different sites on the frog mucosa.

But both these (and all previous studies) made no provision for examining responses to odors in isolation from sorptive (i.e., imposed) effects. This was attempted by Kauer and Moulton (1974), who used a pipette with vacuum surround to restrict odor spread to a circle of about 350 μm in diameter on the epithelium. Using this device in the tiger salamander, they recorded responses of single bulbar units to different odors. Two types of units were found. In the first type, odor stimulation of any restricted mucosal area suppressed ongoing (or "spontaneous") activity. The other type of unit was maximally excited by stimulation of one or—in the case of amyl acetate—two areas. For a given odor, these fields remained surprisingly constant from animal to animal, but they were not sharply defined. This evidence suggests that specific odors may indeed be represented topographically on the receptor surface. The microstructure of such fields has not been explored to determine if further details of patterning exist which would serve to characterize an odor, or group of odors, more effectively.

Further evidence that spatial patterning may be a component of odor quality coding comes from still another approach. It depends on the fact that increased metabolic activity in a neuron is reflected in changed glucose consumption. This increased glucose consumption, in turn, can be used to locate the active cell by radioactive labeling. For example, if rats are injected with a radioactive derivative of glucose, exposed to amyl acetate for 45 min, and then sacrificed, autoradiographs of sections through the olfactory bulbs show two densely labeled areas on either side of each bulb. This evidence implies that there might be a specific topographic pattern of neuronal activity elicited by amyl acetate (Sharp *et al.*, 1975).

Finally, prolonged exposure of rats to an odor often induces morphological changes in the olfactory bulb which appear to be specific for an odor or group of odors (Døving and Pinching, 1973; Pinching and Døving, 1974). However, because these changes involve what appears to be a form of degeneration, their significance is more difficult to assess. Both of these phenomena could reflect the development of a combination of intrinsic and imposed patterning.

Both types of patterning, intrinsic and imposed, clearly coexist and may act in concert. It is not known whether they are components of odor quality coding. However, the potential power of intrinsic patterning, in particular, is growing more evident and represents a fertile ground for future research.

THE OLFACTORY BULB: SOME STRUCTURAL AND FUNCTIONAL ASPECTS

OVERVIEW

A full account of the synaptic organization and functional properties of the olfactory bulb and the effects of bulbectomy is beyond the scope of this chapter and is, in any case, provided in other reviews (Moulton and Tucker, 1964; Shepherd, 1972; Wenzel, 1974). There are, however, certain features—particularly in relation to extrinsic fibers to the bulb—which have an actual or potential relevance to behavior and which deserve brief consideration. Figure 2 illustrates some basic points.

Analogies have been drawn between the synaptic organization of the olfactory bulb (with or without the olfactory epithelium) and the retina (e.g., Moulton and Tucker, 1964; Shepherd, 1972). But to what extent the interplay of excitation and inhibition in the bulb sharpens and selects the inflow of olfactory information is not clear. What is evident is that the bulb imposes a drastic condensation on the number of channels of information it receives when compared to the number it projects to the olfactory cortex: for every thousand primary neurons entering the bulb only about one second-order neuron leaves it (Allison and Warwick, 1949). If we accept available estimates, each bulb in the rabbit receives 50 million of these primary neurons and more than that in the cat (Allison and Warwick, 1949; Freeman, 1972b). This is about 10 times the number of optic fibers in man, for example. The bulb is also the first point in the olfactory pathway where the afferent inflow is potentially subject to direct modification by signals from fibers of central origin.

All primary neurons end in glomeruli—discrete, roughly spherical regions of neuropil—where they ramify and synapse with the dendrites of mitral, tufted, and periglomular cells. But an important element in providing the vertical and horizontal interconnection within the bulb is the granule cell. This cell is an axonless neuron lying deep in the bulb. Mitral cell axons, and very probably a proportion of tufted cell axons, leave the bulb in the lateral olfactory tract.

EXTRINSIC BULBAR PATHWAYS

Three axonal pathways project to the bulb other than the primary olfactory fibers: centrifugal fibers of central origin, commissural fibers, and axonal collaterals from the anterior olfactory nucleus. All appear to terminate primarily, but not exclusively, on granule cells. They have been the object of much recent experimentation initiated by interest in the potential these fibers have for modifying and comparing olfactory information before it can reach more central destinations. We shall consider evidence for the termination and origin of these pathways before introducing some interpretations of their possible role.

Although long a matter of controversy, it now appears that centrifugal fibers of central origin form two distinct projections to the main bulb: one group terminates on several cell types at the glomerular level while another terminates in deeper layers (Powell and Cowan, 1963; Powell *et al.*, 1965; Heimer, 1968; Price, 1968, 1969*a*; Price and Powell, 1970*a*; Mascitti *et al.*, 1971; Pinching and Powell, 1972). Centrifugal fibers to the accessory bulb originate in the corticomedial amygdala (Barber and Field, 1975). In the case of the main bulb, centrifugal fibers appear to originate in the nucleus of the horizontal limb of the diagonal band of Broca (Price, 1969*b*; Price and Powell, 1970*b,c*).

Although the pathways involved are not established, stimulation of a substantial region of the basal rhinencephalon evokes responses in the bulb (Kerr and Hagbarth, 1955; Carreras *et al.*, 1967; Dennis and Kerr, 1968, 1975). For example, Dennis and Kerr (1975) recorded centrifugal influences from the pyriform cortex, anterior olfactory nucleus, nucleus of the lateral olfactory tract, olfactory tubercle, cortical amygdaloid nucleus, and nucleus of the lateral olfactory tract. Since these regions all receive fibers from the bulb, they must provide relatively direct feedback loops onto it.

Since the end of the last century the existence of a direct connection between the bulbs through the anterior commissure has been a point of controversy. Ramon y Cajal (1911), for example, believed that the anterior limb of the anterior commissure originates in the tufted cells of one bulb and ends in the other. While a minor connection may exist in, at least, some species of fish (e.g., Finger, 1975), the bulk of the evidence now indicates that such a connection does not exist (e.g., Heimer, 1968; Broadwell, 1975*a*). For example, electrical stimulation of one bulb elicits a slow monophasic potential in the other with a latency too long to reflect a direct interbulbar connection (e.g., Dennis and Kerr, 1968; Daval and Leveteau, 1974). The main effect of stimulation is to depress contralateral bulbar activity. Consistent with this effect, ablation of one bulb increases excitability of the other (e.g., Callens, 1967; see also Moulton, 1963).

It now seems clear that, with the unlikely exception of a minor interbulbar component, fibers crossing in the anterior limb of the anterior commissure and reaching the contralateral bulb originate in the anterior olfactory nucleus. This nucleus also sends fibers to the ipsilateral bulb (Lohman and Mentink, 1969; Price and Powell, 1970*a*; Daval and Leveteau, 1974).

There are several aspects of olfactory function that might be influenced by the action of extrinsic fibers. Recent work has focused on odor detection and localization, olfactory adaptation, and facilitation of response to food-related odors in hungry animals. In one study, Bennett (1968) found that rats lose their ability to perform a learned odor detection task following bilateral commissural transection, unilateral bulb removal, and bilateral commissural transection. All three procedures decreased the degree of adaptation to a test odor nondifferentially. He concluded that the anterior limb of the anterior commissure contains two anatomically and functionally discrete systems: one sums intensive functions of each half of the olfactory system while the second mediates a central component of olfactory adaptation.

On analogy with directional hearing, it is possible that odors can be localized by comparing the time of arrival of odorous molecules at the two nares. While there are reports that this is possible, there is little agreement about the extent to which olfaction alone is involved (von Skramlik, 1925; von Békésy, 1964; Schneider and Schmidt, 1967). In particular, there has been no confirmation, as yet, of von Békésy's remarkable claim that a human subject can detect an interval of the order of 1 msec between birhinal stimuli.

Leveteau et al. (1969) sought a possible basis for this phenomenon in neural events controlled by interbulbar interactions. They stimulated a rabbit birhinally, varying the interval between odorant arrival at each naris. The criterion of response was the degree of inhibition elicited in the slow voltage shift recorded from the glomerular layer of the olfactory bulb. On this basis, they report that a 3 msec interval could be detected. The inhibition was abolished by sectioning the anterior commissure. They suggest that interbulbar connections may amplify slight differences or contrasts in the interval between birhinally delivered stimuli through a mechanism of reciprocal inhibition.

It is conceivable that centrifugal fibers could effect a selective enhancement of bulbar unit response to an odor that had acquired, or already possessed, particular significance for the animal. (If we accept the view that these fibers exert a tonic inhibitory influence on bulbar excitability, then a release from this inhibition could serve as a mechanism for achieving enhancement.) To test this possibility, Pager (1974) has used chronically implanted electrodes to record summated multiunit responses from second-order neurons in the bulb of rats in different nutritional states. Enhanced responses to food odors (but not amyl acetate) were more frequent in hungry as opposed to satiated rats. After unilateral section of the anterior limb of the anterior commissure, however, the effect disappeared on the side of the section but not contralaterally.

Clearly, these pioneering studies raise many questions in cracking the surface of a relatively unexplored field. None was concerned with single-unit responses, and much more work will have to be done before we can attempt to define the role of centrifugal fibers to the bulb.

Secondary Olfactory Connections

Introduction

There was a time when the "olfactory brain" or rhinencephalon—the cortical region receiving olfactory bulb fibers—was assumed to cover much of the cerebral hemisphere of primitive vertebrates and up to the medial rim in mammals. (It included, for example, the hippocampus, the septum, and the cingulum.) Toward the middle of this century the assumed extensiveness of cortical commitment to olfaction came under attack. Much of the momentum stemmed from a critical review by Brodal (1947), but other work reinforced the view. The much shrunken remnants of the "olfactory" brain were delineated in a review by Pribram and Kruger (1954) which reclassified the territory vacated by olfaction as part of the limbic system. But with the application of improved techniques for impregnating degenerating axons (particularly the Fink-Heimer method) and the availability of electron microscopy to identify degenerating boutons it became clear that the earlier studies could not have been definitive (e.g., Heimer, 1968; Ebbesson and Northcutt, 1975). In fact, the new evidence showed that the retreat had gone too far and in the subsequent years much lost ground was reclaimed. This development has now been taken a stage further with the introduction of horseradish peroxidase and autoradiographic techniques. Interpretation of results obtained with these methods—unlike those obtained with degeneration techniques—is not complicated by fibers of passage. Application of these methods has not only confirmed previous findings but also revealed additional and more extensive olfactory projections than were previously accepted (Price, 1973; Barber and Raisman, 1974; Broadwell, 1975a,b; Barber and Field, 1975).

A further development—no doubt stimulated in part by evidence that the vomeronasal organ is implicated in mammalian reproductive behavior—has been the recognition that the projections of the main and accessory olfactory bulbs should be examined separately—not confounded as in earlier studies. The differing afferent and efferent projections of the bulbs that this has revealed have led to the concept of a dual olfactory system (Winans and Scalia, 1970; Raisman, 1972; Scalia and Winans, 1975).

PRIMARY PROJECTIONS OF THE MAIN BULB

Despite some minor areas of uncertainty it is now generally agreed that the main bulb of most mammals probably projects to the prepyriform cortex, the nucleus of the lateral olfactory tract, the anterior olfactory nucleus, the olfactory tubercle, anterior and posterolateral cortical amygdaloid nuclei, the rostroventral end of the anterior hippocampus (tenia tecta or hippocampal rudiment), and the dorsomedial and lateral entorhinal area. Finally, there is one report of a projection to a transition area between the prepyriform cortex and the horizontal limb of the nucleus of the diagonal band of Broca (e.g., Heimer, 1968; Price, 1973; Scalia and Winans, 1975; Broadwell, 1975a). Most of these divisions are shown in Fig. 3.

The chief afferents of the olfactory bulb are through the lateral olfactory tract, sectioning of which appears to produce anosmia. It is a surprisingly complex structure and, in terms of fiber size, has a dual projection: fine collateral branches reach the posterior olfactory cortex while mainly larger-diameter (faster-conducting) fibers supply the anterior olfactory cortex (largely corresponding to the prepyriform cortex) (Price and Sprich, 1975; Dennis and Kerr, 1975). It might be argued that this dichotomy could provide for a separation of information: input requiring rapid processing going to the anterior olfactory cortex with the remainder passing more slowly posteriorly. One possible complication, however, is that nearly all cortical structures of the basal forebrain to which the bulb projects directly also receive an association projection from the prepyriform cortex (Price, 1973).

PROJECTIONS OF THE ACCESSORY OLFACTORY BULB

Until recently it was assumed that the projections of the accessory bulb were distributed to the same sites as those of the olfactory bulb. It now appears that their efferent connections are quite distinct. The accessory bulb projects by way of the accessory olfactory tract (running on the dorsal surface of the ipsilateral lateral olfactory tract), to terminate in the corticomedial amygdala, the bed nucleus of the accessory olfactory tract, and the bed nucleus of the stria terminalis. Of these, the

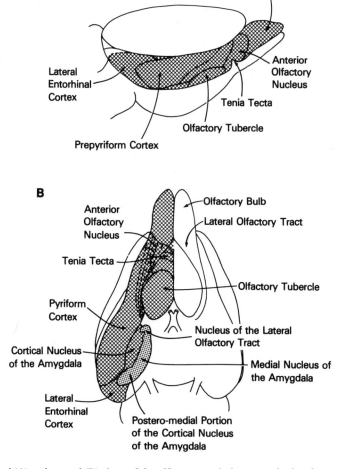

Fig. 3. Lateral (A) and ventral (B) views of the olfactory cortical areas and related structures of the rat. The heavy dashed line in A represents the outline of the lateral olfactory tract. The stippled area in B covers the nuclei receiving fibers from the accessory olfactory bulb. The hatched areas in A and B cover the olfactory bulb and its projection field. The tenia tecta is the anterior rudiment of the hippocampus. Modified from Price (1973).

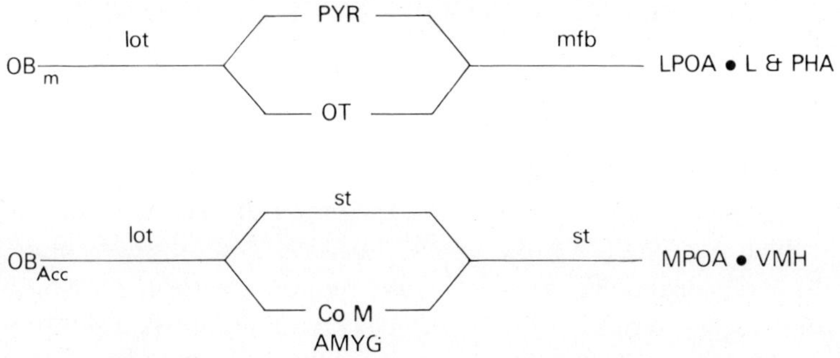

Fig. 4. Differences in the projections of the main (m) and accessory (Acc) olfactory bulbs (OB). CoM AMYG, Corticomeidal group of amygdaloid nuclei; lot, lateral olfactory tract; LPOA, lateral preoptic area; L & PHA, lateral and posterior hypothalamus; mfb, median forebrain bundle; MPOA, medial preoptic area; OT, olfactory tubercle; PYR, pyriform cortex; St, stria terminalis; VMH, ventromedial hypothalamus. Modified from Raisman (1972).

projection to the amygdala is the major one. Specifically, the target sites are the medial amygdaloid nucleus and the posteromedial part of the cortical amygdaloid nucleus (Winans and Scalia, 1970; Price, 1973; Broadwell, 1975a; Scalia and Winans, 1975). The separate centrifugal supply from the corticomedial amygdala to the accessory bulb also passes through the stria terminalis (Raisman, 1972; Barber and Field, 1975).

A significant point of difference between the projections of the main and accessory bulbs, emphasized in Fig. 4, is that whereas both project to the basal telencephalic centers, only the accessory bulb connects directly with the diencephalon (i.e., the bed nucleus of the stria terminalis).

Tertiary Olfactory Connections

Olfactory information probably has access to diencephalic and mesencephalic structures through several parallel pathways and thus may influence many of the wide range of behavioral activities with which these structures are involved. Through its connection with the prefrontal lobe via the dorsomedial nucleus of the thalamus, the main bulbar system has access to neocortical mechanisms. In this section we shall consider evidence for connections between the olfactory system and a few other structures.

Preoptic-Hypothalamic Continuum

The growing evidence of relatively direct olfactory connections to the preoptic-hypothalamic continuum is particularly significant in the context of much recent work documenting the involvement of olfaction in reproductive physiology and sexual behavior (see Doty, 1976). But the degree of involvement of the main and the accessory olfactory systems in these functions may be rather different, if not distinct. This much can be deduced from anatomical evidence suggesting that they project to distinct regions of the hypothalamus. Thus fibers originating in the prepyriform cortex and olfactory tubercle apparently pass in and through the median forebrain bundle to the nuclei gemini of the hypothalamus (Cowan *et al.*, 1965; Heimer, 1972; Scott and Chafin, 1975). Heimer (1972), however, was unable to verify an earlier report of a significant projection from the olfactory cortex to the lateral hypothalamus. On the other hand, that portion of the amygdala which receives its input from the accessory olfactory bulb projects through the stria terminalis to the medial preoptic area and the ventromedial hypothalamic nuclei (Leonard and Scott, 1971). Unfortunately, the fiber connections of those amygdaloid nuclei to which the main bulb projects are not known. This leaves the possibility that the terminations of pathways of the accessory and main bulbs to the preoptic nucleus and the hypothalamus may ultimately be found to overlap extensively. (In this sense, current emphasis on the existence of dual olfactory systems could be premature.) However, on the basis of existing evidence the projections of the two systems may show some minor overlap but are essentially distinct. The significance of this lies partly in reports that the accessory (rather than the main) olfactory projection pathway distributes fibers to an area of the preoptic nucleus which may be involved in the generation of the cyclic preovulatory surge of gonadotropins and thus play a role in sexual behavior (Raisman and Field, 1971). Behavioral evidence concerning the separateness of function of the two olfactory systems is inconclusive (Devor and Murphy, 1973; Powers and Winans, 1975).

In view of the anatomical evidence it is not surprising that both odor and electrical stimulation of the olfactory bulb elicit responses from units in the lateral and medial hypothalamus. Evoked responses show a range of latencies (3–80 msec) probably indicating multisynaptic pathways (Scott and Pfaffman, 1967, 1972; Pfaff and Pfaffmann, 1969; Komisaruk and Beyer, 1972; Scott and Chafin, 1975). In the preoptic area of male rats a high proportion of single units respond differentially to urine vs. nonurine odors. In addition, more preoptic units respond differentially to estrous vs. ovariectomized female urine odors than do olfactory bulb units (Pfaff and Gregory, 1971).

HIPPOCAMPUS

When Brodal (1947) exposed the weakness underlying earlier assumptions of the extensiveness of the "olfactory" brain, he focused criticism on inclusion of the hippocampus. As a result, it became generally accepted that the hippocampus has little to do with olfaction. Nevertheless, a few studies continue to suggest that a significant connection might exist (e.g., Berry *et al.*, 1952; Cragg, 1960; Way, 1962). With the demonstration of a projection from the entorhinal area to the hippocampus, as well as evidence of a direct bulbar projection to the anterior rudiment of the hippocampus, it is beginning to appear that the earlier views of a close relation between the hippocampus and the olfactory system may yet prove to have some validity (Hjorth-Simonsen, 1972; Woods *et al.*, 1969). Evidence that large bilateral lesions of the hippocampus do not impair acquisition of an olfactory discrimination does not necessarily eliminate this possibility in view of the multiplicity of potential pathways for olfactory information (Kimble and Zack, 1967).

Indeed, the hippocampus itself may provide one of several pathways for olfactory information to the hypothalamus since it projects to the paraventricular nucleus via the fornix (Woods *et al.,* 1969).

HABENULA

There is some evidence for olfactory pathways to the habenula, another structure implicated in a wide range of functions. Electrical stimulation of the olfactory bulb elicits responses in the habenula with latencies as short as 7 msec. Odors are also effective stimuli in eliciting habenular responses. However, the route of fibers connecting the olfactory system to the habenula is unknown. One possible pathway may be through the anterior olfactory nucleus since lesions here cause anterograde degeneration in the habenula of the opossum (Ferrer, 1969; Price and Powell, 1971; Heimer, 1972: Wedgewood, 1974; Mok and Mogenson, 1974). It has been suggested on the basis of behavioral evidence—involving lesions of the habenula which led to elevation of olfactory thresholds—that the habenula serves as an important link between olfactory input and somatic motor systems in the rat (Rausch and Long, 1971, 1974).

THALAMUS

It used to be assumed that olfaction is unique among sensory modalities in that the main ascending afferent flow does not pass through a thalamic relay to neocortex. However, fibers originating in the olfactory cortex of the pyriform lobe have been traced to the dorsomedial nucleus of the thalamus, and stimulation of the olfactory bulb elicits responses in the nucleus with latencies as short as 4 msec. (The same cells do not respond to visual, auditory, or somatosensory stimuli.) In one report 43% of the units studied responded to odor stimulation. The route of olfactory input to the dorsomedial nucleus is still unknown. There is some electrophysiological evidence for a pathway to the dorsomedial thalamus from the medial amygdaloid nuclei. This raises the possibility that the accessory bulb may also have a pathway to the thalamus (Powell *et al.,* 1965; Ferrer, 1969; Scott and Leonard, 1971; Heimer, 1972; DeMolina and Ispizu, 1972; Jackson and Benjamin, 1974; Benjamin and Jackson, 1974; Wedgwood, 1974; Motokizawa, 1974*a,b*; Tanabe *et al.,* 1975*a*).

Olfaction, then, is less unique than once supposed: it possesses a thalamic projection. But what pathway provides it with access to the neocortex? There are reports of a projection from the thalamic medial nucleus to the orbitofrontal cortex (e.g., Leonard, 1972). More recently, Tanabe *et al.* (1975*b*) have recorded potentials in the monkey orbitofrontal cortex following electrical stimulation of the dorsomedial nucleus. However, they also found units in a separate (lateroposterior) region of the orbitofrontal cortex that responded to stimulation of the olfactory bulb (see below). These responses could still be evoked following massive destruction of the medial thalamus. Thus, although the question of whether the olfactory input to the thalamus provides the only route to the neocortex remains unresolved, it has become less critical. By one route or another olfactory information does reach the neocortex.

Using both ablation and evoked potential techniques, Allen (1940, 1943*a*) found evidence for an olfactory projection area in the prefrontal cortex of the dog. Although these results were not believed at the time, they have since been confirmed by Tanabe *et al.* (1975*a*), who evoked potentials in the lateroposterior portion of the orbitofrontal cortex (LPOF) of monkeys by stimulating the olfactory bulb. Bilateral ablation of the LPOF—but not other areas of the prefrontal cortex—markedly impaired conditioned discrimination between two odors (although not for all). Again, these results confirm and extend an earlier study by Allen (1943*b*) in the dog. In seeking possible connections between the olfactory bulb and the LPOF, the authors were able to evoke potentials in the LPOF upon stimulation of the anterior pyriform cortex, entorhinal cortex, the medial amygdala, and the anterolateral and dorsoposterior hypothalamus. Since lesions in the hypothalamus eliminated responses in the LPOF evoked by stimulating the olfactory bulb, the authors concluded that there is a pathway between these structures which passes through the pyriform lobe and hypothalamus.

In a further study recordings were made from single LPOF units in awake but restrained monkeys (Tanabe *et al.*, 1975*b*). Thirty-seven percent of the cells responded to at least one of a group of eight odors and of these cells 50% responded to only one odor. (Cells in the dorsal portion of the prefrontal cortex did not respond to odors.) For comparison, responses to the same group of odors were recorded from units in the anterior pyriform cortex, the medial portion of the amygdala, and the olfactory bulb. Although the proportion of cells responding to odors was higher (50–60%) in these latter structures, their response spectra were broader than those of LPOF units. The influence of concentration on these relations has yet to be determined, but it is quite possible that fine and specific discrimination of odors is completed at the level of the orbitofrontal cortex.

In addition to the prefrontal lobe, potentials have been evoked after 15–20 msec in the gustatory cortical area following stimulation of the olfactory bulb (Giachetti and MacLeod, 1975), while odor detection thresholds were increased following removal of the temporal lobe in human patients (Rausch and Serafetinides, 1975).

MESENCEPHALIC RETICULAR FORMATION

The capacity of odorous stimuli to induce arousal reactions may stem, in part, from olfactory connections with the mesencephalic reticular formation (MRF). The median forebrain bundle, which receives axons from olfactory areas, projects to the mesencephalic tegmentum (Millhouse, 1969). In addition, single MRF units respond to odor stimulation in both rats and cats (Pfaff and Pfaffmann, 1969; Motokizawa, 1974*b*). In one study, 58% of units responded in this way. Potentials evoked in the MRF by stimulating the olfactory bulb had latencies of 10–30 msec. A lesion in the median forebrain bundle at the preoptic level abolished this response completely (Motokizawa, 1974*b*).

These studies also indicate that olfactory influences on the MRF are nonspecific and unexceptional in the proportion of units they excite as compared with somatic visual and auditory stimulation.

Conclusions

In addition to the olfactory organ, many vertebrates possess two or three different chemosensitive areas in the nasal region: the vomeronasal organ, the septal organ, and the nasal mucosa supplied by the trigeminal nerve. The relative contribution of these systems to the control of different behavior patterns is not clear in most cases. However, odors play a major role in the control of social and sexual behavior, trail following, feeding behavior, and the identification of territory. In addition, they may directly influence certain physiological functions including some mediated by endocrine activity. In general, the olfactory system appears to be implicated in many functions attributed to limbic and hypothalamic structures.

The organization of the olfactory epithelium is relatively uniform throughout the vertebrates. Odorants are apparently recognized by receptor molecules—probably proteinaceous—forming receptor sites. Several types of sites may occur on a single receptor. There is no generally accepted theory to account for the odor transduction process. Individual receptors possess a relatively low degree of odor specificity. While this in itself might provide a sufficient basis for odor quality discrimination, there is also evidence that different odors elicit different spatial patterns of excitation across the receptor sheet. Since there is some degree of topographic representation of the olfactory epithelium on the olfactory bulb, this pattern should persist at the bulbar level. There appear, however, to be two types of spatial pattern: imposed and inherent. The imposed pattern is generated by differential sorption of molecules as they cross the receptor sheet, while the imposed pattern depends on the tendency for receptors possessing similar odor specificities to be more concentrated in certain regions of the receptor sheet. Either, neither, or both of these patterns may contribute information used in odor quality discrimination.

The olfactory bulb imposes a sharp condensation on the input it receives from the receptors. Transmission and processing of olfactory information proceed in vertical and horizontal neural networks within the bulb. Fibers originating in the nucleus of the horizontal limb of the diagonal band of Broca terminate in the bulb, where they can control excitability levels of neural elements. Bulbar interactions also occur, although they are probably not mediated by direct interbulbar connection. There is some evidence that they may influence adaptation to odors.

The main bulb of most mammals projects by way of the lateral olfactory tract to the prepyriform cortex, nucleus of the lateral olfactory tract, anterior olfactory nucleus, olfactory tubercle, anterior and posterolateral cortical amygdaloid nuclei, rostroventral end of the anterior hippocampus, and dorsomedial and lateral entorhinal area. The accessory olfactory bulb, which receives input from the vomeronasal organ, projects to the corticomedial amygdala and the bed nucleus of the stria terminalis. Of these, the projection to the amygdala is the major one.

Olfactory information probably has access to diencephalic and mesencephalic structures through several parallel pathways and thus may influence many of a wide range of behavioral activities with which these structures are involved. Through its connection with the prefrontal lobe via the dorsomedial nucleus of the thalamus, the main bulbar system has access to neocortical mechanisms. An important connection is with the preoptic–hypothalamic continuum in view of much recent work documenting the involvement of olfaction in reproductive physiology and sexual behavior.

REFERENCES

Adams, D. R., and McFarland, L. Z. Septal olfactory organ in *Peromyscus. Comp. Biochem. Physiol.*, 1971, *40A*, 971–974.

Adrian, E. D. Sensory discrimination: With some recent evidence from the olfactory organ. *Br. Med. Bull.*, 1950, *6*, 330–333.

Adrian, E. D. The action of the mammalian olfactory organ. *J. Laryngol. Otol.*, 1956, *70*, 1–14.

Adrian, E. D. Des réactions électriques du système olfactif. *Act. Neurophysiol.*, 1959, *1*, 11–18.

Alberts, J. R. Producing and interpreting olfactory deficits. *Physiol. Behav.*, 1974, *12*, 657–670.

Allen, W. F. Effect of ablating the frontal lobes, hippocampi, and occipito-parieto-temporal (excepting pyriform areas) lobes on positive and negative conditioned reflexes. *Am. J. Physiol.*, 1940, *128*, 754–771.

Allen, W. F. Distribution of cortical potentials resulting from insufflation of vapors into the nostrils and from stimulation of the olfactory bulbs and the pyriform lobe. *Am. J. Physiol.*, 1943a, *139*, 553–555.

Allen, W. F. Results of prefrontal lobectomy on acquired and acquiring correct conditioned differential responses with auditory general cutaneous and optic stimuli. *Am. J. Physiol.*, 1943b, *139*, 525–531.

Allison, A. C., and Warwick, T. R. R. Quantitative observations of the olfactory system of the rabbit. *Brain*, 1949, *72*, 186–197.

Altner, H., and Boeckh, J. Über das Reaktionsspektrum von Wasser fröschen *(Rana esculenta). Z. Vergleich. Physiol.*, 1967, *55*, 299–306.

Altner, H., and Kolnberger, I. The application of transmission electron microscopy to the study of the olfactory epithelium of vertebrates. In D. G. Moulton, A. Turk, and J. W. Johnston (eds.), *Methods in Olfactory Research*. Academic Press, New York, 1975, pp. 163–190.

Anderson, P. Inhibitory reflexes elicited from the trigeminal and olfactory nerves in rabbits. *Acta Physiol. Scand.*, 1954, *30*, 137–148.

Barber, P. C., and Field, P. M. Autoradiographic demonstration of afferent connections of the accessory olfactory bulb in the mouse. *Brain Res.*, 1975, *85*, 201–203.

Barber, P. C., and Raisman, G. An autoradiographic investigation of the projection of the vomeronasal organ to the accessory olfactory bulb in the mouse. *Brain Res.*, 1974, *81*, 21–30.

Baylin, F., and Moulton, D. G. Adaptation and cross-adaptation to odor stimulation of olfactory receptors in the tiger salamander. *Fed. Proc.*, 1975, *34*, 388 (abstr.).

Benjamin, R. M., and Jackson, J. C. Unit discharges in the mediodorsal nucleus of the squirrel monkey evoked by electrical stimulation of the olfactory bulb. *Brain Res.*, 1974, *75*, 181–191.

Bennett, M. H. The role of the anterior limb of the anterior commissure in olfaction. *Physiol. Behav.*, 1968, *3*, 507–515.

Berry, C. M., Hagamen, W. D., and Hinsey, J. C., Distribution of potentials following stimulation of the olfactory bulb in cat. *J. Neurophysiol.*, 1952, *15*, 139–148.

Blank, D. L. Mechanisms underlying the analysis of odorant quality at the level of the olfactory mucosa. II. Receptor selective sensitivity. *Ann. N.Y. Acad. Sci.*, 1974, *237*, 91–101.

Bojsen-Møller, F. Demonstration of terminals, olfactory, trigeminal and perivascular nerves in the rat nasal septum. *J. Comp. Neurol.*, 1975, *159*, 245–256.

Broadwell, R. D. Olfactory relationships of the telencephalon and diencephalon in the rabbit. I. An autoradiographic study of the efferent connections of the main and accessory olfactory bulbs. *J. Comp. Neurol.*, 1975a, *163*, 329–346.

Broadwell, R. D. Olfactory relationships of the telencephalon and diencephalon in the rabbit. II. An autoradiographic and horseradish proxidase study of the efferent connections of the anterior olfactory nucleus. *J. Comp. Neurol.*, 1975*b*, *164*, 389–410.

Brodal, A. The hippocampus and the sense of smell. *Brain*, 1947, *70*, 179–222.

Broman, J. Das Organon vomeronasale Jacobsoni: ein Wassergeruchsorgan *Anat. Hefte*, 1920, *58*, 137–192.

Broman, J. Über die Entwickelung der constanten grösseren Nasenhöhlendrüsen der Nagetiere. *Z. Anat. Entwicksl.-Gesch.*, 1921, *60*, 439–586.

Bruce, H. M. Pheromones. *Br. Med. Bull.*, 1970, *26*, 10–13.

Burghardt, G. M. Chemical perception in reptiles. In J. W. Johnston, Jr., D. G. Moulton, and A. Turk (eds.), *Communication by Chemical Signals*. Appleton-Century-Crofts, New York, 1970, pp. 241–308.

Cain, W. S. Contribution of the trigeminal nerve to perceived odor magnitude. *Ann. N.Y. Acad. Sci.*, 1974, *237*, 28–34.

Callens, M. Peripheral and central regulatory mechanisms of the excitability of the olfactory system. Thesis, Universite de Louvain, 1967, 131 pp.

Carreras, M., Mancia, D., and Mancia, M. Centrifugal control of the olfactory bulb as revealed by induced DC potential changes. *Brain Res.*, 1967, *6*, 548–560.

Costanzo, R. M., and Mozell, M. M. Electrophysiological evidence for a topographical projection of the nasal mucosa onto the olfactory bulb of the frog. *Soc. Neurosci. Abstr.*, 1974, 178.

Cowan, W. M., Raksman, G., and Powell, T. P. S. The connexions of the amygdala. *J. Neurol. Neurosurg. Psychiat.*, 1965, *28*, 137–151.

Cragg, B. G. Responses of the hippocampus to stimulation of the olfactory bulb and of various afferent nerves in mammals. *Exp. Neurol.*, 1960, *2*, 547–572.

Daval, G., and Leveteau, J. Electrophysiological studies of centrifugal and centripetal connections of the anterior olfactory nucleus. *Brain Res.*, 1974, *78*, 395–410.

DeMolina, A. F., and Ispizu, A. Neuronal activity evoked in nucleus medialis dorsalis of the thalamus after stimulation of the amygdala. *Physiol. Behav.*, 1972, *8*, 135–138.

Dennis, B. J., and Kerr, D. I. B. An evoked potential study of centripetal and centrifugal connections of the olfactory bulb. *Brain Res.*, 1968, *11*, 373–396.

Dennis, B. J., and Kerr, D. I. B. Olfactory bulb connections with basal rhinencephalon in the ferret: An evoked potential and neuroanatomical study. *J. Comp. Neurol.*, 1975, *159*, 129–148.

Devor, M., and Murphy, M. R. The effect of peripheral olfactory blockade on the social behavior of the male golden hamster. *Behav. Biol.*, 1973, *9*, 31–42.

Digiesi, V., Palchetti, R., and Tortoli, V. Influenza di odori non alimentari sull' accresciemento corporea del ratto. *Rass. Neurol. Vegetat. (Florence)*, 1963, *17*, 55–66.

Doty, R. L. Intranasal trigeminal detection of chemical vapors by humans. *Physiol. Behav.*, 1975, *14*, 855–859.

Doty, R. L. (ed.). *Mammalian Olfaction, Reproductive Processes and Behavior*. Academic Press, New York, 1976.

Doving, K. B., and Pinching, A. J. Selective degeneration of neurones in the olfactory bulb following prolonged odour exposure. *Brain Res.*, 1973, *52*, 115–129.

Duchamp, A., Revial, M. F., Holley, A., and MacLeod, P. Odor discrimination by frog olfactory receptors. *Chem. Senses Flav.*, 1974, *1*, 213–233.

Ebbesson, S. O. E., and Northcutt, R. G. Neurology of anamniotic vertebrates. In R. B. Masterton (ed.), *Evolution of the Nervous System & Behavior*. Winston, Washington, D.C., 1975.

Edwards, D. A., and Roberts, R. L. Olfactory bulb removal produces a selective deficit in behavioral regulation. *Physiol. Behav.*, 1972, *9*, 747–752.

Eichelman, B., Thoa, N. B., Bugbee, N. M., and Ng, K. Y. Brain amine and adrenal enzyme levels in aggressive bulbectomized rats. *Physiol. Behav.*, 1972, *9*, 483–485.

Estes, R. D. The role of the vomeronasal organ in mammalian reproduction. *Mammalia*, 1972, *36*, 315–341.

Ferrer, N. G. Efferent projections of the anterior olfactory nucleus. *J. Comp. Neurol.*, 1969, *137*, 309–320.

Finger, T. E. The distribution of the olfactory tracts in the bullhead catfish *(Ictalurus nebulosus)*. *J. Comp. Neurol.*, 1975, *161*, 125–142.

Freeman, W. J. Spatial divergence and temporal dispersion in primary olfactory nerve of cat. *J. Neurophysiol.*, 1972*a*, *35*, 733–744.

Freeman, W. J. Linear analysis of the dynamics of neural masses. *Ann. Rev. Biophys.* 1972*b*, *1*, 225–256 (Page 226).

Freeman, W. J. Topographic organization of primary olfactory nerve in cat and rabbit as shown by evoked potentials. *Electroencephalog. Clin. Neurophysiol.*, 1974, *36*, 33–45.

Gesteland, R. C., Lettvin, J. Y., Pitts, W. H., and Rojas, A. Odor specificities of the frog's olfactory receptors. In Y. Zotterman (ed.), *Olfaction and Taste*, Vol. I. Pergamon Press, Oxford, 1963, pp. 19–34.

Gesteland, R. C., Lettvin, J. Y., and Pitts, W. H. Chemical transmission in the nose of the frog. *J. Physiol. (London)*, 1965, *181*, 525–559.

Getchell, M. L., and Gesteland, R. C. The chemistry of olfactory reception: stimulus-specific projection from sulfhydryl reagent inhibition. *Proc. Natl. Acad. Sci. (USA)*, 1972, *69*, 1494–1498.

Getchell, T. V. Unitary responses in frog olfactory epithelium to sterically related molecules at low concentrations. *J. Gen. Physiol.*, 1974a, *64*, 241–261.

Getchell, T. V. Electrogenic sources of slow voltage transients recorded from frog olfactory epithelium. *J. Neurophysiol.*, 1974b, *37*, 1115–1130.

Getchell, T. V. Intracellular recordings from salamander olfactory epithelium. *Neurosci. Abstr.*, 1975, *1*, 2.

Getchell, T. V., and Getchell, M. L. Signal-detecting mechanisms in the olfactory epithelium: Molecular discrimination. *Ann. N.Y. Acad. Sci.*, 1974, *237*, 62–75.

Giachetti, I., and MacLeod, P. Cortical neuron responses to odours in the rat. In D. A. Denton and J. P. Coghlan (eds.), *Olfaction and Taste*, Vol. V. Academic Press, New York, 1975, pp. 303–307.

Graziadei, P. The olfactory mucosa of vertebrates. In L. M. Beidler (ed.), *Handbook of Sensory Physiology*, Vol. IV: *Olfaction*. Springer-Verlag, New York, 1971, pp. 27–58.

Hamlin, H. E. Working mechanism for the liquid and gaseous intake and output of the Jacobson's organ. *Am. J. Physiol.*, 1929, *91*, 201–205.

Heimer, L. Synaptic distribution of centripetal and centrifugal nerve fibres in the olfactory system of the rat: An experimental anatomical study. *J. Anat.*, 1968, *103*, 413–432.

Heimer, L. The olfactory connections of the diencephalon in the rat. An experimental light- and electromicroscopic study with special emphasis on the problem of terminal degeneration. *Brain Behav. Evol.*, 1972, *6*, 484–523.

Henton, W. W., Smith, J. C., and Tucker, D. Odor discrimination in pigeons following section of the olfactory nerves. *J. Comp. Physiol. Psychol.*, 1969, *69*, 317–323.

Herrick, C. J. The functions of the olfactory parts of the cerebral cortex. *Proc. Natl. Acad. Sci. (USA)*, 1933, *19*, 7–14.

Hjorth-Simonsen, A. Projection of the lateral part of the entorhinal areas to the hippocampus and fascia dentata. *J. Comp. Neurol.*, 1972, *65*, 606–711.

Hornung, D. E., Lansing, R. D., and Mozell, M. M. Distribution of butanol molecules along bullfrog olfactory mucosa. *Nature*, 1975, *254*, 617–618.

Jackson, J. C., and Benjamin, R. M. Unit discharges in the mediodorsal nucleus of the rabbit evoked by electrical stimulation of the olfactory bulb. *Brain Res.*, 1974, *75*, 193–201.

Jacobson, L. Description anatomique d'un organe observé dans les mammifères. *Ann. Mus. Hist. Nat. Paris*, 1811, *18*, 412–424.

Kauer, J. S., and Moulton, D. G. Responses of olfactory bulb neurones to odour stimulation of small nasal areas in the salamander. *J. Physiol. (London)*, 1974, *243*, 717–737.

Kerr, D. I. B., and Hagbarth, K.-E. An investigation of olfactory centrifugal system. *J. Neurophysiol.*, 1955, *18*, 362–374.

Kimble, D. P., and Zack, S. Olfactory discrimination in rats with hippocampal lesions. *Psychon. Sci.*, 1967, *8*, 211–212.

King, M. G., and Cairncross, K. D., Effects of olfactory bulb section on brain noradrenaline, corticosterone and conditioning in the rat. *Pharmacol. Biochem. Behav.*, 1974, *2*, 347–353.

Kölliker, A. Über das Jacobsonsche Organ des Menschen. Gratulationsschrift d. Med. Facultät in Würzburg, Leipzig, 1877. Cited by Mann (1961).

Kolnberger, I. Vergleichende Untersuchungen am Riechepithel, insbesondere des Jacobsonschen Organs von Amphibien, Reptilien, und Säugetieren. *Z. Zellforsch.*, 1971, *122*, 53–67.

Komisaruk, B. R., and Beyer, C. Responses of diencephalic neurons to olfactory bulb stimulation, odor and arousal. *Brain Res.*, 1972, *36*, 153–170.

Kratzing, J. E. The fine structure of the sensory epithelium of the vomeronasal organ in suckling rats. *Aust. J. Biol. Sci.*, 1971, *24*, 787–796.

Land, L. J. Localized projection of olfactory nerves to rabbit olfactory bulb. *Brain Res.*, 1973, *63*, 153–166.

Land, L. J., and Shepherd, G. M. Autoradiographic analysis of olfactory receptor projections in the rabbit. *Brain Res.*, 1974, *70*, 506–510.

Le Gros Clark, W. E. The projection of the olfactory epithelium on the olfactory bulb in the rabbit. *J. Neurol. Neurosurg. Psychiat.*, 1951, *14*, 1–10.

Le Gros Clark, W. E. Observations on the structure and organization of the olfactory receptors of the rabbit. *Yale J. Biol. Med.*, 1956, *29*, 83–95.

Le Gros Clark, W. E. Inquiries into the anatomical basis of olfactory discrimination. *Proc. Roy. Soc. London Ser. B*, 1957, *146*, 299–319.

Leonard, C. M. The connections of the dorsomedial nuclei. *Brain Behav. Evol.*, 1972, *6*, 524–541.

Leonard, C. M., and Scott, J. W. Origin and distribution of the amygdalofugal pathways in the rat: An experimental neuroanatomical study. *J. Comp. Neurol.*, 1971, *141*, 313–330.

Leveteau, J., MacLeod, P., and Daval, G. Etude électrophysiologique de la discrimination latérale en olfaction. *Physiol. Behav.*, 1969, *4*, 479–482.

Lohman, A. H. M., and Mentink, G. M. The lateral olfactory tract, the anterior commissure and the cells of the olfactory bulb. *Brain Res.*, 1969, *12*, 299–318.

Mann, G. Bulbus olfactorius accessorius in Chiroptera. *J. Comp. Neurol.*, 1961, *116*, 135–144.

Mascitti, T. A., Vaccarezza, R. R., Caruso, R. A., and Pavia, M. A. Centrifugal olfactory fibers in the cat. 1. Site of termination. An experimental study with silver impregnation methods. *Acta Physiol. Latino Am.*, 1971, *21*, 216–228.

Mathews, D. F. Response patterns of single neurones in the tortoise olfactory epithelium and bulb. *J. Gen. Physiol.*, 1972, *60*, 166–180.

Millhouse, D. E. A Golgi study of the descending medial forebrain bundle. *Brain Res.*, 1969, *15*, 341–363.

Mok, A. C. S., and Mogenson, C. J. Effects of electrical stimulation of the lateral hypothalamus, hippocampus, amygdala and olfactory bulb on unit activity of the lateral habenular nucleus in the rat. *Brain Res.*, 1974, *77*, 417–429.

Motokizawa, F. Olfactory input to the thalamus: Electrophysiological evidence. *Brain Res.*, 1974*a*, *67*, 334–337.

Motokizawa, F. Electrophysiological studies of olfactory projection to the mesencephalic reticular formation. *Exp. Neurol.*, 1974*b*, *44*, 135–144.

Moulton, D. G. Electrical activity in the olfactory system of rabbits with indwelling electrodes. In Y. Zotterman (ed.), *Olfaction and Taste*. Pergamon Press, Oxford, 1963, pp. 71–84.

Moulton, D. G. Interrelation of the chemical senses. In M. R. Kare and O. Maller (eds.), *The Chemical Senses and Nutrition.* 1967*a*, Johns Hopkins, Baltimore, pp. 19–67.

Moulton, D. G. Spatio-temporal patterning of response in the olfactory system. In T. Hayashi (ed.), *Olfaction and Taste*, Vol. II. Pergamon Press, Oxford, 1967*b*, pp. 109–116.

Moulton, D. G. In C. Pfaffmann (ed.), *Olfaction and Taste*, Vol. III. Rockefeller University Press, New York, 1969, p. 231.

Moulton, D. G. Dynamics of cell populations in the olfactory epithelium. *Ann. N.Y. Acad. Sci.*, 1974, *237*, 52–61.

Moulton, D. G. Cell renewal in the olfactory epithelium of the mouse. In D. A. Denton and J. P. Coghlan (eds.), *Olfaction and Taste*, Vol. V. Academic Press, New York, 1975, pp. 111–114.

Moulton, D. G. Spatial patterning of response in the peripheral olfactory system. *Physiol. Rev.*, 1976, *56*, 478–593.

Moulton, D. G., and Beidler, L. M. Structure and function in the peripheral olfactory system. *Physiol. Rev.*, 1967, *47*, 1–52.

Moulton, D. G., and Tucker, D. Electrophysiology of the olfactory system. *Ann. N.Y. Acad. Sci.*, 1964, *116*, 380–428.

Mozell, M. M. Olfactory discrimination: Electrophysiological spatiotemporal basis. *Science*, 1964, *143*, 1336–1337.

Mozell, M. M. The spatiotemporal analysis of odorants at the level of the olfactory receptor sheet. *J. Gen. Physiol.*, 1966, *50*, 25–41.

Mozell, M. M., and Jagodowicz, M. Chromatographic separation of odorants by the nose: Retention times measured across *in vivo* olfactory mucosa. *Science*, 1973, *181*, 1247–1249.

Mustaparta, H. Spatial distribution of receptor-responses to stimulation with different odours. *Acta Physiol. Scand.*, 1971, *82*, 154–166.

Nováková, V., and Dlouhá, H. Effect of severing the olfactory bulbs on the intake and excretion of water in the rat. *Nature*, 1960, *186*, 638–639.

O'Connell, R. J., and Mozell, M. M. Quantitative stimulation of frog olfactory receptors. *J. Neurophysiol.*, 1969, *32*, 51–63.

Okano, M., Weber, A. F., and Frommes, S. P. Electron microscopic studies of the distal border of the canine olfactory epithelium. *J. Ultrastruct. Res.*, 1967, *17*, 487–502.

Ottoson, D. Analysis of the electrical activity of the olfactory epithelium. *Acta Physiol. Scand.,* 1956, *35*, Suppl. 122, 1–83.

Pager, J. A selective modulation of the olfactory bulb electrical activity in relation to the learning of palatability in hungry and satiated rats. *Physiol. Behav.,* 1974, *12*, 189–195.

Parkes, and Bruce, 1961, Olfactory stimuli in mammalian reproduction. *Science, 134,* 1049–1054.

Pfaff, D. W., and Gregory, E. Olfactory coding in olfactory bulb and medial forebrain bundle of normal and castrated male rats. *J. Neurophysiol.,* 1971, *34*, 208–216.

Pfaff, D. W., and Pfaffmann, C. Behavioral and electrophysiological responses of male rats to female rat urine odors. In C. Pfaffmann (ed.), *Olfaction and Taste,* Vol. III. Rockefeller University Press, New York, 1969, pp. 258–267.

Pinching, A. J., and Døving, K. B. Selective degeneration in the rat olfactory bulb following exposure to different odours. *Brain Res.,* 1974, *82*, 195–204.

Pinching, A. J., and Powell, T. P. S. The termination of centrifugal fibres in the glomerular layer of the olfactory bulb. *J. Cell Sci.,* 1972, *10*, 621–635.

Pohorecky, L. A., Zigmond, M. J., Heimer, L., and Wurtman, R. J. Olfactory bulb removal: Effects on brain norepinephrine. *Proc. Natl. Acad. Sci. (USA),* 1969, *62*, 1052–1055.

Powell, T. P. S., and Cowan, W. M. Centrifugal fibres in the lateral olfactory tract. *Nature,* 1963, *199*, 1296–1297.

Powell, T. P. S., Cowan, W. M., and Raisman, G. The central olfactory connections. *J. Anat.,* 1965, *99*, 791–813.

Powers, J. B., and Winans, S. S. Vomeronasal organ: Critical role in mediating sexual behavior of the male hamster. *Science,* 1975, *187*, 961–963.

Pribram, K. H., and Kruger, L. Functions of the "olfactory brain." *Ann. N.Y. Acad. Sci.,* 1954, *58*, 109–138.

Price, J. L. The termination of centrifugal fibers to the olfactory bulb. *Brain Res.,* 1968, *14*, 542–545.

Price, J. L. The structure and connexions of the granule cells of the olfactory bulb: An electronmicroscopic study. *J. Physiol. (London),* 1969a, *204*, 77–78.

Price, J. L. The origin of the centrifugal fibers to the olfactory bulbs. *Brain Res.,* 1969b, *14*, 542–545.

Price, J. L. An autoradiographic study of the complementary laminar patterns of termination of afferent fibers to the olfactory cortex. *J. Comp. Neurol.,* 1973, *150*, 87–108.

Price, J. L., and Powell, T. P. S. An electronmicroscopic study of the termination of the afferent fibers to the olfactory bulb from the cerebral hemisphere. *J. Cell Sci.,* 1970a, *7*, 157–187.

Price, J. L., and Powell, T. P. S. An experimental study of the site of origin and the course of the centrifugal fibers to the olfactory bulbs in the rat. *J. Anat.,* 1970b, *107*, 215–237.

Price, J. L., and Powell, T. P. S. The afferent connections of the nucleus of the horizontal limb of the diagonal band. *J. Anat.,* 1970c, *107*, 239–256.

Price, J. L., and Powell, T. P. S. Certain observations on the olfactory pathway. *J. Anat.,* 1971, *110*, 105–126.

Price, J. L., and Sprich, W. W. Observations on the lateral olfactory tract of the rat. *J. Comp. Neurol.,* 1975, *162*, 321–336.

Raisman, G. An experimental study of the projection of the amygdala to the accessory olfactory bulb and its relationship to the concept of a dual olfactory system. *Exp. Brain. Res.,* 1972, *14*, 395–408.

Raisman, G., and Field, P. M. Sexual dimorphism in the preoptic area of the rat. *Science,* 1971, *173*, 731–733.

Ramon y Cajal, S. R. Y. *Histologie du Système Nerveux de l'Homme et des Vertébres,* Tome 11. A. Maloire, Paris, 1911.

Rausch, L. J., and Long, C. J. Habenular-nuclei: A crucial link between the olfactory and motor systems. *Brain Res.,* 1971, *29*, 146–150.

Rausch, L. J., and Long, C. J. Habenular lesions and discrimination responding to olfactory and visual stimuli. *Physiol. Behav.,* 1974, *13*, 357–364.

Rausch, R., and Serafetinides, E. A. Specific alterations of olfactory function in humans with temporal lobe lesions. *Nature,* 1975, *255*, 557–558.

Rodolfo-Masera, T. Su l'esistenza di un particolare organo olfattivo nel setto nasale della cavia e di altri rodentori. *Arch. Ital. Anat. Embriol.,* 1943, *48*, 157–212.

Scalia, F., and Winans, S. S. The differential projections of the olfactory bulb and accessory olfactory bulb in mammals. *J. Comp. Neurol.,* 1975, *161*, 31–56.

Schneider, R. A., and Schmidt, C. E. Dependency of olfactory localization on non-olfactory cues. *Physiol. Behav.,* 1967, *2*, 305–309.

Scott, J. W., and Chafin, B. R. Origin of olfactory projection to lateral hypothalamus and nuclei gemini of the rat. *Brain Res.,* 1975, *88*, 64–68.

Scott, J. W., and Leonard, C. M. The olfactory connections of the lateral hypothalamus in the rat mouse and hamster. *J. Comp. Neurol.*, 1971, *141*, 331–344.

Scott, J. W., and Pfaffmann, C. Olfactory input to the hypothalamus: Electrophysiological evidence. *Science*, 1967, *158*, 1592–1594.

Scott, J. W., and Pfaffmann, C. Characteristics of responses of lateral hypothalamic neurons to olfactory stimulation in the rat. *Brain Res.*, 1972, *48*, 251–264.

Sharp, F. R., Kauer, J. S., and Shepherd, G. M. Local sites of activity-related glucose metabolism in the rat olfactory bulb during olfactory stimulation. *Brain Res.*, 1975, *98*, 596–600.

Shepherd, G. M. Synaptic organization of the mammalian olfactory bulb. *Physiol. Rev.*, 1972, *52*, 864–917.

Shibuya, T., and Shibuya, S. Olfactory epithelium: Unitary responses in the tortoise. *Science*, 1963, *140*, 495–496.

Sieck, M. H., and Daumbach, H. D. Differential effects of peripheral and central anosmia producing techniques on spontaneous behavior patterns. *Physiol. Behav.*, 1974, *13*, 407–425.

Takagi, S. F. Degeneration and regeneration of the olfactory epithelium. In L. M. Beidler (ed.), *Olfaction: Handbook of Sensory Physiology*. Springer-Verlag, New York, 1971, pp. 75–94.

Takagi, S. F., and Omura, K. Responses of the olfactory receptor cells to odours. *Proc. Japan Acad.*, 1963, *36*, 253–255.

Tanabe, T., Yarita, H., Iino, Y., Ooshima, Y., and Takagi, S. F. An olfactory projection area in orbitofrontal cortex of the monkey. *J. Neurophysiol.*, 1975a, *38*, 1269–1283.

Tanabe, T., Iino, M., and Takagi, S. F. Discrimination of odors in olfactory bulb, pyriform-amygdaloid areas and orbitofrontal cortex of the monkey. *J. Neurophysiol.*, 1975b, *38*, 1284–1296.

Tucker, D. Physical variables in the olfactory stimulation process. *J. Gen. Physiol.*, 1963a, *46*, 453–489.

Tucker, D. Olfactory, vomeronasal and trigeminal receptor responses to odorants. In Y. Zotterman (ed.), *Olfaction and Taste*, Vol. I. New York, Pergamon Press, 1963b, pp. 45–69.

Tucker, D. Nonolfactory responses from the nasal cavity: Jacobson's organ and the trigeminal system. In L. M. Beidler (ed.), *Handbook of Sensory Physiology*, Vol. IV. Springer-Verlag, New York, 1971, pp. 151–177.

Tucker, D., and Beidler, L. M. Efferent impulses to the nasal area. *Fed. Proc.*, 1956, *15*, 613.

Tucker, D., Graziadei, P. P. C., and Smith, J. C. Recovery of olfactory function in pigeons after bilateral transection of the olfactory nerves. In D. A. Denton and J. P. Coghlan (eds.), *Olfaction and Taste*, Vol. V. Academic Press, New York, 1975, pp. 369–373.

von Békésy, G. Olfactory analogue to directional hearing. *J. Appl. Physiol.*, 1964, *19*, 369–373.

von Brunn, A. Beiträge zur mikroskopischen Anatomie der menschlichen Nasenhöhle. *Arch. Mikrosk. Anat.*, 1892, *39*, 632–651.

von Skramlik, E. Über die Lokalisation der Empfindungen bei den niederen Sinnen. *Z. Sinnesphysiol.*, 1925, *56*, 69–100.

Way, J. S. An oscillographic study of afferent connections to the hippocampus in the cat *(Felis domesticus)*. *Electroencephalog. Clin. Neurophysiol.*, 1962, *14*, 78–89.

Wedgwood, M. Connexions between the olfactory bulb and the habenula and dorsomedial thalamic nuclei. *J. Physiol. (London)*, 1974, *239*, 88–89.

Wenzel, B. M. The olfactory system and behavior. In L. V. DiCara (ed.), *Limbic and Autonomic Nervous Systems Research*. Plenum, New York, 1974, pp. 1–40.

Whitten, W. K. Occurrence of anoestrous in mice caged in groups. *J. Endocrinol.*, 1959, *18*, 102–107.

Willey, J. Ultrastructure of the cat olfactory bulb. *J. Comp. Neurol.*, 1973, *152*, 211–232.

Winans, S., and Scalia, F. Amygdaloid nucleus: New afferent input from the vomeronasal organ. *Science*, 1970, *170*, 330–332.

Woods, W. H., Holland, R. C., and Powell, E. W. Connections of cerebral structures functioning in neurohypophysial hormone release. *Brain Res.*, 1969, *12*, 26–46.

5

Visual System: Superior Colliculus

MICHAEL E. GOLDBERG AND DAVID LEE ROBINSON

INTRODUCTION

The primary visual brain of lower vertebrates is the optic lobe or optic tectum, an organ which receives visual input and helps generate visually guided behavior. The evolution of the cerebral cortex did not result in the elimination of the tectum, but instead, as the superior colliculus, the visual organ in the midbrain continues to play some function in the organization of visually motivated behavior (Sprague *et al.*, 1972; Ingle, 1973). This chapter will discuss the anatomy and physiology of the mammalian superior colliculus, the effects of collicular lesions on behavior, and the various current hypotheses of the role of the superior colliculus in visually motivated behavior.

ANATOMY

The mammalian superior colliculus is a laminar structure in the midbrain bordered rostrally by the pretectum, caudally by the inferior colliculus, ventrally by the mesencephalic central gray and reticular formation, and dorsally by the ambient cistern. The brachium of the superior colliculus forms the dorsolateral border.

MICHAEL E. GOLDBERG AND DAVID LEE ROBINSON   Neurobiology Department, Armed Forces Radiobiology Research Institute, Bethesda, Maryland 20014.

MICHAEL E.
GOLDBERG AND
DAVID LEE ROBINSON

The superior colliculus contains three general subdivisions, the superficial, intermediate, and deep layers. These layers in turn have further subdivisions. Kanaseki and Sprague (1974) adopted a numbering system based on studies of the cat superior colliculus (Fig. 1), but similar subdivisions are found in all mammals studied (Ramon y Cajal, 1911; Olszewski and Baxter, 1954; Viktorov, 1966; Lund, 1972).

The superficial layers contain the stratum zonale (lamina I of Kanaseki and Sprague), the stratum griseum superficiale (superficial gray, stratum cincerium, or lamina II), and stratum opticum (optic layer or lamina III). The intermediate layers consist of the stratum griseum intermediale (intermediate gray or lamina IV) and stratum album intermediale (intermediate white, stratum lemnisci, or

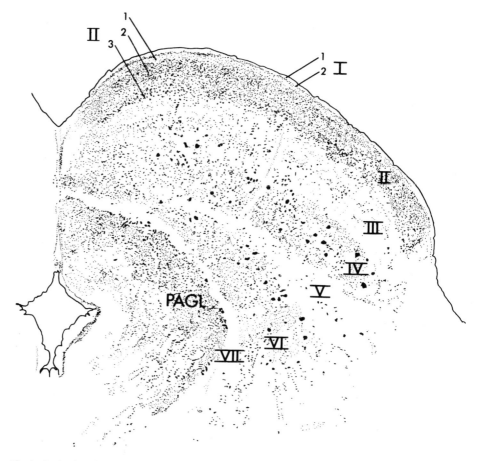

Fig. 1. Projection drawing of Nissl-stained section of cat superior colliculus illustrating laminar organization. Dots correspond to collicular neurons and approximate size. I is stratum zonale with sublaminae 1 and 2; II is stratum griseum superficiale with sublaminae 1, 2 , and 3; III, stratum opticum; IV, stratum griseum intermediale; V, stratum lemnisci; VI, stratum griseum profundum; VII, stratum album profundum; PAGL, periaqueductal gray, pars lateralis. Reproduced with permission from Kanaseki and Sprague (1974).

lamina V). The deep layers are made of the stratum griseum profundum (deep gray or lamina VI) and the stratum album profundum (deep white or lamina VII).

The stratum zonale contains a limited number of medium- and small-sized neurons (Ramon y Cajal, 1911; Olszewski and Baxter, 1954; Viktorov, 1966, 1968; Sterling, 1971; Kanaseki and Sprague, 1974). The medium-sized cells have sparsely ramified dendrites which are horizontally oriented and remain within the layer. The small cells have dendrites which dip into the subjacent laminae (Sterling, 1971). Neurons are generally found more regularly in the lower border of zonale, although some are present scattered among the glial cells and fine myelinated axons of the most dorsal area.

Between laminae I and II there is a clear area with relatively few neurons. Ventral to this gap there is a dense packing of medium-sized cells (Sterling, 1971; Kanaseki and Sprague, 1974). These neurons are very diverse in size and shape; their dendrites ramify throughout the layer but do not leave it. Near the ventral border these medium-sized cells become somewhat more loosely packed. Axons of cells in these parts of the superficial gray layer descend to deeper layers of the colliculus and also provide ascending thalamic afferents (Harting *et al.,* 1973; Sprague, 1975).

The stratum opticum contains predominantly afferent and efferent fibers, and in fact blends into the brachium of the superior colliculus, the great bundle of afferent and efferent tracts of the colliculus. The optic layer does contain a few small- and medium-sized neurons with dendrites restricted to this layer and axons projecting to deeper layers (Viktorov, 1968; Sterling, 1971).

The stratum griseum intermediale is a thick, clearly defined cellular layer composed of some neurons similar to those in the dorsal layers and some large multipolar neurons (Kanaseki and Sprague, 1974). The large cells here and in deeper layers project to the brain stem (Sprague *et al.,* 1963). The intermediate white layer is formed by a collection of fibers ascending to the colliculus from spinal and brain stem centers as well as fibers that pass through the colliculus on their way to the pretectum and thalamus. This lamina also contains many small-sized cells and a few medium-sized cells.

SYNAPTIC ORGANIZATION

Sterling (1971) and Lund (1972) have studied the synaptic organization of the superficial layers of the cat and monkey superior colliculus. Although the cat and monkey superficial layers differ strikingly in their physiology, the anatomy as studied in the electron microscope is quite similar in the two species.

In the cat there are two types of terminals (Sterling, 1971). The first is large and filled with vesicles and pale mitochondria. A single one of these terminals will frequently make several synaptic contacts onto postsynaptic elements, so that although this form accounts for only one-fourth of the terminals in the superficial layers, it supplies about half of the synapses. The remaining terminals are densely filled with synaptic vesicles and contain dark mitochondria. These terminals have no other consistently demonstrated morphological features.

Within the strata zonale and griseum superficiale of both cat and monkey the vast majority of the synapses are axodendritic, onto both spines and trunks, and only very few are axosomatic. Although many of the presynaptic elements in the colliculus arise from axons, there are a significant but undetermined proportion of dendrodendritic connections (Sterling, 1971; Lund, 1972).

AFFERENTS

There is a general organization of the projections to the colliculus. The more dorsal (superficial) layers receive their densest projections from primary visual structures in a laminar and retinotopic pattern. Afferents to more ventral (deeper) layers come from cortical areas which are progressively less important to the visual system, and these projections are less strictly laminated and their topography is less clear (Fig. 2). (The following data on retinal and cortical afferents, except where noted otherwise, come from reports by Altman, 1962; Sprague, 1963; Myers, 1963b; Kuypers, 1962; Kuypers and Lawrence, 1967; Garey et al., 1968; Spatz et al., 1970; Wilson and Toyne, 1970; Astruc, 1971; Sterling, 1971; Paula-Barbosa and Sousa-Pinta, 1973; Kawamura et al., 1974b).

Retinal afferents end most superficially, followed by fibers from occipital cortex which end in the superficial gray layer. Temporal cortex projects primarily to the subjacent optic layer. Parietal cortex projects to the intermediate white layer. Frontal cortex projects predominantly to the deep and intermediate layers. This scheme outlines the major collicular projections from these areas. However, various afferents overlap, and it is useful to examine the inputs to individual layers.

Although both retina and striate cortex project to the superior colliculus, foveal fibers come predominantly from the foveal cortical areas rather than directly from the retinal fovea. Since the foveal representation is the most rostral portion of the superior colliculus, there is a definite asymmetry between the cortical and retinal projections. Following enucleation of an eye, the only significant terminal degeneration found in the stratum zonale is in the caudal regions. This is dramatic in the monkey and less apparent in the cat. Several investigators (Wilson and Toyne, 1970; Lund, 1972) have observed a sparse terminal degeneration in rostral colliculus following enucleation; however, autoradiographic (Hubel et al., 1975) and physiological experiments (Schiller et al., 1974) provide support for some input from the fovea to the superior colliculus. Ablation of striate or prestriate cortex results in degeneration throughout the stratum zonale. A limited amount of degeneration in ipsilateral or contralateral stratum zonale is seen after damage to the temporal lobe. Frontal and parietal lobe have little or no afferent input to the stratum zonale. Graybiel (1975) and Hubel et al. (1975) used intraocular injection of radioactively labeled amino acids to study the retinotectal projections. In both cat (Graybiel, 1975) and monkey (Hubel et al., 1975) the contralateral and ipsilateral projections were found to be anatomically separate. The contralateral projection is more dense, forming a "sheet" of terminals in the superficial gray layer. The sheet is interrupted by 200-μm "holes." Input from the ipsilateral eye is distributed in discrete "puffs" in the superficial gray. It is likely that the ipsilateral puffs correspond to the contralateral holes.

The stratum griseum superficiale receives a pattern of afferent input similar to that of the stratum zonale: striate cortical input predominating rostrally, retinal and visual cortical input predominating caudally, sparse temporal input, very limited frontal projections, and no parietal projections.

The stratum opticum has sparser input from retina and occipital cortex than have the more superficial areas. It has a strong bilateral temporal projection and a limited frontal projection. The intermediate layers have no primary visual input, from either occipital cortex or retina, and the predominant cortical input comes from temporal, frontal, and parietal lobes. In particular, a powerful input to the stratum griseum intermediale of the monkey comes from area 8, the frontal eye

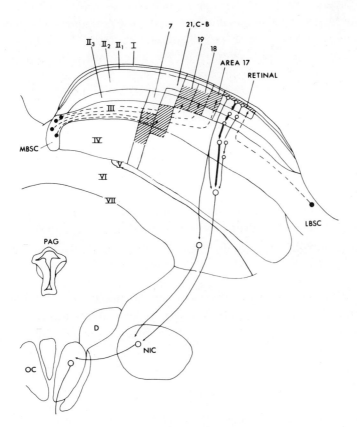

Fig. 2. Laminar organization and afferent inputs to cat superior colliculus. Laminar segregation and Roman numerals indicating such are taken from normal histological material such as in Fig. 1. Laminar terminations of collicular afferents are based on orthograde degeneration studies. Boxes are included for clarity to illustrate representative slices through layers and show terminal fields for afferents from retina and various cortical fields (areas 17, 18, 19, 21, C-B, and 7). Diagonal stripes indicate major concentrations of degeneration. MBSC, Medial brachium of superior colliculus; LBSC, lateral brachium of superior colliculus; NIC, interstitial nucleus of Cajal; C-B, Clare-Bishop cortical area; D, nucleus of Darkshevitsch; OC, oculomotor nuclei; PAG, periaqueductal gray matter. Reproduced with permission from Sprague (1975).

MICHAEL E.
GOLDBERG AND
DAVID LEE ROBINSON

fields. The stratum profundum receives significantly less cortical input than the more superficial colliculus and those afferents which do project from cortex arise from the frontal and parietal lobes.

Although subcortical afferents to the colliculus have not been studied as thoroughly as those from cortex and retina, they fit into the same scheme: more visual structures project to superficial colliculus than do structures related to other modalities. The superficial layers receive a dense projection from the pulvinar (Altman, 1962) and a light input from the ventral lateral geniculate nucleus (Graybiel, 1974; Edwards *et al.*, 1974). Subcortical afferents to the intermediate layers arise from the ventral lateral geniculate nucleus (Graybiel, 1974; Edwards *et al.*, 1974), inferior colliculus (Moore and Goldberg, 1963, 1966; Powell and Hatton, 1969; Mehler, 1969), and medullary and pontine reticular formations (Nauta and Kuypers, 1958). These reticular regions also project to the deep collicular layers (Nauta and Kuypers, 1958) as does the fastigial nucleus of the cerebellum (Angaut, 1969). Finally, axons from the periaqueductal gray project to an as yet unspecified region of the colliculus (Hamilton, 1973). There are conflicting data concerning a projection from the pretectum to the superior colliculus (Kuhlenbeck and Miller, 1942; Casagrande *et al.*, 1972; Carpenter and Pierson, 1973). This controversy arises because pretectal lesions could damage other afferents to the superior colliculus, and degeneration in the colliculus from pretectal lesions need not arise from damage to cell bodies lying in the pretectum.

Efferents

Altman and Carpenter (1961) suggested that the efferents of the superior colliculus in the cat separate on the basis of their laminar origin. They stated that descending efferents arise primarily from the deeper layers and that these projections could be separated into three groups: tectopontine, tectoreticular, and predorsal bundle. The tectopontine pathway constitutes the largest descending branch, and in contrast to other descending pathways receives a small part of its fibers from the superficial layers (Kawamura and Brodal, 1973). During its travel to the contralateral pons, this bundle sends efferents to the mesencephalic reticular formation and magnocellular part of the medial geniculate nucleus. The bulk of the tectopontine projection, however, ends in the dorsolateral and lateral pontine nuclei. The tectoreticular fibers end primarily in the ipsilateral dosolateral mesencephalic reticular formation. No terminal degeneration has been found in the extraocular muscle motor nuclei (Altman and Carpenter, 1961; Sprague *et al.*, 1963; Kawamura and Brodal, 1973; Kawamura *et al.*, 1974*a*).

The predorsal bundle sends terminations bilaterally to the interstitial nucleus of Cajal, the nucleus of Darkschewitsch, and the superior central nucleus of the mesencephalon. More caudally there is a suggestion of degeneration in the paramedian pontine reticular formation (Kawamura *et al.*, 1974*a*), a reticular group implicated in the control of eye movements (Cohen and Henn, 1972; Cohen and Komatsuzaki, 1972; Luschei and Fuchs, 1972; Keller, 1974). The predorsal bundle also projects to the inferior olive (Escobar and de Cárdenas, 1968) and sends a diffuse projection into the spinal cord which is found predominantly in the contralateral upper cervical segments (Nyberg-Hansen, 1964).

Descending efferents of the monkey superior colliculus are generally similar to those described in the cat (Myers, 1963*a*). All of the connections demonstrated in the cat and monkey have been found in the tree shrew (Harting *et al.*, 1973). In addition, this species has projections from the deep collicular layers to the parabigeminal nucleus and the motor facial nucleus.

Although the bulk of the descending collicular efferents arise from the deep collicular layers, ascending projections originate from both the superficial and deep layers. As a result, several experiments have attempted to segregate ascending collicular targets on the basis of differential projections of the superficial and deep layers (Graybiel, 1972*a,b*; Harting *et al.*, 1973; Benevento and Fallon, 1975). Interpretation of such experiments is difficult since lesions of the superficial layers may damage efferents of the deep layers, and electrode tracks into the deep layers could damage superficial elements. However, this approach has been applied to the monkey, cat, and tree shrew, and the results have suggested that the different layers of the colliculus have different targets.

Degeneration studies based on removing the entire superior colliculus of the cat (Altman and Carpenter, 1961; Niimi *et al.*, 1970; Graybiel, 1972*a,b*) have shown connections to the pretectum and several thalamic nuclei including the pulvinar, the lateral posterior nucleus, the posterior group of Rose and Woolsey (1958)—which includes the suprageniculate and magnocellular division of the medial geniculate—and the posterior group of Rioch (1929)—which includes the intralaminar nuclear group, and the dorsal and ventral lateral geniculate nuclei.

In the tree shrew (Harting *et al.*, 1973) the superficial layers project to those of the above regions that are more classically visual: the dorsal and ventral lateral geniculate nuclei, the pretectum, and the pulvinar. The deep layers project to the posterior group of Rose and Woolsey, the intralaminar group, and the subthalamic region. In the rhesus monkey (Benevento and Fallon, 1975) the superficial layer projections are similar to those of the tree shrew but also include the intralaminar nuclei. Efferents of the deep layers in the rhesus monkey include the medial and oral pulvinar, the medial part of the lateral posterior nucleus, and the intralaminar nucleus. Strangely, the total squirrel monkey colliculus projects only to the inferior pulvinar and the suprageniculate nucleus (Mathers, 1971). It is interesting to note that there is no evidence from any species showing that the superior colliculus projects to the cerebral cortex.

Although comparably detailed experiments have not been conducted in the cat, Graybiel (1972*a,b*) has suggested a segregation of efferents since the superficial layers of the cat project to the medial lateral posterior nucleus, and the deep layers project to the ventral lateral posterior nucleus. In addition to efferents similar to those discussed above, the cat superior colliculus sends ascending efferents into the optic tract. The termination of these fibers is as yet unknown (Altman and Carpenter, 1961).

MICHAEL E.
GOLDBERG AND
DAVID LEE ROBINSON

The mammalian superior colliculus has been shown to have both sensory- and motor-related properties. The superficial layers have predominantly visual responses. The intermediate and deeper layers have visual responses, but they also have properties related to other sensory modalities, and, more importantly, properties related to movement. In this section we discuss first the visual, then the other sensory, and finally the motor aspects of the physiology of the mammalian superior colliculus.

VISUAL PHYSIOLOGY

Apter demonstrated in 1945 that the cat superior colliculus has an evoked response to stimulation of the contralateral visual field, and that this response has a retinotopic map. This work has been amplified and extended by workers who have demonstrated visual receptive fields in single neurons in the superior colliculus of many species, including mouse (Dräger and Hubel, 1975), rat (Humphrey, 1968), gray squirrel (Lane *et al.*, 1971), tree shrew (Lane *et al.*, 1971), ground squirrel (Michael, 1972*a*), rabbit (Schaeffer, 1966; Masland *et al.*, 1971), cat (Marchifava and Pepeu, 1966; Straschill and Taghavy, 1967; McIlwain and Buser, 1968; Sprague *et al.*, 1968; Sterling and Wickelgren, 1969; Straschill and Hoffmann, 1969; Feldon *et al.*, 1970; Berman and Cynader, 1972; Dreher and Hoffmann, 1973; Hoffmann and Dreher, 1973), and several different species of primates including galago (Lane *et al.*, 1973), owl monkey (Lane *et al.*, 1973), cebus monkey (Updyke, 1974), rhesus monkey (Humphrey, 1968; Schiller and Koerner, 1971; Cynader and Berman, 1972; Goldberg and Wurtz, 1972*a*), and squirrel monkey (Kadoya *et al.*, 1971*a*). From this great amount of data several clear patterns emerge concerning the topology of the representation of the visual field on the superior colliculus and the nature of the visual responses of single neurons in the superior colliculus.

VISUAL MAP. There are two different patterns of topological map of the visual field onto the superior colliculus. In the primate the map is clearly one of the contralateral hemifield onto the ipsilateral colliculus, and although individual cells show some overlap of the vertical meridian, cells which are occupied exclusively with ipsilateral stimuli have not been described (Lane *et al.*, 1973) (Fig. 3). In nonprimate animals, such as carnivore, rodent, and marsupial, the superior colliculus does have a representation of at least part of the ipsilateral field (Feldon *et al.*, 1970; Lane *et al.*, 1973). The ipsilateral field may be as large as the nasal field of the contralateral retina (Fig. 4) (Lane *et al.*, 1974). This representation is located in the rostral portion of the superior colliculus, a technically difficult area to study, and this may explain why earlier studies (e.g., Apter, 1945) did not describe the large ipsilateral representation.

RECEPTIVE FIELDS: SPECIES DIFFERENCES. The responses of single neurons to visual stimuli also show a large interspecies variability, but there are several trends that obtain for all species: (1) where such comparisons have been made, cells in the superior colliculus have much larger visual receptive fields than cells in striate cortex with visual receptive fields in the same area of the retina; (2) although most cells have some degree of center-surround organization, neurons in the superior colliculus do not have the fastidious requirements for stimulus trigger features that are the most characteristic feature of visual cortical neurons (Hubel and Wiesel, 1965, 1968); (3) neurons in the superior colliculus generally give transient rather than sustained responses. Changing stimuli—either moving stimuli or the onset or disappearance of stationary stimuli—are better than sustained static stimuli.

The interspecies differences in receptive field properties are significant enough that extrapolating data from one species to another is difficult. Although the purpose of this chapter is not to catalogue the properties of visually responsive neurons in the superior colliculus of every species in which they have been studied, it is useful to examine the sorts of receptive field properties of several different species in some detail.

Ground Squirrel. In a survey of over a thousand neurons in the superior colliculus of the ground squirrel, Michael (1972*a*) found two different classes of cells which he labeled "directionally selective" and "hypercomplex." Directionally selective cells have an excitatory center and an inhibitory surround. They give on- and off-responses to lights flashed in their center, but give the most sustained responses to similar stimuli traveling through the receptive field in a preferred direction. Hypercomplex cells do not respond to the onset of any stationary stimulus, and respond best to the movement of a specifically oriented edge, light bar, or dark bar which must be limited in its length at both ends. Michael found that the directionally selective cells are located predominantly in the superficial layers, and the hypercomplex cells are located in the deep layers.

Cat. Several investigators have examined the properties of neurons in the superficial layers of the cat superior colliculus. Most cells respond better to moving stimuli than to the onset of stationary stimuli, and most cells exhibit a broadly

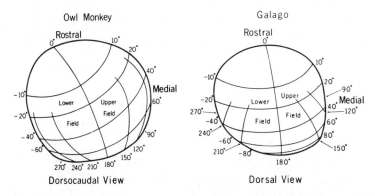

Fig. 3. Projection of visual field onto primate superior colliculus. Surface of superior colliculus of owl monkey (left) and galago (right) with polar coordinates superimposed. The horizontal meridian lies on the anterior border. From −90° to +90° of elevation, from 90° to 270° of azimuth. Reproduced with permission from Lane *et al.* (1973).

tuned preference for stimulus direction (Sterling and Wickelgren, 1969) (Fig. 5). The population of cells as a whole shows a preference for stimuli moving centrifugally with respect to the fovea, and the most favored direction is horizontal-temporal.

Most cells have excitatory regions with inhibitory surrounds. Within the excitatory regions the cells are not fastidious about the shape or orientation of the leading edge of the stimulus, although some workers have found a smaller population of orientation-specific cells (Sterling and Wickelgren, 1969). The area of the excitatory receptive field is approximately 3 times the area of receptive fields of cortical cells subtending the same area of the visual field. Ninety-seven percent of the cells receive binocular input, although the ocular dominance population is skewed slightly toward the contralateral eye.

Hayaishi *et al.* (1973) examined the binocular interaction in the cat's superior colliculus and found that although almost all cells could be well driven with either

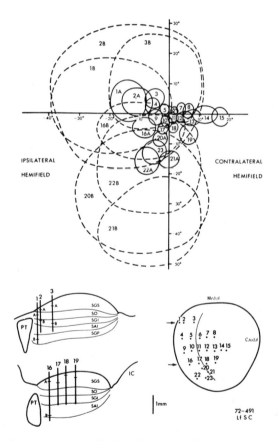

Fig. 4. Visual map in the cat superior colliculus. Note the significant ipsilateral representation. Each receptive field in the upper figure corresponds to a location in the superior colliculus outlined in the two lower figures. The arrows in the lower right mark the positions of the parasagittal sections shown in the lower left. SGS, stratum griseum superficiale; SO, stratum opticum; SGI, stratum griseum intermediale; SAI, stratum album intermediale; PT, pretectum; IC, inferior colliculus. Reproduced by permission from Lane *et al.* (1974).

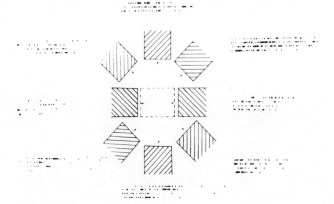

Fig. 5. Directional selectivity of cat superior colliculus neuron. The response of a single neuron is shown as a dark tongue entering its receptive field from different directions. Note there is a definite maximum and a definite minimum response. The cell does respond slightly to the stimulus traveling in even the least effective direction. Reproduced with permission from Sterling and Wickelgren (1969).

eye, most cells had some binocular interaction. This interaction had several different forms: facilitation, where the binocular response exceeded the sum of the two monocular responses; summation and occlusion, where the binocular response was greater than the monocular response but did not exceed the sum of the monocular responses; inhibition, where the binocular response was less than the maximal monocular response; and disinhibition, where an inhibitory monocular effect was weakened by binocular stimulation. In general, binocular interaction was stronger in directionally selective cells with some ocular dominance. Berman *et al.* (1975) investigated the effect of retinal disparity on the binocular interaction in cat superior colliculus. They found that some cells responded better when there was a small degree of disparity between the locations of the stimuli on the retinas. The range of disparity was 5° horizontally, 2.7° vertically, and did not tend to increase with increasing retinal eccentricity.

Monkey. The receptive fields of cells in the rhesus monkey superior colliculus differ in several significant ways from those in cat and ground squirrel. Cynader and Berman (1972) using a barbiturate-anesthetized rhesus monkey, Schiller and Koerner (1971) and Schiller and Stryker (1972) using an awake monkey with a paralyzed eye, and Goldberg and Wurtz (1972a) using an awake, behaving monkey, all noted that the majority of cells in the superficial layers of the superior colliculus did not show a directional preference for moving stimuli (Fig. 6). In fact, most cells could easily be driven by the onset of a stationary stimulus and gave an equally brisk off-response. Stimuli small relative to the total excitatory receptive field were generally most effective. Many cells have an inhibitory surround (Fig. 7) but some cells clearly do not. Cells without an inhibitory region respond very well to changes in diffuse illumination. As in the cat, rhesus monkey superior collicular neurons have receptive fields that are larger than comparable cortical receptive fields. The collicular neurons in the monkey are also far less fastidious about trigger features again than are cortical neurons (Hubel and Wiesel, 1968).

MICHAEL E.
GOLDBERG AND
DAVID LEE ROBINSON

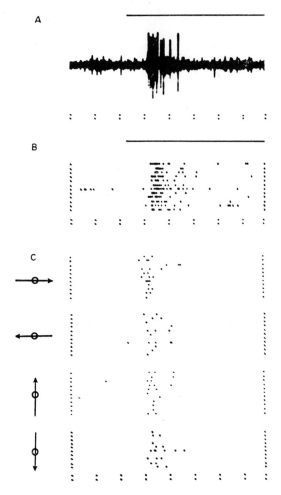

Fig. 6. Response of cell in superficial layer of monkey superior colliculus. The cell responds well to the onset of a stationary spot (A and B) but less well to the same spot moving through its field. It does not show a significant directional preference (C). The time dots are 50 msec apart. Reproduced by permission from Goldberg and Wurtz (1972a).

RECEPTIVE FIELDS: OTHER ASPECTS

Directional Selectivity. Both squirrel monkey (Kadoya *et al.*, 1971a) and cebus monkey (Updyke, 1974) have a higher number of cells with directional selectivity than does the rhesus monkey. In the squirrel monkey the directionally selective cells are clustered in the lower portion of the stratum opticum.

The scatter of directionally selective cells among species must lead to the conclusion that directional selectivity is probably not a very important clue to the general understanding of collicular function. There is not only a wide variability of the presence or absence of directional selectivity but also a species-to-species difference in the nature of the preferred directions. The ground squirrel seems to have no preferred direction for its high number of directional cells (Michael, 1972a). The cat seems to prefer the horizontal-temporal direction (Sterling and Wickelgren, 1969) and the mouse, curiously, the upward and nasal direction (Dräger and Hubel, 1975).

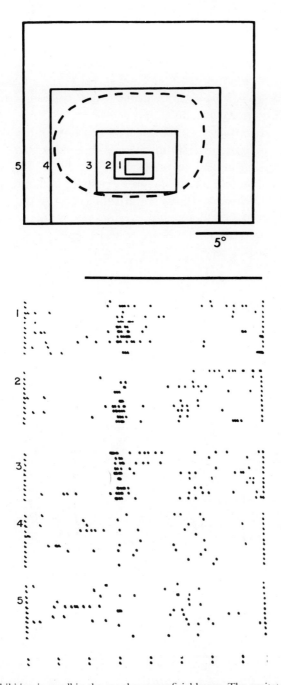

Fig. 7. Surround inhibition in a cell in the monkey superficial layers. The excitatory receptive field as determined by a response to small spots is outlined by the dashed line. The solid lines show the stimuli corresponding to responses 1–5. Note that the cell responds roughly equally to stimuli of different sizes that remain within the excitatory field (1,2,3) but does not respond to stimuli that overlap the inhibitory surround (4,5). The stimuli are flashed on for the time shown by the black stimulus indicator. The time dots are 50 msec apart. Reproduced by permission from Goldberg and Wurtz (1972a).

Color. Most investigators have been satisfied with white light as a visual stimulus adequate to drive all cells. Michael (1972*a*) looked for color responses in the ground squirrel because he was interested in defining differences between the geniculocortical and retinocollicular systems. He was unable to show any color-sensitive neurons in the superior colliculus as opposed to the lateral geniculate in an animal with an all cone retina. Kadoya *et al.* (1971*b*) were able to show some monochromatic responses using both evoked and single-unit responses in the squirrel monkey superior colliculus.

Size. In rat (Humphrey, 1968), cat (Harutiunian-Kozak *et al.*, 1970; McIlwain, 1975), and monkey (Humphrey, 1968; Goldberg and Wurtz, 1972*a*), the size of the receptive field increases with depth in the superficial layers. McIlwain (1975) pointed out that if one uses a retinal position map, the centers of the nested receptive fields are skewed toward the center of the gaze. However, if one uses a coordinate system based on the representation of the visual field on the collicular surface, the receptive fields are concentric (Fig. 8).

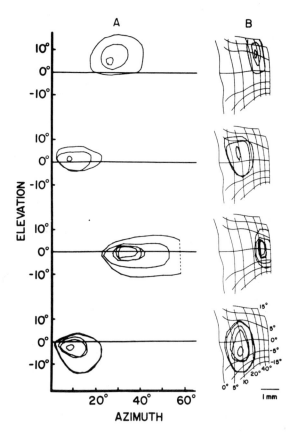

Fig. 8. Remapping of collicular fields. Column A shows four sets of visual receptive fields of neurons in the superficial layers of cat superior colliculus. Each set includes the fields from a single electrode penetration. In each case the fields grow larger as the penetration becomes deeper. Note that the center of each field moves peripherally as the field becomes larger. Column B shows the same fields displayed in a coordinate system that is distorted in the same way that the visual field is distorted in its map on the collicular surface. Now fields within a given penetration are concentric. Reproduced with permission from McIlwain (1975).

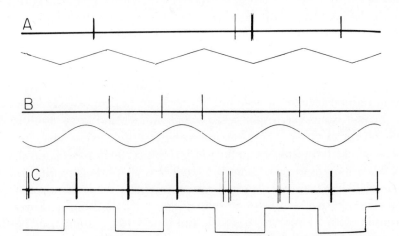

Fig. 9. Jerk detector in intermediate layers of the monkey superior colliculus. A and B show the response of a neuron to smoothly moving stimuli (ramp, A; sine wave, B). C shows the much better response of the neuron to the stimulus being jerked across the same receptive field. Reproduced by permission from Cynader and Berman (1972).

INTERMEDIATE LAYER VISUAL RESPONSES. Some cells in the intermediate gray and white layers of the cat superior colliculus have visual responses, but the visual responses are more difficult to study than those in the superficial layers. The cells have larger receptive fields than those in the overlying superficial layers, and these receptive fields have less well-defined borders (Gordon, 1973). The cells tend to habituate very rapidly, responding much better to novel stimuli than to stimuli that had previously been effective. The cells are very sensitive to anesthesia (Straschill and Hoffmann, 1970) and are best studied in an unanesthetized preparation (Gordon, 1973). They seem to have similar feature detection properties to cells in the superficial layers, but the rapidity of habituation makes detailed study difficult.

In the monkey the intermediate and deep layer neurons also have visual responses. Although they share the feature detection properties of the superficial neurons (in the rhesus monkey a lack of directional specificity), they have larger receptive fields, and are much more difficult to drive with repetitive stimuli. Thus Cynader and Berman (1972) described 20% of the cells they studied in the intermediate layers as "novelty detectors." This class of neuron was particularly easy to drive with the first presentation of any visual stimulus, and particularly hard to drive with subsequent presentations of the same stimulus. Another class of neurons responded much better to jerkily moved stimuli as opposed either to sinusoidally or smoothly moved stimuli (Fig. 9).

PHYSIOLOGY OF COLLICULAR CONNECTIONS. Since visual input to the superior colliculus comes via the retina and the visual cortex, it has been a matter of interest to determine what properties of collicular cells are retinal and what properties are cortical in origin.

Retinotectal Connections. Recent electrophysiological studies have suggested that most cat retinal ganglion cells fall into one of three major categories called W, X, and Y cells (Cleland and Levick, 1974*b*). The separation into X and Y groups

MICHAEL E.
GOLDBERG AND
DAVID LEE ROBINSON

was originally based on the linear and nonlinear spatial summation of ganglion cells (Enroth-Cugell and Robson, 1966). Since subsequent investigators have not used these criteria for initial classification, generalization of other properties of these cells may not be possible; however, enough work has been done to establish a general schema that pertains to most retinal ganglion cells and is useful for analyzing retinocollicular projections. Y cells have fast-conducting axons (35–45 m/sec), phasic (transient) responses to visual stimuli, and large nondirectionally selective receptive fields. They respond to high stimulus velocities (greater than 200°/sec). X cells have slower conduction velocities (20–25 m/sec), and have tonic (sustained) responses to visual stimuli. W cells have the slowest conduction velocity (3–15 m/sec), have several types of visual receptive fields some of which are directionally selective, and respond only to slowly moving stimuli (Enroth-Cugell and Robson, 1966; Fukuda, 1971; Cleland et al., 1971; Stone and Hoffmann, 1972; Ikeda and Wright, 1972; Fukuda and Stone, 1973; Boycott and Wässle, 1974).

These cell classes project differentially to the central nervous system (Clare et al., 1969; Hoffmann, 1973; Cleland and Levick, 1974a,b). W cells project to the superior colliculus (Hoffmann, 1972, 1973). [Recent anatomical evidence for the monkey and electrophysiological data for the cat suggest that W cells also project to the lateral geniculate nucleus (Bunt et al., 1975; Cleland et al., 1975; Wilson and Stone, 1975]. The collicular cells that receive efferents from W cells (as determined by the conduction velocities of the retinal shock required to activate the collicular cell) respond to low stimulus velocities and are frequently directionally selective (Hoffmann, 1973).

There is no evidence that X cells project to the superior colliculus. Y cells project to both the superior colliculus and the lateral geniculate. Collicular cells which receive a direct input from Y cells (as judged by conduction velocity) respond to high stimulus velocities and are not generally directionally selective. Hoffmann (1973) has described another series of cells with properties similar to those of Y cells but with longer latency of response to shock of optic tract. He postulated that these cells received retinal input from Y cells via the cortex, and, in fact, such cells can be driven with shorter latency by cortical stimulation. Hoffmann found a few cells with both direct and indirect Y cell input. His results are not in keeping with those of McIlwain and Fields (1971), who found a higher percentage of cells with combined cortical and retinal input.

Corticotectal Connections. Anatomical studies have demonstrated that the striate cortex of the cat provides one of the largest projections to the superficial layers of the colliculus. A second major cortical projection comes from the Clare-Bishop area; weaker afferents arise from areas 18 and 19 (Kawamura et al., 1974b; Holländer, 1974). Both electrophysiological (Hayaishi, 1969; Toyama et al., 1969; Palmer and Rosenquist, 1974) and histological (Holländer, 1974) studies have demonstrated that the cells in cortical layer V are the primary source of this projection. These cells have binocular, directionally selective, oriented, complex receptive fields (Palmer and Rosenquist, 1974). In contrast to other cortical complex cells, these neurons lack clear summation over the length of their receptive fields, and respond very well to the movement of small spots of light, a characteristic property of collicular neurons.

Corticotectal Interactions. Not only do both retina and striate cortex project to the superior colliculus, they also project in many cases to the same cell (McIlwain and Fields, 1971; Hoffmann and Straschill, 1971; Hoffmann, 1973). Cortical effects are both excitatory and inhibitory. No striate cortical effects seem to be mediated by areas 18 and 19, since ablation of these areas does not alter the effects of stimulating area 17 (McIlwain, 1973*a*). The inputs from area 17 and the retina are retinotopically organized. A point on the cortical surface which is most effective in influencing a neuron in the superior colliculus will contain neurons with receptive fields that are in the part of the visual field covered by the receptive field of the collicular neuron (McIlwain, 1973*b*). There is, however, much overlap in the projection from area 17, and neighboring collicular cells can receive striate inputs from a wide area. A retinotopic input from area 17 to the superficial layers of the ipsilateral superior colliculus has also been demonstrated physiologically in the squirrel monkey (Kadoya *et al.,* 1971).

Removal of Cortical Input. Since single collicular neurons can contain both cortical and retinal input, it has been of interest to determine what properties are due to direct retinal input and what properties are mediated by striate cortex.

Rodent. In the ground squirrel (Michael, 1972*b*) directionally selective cells lie predominantly in the upper layers and hypercomplex cells predominantly in the lower layers. Directionally selective cells are not affected by chronic ablation of striate cortex, but the lower-layer cells become unresponsive. Cooling the visual cortex also eliminates the visual responsiveness of hypercomplex cells. Thus it appears that hypercomplex cells require visual cortex, whereas the directionally selective cells depend entirely on retinal input for their visual properties (Fig. 10). It must be emphasized, however, that the directional selectivity is fixed in the retina and not generated in the superior colliculus of the ground squirrel.

In the rabbit (Masland *et al.,* 1971; Stewart *et al.,* 1973), there does not seem to be any effect of cortical ablation or cooling on collicular neurons.

Cat. In the cat there is also a differential contribution of cortical and retinal inputs to the visual properties of neurons in the superior colliculus. Wickelgren and Sterling (1969) first reported that cooling or chronic ablation of occipital

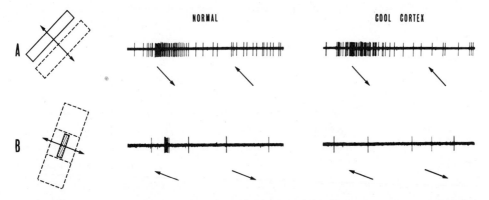

Fig. 10. Effect of cortical cooling on hypercomplex and directionally selective neurons in ground squirrel superior colliculus. A: Response of a directionally selective cell to cooling. There is no effect. B: Response of a hypercomplex cell to cooling. The discharge is eliminated. Time of sweep is 3 sec. Reproduced with permission from Michael (1972*b*).

MICHAEL E.
GOLDBERG AND
DAVID LEE ROBINSON

cortex caused cells in the ipsilateral superior colliculus to lose their directional selectivity. They also showed that although collicular cells in the intact cat are binocularly driven, destruction of the visual cortex results in cells which can be driven only by the contralateral eye. Furthermore, these cells respond to stationary spots of light much better than in the intact animal. Similar experiments have confirmed these results (Rosenquist and Palmer, 1971; Richard *et al.,* 1973; Berman and Cynader, 1975). Other investigators have failed to eliminate directional selectivity by cortical ablation (Marchiafava and Pepeu, 1966; Hoffmann and Straschill, 1971; Rizzolatti *et al.,* 1973).

Berman and Cynader (1975) examined the properties of corticotectal interactions in the context of the classification of retinal inputs to the colliculus. They found three classes of cells after cortical ablation. The largest class (83%) responded best to small stimuli, and responded only to slow stimulus velocities. The cells had strong inhibitory surrounds that were sensitive to high stimulus velocities. Thus these cells behaved as if they had W cell input to their centers and Y and W cell inputs to their surrounds. The second class of cells (12%) responded clearly to high stimulus velocities. These cells behaved as if they had exclusive Y cell input. A small class of cells (15%) had concentric visual receptive fields, with surround and center having properties consistent with inputs from identical ganglion cell classes. The authors showed that the cells with only presumed Y cell excitatory input responded well to flicker and called these cells "flicker" cells. The cells with presumed W cell excitatory and Y cell inhibitory input were strongly inhibited by flicker, even in the presence of maximal stimuli for their W cell excitatory regions. Since the class of cells inhibited by flicker makes up the great majority of cells in the colliculus, the authors postulated that a cat with bilateral striate lesions would have a relatively harder time seeing in a dim, flickering environment.

Monkey. Cells in the superficial layers of the monkey superior colliculus are much less vulnerable to cortical ablation than are those in the cat and ground squirrel. Schiller *et al.* (1974) showed that the balanced on- and off-responses of cells in the intact monkey are disturbed by cooling the cortex. Some cells in the stratum opticum and the border between stratum opticum and stratum griseum superficiale have patches of unresponsiveness intermixed with responsive patches in their visual receptive fields, whereas the intact animal has cells with relatively smooth responsiveness throughout the receptive field. Surprisingly, binocularity is left undisturbed by cortical ablation, and there is little directional selectivity to disrupt. Cortical cooling does, however, entirely eliminate the visual responsiveness of cells in the intermediate layers. These cells continue to discharge before eye movements in the absence of a cortical input. Schiller *et al.* were unable to find a differential effect on foveal and parafoveal receptive fields on cortical disruption. This implies that whatever sparse projection there is from the retinal fovea to the colliculus is sufficient to maintain collicular function in the absence of striate cortex.

Nonvisual Influences

Auditory and Tactile. In the cat and monkey, cells in the intermediate layers respond to auditory and tactile stimuli as well as to visual stimuli (Jassik-

Gerschenfeld, 1966; Stein and Arigbede, 1972; Cynader and Berman, 1972; Gordon, 1973; Updyke, 1974). Using an unanesthetized cat, Gordon (1973) showed that the most effective acoustic stimulus was a hiss emitted by a moving air hose. The optimal direction of movement of the sound source was similar to the optimal directional movement for a visual stimulus in the same cell, and effective acoustic stimuli were limited to a region similar to the visual receptive field of the cell (Fig. 11). There is a similar correspondence between laterality of visual and tactile responses. Stein *et al.* (1975) showed that the collicular neurons with trigeminal representation lie in an area of the colliculus with a central visual representation and that limb representations lie in collicular areas with more preipheral visual representations.

Dräger and Hubel (1975) found that the somatosensory representation of the mouse vibrissa system also lies in an area of the colliculus with a visual representation that includes the area of space traversed by the whiskers (Fig. 12). Cebus (Upkyde, 1974) and rhesus (Cynader and Berman, 1972) monkeys also show acoustic and tactile responses in the deeper layers of the superior colliculus, and trimodal cells are not difficult to find.

EXTRARETINAL MODIFICATION OF VISUAL RESPONSE. *Proprioceptive.* Abrahams and Rose (1975a) showed that visually responsive neurons, particularly those in the intermediate layers, could be driven by stimulation of extraocular and neck proprioceptor nerves. Nearly two-thirds of the visually responsive cells showed some response to muscle afferent stimulation. The response was either a short-latency burst that could follow stimulation at 1 Hz or a long-latency discharge that followed at 0.25 Hz. Some cells responded with both long- and short-latency discharges. The majority of cells studied responded to both. Since the superior colliculus has been shown to receive input from eye muscle stretch

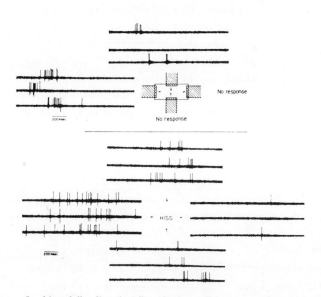

Fig. 11. Responses of a bimodally directionally selective cell in intermediate layers of cat superior colliculus. The upper portion shows the neuron's response to a visual stimulus moving in four orthogonal directions. The lower section shows the neuron's discharge in response to a hissing air hose traveling in the directions marked. Note that the optimum direction is the same for both the visual and auditory stimuli. Reproduced with permission from Gordon (1973).

MICHAEL E.
GOLDBERG AND
DAVID LEE ROBINSON

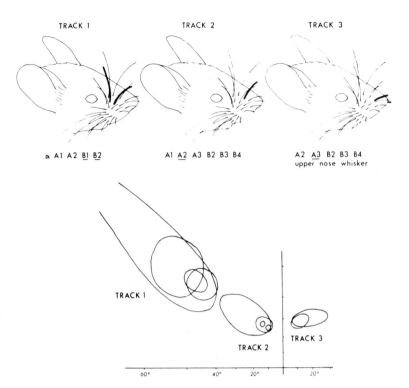

Fig. 12. Superimposition of visual and tactile functions in a given area of the mouse superior colliculus. Each upper diagram shows the vibrissae which activated neurons in a given penetration in the mouse superior colliculus. Each lower diagram shows the visual receptive fields encountered in the same penetration. Note that the vibrissae activated in a given penetration project into the visual receptive fields of the neurons in that penetration. Reproduced with permission from Dräger and Hubel (1975).

receptors in goat (Cooper *et al.*, 1953), cat, monkey (Cooper and Fillenz, 1955; Fillenz, 1955), and sheep (Manni *et al.*, 1972), it is not unreasonable to postulate that the muscle afferent effect comes from stretch receptors.

Abrahams and Rose (1975*b*) subsequently investigated the effects of passive eye movements on neurons in the superior colliculus. They found that cells discharged after passive eye movements with latencies of 7–100 msec, and that the cells responded best at rapid velocities of eye movement. Each cell had a minimum eye movement distance, and the displacement threshold seemed independent of eye position, although this question was not adequately studied for cells with small displacement thresholds. This independence of orbital position would make the passive displacement responses seem similar to the active eye movement response, and the possibility exists that passive eye movements are mapped onto the colliculus in a retinotopic manner as are saccadic eye movements. This question warrants further investigation.

Vestibular. Bisti *et al.* (1974) investigated the effects of body tilt on the activity of neurons in the superficial layers of the superior colliculus of the unanesthetized, paralyzed cat. They found that the response intensity of half of the directionally selective neurons and a quarter of the directionally nonselective neurons varied as a function of tilt. Rieger and Straschill (1973) were unable to duplicate these results.

Oculomotor. One of the more interesting properties of the visually responsive neurons in the superficial layers of the superior colliculus is the ease with which such responses can be inhibited or otherwise modified, by both visual and nonvisual means. Goldberg and Wurtz (1972a) noted that in the awake monkey visual neurons with high background rates could have their activity suppressed by saccadic eye movements in total darkness, regardless of the direction of the eye movement. D. L. Robinson and Wurtz (1976) showed that this extraretinal input enables collicular neurons to distinguish between externally generated stimulus movement and self-induced stimulus movement evoked by an eye movement. A cell giving a brisk response to stimulus movement across a stationary retina does not respond to comparable retinal stimulus movement evoked by an eye movement of equal magnitude and opposite direction. The cell receives an extraretinal signal to suppress what would otherwise be an excellent stimulus (Fig. 13).

Rizzolatti *et al.* (1975) found that moving stimuli in an area that had neither direct excitatory nor inhibitory effects on neurons in the superficial layers inhibited the response of those neurons to stimuli in the receptive field. This effect was demonstrable in paralyzed, awake cats with unsynchronized EEGs. It is possible that this inhibition may be related to the extraretinal input described by Goldberg and Wurtz (1972a) and D. L. Robinson and Wurtz (1976). Possibly the paralyzed and aroused animal attempts to fixate the new stimulus and the resultant extraretinal input inhibits the response to stimuli in the receptive field. Wurtz and Mohler (1976a) were unable to duplicate the results in an awake monkey. In such an animal which was voluntarily fixating a target outside the excitatory area of a cell, moving a second stimulus anywhere in the visual field did not affect the response of the neuron to a stimulus in its receptive field.

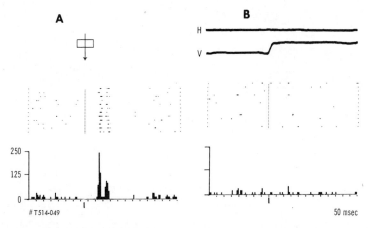

Fig. 13. Cell in monkey superior colliculus that differentiates between externally generated and self-induced stimulus movement. A: Response of the neuron to stimulus movement evoked by the stimulus moving across the tangent screen while the monkey's eye is still. B: Response of the neuron to stimulus movement evoked by the eye moving across the tangent screen while the stimulus is still. Note that although the retinal event—stimulus sweeping across the retina—is comparable in both cases, the response is markedly suppressed in B. An extraretinal signal prevents the cell from responding to stimulus movement evoked by an eye movement. H and V are, respectively, horizontal and vertical electrooculograms illustrating a representative eye movement. From D. L. Robinson and R. H. Wurtz (unpublished data).

MICHAEL E.
GOLDBERG AND
DAVID LEE ROBINSON

Behavioral Enhancement. Half of the visually responsive neurons in the superficial layers of the rhesus monkey colliculus can have their responses to visual stimuli modified by the behavioral significance of those stimuli. Goldberg and Wurtz (1972*b*) showed that the response of these cells to a visual stimulus could be enhanced when the monkey made a saccadic eye movement to fixate the stimulus (Fig. 14). The enhancement can occur in two different ways: either the on-response becomes brisker and more regular (the early response) or the discharge becomes prolonged until close to the start of the eye movement (the late response) (Fig. 15). The late response occurs independently of the on-response: when an animal fixates a stimulus that has been present in the visual field for a long time, the response begins after the signal to make the eye movement, and ends at the eye movement. The late response is not merely a premovement discharge, because cells which show the enhancement effect do not discharge before eye movements in the dark.

The enhancement effect has only a minor influence on the spatial organization of the receptive field. For many neurons the size of the receptive field is

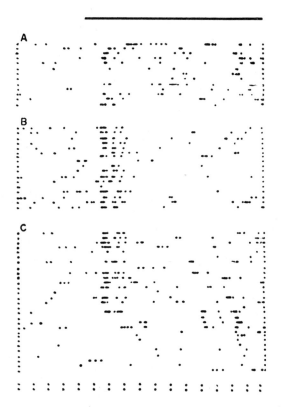

Fig. 14. Enhancement of visual response. A: Response of a neuron in superficial layers of rhesus monkey superior colliculus to the onset of a spot of light (shown by bar). During this series of trials the animal does not make any eye movement. B: Response of the same neuron to the same stimulus when that stimulus is to be used as the target for a saccadic eye movement. Note that the response is both more vigorous and more regular than in A. In this series the monkey makes eye movements 250 msec after the stimulus onset, well after the enhanced response. C: Falloff of enhancement after the monkey ceases to make the eye movement. Time line dots are 50 msec apart. Reproduced with permission from Goldberg and Wurtz (1972*b*).

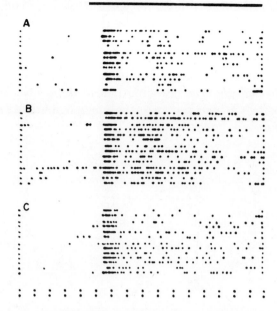

Fig. 15. Late enhancement of visual response before an eye movement. A: Response of a neuron in superficial layers of rhesus monkey superior colliculus to a spot of light. There is no associated eye movement. B: Response of the same neuron to the same spot when the monkey is going to use the spot as a target for an eye movement. The response of the neuron continues long after the on-burst in B. C: Immediate absence of the late response when the monkey no longer makes the eye movement. Time line dots are 50 msec apart. Indicator bar shows the onset of the stimulus. Reproduced by permission from Goldberg and Wurtz (1972*b*).

increased when the response is enhanced, while for others the response of the neuron is smoothed out within the borders of the excitatory area.

The enhancement effect is not merely arousal related to making an eye movement, because it is specific to the general receptive field area of the neuron involved; enhancement of a visual response does not occur when the animal makes an eye movement to a target distant from the receptive field of the cell (Fig. 16). However, the enhancement is not absolutely related to the receptive field of the cell, because it can be demonstrated when the animal makes an eye movement to a target near to but not in the receptive field of the cell. The enhancement does seem to require an eye movement. Wurtz and Mohler (1976*a*) trained animals to make a response to a target in the peripheral field without making an eye movement to fixate the target, and they found that the cells did not show the enhancement when the animals responded to but did not fixate the stimulus. The enhancement is not mediated by striate cortex. In fact, Mohler and Wurtz (1976*b*) found that after a striate cortex lesion more cells in the colliculus ipsilateral to the lesion show the effect than in the contralateral colliculus.

Habituation and Enhancement. A problem in studying some collicular neurons has been their propensity to habituate (Horn, 1969). Although this is more true of neurons in the deeper layers (Cynader and Berman, 1972; Gordon, 1973), it is true of most neurons in the superior colliculus. The habituation is more dramatic for suboptimal stimuli (Cynader and Berman, 1972) and can be found for all

MICHAEL E.
GOLDBERG AND
DAVID LEE ROBINSON

modalities that can stimulate a multimodal cell (Horn and Hill, 1966). For cells which show the enhancement effect, increasing the behavioral significance of the stimulus dramatically reverses habituation (Fig. 17). As long as a monkey can be made to make a saccade to fixate a spot of light in the receptive field of a neuron, the spot will elicit a maximal response from the neuron. If the response has habituated before the spot becomes important to the animal, the habituation is reversed. As soon as the spot no longer becomes significant to the animal, the response habituates.

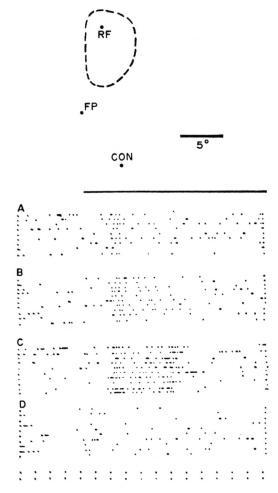

Fig. 16. Effects of eye movements to points distant from the receptive field of an enhancible neuron on the discharge of the neuron. The animal was presented with two stimuli, one within the receptive field (labeled RF) and one distant from the receptive field (labeled CON) but both approximately the same distance from the fixation point (FP). The animal was rewarded for fixating either of the two spots, and tended to alternate randomly between the two. A: Discharge of the neuron when the animal did not make a saccade. B: Discharge of the neuron when the animal chose to fixate the control spot. C: Enhanced discharge of the neuron when the animal fixated the receptive field spot. D: Discharge of the neuron when only the control spot was flashed on the screen. Reproduced by permission from Goldberg and Wurtz (1972b).

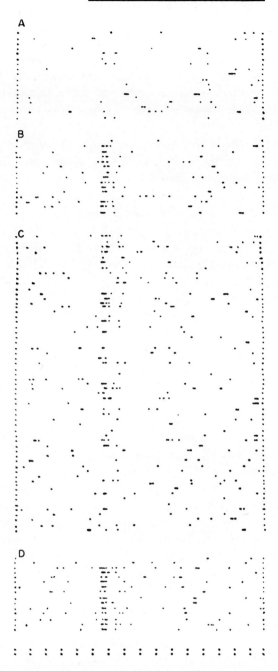

Fig. 17. Habituation of a neuron in the monkey superior colliculus reversed by enhancement. A: Response of a neuron in superficial layers of monkey superior colliculus in the absence of an eye movement. The response has habituated to the point that it is barely present. B: Immediate enhancement of the neuronal response when the animal is going to use the stimulus as the target for an eye movement. There is an enhanced response and no decrement. C: Habituation of the enhanced response when the animal no longer will use the stimulus as a target for an eye movement. D: Immediate dishabituation when the animal again uses the stimulus as a target for the eye movement. Time line dots are 50 msec apart. Indicator bar shows the onset of target. Reproduced with permission from Goldberg and Wurtz (1972b).

MICHAEL E.
GOLDBERG AND
DAVID LEE ROBINSON

In 1870 Adamük stimulated the superior colliculus and observed eye movements to the contralateral side. Since then, many investigators have amplified and refined his basic observation, and the weight of evidence overwhelmingly implicates the superior colliculus as having some role in the neural generation of eye movements (Apter, 1946; Hess *et al.,* 1946; Akert, 1949). However, the nature of this role is yet to be established.

STIMULATION. Apter (1946) used local application of strychnine to increase the excitability of the superior colliculus. Although the strychnine alone did not have an effect, she found that if she then flashed a light in a particular area of the visual field the anesthetized cat would make a slow eye movement to fixate it. Longer periods of strychninization resulted in head and eye movements and even limb movements toward the light. The map of target points for eye movements was roughly congruent with the representation of the contralateral retina on the surface of the colliculus. Precht *et al.* (1974) have shown that collicular stimulation in the cat produces di- and polysynaptic excitatory potentials in contralateral abducens motoneurons and reciprocal effects in the ipsilateral motoneurons.

Most recently, D. A. Robinson (1972) and Schiller and Stryker (1972) have shown that microstimulation of the awake rhesus monkey superior colliculus results in the generation of a saccadic eye movement toward a specific area of the visual field. Stimulation of different points in the colliculus results in a map of eye movement targets that is congruent with the map of the retina onto the colliculus (Fig. 18). Prolonged stimulation of a given point in the colliculus results in a series of saccades each of the same magnitude and direction. Simultaneous stimulation of two points results in a saccade whose magnitude and direction are between those elicited by stimulation of each point alone.

In these experiments, therefore, stimulation of the colliculus results in an eye movement that is retinotopically organized and independent of the position of the eye in the head. A diametrically opposite result was obtained by Straschill and Rieger (1973), who found that, in the cat, stimulation of the superior colliculus results in eye movements organized to fixate a point in space and that the position of the eye in the orbit is a crucial determinant of saccade direction and amplitude. The differences between these results, either species or technical, must be resolved by further work.

SINGLE-NEURON RECORDING. Single-neuron analogies to the stimulation data have been found. Straschill and Hoffmann (1970) described neurons in the cat superior colliculus that are excited or suppressed by eye movements in the dark. Goldberg and Wurtz (1970) and Wurtz and Goldberg (1971, 1972*a*) described a class of neurons histologically located in the intermediate layers of the monkey superior colliculus that discharge before eye movements in a given direction and distance. These neurons discharge before all kinds of rapid eye movements: saccades to fixate visual targets, spontaneous saccades in total darkness, and the eye movements of the quick phase of vestibular nystagmus. Each neuron discharges when the animal makes a saccade only to targets in a specific area of the visual field, an area called the movement field of the neuron. The representation of movement fields of cells in the intermediate layers forms a map on the collicular anatomy congruent with the visual receptive field maps and the eye movement stimulation maps described above (Schiller and Koerner, 1971; Wurtz and Goldberg, 1972a). The discharge of the neurons is unrelated to the eye's orbital position, although there are a few neurons deep in the superior colliculus that do have a discharge related to static orbital position (Wurtz and Goldberg, 1972a). Although discharge of the neurons always takes place when the animal makes an appropriate saccade, discharge of the neuron does not necessarily imply that the saccade must take place (Mohler and Wurtz, 1976a). If the animal aborts the eye movement because the stimulus has changed, the neuron will discharge as if the

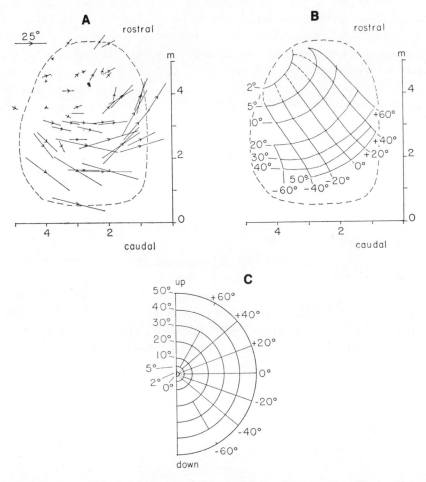

Fig. 18. Map of saccadic eye movements induced by stimulation of the superior colliculus of an awake rhesus monkey. A: Eye movements induced from stimulation of various points in the colliculus. Each arrow shows the magnitude and direction of the eye movement evoked from that point in the colliculus. B: Map of the polar coordinates of the eye movement targets induced from stimulating the superior colliculus transformed onto the collicular surface. C: Same map as it appears in the visual field. Reproduced with permission from D. A. Robinson (1972).

MICHAEL E.
GOLDBERG AND
DAVID LEE ROBINSON

eye movement were going to take place. If the animal fixates a very peripheral target by means of two successive saccades, the neuron discharges as if the animal were going to make one large saccade.

In an elegant experiment, Schiller and Stryker (1972) showed that stimulation through a recording microelectrode reached a threshold minimum in the intermediate layers of the rhesus monkey colliculus, and that microstimulation resulted in a saccade to the movement field of neurons recorded by the microelectrode (Fig. 19).

One of the intriguing features of the neurons in the intermediate layers of the superior colliculus is the large size of their movement fields. A monkey can make an eye movement at 20° with an accuracy of ½°. The movement fields of individual collicular neurons are an order of magnitude larger than that, and the question has arisen whether or not the neurons in the intermediate layers could be specifying the locus of an eye movement. In an attempt to analyze this question, Sparks (1975) made a computer analysis of movement fields. He determined that the tuning curves of the collicular neurons are rather flat compared with the accuracy of eye movements. Although the magnitude and direction of the eye movement cannot be predicted from the discharge properties of any single neuron in the superior colliculus, the prediction might be accurately generated from a knowledge of where in the colliculus the maximum activity is.

Mohler and Wurtz (1976a) showed that there is a tendency for movement fields to grow larger with depth in the colliculus (Fig. 20). However, the assumption that the large movement fields are assembled serially from more superficial cells with smaller movement fields cannot be true since the deeper cells start to discharge before the more superficial ones. This arrangement also proves that the more superficial cells in the intermediate layers do not cause the deeper cells to discharge (Fig. 20).

Many of the intermediate-layer neurons with movement related discharge also have visual receptive fields (Schiller and Koerner, 1971; Wurtz and Goldberg, 1972a). The visual and movement responses are clearly separable, and although the visual receptive field and the movement field lie in the same general area of the visual field, they are not usually superimposable. In cells with both visual and movement responses, the movement response is usually more vigorous (Fig. 21).

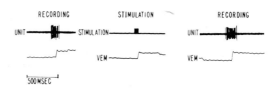

Fig. 19. Comparison of microstimulation and recording of movement cell in monkey superior colliculus. The recording examples show the discharge of the neuron in monkey superior colliculus before an eye movement. Upper trace is unit recording, lower trace is vertical electrooculogram. The stimulation example shows the eye movement evoked by stimulating through the same microelectrode used to record the discharge in the previous example. Note that the eye movement evoked by the stimulation is similar to that which is naturally preceded by the discharge of the neuron. Reproduced by permission from Schiller and Stryker (1972).

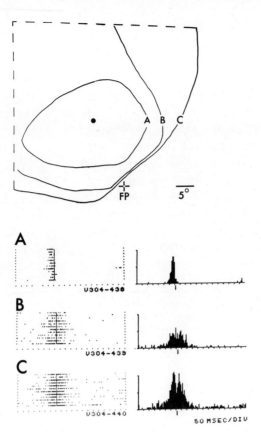

Fig. 20. Increasing size of movement fields and earlier onset of eye movement discharge in association with increasing depth in the intermediate layers of the colliculus. The areas enclosed in the upper part of the figure represent movement fields of cells recorded in a single penetration through the colliculus. A: Movement field for the first movement cell recorded. B, C: Movement fields for cells 1/4 mm and 1/4–1/2 mm below the first cell, respectively. The size of the movement fields increases with depth in the colliculus. The rasters and histograms at the bottom of the firgure show the discharge of the cell in association with eye movements from the fixation point (FP) to the dot within the fields. Deeper cells begin to dishcarge earlier before the eye movement. The histogram sums the individual trials of the adjacent rasters and the vertical axis is 250 spikes/sec/trial. Triggers for all displays are the onset of the eye movement.

No cells with eye movement related discharge and acoustic or tactile responses have been demonstrated. It is interesting to speculate that since acoustic and tactile responses have been demonstrated only in the intermediate and deep layers in animals that because of anesthesia or paralysis could not move their eyes, the responses could be more related to eye movements to look at the stimulus than to analysis of the stimulus itself.

HEAD MOVEMENT. Stimulation of the superior colliculus in animals free to move their heads results in combined head and eye movement (Hess *et al.*, 1946; Akert, 1949; Syka and Radil-Weiss, 1971; Schaffer, 1972; Straschill and Rieger, 1973; Stryker and Schiller, 1975).

Wilson and his co-workers (Anderson *et al.*, 1971; Peterson *et al.*, 1971) have investigated the connections between the cat superior colliculus and cervical motoneurons, and have found mono- and disynaptic connections, the intermediate synapse occurring in the origins of the reticulospinal path. Abrahams and Rose (1975a) showed that neck muscle afferents project to the cells of origin of the tectospinal tract in the cat.

Bizzi *et al.* (1971, 1972) have shown that, in the monkey, head and eye movements occur synchronously and that in the absence of free head movement the neck muscles discharge in a regular fashion.

It is therefore not unreasonable to postulate that the superior colliculus is involved in the central control of head movements. However, when D. L. Robinson and Jarvis (1974) studied this question in the rhesus monkey, they could not find cells that discharge in synchrony with the head movement component of an eye and head movement, although many cells in the intermediate layers are clearly related to eye movement (Fig. 22). A more surprising finding was that the discharge of the cell is not related to the magnitude of the final eye movement

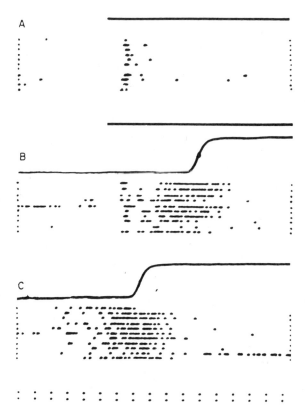

Fig. 21. Neuron in monkey superior colliculus with both visual and eye movement related responses. A: Response of the neuron to the onset of a spot of light in the absence of an eye movement. The indicator shows the duration of the stimulus presentation. B: Response of the same neuron during a visually evoked eye movement. The straight indicator bar shows the duration of the target presentation. The second line is the horizontal electrooculogram. The sweeps are triggered on the stimulus and the response to the stimulus can be easily seen. C: Same responses triggered on the eye movement. Note that the movement-related discharge is well synchronized but that the stimulus-related burst is no longer well seen. The movement-related discharge is much more vigorous than the stimulus-related discharge. Reproduced with permission from Wurtz and Goldberg (1972a).

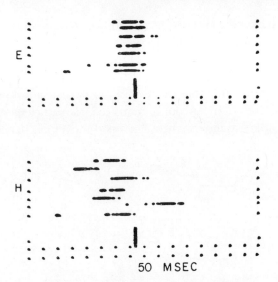

Fig. 22. Comparison of discharge pattern of single neuron of monkey superior colliculus with eye and head movements. The monkey has been allowed to make a combined head and eye movement. The upper figure shows the discharge of a single neuron in intermediate layers in relation to the eye movement component of the combined movement (shown by the vertical indicator bar). The lower figure shows the same neuronal discharges displayed in synchrony with the neck movement. Note that there is an excellent correlation between neuronal discharge and eye movement, and no correlation between neuronal discharge and neck movement. Reproduced with permission from D. L. Robinson and Jarvis (1974).

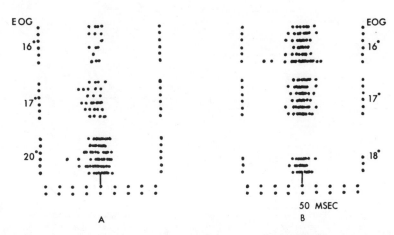

Fig. 23. Discharge of neuron with saccades which are part of a combined head and eye movement compared to saccades when the head is held. The left column shows the head-held data. Actual eye movement length is shown at far left. The right column shows the head-free data. In these trials the monkey made a combined head and eye movement; the size of eye movement adjusted because of the concurrent head movement is shown in the column at the far right. The target in all the head-free trials was 20° from the fixation point. Although this cell discharges differentially for programmed eye movements of various sizes (head held), its burst is consistent with the programmed eye movement but not the accomplished movement when the head is free to modify the saccade. Reproduced with permission from D. L. Robinson and Jarvis (1974).

when the animal makes a combined head and eye movement but is related to the distance the eye movement would have been had there been no head movement (Fig. 23).

Stryker and Schiller (1975) analyzed the effect of collicular stimulation on head movement. They found that short-duration pulse trains do not reliably elicit head movements, although the pulse trains are of sufficient intensity to elicit reproducible saccadic eye movements. The head movements elicited are variable

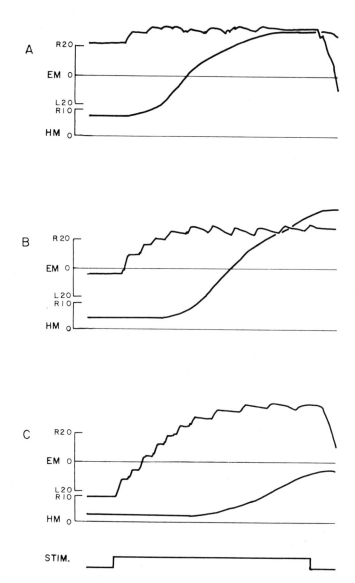

Fig. 24. Effect of stimulating the superior colliculus on combined eye and head movements. Upper trace in each figure is eye movement. Lower trace in each figure is neck movement. The stimulating electrode is in the left superior colliculus. When the eye deviates to the right (contralateral, A), there is an earlier onset of head movement and a less regular staircase of saccades than when the eye is in a midorbital (B) or ipsilateral (C) initial position. Reproduced with permission from Stryker and Schiller (1975).

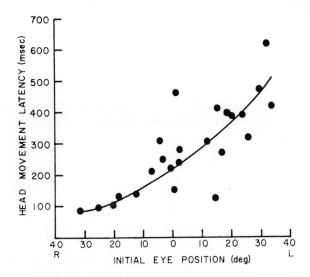

Fig. 25. Relationship of onset of head movement to position of the eye in the orbit. Ordinate is the latency of the beginning of the head movement in response to microstimulation of the contralateral superior colliculus. The abscissa is the position of the eye in the orbit at the time of stimulation. Note that head movement was more readily elicited when the eye was at the extreme of the orbit. Reproduced by permission from Stryker and Schiller (1975).

in length and latency, and are followed by compensatory (presumably vestibular induced) eye movements which follow the saccades originally elicited by the pulse trains. Longer-duration pulse trains, which elicit staircase sequences of saccades (Fig. 24), elicit head movements. The latency of the head movements is a function of the orbital position of the eye: latency decreases the farther the eye is displaced in the orbit in the direction of eye movement (Fig. 25).

From the foregoing it is apparent that, in the monkey, the superior colliculus cannot be important in the programming of head movements. However, similar experiments remain to be done for the cat where the physiology of tectospinal connections has best been worked out.

Behavioral Effects of Ablation

The effects of ablation of the superior colliculus have been studied in several mammals, and, like the results of single-unit studies, tend to vary from species to species. The drama of the deficit tends to increase with the relative size of the colliculus in the visual system, but even animals with large and intricately developed visual cortices show significant deficits.

Hamster

Schneider (1969), comparing collicular and cortical lesions in the golden hamster, noted a qualitative difference between the effects of the two lesions. Animals with collicular lesions had great difficulty orienting themselves in space,

MICHAEL E.
GOLDBERG AND
DAVID LEE ROBINSON

and could not turn toward food held in front of them. They could, however, solve pattern discriminations that did not require them to base any behavior on the position of the test objects in space. Animals with cortical lesions could easily locate objects in space, but could not solve the pattern discrimination. These data led Schneider to postulate "two visual systems," a cortical one to say "what" an object is and a tectal system to tell "where" it is. Other investigations have shown that this concept is an oversimplification, as one would expect from the extensive anatomical communications between cortex and colliculus, but the concept has proven heuristically useful.

TREE SHREW

Casgrande and Diamond (1974) have shown that in the tree shrew a similar qualitative distinction can be made between lesions involving the entire colliculus and lesions involving only the superficial layers. They found that tree shrews with collicular ablations limited to the superficial layers could acquire simple pattern discrimination habits (such as orientation of stripes) but not more difficult ones (such as orientation of triangles). These animals would respond normally to threat and could follow and orient to visual stimuli. Animals with lesions involving both superficial and deep layers could neither solve pattern discriminations nor respond to threat nor orient to visual stimuli. Discrimination deficits in the animals with the more extensive lesions were similar to those with the superficial lesions. All animals were able to avoid static barriers while walking. These data tend to reinforce the single-unit data concept that there is a significant difference between superficial and deeper layers of the colliculus. The tree shrew is, however, unusual in its reliance upon the colliculus for pattern discrimination.

Jane et al. (1972) showed that bilateral collicular ablation was necessary for a pattern deficit in the tree shrew. Animals with complete unilateral ablations behaved as if blind when the eye ipsilateral to the lesion was occluded.

CAT

Cats with bilateral superior collicular lesions have little difficulty learning or retaining brightness discriminations but have signficant problems learning new pattern discriminations (Blake, 1959; Fischman and Meikle, 1965).

Winterkorn (1975) found that cats with bilateral collicular ablations could make light–dark or horizontal–vertical discriminations in a V maze, and if one examined only the number of times the cat actually pressed the door at the end of the maze, cats with bilateral ablations did as well as normal controls. However, if one instead examined the number of times the animal entered the wrong alley in the maze, cats with bilateral collicular lesions did much less well.

Cats with unilateral collicular lesions show marked deficits both in performing visual tasks and in orienting in space. Sprague and his co-workers (Sprague and Meikle, 1965; Berlucchi et al., 1972) have documented that after unilateral collicu-lectomy cats compulsively circle in a direction ipsilateral to the ablated colliculus, cannot follow objects across the midline, and mislocalize tactile and acoustic stimuli as well as visual ones. Although the intensity of the deficits decreases with time, the cats always maintain a preference for the ipsilateral side, and never explore the contralateral field as much as they attend to the ipsilateral field.

The same group (Berlucchi *et al.*, 1972) analyzed the visual problem-solving abilities of cats with collicular and combined collicular-cortical lesions. They used as a basic preparation cats with split optic chiasm, corpus callosum, anterior commissure, hippocampal commissure, and, in some cases, posterior and habenular commissures. This procedure ensured that each colliculus and cortex received input from the ipsilateral eye almost exclusively. Operation on one side only and monocular testing of the animals made it possible for each animal to act as its own control.

The authors found that removing the superior colliculus resulted in a lengthening of the time that it took the animals to learn a simple pattern discrimination. There was no similar problem with relearning tasks that had been learned before the collicular surgery. Subsequent removal of striate cortex had no further effect, but removal of areas 18 and 19 and suprasylvian gyrus after colliculus and striate ablations remarkably extended the deficits. Animals with damage limited primarily to the pretectum did much better than animals with damage fundamentally in the colliculus. The authors also state that following collicular ablation many animals had a side preference that markedly interfered with training. They did not systematically study the side preference. All of the animals used in this study had some encroachment on the pretectum, and it was the feeling of the authors that pretectal and collicular damage summed in their effects.

There is one case in which collicular ablation results in an augmentation rather than a diminution of behavior: Sprague (1966) and Sherman (1974) showed that cats with striate cortical lesions develop a stable hemianopia. This hemianopia can be reversed by ablating the superior colliculus contralateral to the excised striate cortex. More surprisingly, the same results can be achieved merely by sectioning the collicular commissure. The implication of this study is that the superior colliculus receives some facilitatory input from the ipsilateral striate cortex which is balanced by an inhibitory input from the contralateral colliculus. In the absence of the ipsilateral striate cortex, the superior colliculus can participate in the control of behavior only if the inhibitory effect of the contralateral colliculus can be eliminated. The effect is dependent on the order of ablation. Function recovers more quickly if the superior colliculus is ablated after the striate cortex than if the colliculus is removed first (Wood, 1975).

MONKEY

The results of collicular ablations in the monkey have been less obvious than those in the cat or the hamster. Denny-Brown (1962) made collicular lesions in monkeys and reported dramatic deficits. The animals appeared blind, and did not respond to any kind of sensory stimuli. Visual driving of the electroencephalogram was normal. However, Denny-Brown's lesions included far more of the midbrain than the superior colliculus, and other investigators (Rosvold *et al.*, 1958; Pasik *et al.*, 1966; Anderson and Symmes, 1969; Thompson and Myers,

MICHAEL E.
GOLDBERG AND
DAVID LEE ROBINSON

1971; Wurtz and Goldberg, 1972*b*; Butter, 1974; Keating, 1974) have been unable to duplicate his results with lesions limited to the superior colliculus. Nevertheless, most investigators (Pasik *et al.*, 1966; Anderson and Symmes, 1969) agree that monkeys with lesions in the superior colliculus have a tendency toward a fixed gaze, and in the presence of unilateral lesions are more responsive to stimuli in the visual field ipsilateral to the lesion.

Most studies of visual discrimination performance in monkeys with collicular ablations have been unable to reveal any deficits (Rosvold *et al.*, 1958; Thompson and Myers, 1971). Anderson and Symmes (1969) found that monkeys with bilateral superior collicular ablations had difficulty retaining a task that required them to discriminate between a rapidly revolving disk and one revolving at one-third the speed. The task required that the monkeys make a discrimination within 5 sec, but the authors stated that they could see no difference in the way the normal and experimental monkeys acted in the limited time period. These monkeys had no difficulty with color, form, or flicker-fusion discriminations, nor did they have difficulty discriminating between a stationary and a moving disk.

Butter (1974) found that monkeys with bilateral superior collicular lesions had a slight difficulty learning a discrimination which required them to push a manipulandum separate from the visual patterns they had to discriminate. Since monkeys tend to look at their hands, this stimulus-response separation task forced the animals to analyze extrafoveal space. Animals with lateral striate lesions had no similar difficulty, and animals with collicular lesions could learn the task without any difficulty if there were no stimulus-response separation.

Keating (1974) found that under time pressure rhesus monkeys had difficulty solving a luminous flux problem. He trained the monkeys to press the dimmer of two lighted panels in a 6 × 4 array. The panels remained lighted for 200 msec, shorter than the latency for a saccade. He found that not only did the lesioned animals take longer to regain criterion performance on the task, but they also tended to make reaching errors by hitting panels that had not been lighted. Normal monkeys misreached in 12% of missed trials; operated animals misreached in 47% of missed trials. Monkeys misreached most often when the trial began with the head pointing toward the opposite half of the stimulus array.

Pasik *et al.* (1966) looked at optokinetic nystagmus, vestibular nystagmus, and spontaneous eye movements in rhesus monkeys with bilateral superior collicular ablations, and were unable to find any qualitative deficit in eye movements.

Wurtz and Goldberg (1972*b*) examined the eye movements of monkeys with unilateral or partial superior collicular ablations. They found that the latency of eye movement was markedly lengthened, but the accuracy of the eye movement was not significantly altered, nor were its dynamics. This latency deficit was seen only when the animal made an eye movement into that area of the visual field no longer represented in the colliculus (Fig. 26); it persisted for at least 6 weeks of regular testing. Mohler and Wurtz (1976*b*) subsequently refined these data and showed that in addition to the latency deficit the frequency of small corrective saccades was slightly increased for some but not all monkeys after collicular ablation, implying that the accuracy of some eye movements was mildly impaired.

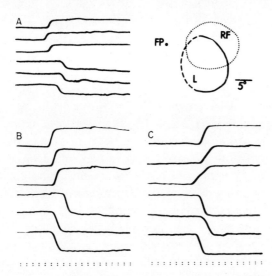

Fig. 26. Effect of a focal lesion in the rhesus monkey superior colliculus on eye movements. Receptive fields of neurons were recorded with a microelectrode to establish location in the superior colliculus. A lesion was then made in the intermediate layers at that point using the same microelectrode. The eye movement latencies were measured the next day. The drawing in the upper right shows the area of the receptive field (marked with a dotted line and labeled "RF"). The area of the visual field to which saccades had a longer latency after the lesion is marked with a solid line and labeled L. A,B, and C: Eye movements to points within the lesion area (A), to its border (B), and outside (C). Each figure consists of three consecutive horizontal electrooculograms to equivalent points in the field ipsilateral (top three) and contralateral (bottom three) to the lesion. Each sweep is triggered by the stimulus to make the eye movement. Time dots are 50 msec apart. Reproduced with permission from Wurtz and Goldberg (1972*b*).

The ablation of striate cortex resulted in a dramatic but transient decrease in accuracy, without a significant increase in latency. Animals with combined collicular and cortical lesions could not perform the saccade task at all.

CONCLUSIONS

Anatomical and physiological evidence shows the superior colliculus to be an organ with complex spatially organized sensory input and ocular and spinal motor output. Lesion studies indicate problems with perception, learning, movement, and eye movement after collicular ablation. However, this prodigious amount of experimental data has not yielded a coherent theory of collicular function.

One difficulty is the clearly changing role of the superior colliculus in the mammalian brain as the cerebral cortex has evolved in complexity. Rodents and insectivores have small lisencephalic neocortices, and large well-developed superior colliculi, and it is therefore not surprising that the colliculus in these animals is responsible for a larger fraction of visually guided behavior. Thus the behavioral lesions following collicular ablation in the golden hamster indicate that the colliculus is crucial for organizing the orientation of the animal to visual and perhaps

MICHAEL E.
GOLDBERG AND
DAVID LEE ROBINSON

other stimuli. In the tree shrew the superficial layers are involved in visual perception and the deeper layers in orientation. Because tree shrews and hamsters with collicular ablations have such difficulty with orientation in space, they appear blind. With increasing encephalization of visual function, deficits are less dramatic. The cat develops ipsiversive circling immediately after collicular ablation, but this disappears, and the stable deficits are a difficulty in learning new visual discriminations and contralateral neglect.

In the primate, lesion studies have been surprising in the lack of dramatic result of collicular ablation. Measures of gross perceptual and oculomotor parameters failed to show any significant results from collicular ablation. Those experiments discussed above that do show significant deficits from collicular destruction all share the requirement of making the monkeys perform difficult tasks requiring visual exploration under time pressure.

Those animals with well-developed visual cortices also have evolved foveate retinas, where one area of the retina has significantly finer grain than the rest of the retina, and most critical perceptual processing must involve bringing the fovea to bear on the object to be analyzed. It is highly likely that in the evolution of the brain of foveate animals the role of the colliculus changed from directly controlling the animal's orientation to participating in the control of the fovea's orientation. This in turn controls how and what the animal sees. Two different hypotheses have been put forth to explain the role that the superior colliculus plays in controlling primate visual orientation and eye movements, the foveation hypothesis and the attention hypothesis.

The foveation hypothesis: Schiller (1972) and D. A. Robinson (1972) have propounded the view that the superior colliculus is an intimate link in the neural machinery underlying eye movements. In their view the colliculus programs the coordinates of the next object to be fixated ("foveated") and initiates the eye movement program that accomplishes the foveation. They use as evidence the congruence of visual and eye movement maps, and the ease and reliability of saccade generation from electrical stimulation in the intermediate layers of the colliculus.

There are several problems with this interpretation, the first of which lies in the nature of the deficits induced by collicular ablation. A monkey with a collicular scotoma can fixate objects perfectly well. The saccades which accomplish the fixation have, in some but not all animals, a slight deficit in accuracy as judged by a mild increase in the number of small corrective saccades. The major deficit is a lag in the onset of the eye movement. If the collicular spatial map were crucial to foveation, then one would expect a larger dislocation of saccadic accuracy, and not so much a deficit in the initiation of a well-controlled eye movement. Since animals with entire unilateral collicular ablations show the same deficits, it is clear that the superior colliculus is not necessary for an accurate saccadic eye movement, although its presence makes the initiation of that eye movement more efficient.

The head movement data are also disturbing in the context of a foveation hypothesis. Bizzi *et al.* (1971, 1972) have shown that in the monkey exploring visual space in a predictive manner, activation of eye musculature is preceded by activation of neck musculature and a head movement. Thus the dimensions of the saccade are adjusted according to the head movement. The activity of eye move-ment related neurons in the superior colliculus, however, is related to the retinal position of the target regardless of the final saccade actually made, and collicular stimulation *per se* does not clearly affect head movement. Therefore, if the colliculus were sending a foveation signal to the brain stem, the signal could not be going directly to the saccade "pulse generator." Rather it must go to some other center which must then take into account other data—presumably including eye orbital position—and then programs a saccade which compensates for the head movement. Only if no head movement is to take place can the saccade parameters suggested by the superior colliculus be translated into the actual saccade dimensions.

Another difficulty with the foveation hypothesis lies in the nature of the movement fields, which are an order of magnitude larger than the eye movement accuracy of a monkey. Clearly a small number of collicular neurons cannot determine an accurate eye movement, although the output of a very large ensemble of them might (McIlwain, 1975). Finally, discharge of a movement-related neuron in the monkey superior colliculus is not obligately linked to the occurrence of the eye movement. Therefore, although there is clear evidence that the superior colliculus is involved in foveation, it is difficult to postulate that the collicular discharge specifies the actual eye movement in any more than a general way.

Attention hypothesis: Wurtz and Goldberg (1972*c*) have fashioned a some-what different hypothesis of collicular function. In their view the colliculus is involved in helping to select the important object in the field for fixation, and initiating the eye movement toward that object, rather than just programming an eye movement. In this view the important phenomenon is the enhancement effect: when an animal is going to make an eye movement to an area of the visual field, collicular neurons with receptive fields in that area have enhanced responses to visual stimuli. For eye movements to points outside of the receptive field, these neurons are suppressed by an extraretinal input so that rapid stimulus movement which would ordinarily be an effective collicular stimulus is not effective. In this hypothesis the critical collicular contribution is in the visual exploration that precedes the eye movement, which is somehow rendered less efficient without the collicular contribution.

This enables one to explain various perceptual deficits that are seen following collicular ablation. Sprague's demonstration of difficulty with pattern discrimina-tion learning in cats can be explained as a deficit of visual exploration, as can Butter's demonstration of slight difficulty with stimulus–response separation tasks in monkeys, Keating's demonstration of spatial localization difficulties with briefly presented stimuli, and Anderson and Symmes's demonstration of difficulty with time-pressured movement discrimination in monkeys. All of the above tasks require the animal to explore the visual world by choosing peripheral stimuli to be fixated. A deficit in the selection process can result in neglect at worst—which is the ipsiversive circling, contralateral neglect, and position habit seen in the cat after unilateral collicular ablation—or delay of eye movement onset, which can be viewed as a deficit in target choice.

MICHAEL E.
GOLDBERG AND
DAVID LEE ROBINSON

This hypothesis would also provide a function for the ascending connections of the superior colliculus. Although the superior colliculus has no direct cortical projection, in the monkey it has a strong projection to the pulvinar nuclei, which in turn project to cortical visual association areas. By facilitating visual input from one area of the visual field via an enhanced visual response, the colliculus could render that area more salient to the pulvinar, and hence to the cortex. There are no data on the role of the pulvinar in eye movements and visual search. However, there is a striking human neurological disorder, Balint's syndrome (Hécaen and de Ajuriaguerra, 1954; Luria, 1959; Tyler, 1968), which has been shown to be a deficit in visual search. Patients with this syndrome have full visual fields as measured by perimetry, yet have great difficulty perceiving complex visual stimuli. Analysis of their eye movements (Tyler, 1968) has shown that they have a paucity of exploratory eye movements and have great difficulty breaking and reestablishing gaze. Nonetheless, they have the full range of eye movements on command. Thus one can view their deficit as a difficulty with visual search and with communication of the results of visual search to the eye movement system. The usual lesion found in patients with this syndrome is a bilateral posterior-parietal, superior temporal, anterior occipital lesion. The area involved includes the cortical projection of the pulvinar, which in turn relays information from the superior colliculus. This enables us to speculate that the colliculus is important in relaying visual search information upward as well as oculomotor information downward. The function which in a golden hamster is simply "There is a target; orient to it" becomes in the monkey "There is an interesting object; think about looking at it."

The attention and foveation hypotheses are not mutually exclusive, because the first part of foveation is noticing the target, and the result of the choice is the eye movement. However, foveation is clearly not a uniquely collicular function, because animals deprived of their colliculus can foveate immediately after their lesions. The deficits of animals with collicular lesions seem rather to involve the interplay of vision and foveation, and it is in this middle ground that the colliculus may be found to have its role in visually guided behavior.

REFERENCES

Abrahams, V. C., and Rose, P. K. Projections of extraocular, neck muscle, and retinal afferents to the superior colliculus in the cat: Their connections to the cells of origin of the tectospinal tract. *J. Neurophysiol.*, 1975a, *38*, 10–18.

Abrahams, V. C., and Rose, P. K. Velocity and displacement characteristics of passive eye movement which initiate unit discharges in the superior colliculus. *J. Physiol. (London)*, 1975b, *246*, 101p.

Adamük, E. Über die Innervation der Augenbewegungen. *Zentr. Med. Wiss.*, 1870, *8*, 65.

Akert, K. Der visuelle Greifreflex. *Helv. Physiol. Acta*, 1949, *7*, 112–134.

Altman, J. Some fiber projections to the superior colliculus in the cat. *J. Comp. Neurol.*, 1962, *119*, 77–95.

Altman, J., and Carpenter, M. B. Fiber projections of the superior colliculus in the cat. *J. Comp. Neurol.*, 1961, *116*, 157–177.

Anderson, K. V., and Symmes, D. The superior colliculus and higher visual functions in the monkey. *Brain Res.*, 1969, *13*, 37–52.

Anderson, M. E., Yoshida, M., and Wilson, V. J. Influence of superior colliculus on cat neck motoneurons. *J. Neurophysiol.*, 1971, *34*, 898–907.

Angaut, P. The fastigio-tectal projections: An anatomical experimental study. *Brain Res.*, 1969, *13*, 186–189.

Apter, J. T. Projection of the retina on superior colliculus of cats. *J. Neurophysiol.*, 1945, *8*, 123–134.

Apter, J. T. Eye movements following strychninization of the superior colliculus of cats. *J. Neurophysiol.*, 1946, *9*, 73–86.

Astruc, J. Corticofugal connections of area 8 (frontal eye field) in *Macaca mulatta*. *Brain Res.*, 1971, *33*, 241–256.

Benevento, L. A., and Fallon, J. H. The ascending projections of the superior colliculus in the rhesus monkey (*Macaca mulatta*). *J. Comp. Neurol.*, 1975, *160*, 339–362.

Berlucchi, G., Sprague, J. M., Levy, J., and DiBerardino, A. C. Pretectum and superior colliculus in visually guided behavior and in flux and form discrimination in the cat. *J. Comp. Physiol. Psychol.*, 1972, *78*, 123–172.

Berman, N., and Cynader, M. Comparison of receptive-field organization of the superior colliculus in Siamese and normal cats. *J. Physiol. (London)*, 1972, *224*, 363–389.

Berman, N., and Cynader, M. Receptive fields in cat superior colliculus after visual cortex lesions. *J. Physiol. (London)*, 1975, *245*, 261–270.

Berman, N., Blakemore, C., and Cynader, M. Binocular interaction in the cat's superior colliculus. *J. Physiol. (London)*, 1975, *246*, 595–615.

Bisti, S., Maffei, L., and Piccolino, M. Visuovestibular interactions in the cat superior colliculus. *J. Neurophysiol.*, 1974, *37*, 146–155.

Bizzi, E., Kalil, R. E., and Tagliasco, V. Eye-head coordination in monkeys: Evidence of centrally patterned organization. *Science*, 1971, *173*, 452–454.

Bizzi, E., Kalil, R. E., Morasso, P., and Tagliasco, V. Central programming and peripheral feedback during eye-head coordination in monkeys. *Bibl. Ophthalmol.*, 1972, *82*, 220–232.

Blake, L. The effect of lesions of the superior colliculus on brightness and pattern discrimination in the cat. *J. Comp. Physiol. Psychol.*, 1959, *52*, 272–278.

Boycott, B. B., and Wässle, H. The morphological types of ganglion cells of the domestic cat's retina. *J. Physiol. (London)*, 1974, *240*, 397–419.

Bunt, A. H., Hendrickson, A. E., Lund, J. S., Lund, R. D., and Fuchs, A. F. Monkey retinal ganglion cells: Morphometric analysis and tracing of axonal projections, with a consideration of the peroxidase technique. *J. Comp. Neurol.*, 1975, *164*, 265–286.

Butter, C. M. Effect of superior colliculus, striate and prestriate lesions on visual sampling in rhesus monkeys. *J. Comp. Physiol. Psychol.*, 1974, *87*, 905–917.

Carpenter, M. B., and Pierson, R. J. Pretectal region and the pupillary light reflex: An anatomical analysis in the monkey. *J. Comp. Neurol.*, 1973, *149*, 271–300.

Casagrande, V. A., and Diamond, I. T. Ablation study of the superior colliculus in the tree shrew (*Tupaia glis*). *J. Comp. Neurol.*, 1974, *156*, 207–238.

Casagrande, V. A., Harting, J. K., Hall, W. C., Diamond, I. T., and Martin, G. F. Superior colliculus of the tree shrew: A structural and functional subdivision into superficial and deep layers. *Science*, 1972, *177*, 444–447.

Clare, M. H., Landau, W. M., and Bishop, G. H. The relationship of optic nerve fiber groups activated by electrical stimulation of the consequent central postsynaptic events. *Exp. Neurol.*, 1969, *24*, 400–420.

Cleland, B. G., and Levick, W. R. Brisk and sluggish concentrically organized ganglion cells in the cat's retina. *J. Physiol. (London)*, 1974a, *240*, 421–456.

Cleland, B. G., and Levick, W. R. Properties of rarely encountered types of ganglion cells in the cat's retina and an overall classification. *J. Physiol. (London)*, 1974b, *240*, 457–492.

Cleland, B. G., Dubin, M. W., and Levick, W. R. Sustained and transient neurones in the cat's retina and lateral geniculate nucleus. *J. Physiol. (London)*, 1971, *217*, 473–496.

Cleland, B. G., Morstyn, R., Wagner, H. G., and Levick, W. R. Rarely encountered receptive field types in the LGN of the cat. Assoc. Res. Vision Ophthal. Spring Meeting, 1975.

Cohen, B., and Henn, V. Unit activity in the pontine reticular formation associated with eye movements. *Brain Res.*, 1972, *46*, 403–410.

Cohen, B., and Komatsuzaki, A. Eye movements induced by stimulation of the pontine reticular formation: Evidence for integration in oculomotor pathways. *Exp. Neurol.*, 1972, *36*, 101–117.

Cooper, S., and Fillenz, M. Afferent discharges in response to stretch from the extraocular muscles of the cat and monkey and the innervation of these muscles. *J. Physiol (London)*, 1955, *127*, 400–413.

Cooper, S., Daniel, P. M., and Whitteridge, D. Nerve impulses in the brainstem of the goat: Responses with long latencies obtained by stretching the extrinsic eye muscles. *J. Physiol. (London)*, 1953, *120*, 491–513.

Cynader, M., and Berman, N. Receptive-field organization of monkey superior colliculus. *J. Neurophysiol.*, 1972, *35*, 187–201.

Denny-Brown, D. The midbrain and motor integration. *Proc. Roy. Soc. Med.*, 1962, *55*, 527–538.

Dräger, U. C., and Hubel, D. H. Responses to visual stimulation and relationship between visual, auditory and somatosensory inputs in mouse superior colliculus. *J. Neurophysiol.*, 1975, *38*, 690–713.

Dreher, B., and Hoffman, K.-P. Properties of excitatory and inhibitory regions in the receptive fields of single units in the cat's superior colliculus. *Exp. Brain Res.*, 1973, *16*, 333–353.

Edwards, S. B., Rosenquist, A. C., and Palmer, L. A. An autoradiographic study of ventral lateral geniculate projections in the cat. *Brain Res.*, 1974, *72*, 282–287.

Enroth-Cugell, C., and Robson, J. G. The contrast sensitivity of ganglion cells in the cat. *J. Physiol. (London)*, 1966, *187*, 517–552.

Escobar, A., and de Cárdenas, M. J. On the connections between the superior colliculus and the inferior olivary nucleus: An experimental study in the cat. *Bol. Estud. Med. Biol.*, 1968, *25*, 281–290.

Feldon, S., Feldon, P., and Kruger, L. Topography of the retinal projection upon the superior colliculus of the cat. *Vision Res.*, 1970, *10*, 135–143.

Fillenz, M. Responses in the brainstem of the cat to stretch of extrinsic ocular muscles. *J. Physiol. (London)*, 1955, *128*, 182–199.

Fischman, M. W., and Meikle, T. H., Jr. Visual intensity discrimination in cats after serial tectal and cortical lesions. *J. Comp. Physiol. Psychol.*, 1965, *59*, 193–201.

Fukuda, Y. Receptive field organization of cat optic nerve fibers with special reference to conduction velocity. *Vision Res.*, 1971, *11*, 209–226.

Fukuda, Y., and Stone, J. Observations on the retinal input to the pupillo-constrictor reflex in the cat. *Proc. Aust. Physiol. Pharmacol. Soc.*, 1973, *4*, 138–139.

Garey, L. J., Jones, E. G., and Powell, T. P. S. Interrelationships of striate and extrastriate cortex with the primary relay sites of the visual pathway. *J. Neurol. Neurosurg. Psychiat.*, 1968, *31*, 135–157.

Goldberg, M. E., and Wurtz, R. H. Effects of eye movement and visual stimulus on units in monkey superior colliculus. *Fed. Proc.*, 1970, *29*, 453.

Goldberg, M. E., and Wurtz, R. H. Activity of superior colliculus in behaving monkey. I. Visual receptive fields of single neurons. J. Neurophysiol., 1972*a*, *35*, 542–559.

Goldberg, M. E., and Wurtz, R. H. Activity of superior colliculus in behaving monkey. II. Effect of attention on neuronal responses. *J. Neurophysiol.*, 1972*b*, *35*, 560–574.

Gordon, B. Receptive fields in deep layers of cat superior colliculus. *J. Neurophysiol.*, 1973, *36*, 157–178.

Graybiel, A. M. Some fiber pathways related to the posterior thalamic region in the cat. *Brain Behav. Evol.*, 1972*a*, *6*, 363–393.

Graybiel, A. M. Some extrageniculate visual pathways in the cat. *Invest. Opthalmol.*, 1972*b*, *11*, 322–332.

Graybiel, A. M. Visuo-cerebellar and cerebello-visual connections involving the ventral lateral geniculate nucleus. *Exp. Brain Res.*, 1974, *20*, 303–306.

Graybiel, A. M. Anatomical organization of retinotectal afferents in the cat: An autoradiographic study, *Brain Res.*, 1975, *96*, 1–23.

Hamilton, B. L. Projections of the nuclei of the periaqueductal gray matter in the cat. *J. Comp. Neurol.*, 1973, *152*, 45–58.

Harting, J. K., Hall, W. C., Diamond, I. T., and Martin, G. F. Anterograde degeneration study of the superior colliculus in *Tupaia glis*: Evidence for a subdivision between superficial and deep layers. *J. Comp. Neurol.*, 1973, *148*, 361–386.

Harutiunian-Kozak, B., Kozak, W., and Dec, K. Visually-evoked potentials and single unit activity in the superior colliculus of the cat. *Acta Neurobiol. Exp.*, 1970, *30*, 211–232.

Hayaishi, Y. Recurrent collateral inhibition of visual cortical cells projecting to superior colliculus in cats. *Vision Res.*, 1969, *9*, 1367–1380.

Hayaishi, Y., Nagata, T., Tamaki, Y., and Iwama, K. Binocular interaction in the superior colliculus of chronic cats. *Exp. Brain Res.*, 1973, *18*, 531–547.

Hécaen, H., and de Ajuriaguerra, J. Balint's syndrome (psychic paralysis of visual fixation) and its minor forms. *Brain*, 1954, *77*, 373–400.

Hendrickson, A., Wilson, M. E., and Toyne, M. J. The distribution of optic nerve fibers in *Macaca mulatta*. *Brain Res.*, 1970, *23*, 425–427.

Hess, W. R., Bürgi, S., and Bucher, V. Motorische Funktion des Tectal- und Tegmentalgebietes. *Psychiat. Neurol.*, 1946, *112*, 1–52.

Hoffman, K.-P. The retinal input to the superior colliculus in the cat. *Invest. Ophthalmol.*, 1972, *11*, 467–470.

Hoffman, K.-P. Conduction velocity in pathways from retina to superior colliculus in the cat: A correlation with receptive-field properties. *J. Neurophysiol*, 1973, *36*, 409–424.

Hoffman, K.-P., and Dreher, B. The spatial organization of the excitatory region of receptive fields in the cat's superior colliculus. *Exp. Brain Res.*, 1973, *16*, 354–370.

Hoffman, K.-P., and Straschill, M. Influences of corticotectal and intertectal connections on visual responses in the cat's superior colliculus. *Exp. Brain Res.*, 1971, *12*, 120–131.

Holländer, H. On the origin of the corticotectal projections in the cat. *Exp. Brain Res.*, 1974, *21*, 433–439.

Horn, G. Novelty, attention and habituation. In C. R. Evans and T. B. Mulholland (eds.), *Attention in Neurophysiology.* Appleton-Century-Crofts, New York, 1969, pp. 230–246.

Horn, G., and Hill, R. H. Responsiveness to sensory stimulation of units in the superior colliculus and subjacent tectotegmental regions of the rabbit. *Exp. Neurol.*, 1966, *14*, 199–223.

Hubel, D. H., and Wiesel, T. N. Receptive fields and functional architecture in two nonstriate visual areas (18 and 19) of the cat. *J. Neurophysiol.*, 1965, *28*, 229–289.

Hubel, D. H., and Wiesel, T. N. Receptive fields and functional architecture of monkey striate cortex. *J. Physiol. (London)*, 1968, *195*, 215–243.

Hubel, D. H., LeVay, S., and Wiesel, T. N. Mode of termination of retinotectal fibers in macaque monkey: An autoradiographic study, *Brain Res.*, 1975, *96*, 25–40.

Humphrey, N. K. Responses to visual stimuli of units in the superior colliculus of rats and monkeys. *Exp. Neurol.*, 1968, *20*, 312–340.

Ikeda, H., and Wright, M. J. The outer disinhibitory surround of the retinal ganglion cell receptive field. *J. Physiol. (London)*, 1972, *226*, 511–544.

Ingle, D. Evolutionary perspectives on the function of the optic tectum. *Brain Behav. Evol.*, 1973, *8*, 211–237.

Jane, J. A., Levey, N., and Carlson, N. J. Tectal and cortical function in vision. *Exp. Neurol.*, 1972, *35*, 61–77.

Jassik-Gerschenfeld, D. Activity of somatic origin evoked in the superior colliculus of the cat. *Exp. Neurol.*, 1966, *16*, 104–118.

Kadoya, S., Wolin, L. R., and Massopust, L. C., Jr. Photically evoked unit activity in the tectum opticum of the squirrel monkey. *J. Comp. Neurol.*, 1971*a*, *142*, 495–508.

Kadoya, S., Wolin, L. R., and Massopust, L. C., Jr. Collicular unit responses to monochromatic stimulation in squirrel monkey. *Brain Res.*, 1971*b*, *32*, 251–254.

Kadoya, S., Massopust, L. C., Jr., and Wolin, L. R. Striate cortex–superior colliculus projections in squirrel monkey. *Exp. Neurol.*, 1971*c*, *32*, 98–110.

Kanaseki, T., and Sprague, J. M. Anatomical organization of pretectal and tectal laminae in the cat. *J. Comp. Neurol.*, 1974, *158*, 319–337.

Kawamura, K., and Brodal, A. The tectopontine projection in the cat: An experimental anatomical study with comments on pathways for teleceptive impulses to the cerebellum. *J. Comp. Neurol.*, 1973, *149*, 371–390.

Kawamura, K., Brodal, A., and Hoddevik, G. The projection of the superior colliculus onto the reticular formation of the brain stem: An experimental anatomical study in the cat. *Exp. Brain Res.*, 1974*a*, *19*, 1–19.

Kawamura, S., Sprague, J. M., and Niimi, K. Corticofugal projections from the visual cortices to the thalamus, pretectum and superior colliculus in the cat. *J. Comp. Neurol.*, 1974*b*, *158*, 339–362.

Keating, E. G. Impaired orientation after primate tectal lesions. *Brain Res.*, 1974, *67*, 538–541.

Keller, E. L. Participation of medial pontine reticular formation in eye movement generation in monkey. *J. Neurophysiol.*, 1974, *37*, 316–332.

Kuhlenbeck, H., and Miller, R. N. The pretectal region of the rabbit's brain. *J. Comp. Neurol.*, 1942, *76*, 323–365.

Kuypers, H. G. J. M. Discussion. In V. B. Mountcastle (ed.), *Cerebral Dominance and Interhemispheric Relations.* 1962, pp. 114–116. Johns Hopkins Press, Baltimore.

Kuypers, H. G. J. M., and Lawrence, D. G. Cortical projections to the red nucleus and the brain stem in the rhesus monkey. *Brain Res.*, 1967, *4*, 151–188.

Lane, R. H., Allman, J. M., and Kaas, J. H. Representation of the visual field in the superior colliculus of the gray squirrel (*Sciurus carolinensis*) and the tree shrew (*Tupaia glis*). *Brain Res.*, 1971, *26*, 277–292.

Lane, R. H., Allman, J. M., Kaas, J. H., and Miezin, F. M. The visuotopic organization of the superior colliculus of the owl monkey (*Aotus trivirgatus*) and the bush baby (*Galago senegalensis*). *Brain Res.*, 1973, *60*, 335–349.

Lane, R. H., Kaas, J. H., and Allman, J. M. Visuotopic organization of the superior colliculus in normal and siamese cats. *Brain Res.*, 1974, *70*, 413–430.

Lund, R. D. Synaptic patterns in the superficial layers of the superior colliculus of the monkey. *Macaca mulatta. Exp. Brain Res.*, 1972, *15*, 194–211.

Luria, A. R. Disorders of "simultaneous perception" in a case of bilateral occipito-parietal brain injury. *Brain*, 1959, *82*, 437–449.

Luschei, E. S., and Fuchs, A. F. Activity of brain stem neurons during eye movements of alert monkeys. *J. Neurophysiol.*, 1972, *35*, 445–461.

Manni, E., Palmieri, G., and Marini, R. Mesodiencephalic representation of the eye muscle proprioception. *Exp. Neurol.*, 1972, *37*, 412–421.

Marchiafava, P. L., and Pepeu, G. The responses of units in the superior colliculus of the cat to a moving visual stimulus. *Experientia*, 1966, *22*, 51–53.

Masland, R. H., Chow, K. L., and Stewart, D. L. Receptive-field characteristics of superior colliculus neurons in the rabbit. *J. Neurophysiol.*, 1971, *34*, 148–156.

Mathers, L. H. Tectal projection to the posterior thalamus of the squirrel monkey. *Brain Res.*, 1971, *35*, 295–298.

McIlwain, J. T. Topographic relationships in projection from striate cortex to superior colliculus of the cat. *J. Neurophysiol.*, 1973a, *36*, 690–701.

McIlwain, J. T. Retinotopic fidelity of striate cortex–superior colliculus interactions in the cat. *J. Neurophysiol.*, 1973b, *36*, 702–710.

McIlwain, J. T. Visual receptive fields and their images in superior colliculus of the cat. *J. Neurophysiol.*, 1975, *38*, 219–230.

McIlwain, J. T., and Buser, P. Receptive fields of single cells in the cat's superior colliculus. *Exp. Brain Res.*, 1968, *5*, 314–325.

McIlwain, J. T., and Fields, H. L. Interactions of cortical and retinal projections on single neurons of the cat's superior colliculus. *J. Neurophysiol.*, 1971, *34*, 763–772.

Mehler, W. R. Some neurological species differences—*a posteriori*. *Ann. N.Y. Acad. Sci.*, 1969, *167*, 424–468.

Michael, C. R. Visual receptive fields of single neurons in superior colliculus of the ground squirrel. *J. Neurophysiol.*, 1972a, *35*, 815–832.

Michael, C. R. Functional organization of cells in superior colliculus of the ground squirrel. *J. Neurophysiol.*, 1972b, *35*, 833–846.

Mohler, C. W., and Wurtz, R. H. Organization of monkey superior colliculus: Intermediate layer cells discharging before eye movements. *J. Neurophysiol.*, 1976a, *39*, 722–744.

Mohler, C. W., and Wurtz, R. H. Role of striate cortex and superior colliculus in the visual guidance of saccadic eye movements in the monkey. *J. Neurophysiol.*, 1976b, *40*, 74–94.

Moore, R. Y., and Goldberg, J. M. Ascending projections of the inferior colliculus in the cat. *J. Comp. Neurol.*, 1963, *129*, 109–135.

Moore, R. Y., and Goldberg, J. M. Projections of the inferior colliculus in the monkey. *Exp. Neurol.*, 1966, *14*, 429-438.

Myers, R. E. Projections of superior colliculus in monkey. *Anat. Rec.*, 1963a, *145*, 264.

Myers, R. E. Cortical projections to midbrain in monkey. *Anat. Rec.*, 1963b, *145*, 337–338.

Nauta, W. J. H., and Kuypers, H. G. J. M. Some ascending pathways in the brainstem reticular formation. In H. H. Jasper, L. D. Proctor, R. S. Knighton, W. C. Noshay, and R. T. Costello (eds.), *Reticular Formation of the Brain*. Little, Brown, Boston, 1958, pp. 3–30.

Niimi, K., Miki, M., and Kawamura, S. Ascending projections of the superior colliculus in the cat. *Okajimas Fol. Anat. Jap.*, 1970, *47*, 269–287.

Nyberg-Hansen, R. The location and termination of tectospinal fibers in the cat. *Exp. Neurol.*, 1964, *9*, 212–227.

Olszewski, J., and Baxter, D. *Cytoarchetecture of the Human Brain Stem.* Karger, Basel, 1954.

Palmer, L. A., and Rosenquist, A. C. Visual receptive fields of single striate cortical units projecting to the superior colliculus in the cat. *Brain Res.*, 1974, *67*, 27–42.

Pasik, T., Pasik, P., and Bender, M. B. The superior colliculi and eye movements. *Arch. Neurol.*, 1966, *15*, 420–436.

Paula-Barbosa, M. M., and Sousa-Pinto, A. Auditory cortical projections to the superior colliculus in the cat. *Brain Res.,* 1973, *30*, 47–61.

Peterson, B. W., Anderson, M. E., Fillion, M., and Wilson, V. J. Responses of reticulospinal neurons to stimulation of the superior colliculus. *Brain Res.*, 1971, *33*, 495–498.

Powell, E. W., and Hatton, J. B. Projections of the inferior colliculus in cat. *J. Comp. Neurol.*, 1969, *136*, 183–192.

Precht, W., Schwindt, P. C., and Magherini, P. C. Tectal influences on cat ocular motoneurons. *Brain Res.*, 1974, *82*, 27–40.

Ramon y Cajal, S. *Histologie du Systeme de l'Homme et des Vertebres,* Vol. 2. A. Maloine, Paris, 1911.

Richard, D., Thiery, J.-C., and Buser, P. Cortical control of the superior colliculus in awake non-paralyzed cats. *Brain Res.*, 1973, *58*, 524–528.

Rieger, P., and Straschill, M. The effect of body tilt upon the transfer and output function of the cat's superior colliculus. *Pflügers Arch.*, 1973, *344*, 187–193.

Rioch, D. M. Studies on the diencephalon of carnivora. Part I. The nuclear configuration of the dog and cat. *J. Comp. Neurol.*, 1929, *49*, 1–119.

Rizzolatti, G., Tradardi, V., and Camarda, R. Unit responses to visual stimuli in the cat's superior colliculus after removal of the visual cortex. *Brain Res.*, 1973, *24*, 336–339.

Rizzolatti, G., Camarda, R., Grupp, L. A., and Pisa, M. Inhibitory effect of remote visual stimuli on visual responses on cat superior colliculus: Spatial and temporal factors. *J. Neurophysiol.*, 1975, *37*, 1262–1275.

Robinson, D. A. Eye movements evoked by collicular stimulation in the alert monkey. *Vision Res.*, 1972, *12*, 1795–1808.

Robinson, D. L., and Jarvis, C. D. Superior colliculus neurons studied during head and eye movements of the behaving monkey. *J. Neurophysiol.*, 1974, *37*, 933–940.

Robinson, D. L., and Wurtz, R. H. Use of an extraretinal signal by monkey superior colliculus neurons to distinguish real from self-induced stimulus movement. *J. Neurophysiol.*, 1976, *39*, 852–870.

Rose, J. E., and Woolsey, C. N. Cortical connections and functional organization of the thalamic auditory system in the cat. In H. F. Harlow and C. N. Woolsey (eds)., *Biological and Biochemical Bases of Behavior.* University of Wisconsin Press, Madison, Wis., 1958, pp. 127–150.

Rosenquist, A. C., and Palmer, L. A. Visual receptive fields of cells of the superior colliculus after cortical lesions in the cat. *Exp. Neurol.*, 1971, *33*, 629–652.

Rosvold, H. E., Mishkin, M., and Szwarcbart, M. K. Effects of subcortical lesions in monkeys on visual-discrimination and single alternation performance. *J. Comp. Physiol. Psychol.*, 1958, *51*, 437–444.

Schaeffer, K.-P. Mikroableitungen in Tectum opticum des frie beweglichen Kaninchens. *Arch. Psychiat. Ges. Neurol.*, 1966, *208*, 120–146.

Schaeffer, K.-P. Neuronal elements of the orienting response: Microrecordings and stimulation experiments in rabbits. *Bibl. Ophthalmol.*, 1972, *82*, 139–148.

Schiller, P. H. The role of the monkey superior colliculus in eye movement and vision. *Invest. Opthalmol.*, 1972, *11*, 451–460.

Schiller, P. H., and Koerner, F. Discharge characteristics of single units in superior colliculus of the alert rhesus monkey. *J. Neurophysiol.*, 1971, *34*, 920–936.

Schiller, P. H., and Stryker, M. P. Single-unit recording and stimulation in superior colliculus of the alert rhesus monkey. *J. Neurophysiol.*, 1972, *35*, 915–924.

Schiller, P. H., Stryker, M. P., Cynader, M., and Berman, N. Response characteristics of single cells in the monkey superior colliculus following ablation or cooling of visual cortex. *J. Neurophysiol.*, 1974, *37*, 181–194.

Schneider, G. E. Two visual systems: Brain mechanisms for localization and discrimination are dissociated by tectal and cortical lesions. *Science*, 1969, *163*, 895–902.

Sherman, S. M. Visual fields of cats with cortical and tectal lesions. *Science*, 1974, *185*, 355–357.

Sparks, D. L. Response properties of eye movement-related neurons in the monkey superior colliculus. *Brain Res.*, 1975, *90*, 147–152.

Spatz, W. B., Tigges, J., and Tigges, M. Subcortical projections, cortical association and some intrinsic interlaminar connections of the striate cortex in the squirrel monkey (*Saimiri*). *J. Comp. Neurol.*, 1970, *140*, 155–174.

Sprague, J. M. Corticofugal projections to the superior colliculus in the cat. *Anat. Rec.*, 1963, *145*, 288.

Sprague, J. M. Interaction of cortex and superior colliculus in mediation of visually guided behavior in the cat. *Science*, 1966, *153*, 1544–1547.

Sprague, J. M. Mammalian tectum: Intrinsic organization, afferent inputs and integrative mechanisms. Anatomical substrate. *Neurosci. Res. Progr. Sensorimotor Function the Midbrain Tectum*, 1975, *13*, 204–213.

Sprague, J. M., and Meikle, T. H., Jr. The role of the superior colliculus in visually guided behavior. *Exp. Neurol.*, 1965, *11*, 115–146.

Sprague, J. M., Levitt, M., Robson, K., Liu, C. N., Stellar, E., and Chambers, W. W. A neuroanatomical and behavioral analysis of the syndromes resulting from midbrain lemniscal and reticular lesions in the cat. *Arch. Ital. Biol.*, 1963, *101*, 225–295.

Sprague, J. M., Marchiafava, P. L., and Rizzolatti, G. Unit responses to visual stimuli in the superior colliculus of the unanesthetized, mid-pontine cat. *Arch. Ital. Biol.*, 1968, *106*, 169–193.

Sprague, J. M., Berlucchi, G., and Rizzolatti, G. The role of the superior colliculus and pretectum in vision and visually guided behavior. In R. Jung (ed.), *Handbook of Sensory Physiology*, Vol. VIII/B. Springer-Verlag, Berlin, 1972, pp. 27–101.

Stein, B. E., and Arigbede, M. O. Unimodal and multimodal response properties of neurons in the cat's superior colliculus. *Exp. Neurol.*, 1972, *36*, 179–196.

Stein, B. E., Magalhaes-Castro, B., and Kruger, L. Superior colliculus: Visuotopic–somatotopic overlap. *Science*, 1975, *189*, 224–226.

Sterling, P. Receptive fields and synaptic organization of the superficial gray layer of the cat superior colliculus. *Vision Res. Suppl. No. 3*, 1971, 309–328.

Sterling, P., and Wickelgren, B. G. Visual receptive fields in the superior colliculus of the cat. *J. Neurophysiol.*, 1969, *32*, 1–15.

Stewart, D. L., Birt, D., and Towns, L. C. Visual receptive-field characteristics of superior colliculus neurons after cortical lesions in the rabbit. *Vision Res.*, 1973, *13*, 1965–1977.

Stone, J., and Hoffman, K.-P. Very slow-conducting ganglion cells in the cat's retina: A major new, functional type? *Brain Res.*, 1972, *43*, 610–616.

Straschill, M., and Hoffman, K.-P. Functional aspects of localization in the cat's tectum opticum. *Brain Res.*, 1969, *13*, 274–283.

Straschill, M., and Hoffman, K.-P. Activity of movement sensitive neurons of the cat's tectum opticum during spontaneous eye movements. *Exp. Brain Res.*, 1970, *11*, 318–326.

Straschill, M., and Rieger, P. Eye movements evoked by focal stimulation of the cat's superior colliculus. *Brain Res.*, 1973, *59*, 211–227.

Straschill, M., and Taghavy, A. Neuronale Reaktionen im Tectum opticum der Katze auf bewegte und stationäre Lichtreize. *Exp. Brain Res.*, 1967, *3*, 353–367.

Stryker, M. P., and Schiller, P. H. Eye and head movements evoked by electrical stimulation of monkey superior colliculus. *Exp. Brain Res.*, 1975, *23*, 103–112.

Syka, J., and Radil-Weiss, T. Electrical stimulation of the tectum in freely moving cats. *Brain Res.*, 1971, *28*, 567–572.

Thompson, R., and Myers, R. E. Brainstem mechanisms underlying visually guided responses in the rhesus monkey. *J. Comp. Physiol. Psychol.*, 1971, *74*, 479–512.

Toyama, K., Matsunami, K., and Ohno, T. Antidromic identification of association, commissural and corticofugal efferent cells in cat visual cortex. *Brain Res.*, 1969, *14*, 513–517.

Tyler, H. R. Abnormalities of perception with defective eye movements. *Cortex*, 1968, *4*, 154–171.

Updyke, B. V. Characteristics of unit responses in superior colliculus of the cebus monkey. *J. Neurophysiol.*, 1974, *37*, 896-909.

Viktorov, I. V. Neuronal structure of anterior corpora bigemina in insectivora and rodents. *Arkh. Anat. Gistol. Embriol.*, 1966, *51*, 82–89.

Viktorov, I. V. Neuronal structure of superior colliculi of corpora quadrigemina. *Arkh. Anat. Gistol. Embriol.*, 1968, *54*, 45–55.

Wickelgren, B. G., and Sterling, P. Influence of visual cortex on receptive fields in the superior colliculus of the cat. *J. Neurophysiol.*, 1969, *32*, 16–23.

Wilson, P. D., and Stone, J. Evidence of W-cell input to the cat's visual cortex via the C laminae of the lateral geniculate nucleus. *Brain Res.*, 1975, *92*, 472–478.

Wilson, M. E., and Toyne, M. J. Retino-tectal and cortico-tectal projections in *Macaca mulatta*. *Brain Res.*, 1970, *24*, 395–406.

Winterkorn, J. M. S. Similar deficits in visual learning by cats with lesions of the frontal cortex or of the superior colliculus. *Brain Res.*, 1975, *83*, 163-168.

Wood, B. S. Monocular relearning of a dark–light discrimination by cats after unilateral cortical and collicular lesions. *Brain Res.*, 1975, *83*, 156–162.

Wurtz, R. H., and Goldberg, M. E. Superior colliculus cell responses related to eye movements in awake monkeys. *Science*, 1971, *171*, 82–84.

Wurtz, R. H., and Goldberg, M. E. Activity of superior colliculus in behaving monkey. III. Cells discharging before eye movements. *J. Neurophysiol.*, 1972a, *35*, 575–586.

Wurtz, R. H., and Goldberg, M. E. Activity of superior colliculus in behaving monkey. IV. Effects of lesions on eye movements. *J. Neurophysiol.*, 1972b, *35*, 587–596.

Wurtz, R. H., and Goldberg, M. E. The primate superior colliculus and the shift of visual attention. *Invest. Ophthalmol.*, 1972c, *11*, 441–450.

Wurtz, R. H., and Mohler, C. W. Organization of monkey superior colliculus: Enhanced visual response of superficial layer cells. *J. Neurophysiol.*, 1976a, *39*, 745–765.

Wurtz, R. H., and Mohler, C. W. Enhancement of visual response in monkey striate cortex and frontal eye fields. *J. Neurophysiol.*, 1976b, *39*, 766–772.

6

Vision: Geniculocortical System

MARK BERKLEY

INTRODUCTION

This chapter is concerned with the functions of some neural structures involved in vision. It does not cover all aspects of vision nor all the neural structures that may be involved in vision. It is limited to a consideration of a portion of the visual system called the *geniculocortical system*. For the purposes of this chapter, the geniculocortical system is defined as: (1) the peripheral receptor apparatus (retina); (2) the thalamic region receiving input from the retina and (3) the region of cerebral cortex receiving a direct input from the thalamus (cf. Chapters 5 and 7).

The emphasis of the chapter is on the functional aspects of the CNS portions of the system; structure and electrophysiological properties will only be considered insofar as it is useful in assessing the functional analysis. The peripheral portion of this system (retina) will only be incidentally considered. The reader is directed to several excellent sources which consider the retina in anatomical and physiological detail (Polyak, 1948; Dowling and Boycott, 1966; Dowling, 1970; Brindley, 1970; Boycott and Dowling, 1969; Rodieck, 1973). Some details, however, regarding the retina will be presented to provide the framework for the discussion of the CNS structures.

While considerable progress has been made recently in the physiological and anatomical examination of the visual system, there still remains to be developed a general conceptual system that would permit the understanding of the visual process. Recent electrophysiological findings have indicated that a simple pictorial representation in the brain is an unsatisfactory model both on logical and on physiological grounds (Pitts and McCulloch, 1947; Barlow, 1969, 1972*a,b*). Most investigators and theorists now agree that some sort of abstraction process occurs

---

MARK BERKLEY   Department of Psychology, Florida State University, Tallahassee, Florida 32306.

within the nervous system so that only certain features or invariants of the visual scene are extracted from the image on the retina, passed on to the central nervous system, and then "reconstructed" into a visual percept. For the most part, there is general agreement that vision represents such a process within the neural visual system. The major disagreement among investigators appears to be with regard to the type of features being abstracted. Thus some claim that the abstracted features consist of the contours of the images (e.g., Barlow, 1972*b*; Hubel and Wiesel, 1965*b*) while others believe that the features may be spatial frequency components of the image (Campbell and Robson, 1968; Pollen *et al.*, 1971). While it is probably true that none of the theories currently being proposed is correct, they are not mutually exclusive and all have in common the idea of feature abstraction.

Anatomy of the Geniculocortical System

Retina

The synaptic networks and cells prior to the *ganglion cells* in the retina are not covered in this chapter and the reader is referred to several excellent sources on this subject (e.g., Dowling and Boycott, 1966; Boycott and Dowling, 1969). The discussion begins with ganglion cells. In his pioneering studies, Ramon y Cajal (1892) classified the output cells of the retina, ganglion cells, into several morphological types based on Golgi stained material. His classification scheme remained dormant for a considerable number of years until the recent attempts at morphological classification made by Dowling and Boycott (1966) and Boycott and Dowling (1969), Boycott and Wässle (1974). These studies are particularly interesting because of recent electrophysiological discoveries indicating at least a three-way differentiation among ganglion cells. This differentiation has encouraged investigators to attempt morphological correlations (Boycott and Wässle, 1974; Cleland and Levick, 1974*a*; Fukuda and Stone, 1975). While Cajal's (1892) early studies distinguished ganglion cell types on cell body size and dendritic arborization and branching levels within the retina, the more recent studies have used these characteristics of ganglion cells but have relied most heavily on cell body and dendritic field size as the major classification criteria (e.g., Leicester and Stone, l967; Boycott and Wässle, 1974; Shkolnik-Yarros, 1971*a*, 1971*b*; Wässle, Levick and Cleland, 1975; Stone and Hollander, 1971).

Fibers Leaving the Retina

The ganglion cells within the retina send axons out of the retina in the optic nerve. Most if not all of the fibers leaving the retina synapse in the *lateral geniculate nucleus* (Polyak, 1957).

In their traverse from the retina into the brain, some fibers cross the midline and some do not, depending on their locus of origin within the retina. Thus in primates all fibers originating from ganglion cells in the nasal retina cross the midline to enter the opposite hemisphere whereas fibers originating from cells residing in temporal retina remain on the same side (Polyak, 1957; Hayhow, 1958;

Stone, 1966). Among mammals in general, the percentage of the total number of fibers which do not cross appears to be related to the percentage of overlap of the visual fields between the two eyes (Walls, 1942). Thus animals with more frontally placed eyes appear to have a greater percentage of fibers not crossing than those with more laterally placed eyes. This rule appears to hold only for mammals and was named the "Newton–Müller–Gudden law" by Walls (1942) in his classic monograph.

Recent work has shown this generalization to be less correct than originally believed in that certain classes of ganglion cells (e.g., "W" ganglion cells; see below) in the cat retina do not follow this decussation rule (Stone and Fukuda, 1974*b*).

LATERAL GENICULATE NUCLEUS

The major recipient of retinal output in the thalamus is the *lateral geniculate nucleus pars dorsalis* (LGN$_D$). The LGN$_D$ is usually a laminated structure, with the number of overt laminae in different animals varying from three to six (Doty *et al.*, 1966; Kanagasuntheram *et al.*, 1969; Kaas *et al.*, 1972*a*; Sanderson, 1974; see also Chapter 2). Differences in cell body size between laminae have been noted by a number of investigators, and serve to differentiate the laminae into those having large cells (magnocellular) and those having small cells (parvocellular) (Kupfer, 1965; Doty *et al.*, 1966; Walls, 1953) (see Fig. 1).

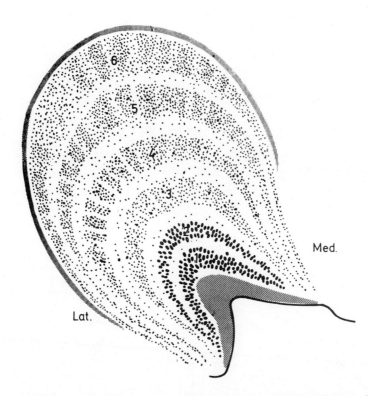

Fig. 1. Semidiagrammatic coronal section of the LGN of the monkey, showing laminar distribution of cells and cell sizes. Note two magnocellular layers (1 and 2) and four parvocellular layers (3,4,5 and 6). From Szentogothai (1973) with permission.

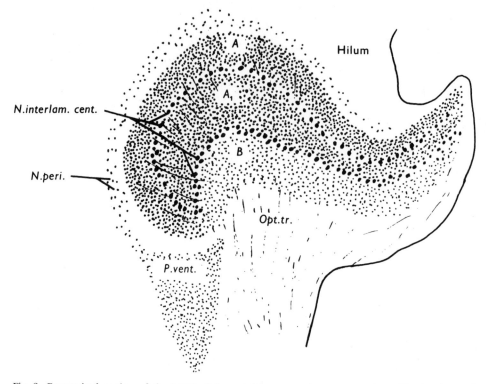

Fig. 2. Parasagittal section of the LGN of the cat. Diagrammatic representation of lamination and distribution of cell sizes. Laminae are labeled A, A₁, and B. Opt.tr., Optic tract; N.peri., nucleus perigeniculatus; P.vent., pars ventralis; N.interlam.cent., nucleus interlaminaris centralis. From Peters and Palay (1966), with permission.

Each lamina receives an input from the retina, and while the exact arrangement of this input is not perfectly understood (e.g., extent of synaptic contact) it is clear that within any particular portion of the LGN the same retinal afferent probably projects to the different laminae along a line perpendicular to the laminae (Kaas *et al.*, 1972*a*) (Fig. 2). Each lamina receives input from only one eye (Stone and Hansen, 1966; Le Gros Clark and Penman, 1934; Glees, 1941; Hayhow, 1958), there being no evidence for direct binocular input from the retina to any of the laminae. Thus in the monkey, which has a six-layered lateral geniculate, layers 2, 3, and 5 receive input from the ipsilateral eye and 1, 4, and 6 receive input from the contralateral eye (Le Gros Clark, 1941; Matthews *et al.*, 1960; Kanagasuntheram *et al.*, 1969).

In the cat, where the layering scheme of Thuma (1928) and of Guillery (1970) is commonly in use, layer A receives input from the contralateral eye while layer A₁ receives input from the ipsilateral eye. Layer B and the subdivisions of C may receive inputs from the ipsilateral eye as well (Garey and Powell, 1968). While there is no evidence that there are binocular inputs from the two retinas in each lamina, there is evidence for binocular interaction mediated by an indirect route, which will be discussed in a later section on electrophysiological properties.

In addition to the retinal inputs discussed above, there is evidence for a major corticofugal input to the lateral geniculate from visual cortex (Szentagothai, 1973;

Beresford, 1962; Guillery, 1966; Updyke, 1975; Wong-Riley, 1972; Holländer and Martinez-Millan, 1975).

169

VISION:
GENICULOCORTICAL
SYSTEM

Cortical Target Zone of LGN Fibers

The fibers originating from cells residing in the dorsal lateral geniculate nucleus project to a restricted zone of neocortex variously known as *striate cortex, area 17,* or *visual cortex.* (For purposes of this discussion, these terms will be used interchangeably, although their precise definitions are quite different.) In primates, the cortical recipient zone of the lateral geniculate fibers is distinguished by a fiber band in layer 4, the *line of Gennari* (Polyak, 1957). This stripe is less obvious in other animals such as the cat (O'Leary, 1941; Otsuka and Hassler, 1962; Sanides and Hoffmann, 1969). It can, however, be distinguished in most mammals.

In most mammals, with the exception of the cat and possibly the rabbit, cells originating in the lateral geniculate nucleus synapse primarily in layer 4 of striate cortex and can be subdivided to some extent in terms of their level of termination within the striate cortex (Hubel and Wiesel, 1969, 1972). In the monkey, for example, there seems to be some differentiation between ipsilateral and contralateral projections within layer 4 (Hubel and Wiesel, 1972). In the tree shrew, however, several investigators have shown that there is a laminar distribution of afferents in the visual cortex rather than a columnar arrangement as has been found in primates and cats (Harting *et al.*, 1973; Casagrande and Harting, 1975; Hubel, 1975). The significance of this laminar organization is yet to be understood.

In the cat, the projection system from lateral geniculate to cortex is quite different from that in primates. In addition to the projection to striate cortex, cells in the LGN project to the adjacent areas 18 and 19 and to a still more lateral zone, the *lateral suprasylvian area* (Garey and Powell, 1967; Glickstein *et al.*, 1967; Glickstein, 1969; Burrows and Hayhow, 1971; Niimi and Sprague, 1970; Wilson and Cragg, 1967). In addition to this peculiarity, the cat has a number of other nuclear groups which behave as separate subdivisions of lateral geniculate and also project to cortex, e.g., nucleus interlaminalis medialis, nucleus interlaminalis centralis, and posterior nucleus (Niimi and Sprague, 1970; Burrows and Hayhow, 1971). The homologues of these nuclei in primates or other mammals are not known.

Physiology of the Geniculocortical System

Properties of Ganglion Cells

While a detailed description of the physiology of ganglion cells is beyond the scope of this chapter, a brief summary of the important features of retinal physiology will be presented. The reader is referred to the excellent review by Rodieck (1973) for more complete details.

In mammals, the majority of ganglion cell receptive fields are of a concentric center-surround type (Kuffler, 1953; Barlow *et al.*, 1957; Rodieck, 1965). Thus a ganglion cell may respond at either the onset or the offset of a stimulus placed on its center while the opposite response will be elicited by stimulation of the surround. While this receptive field type represents the major type found in all mammalian retinas, there are some other types. In rabbits, for example, there are cells that respond differentially to the direction of movement of a visual target (Barlow and Levick, 1965; Barlow *et al.*, 1964). Still other cells respond to changes in levels of illumination and do not have subdivided receptive fields. Such receptive fields have also been described in the cat (e.g., Kuffler, 1953; Barlow and Levick, 1969). In animals with duplex retinas or all-cone retinas, the center-surround receptive field may be further described as color opponent as well as spatially opponent. Thus the center may respond to the onset of a red spot and the surround to offset of a green stimulus. The reader is referred to Gouras (1968) for details of the color organization.

Several investigators have suggested different roles for the "on" center cells and "off" center cells. Jung (1973) has proposed that the temporal response cells may provide information about brightness and darkness while their spatial organization may provide information about contours.

In Kuffler's (1953) original study of the receptive field properties of cat retinal ganglion cells, he described the major features (except for color) of ganglion cell receptive fields as they are currently known. One property which he mentioned has been elaborated recently and has proved to be particularly important (Enroth-Cugell and Robson, 1966). This property may be described as a difference in temporal response characteristics among ganglion cells. Kuffler (1953) described cells that tend to discharge phasically with the stimulus while others respond with a more sustained discharge. Enroth-Cugell and Robson (1966) extended this observation considerably and were able to classify ganglion cells in two major functional groups which they called *X cells* and *Y cells*. Using moving gratings with a sinusoidal luminance profile, they found that X cells tend to respond continuously during the presentation of the drifting grating while Y cells respond in a way that follows the contrast variations in the target. Another criterion that distinguishes these two classes of ganglion cells, is linear summation in the center for the X type but not for the Y type. Using other tests, Fukuda (1971) classified ganglion cells into *type I* and *type II* and Cleland *et al.* (1971*b*, 1973; Cleland and Levick, 1974*a,b*) classified them into *transient* and *sustained* types which are likely correlated with the X and Y classes proposed by Enroth-Cugell and Robson (1966).

Another procedure found to be correlated with the functional classes described above has been used to classify ganglion cell types. Fukuda (1971), for example, and Cleland *et al.* (1971*b*) have found that ganglion cell fibers in the optic tract may be subdivided according to their conduction velocity and that cells with fast conduction velocities (>30 m/sec) are generally of the Y type while fibers with slower conduction velocities (<25 m/sec) tend to be of the X type. Attempts at correlating these properties with ganglion cell morphological characteristics have also been made (Boycott and Wässle, 1974; Wässle *et al.*, 1975).

Recently, a third category of ganglion cells has been recognized and named *W cells* (Stone and Hoffmann, 1972; Levick and Cleland, 1974*a*). Cells of this type have relatively large, unstructured receptive fields, respond to overall luminance changes, and have slow-conducting fibers (Stone and Hoffmann, 1972; Cleland and Levick, 1974a). Such cells had been described before (Stone and Hoffmann, 1972; Stone and Fabian, 1966; Rodieck, 1967; Fukuda, 1971) but not recognized as a separate class. This may have occurred because W-type cells are small and were missed because of sampling biases related to electrode size (Levick and Cleland, 1974b; Stone, 1973).

The earlier classification of receptive fields ("on" center, "off" center) cuts across the X and Y classification scheme as there seem to be all combinations of X and Y and on and off centers (Ikeda and Wright, 1972). Furthermore, the distribution of X and Y cells appears to vary across the retina, there being proportionally more X cells in central vision than in the periphery (Stone and Fukuda, 1974b). But perhaps the most surprising aspect of these recent discoveries concerns the W cells. While all X and most Y cells appear to obey the traditional rules for decussation in the optic chiasma, W cells in the cat do not. W cells from both nasal and temporal retina project to both sides (Stone and Fukuda, 1974b). The significance of this arrangement is not yet known.

PROPERTIES OF LATERAL GENICULATE CELLS

TOPOGRAPHIC ORGANIZATION OF LGN. In all species thus far studied, a systematic, orderly projection has been observed in the retinal input to LGN (Kaas *et al.*, 1972a). The map for the major mammalian species studied, the cat, is shown in Fig. 3. Basically, each lamina of the LGN contains a topographic map of the visual field, and receives its input from only one eye. The laminar maps are all in register so that if a pin were inserted perpendicular to the spatial plane of the layers representing some point in the visual field, the point in visual space would be the same in all layers even though in different eyes. The laminar arrangement of the LGN is, as mentioned in the discussion of its anatomy, limited to the binocular portions of the visual field (Kaas *et al.*, 1972a). Representation of the monocular segment is in the nonlaminar portion of the nucleus. The topographic

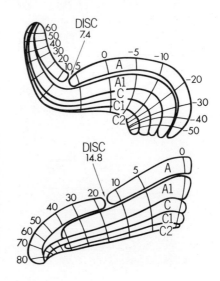

Fig. 3. Schematic representation of the visuotopic organization of the LGN of the cat. Upper: parasagittal section, anterior to right, showing lines of projection corresponding to degrees above and below the horizontal meridian. Layers named according to Guillery (1970). Lower: coronal section, medial to right, showing lines of projection corresponding to degrees of eccentricity along the horizontal meridian. Note break in lamina A locus of optic disk projection. From Kaas *et al.* (1972), with permission.

representation of the visual field is rigidly preserved to the extent that the representation of the retina's optic disk in LGN may be seen as a zone of lowered neuron density (see Fig. 3). The discovery of this landmark is useful in estimating field representations in different animals (Kaas *et al.,* 1972*a*, 1973).

As noted in the anatomical description of LGN, while cell type and density vary somewhat between layers, they are remarkably uniform within a given layer (Thuma, 1928; Doty *et al.,* 1966; Hayhow, 1958; Jones, 1966). Since the input to LGN is derived from ganglion cells whose density is not uniform in the retina, a two-dimensional transform of the visual field occurs such that a larger proportion of LGN is utilized in the central visual field than for the peripheral field (Bishop *et al.,* 1962). This can be expressed as a ratio of a unit distance in the visual field (e.g., degrees of visual angle) to the distance in the LGN representing that visual field distance (e.g., millimeters). This ratio of degrees per millimeter has been called the *magnification ratio* (Talbot and Marshall, 1941; Daniel and Whitteridge, 1961). It is large for central visual field and progressively smaller with increasing eccentricities. It is unfortunate that the phrase "magnification factor" has been used to describe this transform as it leads to the misconception that central vision is "magnified" in the CNS. If the magnification factor is scaled according to the ganglion cell density, instead of degrees per millimeter, it is very nearly a constant. This fact suggests that the number of neurons innervated by a single ganglion cell is constant (see Fig. 4).

Since the density distribution of ganglion cells in the retina is nearly logarith-

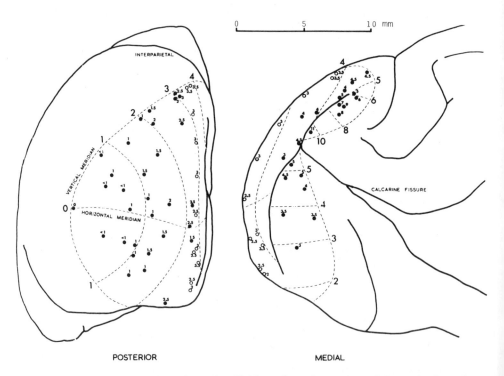

Fig. 4. Visuotopic representation of one hemifield on the striate cortex of the squirrel monkey. Posterior view on the left; mesial view of left hemisphere on right (posterior to the left). Dots and circles are electrode positions used in the mapping procedure. From Cowey (1964), with permission.

mic, the differential representation in LGN can be conceptualized as a log linear transformation of cell density. Such a scheme has been suggested by several investigators, e.g., Bishop *et al.* (1962), Daniel and Whitteridge (1961), Rolls and Cowey (1970), Jacobson (1962), Hubel and Wiesel (1974a), and Berkley (1976), among others. It must be said, however, that this conceptualization will require modification as the details of the distribution of the various cell types, e.g., W cells, in the retina are clarified.

While the visual field is accurately represented in LGN in each lamina, the correspondence of field position between adjacent laminae as well as for adjacent cells within the lamina is not perfect. The representation of a point in visual space has been found to vary slightly from cell to cell in the same column of cells within a lamina. This variation can be described statistically and may have functional consequences in visual cortex (Sanderson, 1971a; Sanderson *et al.*, 1969).

SPATIAL PROPERTIES OF LGN CELLS. For the most part, the spatial characteristics of LGN cells are very similar to the spatial properties of ganglion cells (Hubel and Wiesel, 1961; Wiesel and Hubel, 1966; Sefton and Bruce, 1971). Most receptive fields are of a center-surround type, although there are a significant proportion which are unstructured. At present, it is not clear how the receptive fields of LGN cells are built up from the receptive fields of retinal ganglion cells. Several models have been suggested (Maffei and Fiorentini, 1971, 1972; Cleland *et al.*, 1971a; Singer and Creutzfeldt, 1970) but no one model can account for all the properties currently known to exist for these cells. The simplest model is one that assumes that a single ganglion cell relays onto a single LGN cell and thus invests the LGN cell with its own receptive field properties. Cleland *et al.* (1971a), recording simultaneously from single LGN cells and the input to the cells (e.g., retinal ganglion cells), have demonstrated that at least some LGN cells receive their excitatory input from single ganglion cells while others receive input from only a few ganglion cells.

The surround inhibition in LGN cells is much stronger than that seen in ganglion cells and argues for the presence of an additional mechanism (Wiesel and Hubel, 1966; Singer and Creutzfeldt, 1970). In ganglion cells, surround inhibition drops out when the luminance of the target is lowered (Barlow *et al.*, 1957b) because the threshold for the surround is higher than for the center. However, surround dropout does not occur in LGN cells with luminance reductions (Maffei and Fiorentini, 1972). On the basis of this fact as well as some others, Maffei and Fiorentini (1972) have argued that the surrounds of LGN receptive fields may be made up of the centers of ganglion cells whose response polarity is opposite to that of the ganglion cell(s) feeding the center.

In addition to the traditional surround inhibition, a more extensive suppressive zone has been demonstrated and may extend as much as 5° from the center of the receptive field (McIlwain, 1964, 1966). This suppression is presumed to be mediated by intrageniculate interneurons since such effects cannot be demonstrated in retina. (Several recent reports, however, have claimed distant effects on the receptive fields of retinal ganglion cells, too; e.g., Fischer and Krüger, 1974; Fischer *et al.*, 1975).

TEMPORAL PROPERTIES OF CELLS IN LGN. It is possible to classify groups of cells in LGN according to their temporal response properties just as ganglion cells are classified in the retina. In general, cells have been found in LGN with temporal response properties similar to those described for ganglion cells in the retina (Cleland *et al.,* 1971*b*; Hoffman *et al.,* 1972; Stone and Hoffmann, 1971; Singer and Bedworth, 1973; Ikeda and Wright, 1976). Thus, within each lamina of the LGN of the cat, both X and Y types are found. In the cat, these cell types do not appear to be segregated according to lamina, with perhaps the exception of W cells (Wilson and Stone, 1975). Cells in LGN with X or Y properties have also been described for other animals, e.g., tree shrew (Sherman *et al.,* 1975), monkey (Marrocco and Brown, 1975), and rat (Fukuda, 1973).

Using light sinusoidally modulated in time, the temporal response characteristics of cells in LGN (Maffei and Rizzolatti, 1967; Maffei *et al.,* 1970) have been further described. These studies show that at high modulation frequencies many cells respond like low-pass filters. At low modulation frequencies, however, the simple filter model does not hold in that the response *declines* with still further reduction in frequency, with many cells showing a notch in their response characteristics (e.g., Fukuda and Saito, 1971).

BINOCULAR INTERACTION IN LGN CELLS. Cells in LGN are monocular in the usual sense of the term. That is, there are no excitatory binocular interactions between laminae of LGN (Hubel and Wiesel, 1961; Sanderson, 1971*a,b*). This does not mean, however, that LGN cells are not influenced binocularly. Binocular interactions can be demonstrated by stimulating an LGN cell via one eye and then introducing another stimulus in the same portion of the visual field of the other eye, which, by itself, may not activate the cell. Under such conditions, a reduction in the output of the recorded LGN cell can be observed (Chow *et al.,* 1968; Suzuki and Kato, 1966; Lindsley *et al.,* 1967; Fillenz, 1961; Sanderson *et al.,* 1969, 1971; von Freund *et al.,* 1967). It is not entirely clear whether this effect is mediated via a corticogeniculate pathway or via intrageniculate interlaminar connections (Guillery, 1966; Suzuki and Kato, 1966; Hayhow, 1958; Sanderson *et al.,* 1969, 1971), and there is one report that in unanesthetized preparations, excitatory binocular interactions may be seen (Noda *et al.,* 1972). However, most binocular interactions that have been demonstrated have been inhibitory (e.g., Lindsley *et al.,* 1967; Sanderson *et al.,* 1971). At the present time, it is not known whether these interactions are limited to one cell class or are a common feature of all LGN cells.

COLOR. The color organization found in retinal ganglion cells is also preserved at the LGN (Wiesel and Hubel, 1966; deValois *et al.,* 1967). That is, color opponent cells are common. Both red-green and blue-yellow opponent cells have been found as well as cells that do not respond differentially to color (deValois *et al.,* 1967). These studies have confirmed the view of Walls (1953) that the laminar arrangement in LGN is not concerned with color as suggested by Le Gros Clark (1949). There is some evidence, however, that a large proportion (perhaps all) of the cells in the magnocellular layers of monkey LGN are achromatic (Wiesel and Hubel, 1966).

In the cat, the evidence for color coding in LGN is sparse (Daw and Pearlman, 1970; Pearlman and Daw, l970). The cat has a relatively small number of cones in its retina (Steinberg *et al.,* 1973), and for a long time many workers believed that what color vision the cat did possess was mediated by only one cone type together with the rods (Daw and Pearlman, 1969). Behavioral as well as electrophysiological studies have shown this idea to be incorrect in that two cone types have now been identified (Daw and Pearlman, 1970). The short-wavelength-sensitive cones are, however, very few in number. In cat, unlike monkey, both rods and cones appear to be connected to all ganglion cells (e.g., Barlow *et al.*, 1957*a*).

VARIATION. A common feature among mammals with binocular overlap of the visual fields is lamination of the LGN (Polyak, 1957; Kaas *et al.*, 1972). In some cases the laminar pattern is not obvious and is revealed only through neuroanatomical tracing techniques (e.g., Glickstein, 1967; Doty *et al.*, 1966). In other cases, genetically linked anatomical anomalies obscure the laminar scheme (e.g., Guillery and Kaas, 1971; Guillery *et al.*, 1975). In all cases thus far studied, the segment of LGN in which the monocular segment of the visual field is represented is not laminated (Kaas *et al.*, 1972).

Another common feature of the LGN is the differential distribution of anatomical cell types (Polyak, 1957; Szentogothai, 1973). In most species studied, layers described as magnocellular (as opposed to parvocellular) can be distinguished (Kaas *et al.*, 1972*a*). The reason for this segregation is not known but may represent the anatomical substrate of the segregation of cells according to their response properties, e.g., large cells having transient or Y-type properties and small cells having sustained or X-type properties. The distribution of cell sizes in LGN of the cat is somewhat different. In this animal, the LGN has an intralaminar layer of large cells (called NIM) as well as a group of closely related nuclei that may represent a separate LGN complex (Guillery, 1970; Laties and Sprague, 1966). The two major nuclei that probably should be included in consideration of the LGN are nucleus intralaminaris centralis (NIC, NIM) and the posterior nucleus (Thuma, 1928; Laties and Sprague, 1966; Hayhow, 1958; Kinston *et al.*, 1969; Sanderson, 1971*b*).

PHYSIOLOGY OF CORTICAL RECIPIENT ZONE

As previously mentioned, there are significant differences among species in terms of the cortical areas to which efferents from LGN project. For expository purposes, it will be easier to consider the arrangements in primates before turning to other animals.

VISUOTOPIC ORGANIZATION. Early clinical findings demonstrated that a certain portion of the cerebral cortex was concerned with the processing of visual information. Thus Holmes (1918) and others (see Polyak, 1957) were able to show that injury to certain portions of the occipital pole produced specific visual field defects. More recent and accurate perimetry mapping (e.g., Bender and Furlow, 1945) also permitted the development of a putative map of the projection of the retina upon the cortex in man. Minkowski's (1920) anatomical studies demonstrated an orderly projection from LGN to cortex (see Polyak, 1957), for detailed historical review). But the first successful physiological map of the visual field onto visual cortex in primates was constructed by Marshall *et al.* (1943) using evoked potentials recorded in response to the presentation in the visual field of small, flashed lights. More recent studies by Cowey (1964) and Daniel and Whitteridge (1961) have clarified many of the details of this map.

A representation of one-half of the visual field is found on the occipital pole of monkeys and is shown in Fig. 4. The vertical meridian of the visual half-field is located along the line that separates area 17 from area 18 cytoarchitectonically, while the horizontal meridian of the visual half-field extends from about the middle of the occipital pole backward and slightly upward, ending in the calcarine fissure, see Figure 4 (Cowey, 1964).

The cytoarchitectonic border of areas 17 and 18 has been found to represent the vertical meridian in other animals, also (Kaas *et al.*, 1970, 1972*a,b*). The fovea is represented on the lateral convexity of the occipital pole, with peripheral portions of the visual field being located more posteriorly. The most peripheral portions of the field are located within the calcarine fissure.

In man, the extensive development of the temporal and parietal lobes has pushed the representation of the fovea backward and into the calcarine sulcus. With this transformation, the foveal representation of the visual field is just at the occipital pole, with the more peripheral portions of the visual field being located within the calcarine cortex (Polyak, 1957).

The distortion in the field projection noted in the LGN is also seen in cortex; e.g., central vision is represented in a larger cortical area than peripheral vision (Cowey, 1964; Daniel and Whitteridge, 1961). As pointed out for LGN, however, this is most likely due to the differential distribution of ganglion cells in retina imposed on the uniform cell density found in cortex (Daniel and Whitteridge, 1961; Berkley, 1976; Hubel and Wiesel, 1974*a*).

The projections in the cat are somewhat different from those found in primates or tree shrews. That region of cortex in the cat cytoarchitectonically homologous to area 17 of the primates is located posteriorly on the dorsal posterior and mesial surfaces of the hemispheres (Winkler and Potter, 1914; Otsuka and Hassler, 1962; Bilge *et al.*, 1967; Hubel and Wiesel, 1962; Tusa, 1975). As in primates and tree shrews, the vertical meridian is represented along the area 17–18 architectonic border with the horizontal meridian extending from its perpendicular intersection with the 17–18 border at the bend of the lateral gyrus down along the mesial wall of the hemisphere. However, the cat, unlike the primate, has several other cortical areas receiving direct input from thalamus, e.g., areas 18 and 19 and the lateral suprasylvian area (Glickstein *et al.*, 1967; Garey and Powell, 1967; Wilson and Cragg, 1967; Burrows and Hayhow, 1971; Rosenquist *et al.*, 1974). Furthermore, the lateral suprasylvian area itself may actually contain several independent field representations. It is not entirely clear whether the entire visual hemifield is represented in the areas outside of area 17, but it seems to be in at least several of them (Tusa, 1975).

SPATIAL PROPERTIES OF CORTICAL NEURONS. Electrophysiological study of single cells in visual cortex has shown that these cells have receptive fields that are typically elongated in one dimension and possess various additional properties. Hubel and Wiesel (1959, 1962, 1968) provided the classical description of the properties of these cells. In general, they described three major cell types, which they classified as *simple, complex,* and *hypercomplex.* Simple cells can usually be mapped with small flashing spots of light and the receptive fields subdivided into adjacent elongated zones of on and off responses. Such cells prefer slowly-moving contrast borders oriented parallel to the long axis of their receptive field (Fig. 5).

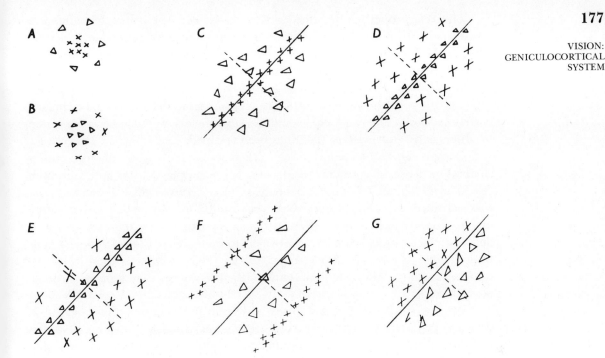

Fig. 5. A and B. Receptive field of typical cell in LGN of cat as mapped with small flashing spots. Triangle indicates a response to light offset; pluses indicate response to light onset. C, D, E and F. Receptive fields of neurons in striate cortex mapped with small flashed lights and classified as simple. Note elongated receptive field shapes and consequent necessity for appropriately oriented contour to optimally stimulate the cells. From Hubel and Wiesel (1962), with permission.

Many single cells are unidirectional, in that they respond to movement in one direction only. All are orientation selective responding poorly to elongated contrast borders which deviate in their orientation from parallel to the long axis of the receptive field by more than a few degrees (e.g., 5–10°) (Hubel and Wiesel, 1959, 1962; Watkins and Berkley, 1974). Such cells rarely have spontaneous activity and rarely respond to whole-field illumination changes (Hubel and Wiesel, 1959, 1962; Pettigrew *et al.*, 1968; Bishop *et al.*, 1971, 1973). Consequently, they are difficult to discover in the central visual field, where they are typically small and tightly tuned.

Cells classified as complex are similar to simple cells (e.g., they are orientation and directionally selective), but they respond poorly to flashed spots of light and thus do not have separable on and off zones. They prefer moving stimuli, have larger fields than simple cells, and respond to movement in the correct direction anywhere within the receptive field. Typically, they show spontaneous activity (Hubel and Wiesel, 1959, 1962; Pettigrew *et al.*, 1968).

Cells classified as hypercomplex are of two general categories: hypercomplex I and II. The first type prefers stimuli which do not exceed a certain length. The second type is more specific, not only requiring stopped edges and correct orientation but also having the unusual property of responding to movement orthogonal to either edge (Hubel and Wiesel, 1965*b*).

The cell properties described above have been confirmed by numerous investigators. Additions and modifications have also been introduced (e.g., Bishop *et al.*, 1971, 1973; Pettigrew *et al.*, 1968). For example, one class of cells not recognized in the early experiments may be described as *nonoriented cells* (Hubel and Wiesel, 1959). These cells were at first believed to be LGN axons but have subsequently been shown to be cortical cells (Joshua and Bishop, 1970; Baumgartner *et al.*, 1965; Hubel and Wiesel, 1968). Nevertheless, the scheme as presented by Hubel and Wiesel (1959, 1962) has been retained.

The precise relationship between cell types in LGN and cells in cortex is currently a topic of considerable debate. For example, Maffei and Fiorentini (1973) have suggested that cells classified as simple receive X LGN cell input while cells classified as complex receive Y cell input; however, other investigators disagree (Ikeda and Wright, 1974, 1975*a,b,c*). Furthermore, there is some evidence, in the cat at least, that Y cells project to both areas 17 and 18 while X cells project only to area 17 (Stone and Dreher, 1973). Although these data are consistent with the Maffei and Fiorentini (1973) view, they do not preclude other possibilities.

Detailed studies of primate cortex addressed to the question of which LGN cells innervate which cortical neurons are not yet available. Anatomical studies have shown that the pattern of termination of LGN cells in cortex is somewhat different for cats and monkeys (LeVay *et al.*, 1975; LeVay and Gilbert, 1976). But the physiological consequence of this difference is also not known.

BINOCULAR INTERACTION. *Ocular Dominance.* One of the most prominent features of the response properties of cortical cells is that a vast majority are binocularly activated (Hubel and Wiesel, 1959, 1962). If inhibitory interocular interactions are included, of the cortical neurons whose receptive fields are in the zone of binocular overlap of the visual fields, perhaps 95% are binocular (Sanderson *et al.*, 1969; Bishop, 1973). The degree of binocular interaction varies between cells but appears to be related, at least partly, to the cortical layer in which the cell resides (Hubel and Wiesel, 1962, 1968, 1972; Albus, 1975*a,b*). Thus, in layer IV, the major recipient zone of afferent terminals from the LGN, the cells are dominated by one or the other eye. In layers above or below this zone, the cells are predominantly binocular (Hubel and Wiesel, 1968).

A useful classification scheme for binocularity is the ocular dominance histogram (Fig. 6) devised by Hubel and Wiesel (1959, 1962, 1963, 1968). In this system, each cell is assigned a number from 1 to 7; cells being driven exclusively by the contralateral eye are given the number 1 while those driven exclusively by the ipsilateral eye are assigned number 7. Cells activated equally by either eye are given the number 4. Intermediate degrees of ocular dominance are given intermediate numbers. Using this scheme, in normal cats and monkeys (ignoring cortical layers) most cells are binocular (i.e., neither 1 nor 7). There is some evidence, however, that the ocular dominance distribution is not uniform for all field positions. Thus Albus (1975*c*) has reported that in the regions of visual cortex representing the central 5–8° of vision there are predominantly monocularly driven cells.

The ocular dominance distributions are also affected by environmental manipulations, e.g., monocular deprivation or strabismus, when applied during a brief and "critical" neonatal period (Hubel and Wiesel, 1970a). These developmental effects are discussed in greater detail in Chapter 3 of this volume.

Recent advances in neuroanatomical techniques have permitted the visualization of ocular dominance columns. Morphologically, an ocular dominance column is defined as a zone, normal to the cortical surface, that receives its afferent input in layer IV from one eye. In the first study to show such columns, Hubel and Wiesel (1969) made small lesions in lamina 6 of the monkey LGN and then traced the pattern of degeneration seen in layer IV of the striate cortex. Study of individual coronal sections showed patches or puffs of degeneration in layer IV spaced at intervals of about 300 μm. Reconstruction of the pattern of degeneration from serial sections showed that when viewed from the cortical surface the patches or puffs formed slabs or stripes of input from LGN (Hubel and Wiesel, 1972). The stripes of degeneration were separated by stripes of nondegenerating regions. The width of these stripes was found to correlate perfectly with the ocular dominance columns in layer IV as measured electrophysiologically.

Subsequent to this initial demonstration, several other techniques have been used to demonstrate ocular dominance columns. In one, the eye of a monkey is injected with [H³]proline and fucose (Wiesel et al., 1974). These substances are axoplasmically transported to the LGN. Furthermore, fucose is transsynaptically transported (Grafstein and Laurens, 1973) and thus eventually appears at the LGN terminals in striate cortex. Autoradiography of sections of striate cortex cut

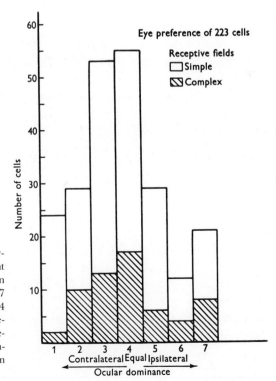

Fig. 6. Ocular dominance histogram showing number of cells activated to different degrees by each eye. Group 1 cells are driven exclusively by contralateral eye, group 7 exclusively by ipsilateral eye, and group 4 equally by both eyes. Open columns represent the number of simple cells in each category while striped columns represent number of complex cells in each category. From Hubel and Wiesel (1962), with permission.

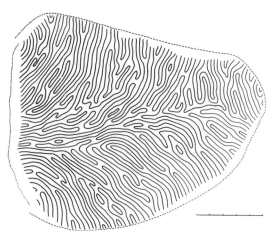

Fig. 7. Reconstruction of planar view of layer IV showing ocular input bands in striate cortex of right hemisphere of monkey. Bands correspond to ocular dominance bands or slabs. Border between area 17 and 18 is indicated by fine dotted line to the left of figure. Horizontal meridian extends from left to right through center of diagram (see Fig. 4). Note that bands intersect vertical meridian region (17–18 border) at right angles and are parallel to horizontal meridian. Reconstructed from tangential sections through layer IV of cortex stained with a modified fiber stain permitting visualization of input to layer IV. From LeVay *et al.* (1975), with permission.

tangential to the surface reveals the pattern of one eye's input to striate cortex, and reconstructions of the tangential sections of striate cortex have shown the pattern of ocular dominance bands or stripes (Wiesel *et al.*, 1974). Similar experiments using a modified fiber stain have also been able to show the complete pattern of ocular dominance bands in the monkey (LeVay *et al.*, 1975). The results are shown in Fig. 7. Note that the stripes intersect the area 17–18 border at right angles and tend to approach the representation of the horizontal meridian in a parallel fashion. A similar LGN input pattern has also been demonstrated in the bushbaby, a prosimian primate (Glendenning and Kofron, 1974).

Anatomical demonstration of ocular dominance bands in cats is somewhat more difficult but has been reported using autoradiographic procedures (Schatz *et al.*, 1975). For the ipsilateral eye in this animal, the monocular input bands are indistinct and broader (500 μm) than in the monkey, although they show essentially the same pattern. The contralateral input zone, however, is more continuous and less bandlike. Furthermore, bands may be seen in area 18 of the cat, but they are coarser than those in area 17 (Schatz *et al.*, 1975).

While these studies might suggest that alternating bands of LGN input to visual cortex are a common feature of the mammalian visual system, such has been found not to be true for several other species. For example, the pattern of input to striate cortex of the tree shrew is laminar rather than columnar. That is, LGN input to layer IV is layered within layer IV (Harting *et al.*, 1973; Hubel, 1975; Casagrande and Harting, 1975). In the mouse, there does not appear to be any banding (columnar) input from the two eyes, the input forming a continuous sheet in layer IV (Grafstein and Laurens, 1973; Dräger, 1975).

Retinal Disparity. A number of binocular cells that have been studied respond best when the receptive field is activated through each eye. Careful measurements have shown that when the eyes are aligned to be in optical correspondence the receptive field of the binocular cells in each eye may not be in precise register. Thus, in order to maximally stimulate the cell, the stimuli have to be slightly offset from each other, a condition called *retinal disparity*. The discovery of these cells in the cat (Pettigrew *et al.*, 1968; Barlow *et al.*, 1967) has led to the speculation that they are the neural substrate of stereopsis (Joshua and Bishop, 1970; Bishop, 1973). While neurons with properties that are consistent with a role in stereopsis have been observed in area 17 of the cat (Pettigrew *et al.*, 1968), they have been observed only in area 18 of the monkey (Hubel and Wiesel, 1970*b*).

ORIENTATION AND MOVEMENT. As previously described, the majority of cortical cells prefer elongated contrast borders (as opposed to small, flashing spots of light) and many of the receptive fields show discrete, separated elongated zones of "on" response and "off" response (e.g., Hubel and Wiesel, 1959, 1962). Almost all cells, simple, complex, and hypercomplex alike, have the requirement of specific contour orientation. In addition, the distribution of orientation preferences between cells is organized in columns. That is, cells encountered in an electrode

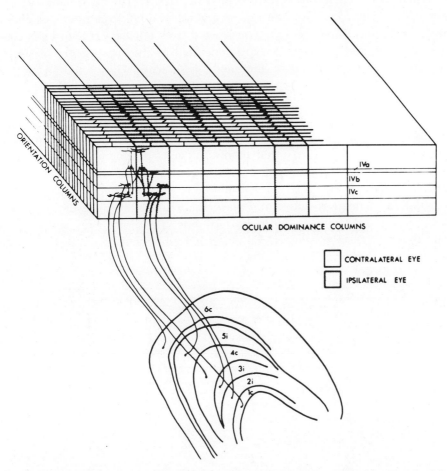

Fig. 8. Possible relationship between ocular dominance columns and orientation columns as proposed by Hubel and Wiesel (1972). Note that width of orientation slab is much less than that of the ocular dominance columns. Lower portion of figure shows possible origin of inputs to cortex from LGN. From Hubel and Wiesel (1972), with permission.

penetration perpendicular to the cortical surface have the same preferred orientation regardless of receptive field type (Hubel and Wiesel, 1963). The precise nature of the arrangement of orientation columns is currently unknown, although it has been suggested that they are orthogonal to the ocular dominance columns (e.g., Hubel and Wiesel, 1974b). This arrangement is depicted in Fig. 8.

While some cells respond to stationary contours, by far the most effective stimulus for cortical cells is a moving contour. However, tuning for movement rate is broad, cells responding over a wide range of stimulus velocities (Pettigrew *et al.*, 1968; Watkins and Berkley, 1974; Movshon, 1975). In general, simple cells respond best to slowly moving contours (<2°/sec) while complex cells respond best to more rapidly moving contours (>5°/sec) (Pettigrew *et al.*, 1968; Movshon, 1975; Watkins and Berkley, 1974).

HIERARCHICAL ORGANIZATION. Hubel and Wiesel (1962) proposed an organizational scheme which attempted to account for the properties of cortical neurons. This scheme suggests that the receptive fields of neurons in visual cortex are constructed by a process of successive convergence of input from more peripheral cells. For example, simple cells are constructed from a linear array of LGN cells' receptive fields, and complex cells are generated by the convergence of simple cells with simple receptive fields. The model is shown in Figs. 9 and 10. Such a plan endows neurons with, at least, the sum of the properties of the individual cells converging on it.

Inherent in this organizational plan is the idea of "feature abstraction." That is, neurons are tuned to specific features in the visual environment (Pitts and McCulloch, 1947). A corollary that follows suggests that neural reconstruction occurs in the visual system utilizing successive convergence of feature abstracting cells. By this means, any visual shape could be represented neurally.

While this scheme is simple and powerful, it suffers from several logical as well as empirical difficulties. On logical grounds, it is difficult to conceive of a system in which every possible visual object is represented by a unique neuron onto which a large number of other neurons selectively sensitive to unique

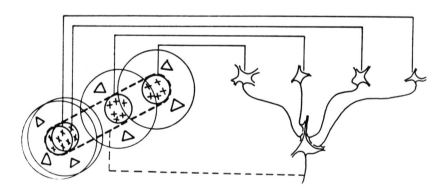

Fig. 9. Proposed model for explaining the organization of simple receptive fields. LGN cells with receptive fields as shown on the left converge onto a single neuron in striate cortex. The receptive field of the striate cortex neuron would have an elongated "on" center as indicated by the interrupted lines surrounding the centers of the LGN cell receptive fields. From Hubel and Wiesel (1962), with permission.

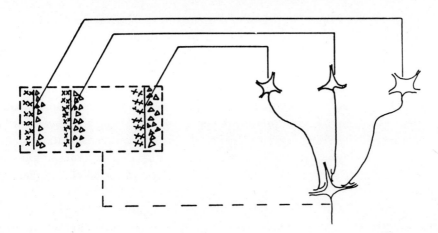

Fig. 10. Possible model for explaining the organization of receptive field of striate cortex neuron classified as complex. Three cells with simple receptive fields, shown on the left, could project onto the neuron shown on the right, investing its receptive field with the sum of the simple receptive fields. Note that the elongated simple receptive fields all have the same orientation. Any appropriately oriented contour, falling within the receptive field, would stimulate at least some of the simple receptive fields and excite the higher-order cell. From Hubel and Wiesel (1962), with permission.

features in the stimulus have converged (Barlow, 1972*b*). Empirically, there is considerable evidence that there are multiple visual pathways in the nervous system, making a simple serial model morphologically unlikely. Some of these shortcomings are discussed in detail in a later section.

VARIATION. The properties of neurons in the visual cortex of many animals are similar to those described in the cat. Thus rhesus monkeys (Hubel and Wiesel, 1968; Wurtz, 1969; Dow and Gouras, 1973), humans (Marg *et al.,* 1968), rats (Wiesenfeld and Kornel, 1975), and mice (Dräger, 1975) have all been found to possess cells with similar properties. There are, however, some notable exceptions. Unlike the animals described above, the rabbit, for example, has directionally selective cells in its retina (Barlow *et al.,* 1964; Barlow and Levick, 1965) as well as in visual cortex (Chow *et al.,* 1971; Arden *et al.,* 1967). Furthermore, nonmammalian species may have evolved a different scheme. These animals have more complex receptive fields in the retina than are found in mammals. Frogs and birds, for example, have retinal ganglion cells with receptive field properties nearly as complex as those found in the cortex of most mammals (Dowling, 1970).

BEHAVIORAL EVALUATION OF SUSPECTED FUNCTIONS

The previous sections have presented a brief overview of the anatomy and electrophysiology of the geniculocortical system. In this section the discussion turns to the behavioral evaluation of those functions suggested by some of the electrophysiological results; namely, the temporal response characteristics of the system, color vision, contour sensitivity, depth perception, and complex spatial vision. The focus will be on ablation-behavior studies.

At the outset, it must be recognized that many behavioral studies of complex spatial vision suffer from the problem of having stimuli with multiple features, any or all of which may be used on one testing occasion and not on another. Thus the conclusions of ablation-behavior studies which do not include careful equivalence tests, or in some other way establish the relevant cue or cues being used by the experimental animal both preoperatively and postoperatively, are very difficult to interpret. For this reason the present review has emphasized those studies which have measured the visual system response to single stimulus dimensions and in this section will emphasize only those behavioral studies designed toward the same end. The utility of this approach can be seen by consideration of the following argument.

The knowledge that the visual system can distinguish between, say, different faces, is an interesting fact but essentially useless in terms of discovering which neural structures are involved in this capacity. The major reason is that a face is a complex visual stimulus, containing many features (e.g., nose, eyes, ears) that could, by themselves, permit accurate discrimination between faces. Thus the loss of the ability to discriminate faces on the basis of different noses does not preclude their discrimination on the basis of different eyes or ears, which means, in turn, that the retention of a "face discrimination" after ablation does not lead to the conclusion that the ablation has had no profound effect. Indeed, it may have completely eliminated the detection of an entire class of features. But because the stimulus has redundant discriminative features, the behavioral discrimination of the stimulus appears to remain without serious deficit. This situation is complicated still further in that the visual system contains parallel information-processing channels and these channels share unknown numbers and classes of individual feature detectors.

Thus survival of a visual discrimination in an ablation-behavior experiment in which complex stimuli are used is at best difficult to interpret, and often impossible. Possible interpretations include the following: (1) the ablated structure is not involved in the discrimination; (2) the ablated structure does not discriminate the stimulus *dimension* being used; and (3) the dimension(s) used postoperatively is different from that used preoperatively. These problems in interpretation can be avoided, of course, by specifying the cue (or dimension) being used by the animal in making the discrimination both pre- and postoperatively. This may be achieved in several ways: (1) by using stimuli with only a single dimension, (2) by determining which of several possible dimensions is being used in the discrimination, or (3) by training the animal to attend to only one specified dimension. The first two of these requirements are often difficult if not impossible to achieve, and the use of nonhuman animal models makes use of the third method difficult. However, using modern animal testing technique and careful stimulus manipulations it can be done—for example, by performing either equivalence tests or psychophysical threshold measurements for the stimulus dimensions in question. This latter procedure permits specifying the dimension or cue being used because the animal is specifically trained to attend to it. Furthermore, the efficacy of the threshold training can be evaluated by the degree to which the animal's behavior is changed by changes in the cue. The visual psychophysical method has two further advantages as a tool in attempting to discover the neural substrates of vision: (1) at suprathreshold values it provides a behavioral control task (to evaluate such variables as memory, motor skills, and motivation) and (2) near threshold it permits the application of the simple assumption that the neural signals produced by the two different stimuli are the same (Brindley, 1970).

Consideration of these problems suggests that certain classes of observation are more useful in discovering the function of various neural structures than others. In the following sections, therefore, ablation-behavior studies using psychophysical measures will be emphasized because of the greater certainty regarding the visual cues that are being used.

TEMPORAL RESPONSE PROPERTIES

As described earlier, there is ample evidence that the geniculocortical system contains units (e.g., Y cells or transient cells) capable of processing more or less rapid temporal changes in visual stimuli. Direct tests of temporal processing in which the geniculocortical system is destroyed have shown that the residual portions of the visual system are capable of detecting temporal changes (flicker), e.g., Teuber *et al.*, 1960; Norton and Clark, 1963*a,b*; Tucker *et al.*, 1968. Thus clinical studies in humans as well as animal studies have demonstrated that flicker can be detected within scotomata due to cortical lesion, and also that flicker can be detected by animals lacking striate cortex. In light of the fact that neural elements capable of processing rapid temporal changes are present outside of geniculocortical part of the visual system, this is not surprising (e.g., Stone and Dreher, 1973; Hoffman, 1973).

However, when flicker *thresholds* are measured in the preparations described above, the results are somewhat less clear. Some studies report that there may or may not be changes in flicker-fusion in a scotoma (Koerner and Teuber, 1973) or differences in the effect depending on the locus of the scotoma (Poppel *et al.*, 1975). Most animal studies, however, have reported a decrease in the flicker-fusion point (Mishkin and Weiskrantz, 1959; Taravella and Clark, 1963; Schwartz and Clark, 1957; Schwartz and Cheney, 1966). If the destriate preparation has neural elements that can process the flicker, it is not clear why thresholds should be elevated. The elevation could be due, for example, either to a loss of the most sensitive elements or to a longer time constant for the residual system, or to a criterion shift.

A more useful evaluation of the role of the geniculocortical system in temporal processing would be obtained if complete temporal modulation transfer functions (TMTF) were obtained from destriate subjects. Unfortunately, these observations have not, as yet, been made.

Several studies have attempted to relate the temporal response properties of various neural elements to comparable behavioral estimates. For example, Lopes da Silva (1970) behaviorally measured the TMTF in dogs and compared it with evoked potentials recorded from various portions of the geniculostriate system. A similar study comparing evoked potentials recorded from area 17 of the cat with behavioral estimates was performed by Loop and Berkley (1975) and Berkley *et al.* (1975). They found reasonable agreement between the shapes of the TMTF determined by each method. They did not, however, determine if *non*-geniculo-cortical-derived potentials also agreed with the behavioral TMTF.

In a more direct study, Spekreijse *et al.* (1971) correlated the temporal modulation response of LGN cells in the monkey with human TMTFs obtained under similar conditions and found excellent agreement between the two measurements.

These studies suggest that the geniculocortical system can participate in the temporal processing of visual information but they do not reveal whether it normally does. Given the fact that the retinotectal system contains Y cell elements which are also capable of processing rapid temporal changes, it is not clear which system participates in the perception of temporal changes.

A visual capacity undoubtedly related to temporal processing is movement discrimination and detection (e.g., Tansley, 1965). Neurophysiological studies have shown neurons in the geniculocortical system to be sensitive to movement and the direction of movement. The retinotectal system appears to be less sensitive to direction of movement. However, the ability to detect movement appears to survive complete removal of the geniculocortical system in the monkey and man. For example, in humans, it has long been known that moving a stimulus within a "blind" field due to cortical damage could elicit responses that some kind of stimulus was in the field (Riddoch, 1917; Denny-Brown and Chambers, 1976; Humphrey and Weiskrantz, 1967; Anderson and Symmes, 1969; Koerner and Teuber, 1973).

Using the optokinetic response, the capacity to detect movement after striate cortex lesions has also been demonstrated in both man (TerBraak *et al.*, 1971) and monkey (TerBraak and van Vliet, 1963; Pasik *et al.*, 1959).

In cats, the ability to detect movement also remains after visual cortex ablation (Kennedy, 1936*a,b,* 1939). These animals, however, show elevated thresholds for the detection of movement; e.g., a greater stimulus velocity is needed after surgery than before. While these results would seem to reinforce the finding in primates, they actually complicate the interpretation in that the lesions in cat and monkey may be comparable on cytoarchitectonic grounds but the cat possesses an extensive geniculocortical projection outside of striate cortex. Thus any residual capacity in this animal cannot safely be attributed to the nongeniculostriate system.

In summary, the findings for flicker and movement detection suggest that these capacities are not unique to the geniculocortical system. Considering the recent electrophysiological studies demonstrating that retinal ganglion cells with properties uniquely suited for the detection of rapid stimulus changes project both to LGN and to tectum, these behavioral findings are not so surprising as they once were.

Color Vision

The question of whether color vision is exclusively mediated by the geniculo-cortical system has been considered by several investigators (Klüver, 1941; Pasik and Pasik, 1970; Malmo, 1966). In well-controlled studies, it has been shown that monkeys without striate cortex cannot discriminate colors (Klüver, 1941). In addition, spectral sensitivity functions derived from such animals show only the operation of rods (Lepore *et al.,* 1975; Malmo, 1966). One study of destriate monkeys did claim finding color vision capacity but the stimuli were not carefully specified, and there is a good possibility that the discrimination was based on a brightness difference (Schilder *et al.*, 1972; Lepore *et al.*, 1975). Taken together, the results of these studies strongly suggest that, in primates, all color information is processed by the geniculocortical system, and that the retinal afferents to tectum are either all rod or have spectral characteristics too broad to mediate color vision (Fig. 11).

In other animals, however, the results appear to show that striate cortex is not necessary for color vision. Snyder *et al.* (1969) have shown that the tree shrew is able to discriminate colors after removal of striate cortex. While seeming to provide negative evidence for the necessity of the geniculocortical system in color vision, this study must be interpreted cautiously because the tree shrew has an essentially all-cone rather than a duplex retina (Walls, 1942; Polyak, 1957). Therefore, the tectum certainly gains cone input.

In rats, Craft and Butter (1968) claim a complete loss of wavelength discrimination after striate cortex ablation. In the ground squirrel, an animal with a mostly cone retina, color vision was found to survive ablation of the geniculocortical system (Kicliter *et al.*, 1974), suggesting that the retinotectal pathway is capable of mediating color vision. This result is puzzling when one considers the electrophysiological results of Michael (1972, 1973), who found only one class of color cell projecting to the tectum. It is not impossible that the ground squirrel has a small rod input to tectum in addition to the one cone type and when striatectomized is discriminating colors with the combination of the two. These studies suggest that in animals with duplex retinas the major geniculocortical input will be derived

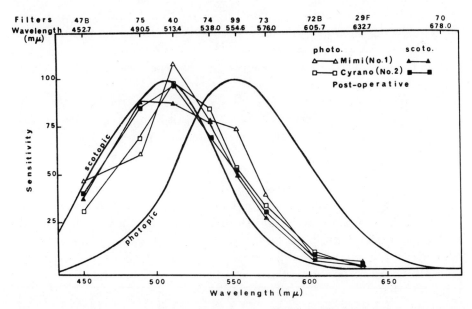

Fig. 11. Spectral sensitivity curves for two monkeys, obtained after removal of striate cortex, at scotopic and photopic luminance levels. Continuous lines show normal primate photopic and scotopic sensitivity functions. From LePore *et al.* (1975), with permission.

from the cone system, with little cone input to tectum. This cannot be true, of course, in animals with all-cone (or predominantly cone) retinas. Thus rats and primates (animals with duplex retinas) lose color vision after geniculocortical ablations while tree shrews and ground squirrels (essentially all-cone retinas) retain their color discrimination capacities after similar lesions.

Contour Sensitivity

Brightness Increment Thresholds. The ability to detect a contour depends first on the ability to detect a difference in brightness. Thus one may consider brightness increment thresholds as being related to contour discrimination. Few studies have examined increment thresholds after geniculocortical ablations. In most relevant studies, a large brightness increment is used, e.g., light vs. no light. There is good agreement in these studies that the geniculocortical system is not necessary to discriminate light from dark (e.g., Klüver, 1941; Lashley, 1931). In some cases, a performance deficit is seen immediately after the lesion but it disappears with continued training (Urbaitis and Meikle, 1968; Baden *et al.*, 1965; Schilder, 1966; Barbas and Spear, 1976; Spear and Braun, 1969*b*; Bekoff *et al.*, 1973; Thompson, 1960; Murphy and Chow, 1974; Schilder *et al.*, 1971). Thus most investigators seem to agree that the geniculocortical system is not necessary for discriminating brightness differences, and this task is often used as a control procedure to assess overall performance ability after a geniculocortical lesion.

While the studies cited above demonstrate that large brightness differences may be discriminated without the geniculocortical system, they did not evaluate a more subtle capacity of brightness vision, the increment threshold. Only a handful of studies have been concerned with this ability. Smith (1936*c*), for example, found that cats without striate cortex show little change in their brightness increment thresholds. In further studies, Mead (1939) found that the increment threshold was elevated at low luminances but was near normal at high levels. He also found an increase in the absolute threshold of his operated cat. Unfortunately, only one animal was used in this study, making the generality of the findings somewhat limited. Except for the studies of Klüver (1941), no increment threshold studies have been performed on primates deprived of striate cortex.

Detail Vision. Both anatomical and physiological data strongly suggest that fine detail vision is mediated by the geniculocortical system. Thus electrophysiological studies of the retina have shown that neurons with the smallest receptive fields are of the X type and project only to the geniculocortical system (Enroth-Cugell and Robson, 1966; Stone and Hoffmann, 1971; Stone and Dreher, 1973). Anatomical studies in which the fovea is damaged and the degenerating axons are followed into the CNS showed that in primates, only a weak input is made to the nongeniculocortical portions of the visual system (Wilson and Toyne, 1969), suggesting that the latter is the lesser of the two major systems concerned with foveal and other fine detail vision.

Ablation studies tend to confirm this view. Thus Smith (1936*d*) showed that cats with massive (but incomplete) lesions of the geniculocortical system have impaired visual acuity. They still have the capacity, however, for detecting large acuity targets. Similar experiments in the monkey showed a complete loss of detail vision (contour acuity) (Weiskrantz and Cowey, 1963, 1967) and earlier experiments with the chimpanzee produced similar effects (Spence and Fulton, 1936). Lesions confined to the central field representation in visual cortex produce losses in acuity in the appropriate portion of the field (Cowey and Ellis, 1969), although the acuity deficit appears to be somewhat less than expected on the basis of the cortical representation of the visual field (Rolls and Cowey, 1970). Studies of humans with striate cortex lesions tend to confirm these findings (Polyak, 1957).

While the results of acuity studies with primates are clear in showing that ability to see fine targets is mediated by the geniculocortical system, the results of similar experiments with other animals are not. Thus in the studies of the cat by Smith (1936*d*) only very extensive lesions produced a significant change in acuity. In more recent studies, Berkley *et al.* (1976) showed that if the cortical lesion was confined to striate cortex, cats suffered only a 20% drop in acuity. Since the cortical region of the cat geniculocortical system is more extensive than the striate cortex (Glickstein *et al.*, 1967; Garey and Powell, 1967; Burrows and Hayhow, 1971), these results are not surprising. It is not clear, however, whether the postoperative visual capacity is being mediated by the residual cortical areas receiving direct LGN input or by midbrain routes (e.g., tecto-LP-cortex). The small acuity loss seems to argue for the residual LGN projection since there is no evidence for X cell projection to the tectum. Lesions which include these other cortical areas produce greater acuity losses (Smith, 1936*d*).

Experiments with the rat confirm the above observations. Thus Lashley and Frank (1934) showed severe impairment of detail vision with striate cortex ablations in this animal. Perhaps more important, they showed that animals that had incomplete lesions had less severe visual defects.

Thus until recently (and with the exception of the cat) the evidence seemed clear that the geniculocortical system was necessary for detail vision. Ablation studies of the tree shrew, however, have shown that this animal retains excellent detail vision after striate cortex ablation (Snyder *et al.*, 1966; Snyder and Diamond, 1968; Ware *et al.*, 1974). It will be recalled that color vision also survives this lesion in the tree shrew. While there is some evidence suggesting that the tree shrew processes visual details in its geniculocortical system (Ward and Masterton, 1970), it is clear that a much greater degree of vision survives striate cortex ablations in this animal than does in monkeys, rats, cats, and man.

The question of why the tree shrew is different is intriguing, and one looks, of course, to the anatomy of its visual system for an explanation. Diamond and his co-workers (Snyder *et al.*, 1966; Snyder and Diamond, 1968) have assumed that the tree shrew has a visual system constructed essentially on the same plan as that of primates, and thus they attribute the high degree of residual vision in this animal after striate cortex ablations to a second system, a system utilizing a tectopulvinar–cortex pathway (Diamond, 1976). Such a pathway has been demonstrated not only in the tree shrew but also in other mammals. The tree shrew, however, may differ in more fundamental ways than simply having an overdeveloped tectopulvinar system. For example, the tree shrew has an essentially all-cone retina as well as a noncolumnar binocular input to striate cortex (e.g., Hubel, 1975; Casagrande and Harting, 1975). These differences may be more important in understanding residual vision in the tree shrew than a consideration of the tectopulvinar system. We shall return to this point after completing the survey of ablation-behavior studies.

CONTRAST SENSITIVITY. The advantages of describing visual capacities in terms of a linear system have been discussed in numerous studies of the physiological properties of retinal ganglion cells. LGN, and cortical neurons, e.g., Campbell *et al.*, 1969, 1970; Pollen and Ronner, 1975. Several workers have advanced visual (neural) processing schemes based on this analysis and postulated the existence of separate "channels" for the processing of spatial information of differing spatial frequencies (Campbell and Robson, 1968; Blakemore and Campbell, 1969). Whether or not this linear system scheme is valid does not detract from the great economy of description that it affords. That is, the family of contrast sensitivity functions (spatial and temporal) can display information about the entire visual system's response to size, contrast, luminance, etc. (e.g., Kelly, 1972). Despite the economy, this type of analysis has, as yet, not seen widespread application in ablation-behavior paradigms or in clinical evaluations of humans with visual system damage. Except for the previously cited studies of acuity, which can be thought of as the high-frequency cutoff of a contrast sensitivity function, no measurements of contrast sensitivity as a function of spatial frequency have been made in animals with geniculocortical damage.

Bodis-Wollner (1972, 1976) has attempted to apply the linear system approach to humans with cerebral damage including portions of visual cortex. He found that human subjects who showed only mild deficits in acuity showed marked departures from normal contrast sensitivity at other spatial frequencies (Bodis-Wollner, 1972, 1976). As of this writing, however, the amount of data on brain-damaged humans is not yet sufficient for any definite conclusion to be drawn regarding the role of the geniculocortical system in contrast sensitivity except for the high-frequency response.

DEPTH PERCEPTION

As discussed previously, neurons selectively sensitive to retinal disparity between the images in the two eyes have been described for cats (Pettigrew *et al.*, 1968; Barlow *et al.*, 1967) and monkeys (Hubel and Wiesel, 1970*b*). The results suggest that these animals possess stereopsis (the ability to judge distance of a visual target using only disparity cues). Of course, even casual observation of the behavior of these animals supports this view. An adequate behavioral demonstration of stereopsis, however, is considerably more difficult to achieve, but it now has been done. Fox and Blake (1971) used a stimulus that provided local disparity cues (a three-rod alignment apparatus) to show that cats are able to discriminate local binocular disparity cues, and Bough (1970) used random dot stereograms to demonstrate stereopsis in the monkey. In a quantitative study, Sarmiento (1975) measured stereoacuity thresholds in the rhesus monkey using an automated version of the classic two-rod Howard-Dolman depth perception apparatus. The monkeys were found to have stereoacuity thresholds essentially identical to those of man if the measured values were corrected for differences in interpupillary distances between the two species.

Depth perception in cats has also been studied quantitatively. Packwood and Gordon (1975) measured the stereopsis capacity of cats using a shadow-casting device (Fox and Blake, 1971) that provided local binocular disparity cues. They found that cats could fuse greater disparities than man but could not use as large unfused disparities as man in making depth judgments (Packwood and Gordon, 1975). Perhaps more interesting was their finding that cats which either congenitally or experimentally do not possess binocularly activated neurons in area 17 do not have stereoscopic vision. Using Siamese cats (with squint) and cats exposed to alternating monocular occlusion during the first 90 days of life (a procedure shown to eliminate binocular cells in area 17; Hubel and Wiesel, 1965a), no signs of stereopsis were found. These animals did, however, possess normal acuity. While these results strongly suggest that area 17 is involved in stereopsis, they do not demonstrate that the disparity-sensitive cells that have been described in area 17 (e.g., Barlow *et al.*, 1967) are the ones responsible for stereopsis.

No direct ablation-behavior tests have as yet been performed in which quantitative measures of stereopsis have been made.

Several ablation studies have utilized the visual cliff apparatus to test for depth discrimination. Several of these studies showed no change in visual cliff behavior after visual cortex ablation (Dalby *et al.*, 1970; Meyer, 1963; Meyer *et al.*, 1966). But studies by Wetzel (1969) and Cornwell *et al.* (1976) report loss of differential responding on the cliff after visual cortex lesions. While these studies are suggestive, they suffer from two serious problems: (1) incomplete lesions of striate cortex and (2) the possibility that judgments could be based on pattern size difference between the two sides of the cliff. Similar results have been obtained in rats (Lewellyn *et al.*, 1969; Meyer *et al.*, 1966; Braun *et al.*, 1970) and rabbits (Stewart and Riesen, 1972). Based on the studies of the effects of visual cortex lesions on visual acuity (see earlier section) it is perhaps not surprising that depth judgments are also affected since it could be argued that a prerequisite for stereopsis is the ability to (1) detect fine contours and (2) align the eyes accurately, both probably heavily dependent upon the fine tuning of neurons in striate cortex.

COMPLEX SPATIAL VISION

As discussed previously one of the major difficulties in the evaluation of potential neural substrates for form vision is that the relevant dimensions of the test stimuli are not known. Thus, although it is interesting to measure the loss of response to complex visual stimuli (e.g., geometric shapes, familiar objects, etc.) these stimuli contain such a variety of stimulus dimensions as to make discovery of the means by which the discrimination is made nearly impossible. One stratagem that may be employed to overcome this problem is to use psychophysical methods and manipulate only one dimension of the stimulus at a time. But the question arises as to which dimensions or in what order? One clue is, of course, provided by electrophysiological studies.

Although the fundamental dimensions of a visual stimulus have been considered in earlier sections, the more global aspects of vision, such as form vision, have not. Form vision is the capacity to discriminate visual objects by their overall shape (or form). (It is important to make the distinction between form and pattern vision stimuli. In the former case, the overall shape of the stimulus is the cue while in the latter, the stimulus contains a repetitive or redundant cue, e.g., grating or texture. This distinction is important because the ability to process these two kinds of stimuli may be different and consequently tap different neural mechanisms.)

A vast literature concerning the role of the geniculocortical system in form vision has accumulated and will only briefly be recounted here. For purposes of clarity, the studies will be divided into two broad categories: (1) losses of form vision capacities with lesions of visual cortex and (2) residual visual capacities after visual cortex lesions.

As mentioned earlier, the data for primates are reasonably clear: complete loss of striate cortex in primates makes them incapable of discriminating objects based on their shape (Klüver, 1941). More recent studies have confirmed these findings (Cowey and Weiskrantz, 1963, 1967; Weiskrantz and Cowey, 1971; Butter, 1969), although some studies seemed to suggest (Weiskrantz, 1963; Humphrey and Weiskrantz, 1967) that some contour vision survives striate cortex ablations. The latter studies have been criticized on the basis of a lack of histological control (Pasik *et al.*, 1969). In studies of incomplete lesions, the results indicate that in the region of reduced vision produced by the cortical lesion no form vision is possible (Polyak, 1957; Humphrey and Weiskrantz, 1967; Teuber *et al.*, 1960; Weiskrantz and Cowey, 1970).

In the course of studying both monkeys and humans after striate cortex ablations, it became clear that while no form vision was possible within the visual field zone of the damaged area, some type of vision other than simple light detection was possible (Humphrey and Weiskrantz, 1967; Riddoch, 1917; Denny-Brown and Chambers, 1976). The precise nature of this residual capacity has been the topic of some debate (Pasik *et al.*, 1969). Some evidence for a weak response to contours has been reported (Weiskrantz, 1963; Pasik and Pasik, 1964), but these stimuli contained large patterns of bars or stripes permitting the discriminations to be made on local flux cues.

There is considerable agreement that primates can detect the position of a stimulus within the blind field even though they cannot identify it (Humphrey and Weiskrantz, 1967; Denny-Brown and Chambers, 1976; Poppel *et al.*, 1973; Weiskrantz *et al.*, 1974). Stimuli presented in the blind field have also been shown to elicit eye movements to the position of the stimulus (Poppel *et al.*, 1973), and a very primitive type of stereopsis has also been described as present in the blind field (Richards, 1973).

While animals have been shown to be contour blind within their blind field after striate cortex lesions, the size of these "blind" areas (scotomata) does not correlate perfectly with the predicted scotomata based on retinocortical topography (Teuber *et al.,* 1960; Cowey and Weiskrantz, 1963; Weiskrantz and Cowey, 1967; Cowey, 1967). Typically, a scotoma is smaller than that predicted by the lesion. Several explanations have been offered such as reorganization (Chow, 1968) or the use of midbrain mechanisms (Weiskrantz and Cowey, 1963). Combined partial lesions of optic tract or retina and visual cortex that presumably together cover the visual field have not produced total blindness in some cases (Galambos *et al.,* 1967; Norton *et al.,* 1967) but has been shown in others (Keating and Horel, 1976). These findings suggest that the topographic organization of the geniculocortical system is not capable of gross reorganization but may be somewhat more diffusely organized than a simple point-for-point topographic plan would suggest.

Variation among Mammals

Numerous studies of complex visual discrimination capacities have been made in cats, and the results are unclear. They range from claims that striate cortex ablations do not impair complex spatial vision (Doty, 1971) to claims that there are severe deficits (Winans, 1967). Some workers claim deficits for simple brightness discriminations as well (Baden *et al.,* 1965). Much of the confusion about the cat's visual capacities after cortical lesions can be traced to four separate difficulties: (1) the definition of the geniculocortical system in the cat, (2) the definition of what constitutes a deficit, (3) the incompleteness of lesions, and (4) the choice of behavioral test problem to be used.

The early studies of Smith (1934*a,b,* 1935, 1936*a,b,c,* 1938; Smith and Warkentin, 1939) strongly suggested that cats retained a considerable ability to discriminate simple contours (e.g., horizontal vs. vertical bars) and had only a moderate decrease in visual acuity after extensive ablations of the geniculocortical system, apparently including all of the striate cortex. Unfortunately, most of these studies used shapes that had large local flux cues, and equivalence tests were not performed to ascertain that the cats were using the shape of the stimulus as the cue. Smith's (1936*c*) findings regarding visual acuity, however, are much more convincing, although he used optokinetic nystagmus as his test. More recent studies have confirmed Smith's findings (e.g., Murphy *et al.,* 1975) and demonstrated that striate cortex ablations alone have relatively little effect on form discrimination in the cat (Winans, 1967, 1971; Doty, 1971; Spear and Braun, 1969*a,b;* Meyer, 1963; Alder and Meikle, 1975; Wood *et al.,* 1974; Dalby *et al.,* 1970). The lesions are not without effect, however, since all the animals used in these studies showed a temporary loss of the preoperative performance and slowed acquisition or reacquisition of the discrimination.

Several workers have suggested that local flux cues or those related to head and/or eye movements may be mediating the behavior (Buchtel, 1969; Dodwell and Freedman, 1968; Winans, 1971). Indeed, Winans (1971) showed that cats will use local flux cues in form discriminations. While this would seem to suggest that cats without striate cortex solve form discriminations on the basis of flux cues, other studies have clearly shown that local cues were probably not significant factors in postoperative behavior (Doty, 1971; Berkley *et al.,* 1976).

As mentioned earlier since the cat possesses a significant extrastriate projection from LGN, it is not clear whether the residual form vision after striate cortex ablation is being mediated by these projections or by the tectal system. Doty (1971) suggests that it is the extrastriate system while Smith (1938) suggests that it is the tectal system. However, one thing is clear: the cat retains a substantially greater visual capacity after striate cortex lesions than does the monkey (see Fig. 12).

Ablation of the geniculocortical system in rats, rabbits, and hedgehogs produces deficits in preoperatively learned pattern discriminations but recovery after prolonged training (Spear and Barbas, 1975; Murphy and Stewart, 1974; Mize *et al.*, 1971; Murphy and Chow, 1974; Hall and Diamond, 1968). Rats, however, have been shown to be unable to learn to discriminate between forms equated for flux (Lashley and Frank, 1934; Bland and Cooper, 1969, Braun *et al.*, 1970; Horel *et al.*, 1966). Spear and Barbas (1975) have shown that striatectomized rats can relearn such problems but only after very extended training and apparently only if extrastriate cortex is intact.

Studies of the tree shrew have suggested that the geniculostriate system in this animal is less involved in form vision than it is in primates. Thus, for example, studies of the tree shrew have shown them to be capable of considerable form vision after removal of striate cortex (Snyder and Diamond, 1968; Ward and Masterton, 1970; Killackey and Diamond, 1971; Killackey *et al.*, 1971, 1972; Ware *et al.*, 1972). As mentioned earlier, color vision survives this ablation as well (Snyder *et al.*, 1969). These results suggest a much more important role for the tectopulvinar–cortex system (Atencio *et al.*, 1975) in this animal than in others.

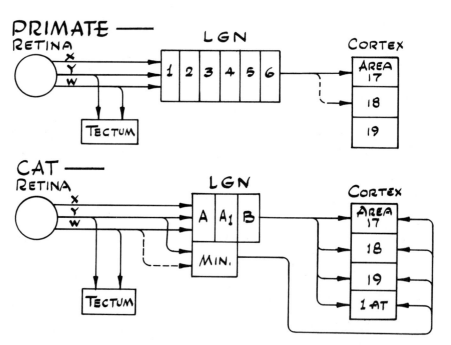

Fig. 12. Schematic diagram summarizing the major pathways from retina into central nervous system for primates (top) and cats (bottom). Note the multiple recipient zones in thalamus and multiple pathways from thalamus to cortex in the cat.

Diamond and his co-workers (Diamond, 1976) suggest that the major difference between the primate visual system and that of the tree shrew (and squirrel) may be the differences in the projection target of the tectopulvinar system. In the monkey area 18 is not a target of the tectopulvinar system, while in the tree shrew it is. An alternative explanation for these differences is presented below.

In summary, most investigators agree that removal of geniculocortical system produces a variety of deficits. No one claims that the animals retain normal visual capacities. Thus, while a cat or monkey can be shown to be capable of responding to contoured stimuli after geniculocortical ablation, both clearly require considerable training and special conditions, e.g., large stimuli.

The vision retained by animals with geniculocortical lesions can be characterized by certain features: (1) the animals appear to respond to movement; (2) they appear to be able to localize the stimuli in space (Weiskrantz and Cowey, 1971; Riddoch, 1917; Denny-Brown and Chambers, 1976); and (3) they may be trained to respond to contoured stimuli but with great difficulty.

Conclusions

In considering all of the findings derived from the studies reviewed above, it is possible to make several conclusions:

1. The geniculocortical system processes visual information containing fine details.
2. The geniculocortical system is responsible for encoding information used in shape discriminations and visual perception.
3. The geniculocortical system is necessary to identify stationary shapes.
4. The geniculocortical system is necessary for accurate eye alignment.
5. The geniculocortical system is probably necessary for at least the first stage of range finding or depth perception based on binocular disparity.

While the majority of the evidence presented in this chapter is consistent with these conclusions, there are several major observations that would seem to be at variance with it and one worth commenting on. Thus the demonstration that monkeys without striate cortex are capable of some vision might be taken as evidence against the conclusions presented above. However, a careful reading of those papers (Pasik and Pasik, 1970; Humphrey and Weiskrantz, 1967) reveals that while these destriate animals have more vision than previously suspected, they still are incapable of discriminating visual stimuli on the basis of shape. Furthermore, there is little or no evidence that they are capable of any degree of depth discrimination.

Other evidence that would seem to contradict the proposed conclusions is derived from studies of the cat. In the cat, ablation of striate cortex reduces visual acuity but has little effect on form vision (Doty, 1971; Winans, 1971; Spear and Braun, 1969a; Berkley et al., 1976). While these findings seem devastating to the proposed functions of the geniculocortical system, consideration of the unusual anatomy of the cat visual system permits a plausible explanation. In the cat, the projections from LGN extend to areas beyond striate cortex (e.g., Glickstein *et al.*, 1967; Garey and Powell, 1967). If all of the LGN projection area is removed in a cat, its residual vision is of about the same quality as that of a destriate monkey.

Perhaps the major piece of evidence that does not fit the conclusions presented above comes from studies of the tree shrew. It will be recalled that ablation of striate cortex in this animal produces little, if any, deficit in simple form discriminations (e.g., Snyder *et al.*, 1966; Snyder and Diamond, 1968). Yet there is no evidence that the projections from LGN to cortex extend beyond striate cortex as in the cat (Harting *et al.*, 1973). The anatomy of the visual system of the tree shrew has been shown to differ from that of both cat and monkey in terms of the pattern of projections from LGN to cortex (Harting *et al.*, 1973; Casagrande and Harting, 1975; Hubel, 1975). This animal also has an essentially all-cone retina and no fovea. These differences suggest that the tree shrew may be unique with regard to its geniculocortical system or that it represents some intermediate evolutionary stage of visual system development.

One speculation about the tree shrew worthy of consideration concerns the possible differences in neural target areas of the X and Y system of ganglion cells in this animal. In the cat and presumably primates, the X system projects to cortex only through the LGN. Thus ablation of the geniculocortical system in these animals eliminates X system function, which is likely to be involved in fine shape discrimination. Residual capacities might include some crude contour sensitivity of the Y system. If in the tree shrew the X system projects to tectum as well as LGN, it could explain the considerable form vision remaining in this animal after geniculocortical ablation. To date, there have been no studies of the cell type projection to tectum in this animal, although cells with Y-type properties and cells with X-type properties have been identified in LGN (Sherman *et al.*, 1975).

REFERENCES

Albus, K. A quantitative study of the projection area of the central and the paracentral visual field in area 17 of the cat. I. The precision of the topography. *Exp. Brain Res.*, 1975a, *24*, 159–179.

Albus, K. A quantitative study of the projection area of the central and the paracentral visual field in area 17 of the cat. II. The spatial organization of the orientation domain. *Exp. Brain Res.*, 1975b, *24*, 181–202.

Albus, K. Predominance of monocularly driven cells in the projection area of the central visual field in cat's striate cortex. *Brain Res.*, 1975c, *89*, 341–347.

Alder, S. W., and Meikle, T. H., Jr. Visual discrimination of flux-equated figures by cats with brain lesions. *Brain Res.*, 1975, *90*, 23–43.

Anderson, K. V., and Symmes, D. The superior colliculus and higher visual functions in the monkey. *Brain Res.*, 1969, *13*, 37–52.

Arden, G. B., Ikeda, H., and Hill, R. M. Rabbit visual cortex: Reaction of cells to movement and contrast. *Nature*, 1967, *214*, 909–912.

Atencio, F. W., Diamond, I. T., and Ward, J. P. Behavioral study of the visual cortex of *Galago senegalensis*. *J. Comp. Physiol. Psychol.*, 1975, *89*, 1109–1135.

Baden, J. Urbaitis, J., and Meikle, T. Effects of serial bilateral neocortical ablations on a visual discrimination by cats. *Exp. Neurol.*, 1965, *13*, 233–251.

Barbas, H., and Spear, P. D. Effects of serial unilateral and serial bilateral visual cortex lesions on brightness discrimination relearning in rats. *J. Comp. Physiol. Psychol.*, 1976, *90*, 279–292.

Barlow, H. B. Pattern recognition and the responses of sensory neurons. *Ann. N.Y. Acad. Sci.*, 1969, *156*, 872.

Barlow, H. B. Visual pattern analysis in machines and animals. *Science*, 1972a, *177*, 567–576.

Barlow, H. B. Single units and sensation: A neuron doctrine for perceptual psychology? *Perception*, 1972b, *1*, 371–394.

Barlow, H. B., and Levick, W. R. The mechanism of directionally selective units in rabbit's retina. *J. Physiol. (London)*, 1965, *178*, 477–504.

Barlow, H. B., and Levick, W. R. Changes in the maintained discharge with adaptation level in the cat retina. *J. Physiol. (London)*, 1969, *202*, 699.

Barlow, H. B., Fitzhugh, R., and Kuffler, S. W. Dark adaptation, absolute threshold and Purkinje shift in single units of the cat's retina. *J. Physiol. (London)*, 1957a, *137*, 327–337.

Barlow, H. B., Fitzhugh, R., and Kuffler, S. W. Change of organization in the receptive fields of the cat's retina during dark adaptation. *J. Physiol.*, 1957b, *137*, 338–354.

Barlow, H. B., Blakemore, C., and Pettigrew, J. D. The neural mechanism of binocular depth discrimination. *J. Physiol. (London)*, 1967, *193*, 327–342.

Barlow, H. B., Hill, R. M., and Levick, W. R. Retinal ganglion cells responding selectively to direction and speed of image motion in the rabbit. *J. Physiol. (London)*, 1964, *173*, 377–407.

Baumgartner, G., Brown, J. L., and Schulz, A. Responses of single units of the cat visual system to rectangular stimulus patterns. *J. Neurophysiol.*, 1965, *28*, 1–18.

Bekoff, M., Lockwood, A., and Meikle, T. H., Jr. Effects of serial lesions in cat visual cortex on a brightness discrimination. *Brain Res.*, 1973, *49*, 190–193.

Bender, M., and Furlow, L. T. Visual disturbances produced by bilateral lesions of the occipital lobes with central scotomas. *Arch. Neurol. Psychiat.*, 1945, *53*, 29–49.

Beresford, W. A. A nauta and gallocyanin study of the cortico-lateral geniculate projection in the cat and monkey. *J. Hirnforsch.*, 1962, *5*, 211–255.

Berkley, M. Cat visual psychophysics: Neural correlates and comparisons with man. *Progr. Psychobiol. Physiol. Psychol.*, 1976, 63–119.

Berkley, M. A., Loop, M. S., and Evinger, C. Temporal modulation sensitivity of the cat. II. Evoked potential estimates. *Vision Res.*, 1975, *15*, 563–568.

Berkley, M., Sprague, J., and Bloom, M. The role of geniculo-cortical system in form vision: Areas 17 and 18 and visual activity in the cat. *Association for Research in Vision and Ophthalmology Annual Meeting*, Sarasota, 1976.

Bilge, M., Bingle, A., Seneviratne, K. N., and Whitteridge. A map of the visual cortex in the cat. *J. Physiol. Soc.*, 1967, *191*, 116–118.

Bishop, P. O. Neurophysiology of binocular single vision and stereopsis. In *Handbook of Sensory Physiology*, Vol. VII, Part A, Chap. 4. 1973.

Bishop, P. O., Kozak, W., Levick, W. R., and Vakkur, G. J. The determination of the projection of the visual field on to the lateral geniculate nucleus in the cat. *J. Physiol. (London)*, 1962, *163*, 503–539.

Bishop, P. O., Coombs, J. S., and Henry, G. H. Responses to visual contours: Spatio-temporal aspects of excitation in the receptive fields of simple striate neurones. *J. Physiol. (London)*, 1971, *219*, 625–657.

Bishop, P. O., Coombs, J. S., and Henry, G. H. Receptive fields of simple cells in the cat striate cortex. *J. Physiol. (London)*, 1973, *231*, 31–60.

Blakemore, C., and Campbell, F. W. On the existence of neurones in the human visual system selectively sensitive to the orientation and size of retinal images. *J. Physiol. (London)*, 1969, *203*, 237.

Bland, B. H., and Cooper, R. M. Posterior neodecortication in the rat: Age at operation and experience. *J. Comp. Physiol. Psychol.*, 1969, *69*, 345–354.

Bodis-Wollner, I. Visual acuity and contrast sensitivity in patients with cerebral lesions. *Science*, 1972, *178*, 769–771.

Bodis-Wollner, I. Vulnerability of spatial frequency channels in cerebral lesions. *Nature*, 1976, *261*, 209–311.

Bough, E. W. Stereoscopic vision in the macaque monkey: A behavioral demonstration. *Nature*, 1970, *225*, 42.

Boycott, B. B., and Dowling, J. E. Organization of the primate retina: Light microscopy. *Phil. Trans. Roy. Soc. London Ser. B*, 1969, *255*, 109–184.

Boycott, B. B., and Wässle, H. The morphological types of ganglion cells of the domestic cat's retina. *J. Physiol. (London)*, 1974, *240*, 397–419.

Braun, J. J., Lundy, E. G., and McCarthy, F. V. Depth discrimination in rats following removal of visual neocortex. *Brain Res.*, 1970, *20*, 283–291.

Brindley, G. S. *Physiology of the Retina and the Visual Pathway.* Monograph Physiological Society, 2nd ed. Edward Arnold, London, 1970.

Buchtel, H. Visual form discrimination on the basis of relative distribution of light. *Science,* 1969, *164,* 857–858.

Burrows, G., and Hayhow, W. R. The organization of the thalamo-cortical visual pathways in the cat. *Brain Behav. Evol.,* 1971, *4,* 220–227.

Butter, C. M. Impairments in selective attention to visual stimuli in monkeys with inferotemporal and lateral striate lesions. *Brain Res.,* 1969, *12,* 374–383.

Campbell, F. W., and Robson, J. G. Application of Fourier analysis to the visibility of gratings. *J. Physiol. (London),* 1968, *197,* 551.

Campbell, F. W., Cooper, G. F., and Enroth-Cugell, C. The spatial selectivity of the visual cells of the cat. *J. Physiol. (London),* 1969, *203,* 223–235.

Campbell, F. W., Cooper, G. F., Robson, J. G., and Sachs, M. B. The spatial selectivity of visual cells of the cat and the squirrel monkey. *Journal Physiol. (London),* 1970, *204,* 120–121.

Casagrande, V. A., and Harting, J. K. Transneuronal transport of tritiated fucose and proline in the visual pathways of tree shrew *Tupaia glis. Brain Res.,* 1975, *96,* 367–372.

Chow, K. L. Visual discrimination after extensive ablation of optic tract and visual cortex in cats. *Brain Res.,* 1968, *9,* 363–366.

Chow, K. L., Lindsley, D. F., and Gollender, M. Modification of response patterns of lateral geniculate neurons after paired stimulation of contralateral and ipsilateral eyes. *J. Neurophysiol.,* 1968, *31,* 729.

Chow, K. L., Masland, R. H., and Steward, D. L. Receptive field characteristics of striate cortical neurons in the rabbit. *Brain Res.,* 1971, *33,* 337.

Cleland, B. G., and Levick, W. R. Brisk and sluggish concentrically organized ganglion cells in the cat's retina. *J. Physiol. (London),* 1974a, *240,* 421–456.

Cleland, B. G., and Levick, W. R. Properties of rarely encountered types of ganglion cells in the cat's retina and an overall classification. *J. Physiol. (London),* 1974b, *240,* 457–492.

Cleland, B. G., Dubin, M. W., and Levick, W. R. Simultaneous recording of input and output of lateral geniculate neurones. *Nature New Biol.,* 1971a, *231,* 191–192.

Cleland, B. G., Dubin, M. W., and Levick, W. R. Sustained and transient neurones in the cat's retina and lateral geniculate nucleus. *J. Physiol. (London),* 1971b, *217,* 473–496.

Cleland, B. G., Levick, W. R., and Sanderson, K. J. Properties of sustained and transient ganglion cells in the cat retina. *J. Physiol. (London),* 1973, *228,* 649–680.

Cornwell, P., Overman, W., Levitsky, C., Shipley, J., and Lezynski, B. Performance on the visual cliff by cats with marginal gyrus lesions. *J. Comp. Physiol. Psychol.,* 1976, *90,* 996–1010.

Cowey, A. Projection of the retina on to striate and prestriate cortex in the squirrel monkey, *Saimiri sciureus. J. Neurophysiol.,* 1964, *27,* 366–393.

Cowey, A. Perimetric study of field defects in monkeys after cortical and retinal ablations. *Q. J. Exp. Psychol.,* 1967, *19,* 232.

Cowey, A., and Ellis, C. M. The cortical representation of the retina in squirrel and rhesus monkeys and its relation to visual acuity. *Exp. Neurol.,* 1969, *24,* 374–385.

Cowey, A., and Weiskrantz, L. A perimetric study of visual field defects in monkeys. *Q. J. Exp. Psychol.,* 1963, *15,* 91–115.

Cowey, A., and Weiskrantz, L. A comparison of the effects of inferotemporal and striate cortex lesions on the visual behavior of rhesus monkey. *Q. J. Exp. Psychol.,* 1967, *19,* 246–253.

Craft, L. H., and Butter, C. M. Effect of striate cortex removal on wavelength discrimination in rats. *Psychol. Rec.,* 1968, *18,* 311.

Dalby, D. A., Meyer, D. R., and Meyer, P. M. Effects of occipital neocortical lesions upon visual discriminations in the cat. *Physiol. Behav.,* 1970, *5,* 727–734.

Daniel, P. M., and Whitteridge, D. The representation of the visual field on the cerebral cortex in monkeys. *J. Physiol. (London),* 1961, *159,* 203–221.

Daw, N. W., and Pearlman, A. L. Cat colour vision: One cone process or several? *J. Physiol. (London),* 1969, *201,* 745.

Daw, N. W., and Pearlman, A. L. Cat colour vision: Evidence for more than one cone process. *J. Physiol. (London),* 1970, *211,* 125–137.

Denny-Brown, D., and Chambers, R. A. Physiological aspects of visual perception. I. Functional aspects of visual cortex. *Arch. Neurol.,* 1976, *33,* 219–227.

deValois, R. L., Abramov, I., and Mead, W. R. Single cell analysis of wavelength discrimination at the lateral geniculate nucleus in the macaque. *J. Neurophysiol.,* 1967, *30,* 415–433.

Diamond, I. T. Organization of the visual cortex: Comparative anatomical and behavioral studies. *Fed. Proc.*, 1976, *35*, 60–67.

Dodwell, P. C., and Freedman, N. L. Visual form discrimination after removal of the visual cortex in cats. *Science*, 1968, *160*, 559–560.

Doty, R. W. Survival of pattern vision after removal of striate cortex in the adult cat. *J. Comp. Neurol.*, 1971, *143*, 341.

Doty, R. W., Glickstein, and Calvin, W. H. Lamination of the lateral geniculate nucleus in the squirrel monkey, *Saimiri sciureus. J. Comp. Neurol.,* 1966, *127*, 335–340.

Dow, B. M., and Gouras, P. Color and spatial specificity of single units in rhesus monkey foveal striate cortex. *J. Neurophysiol.*, 1973, *36*, 79–100.

Dowling, J. E. Organization of vertebrate retinas. *Invest. Ophthalmol.*, 1970, *9*, 655–680.

Dowling, J. E., and Boycott, B. B. Organization of the primate retina: Election microscopy. *Proc. Roy. Soc. London Ser., B* 1966, *166*, 80–111.

Dräger, U. C. Autoradiography of tritiated proline and fucose transported transneuronally from the eye to the visual cortex in pigmented and albino mice. *Brain Res.*, 1974, *82*, 284–292.

Dräger, U. C. Receptive fields of single cells and topography in mouse visual cortex. *J. Comp. Neurol.*, 1975, *160*, 269–289.

Enroth-Cugell, C., and Robson, J. G. The contrast sensitivity of retinal ganglion cells of the cat. *J. Physiol. (London)*, 1966, *187*, 517–552.

Fillenz, M. Binocular interaction in the lateral geniculate body of the cat. In R. Jung and H. Kornhuber (eds.), *The Visual System: Neurophysiology & Psychophysics,* Berlin–Gottingen–Heidelberg: Springer, 1961.

Fischer, B., and Krüger, J. The shift-effect in the cat's lateral geniculate neurons. *Exp. Brain Res.*, 1974, *21*, 225–227.

Fischer, B., Krüger, J., and Droll, W. Quantitative aspects of the shift-effect in cat retinal ganglion cells. *Brain Res.*, 1975, *83*, 391–403.

Fox, R. F., and Blake, R. R. Stereoscopic vision in the cat. *Nature*, 1971, *233*, 55–56.

Fukuda, Y. Receptive field organization of cat optic nerve fibers with special reference to conduction velocity. *Vision Res.*, 1971, *11*, 209.

Fukuda, Y. Differentiation of principal cells of the rat lateral geniculate body into two groups; fast and slow cells. *Exp. Brain Res.*, 1973, *17*, 242–260.

Fukuda, Y., and Saito, H.-A. S. The relationship between response characteristics to flicker stimulation and receptive field organization in the cat's optic nerve fibers. *Vision Res.*, 1971, *11*, 227–240.

Fukuda, Y., and Stone, J. Direct identification of the cell bodies of Y-, X- and W-cells in the cat's retina. *Vision Res.*, 1975, *15*, 1034–1036.

Garey, L., and Powell, T. The projection of the retina in the cat. *J. Anat. (London)*, 1968, *102*, 189–222.

Garey, L. J., and Powell, T. P. S. The projection of the lateral geniculate nucleus upon the cortex in the cat. *Proc. Roy. Soc. London Ser. B*, 1967, *169*, 107–126.

Galambos, R., Norton, T. T., and Frommer, G. P. Optic tract lesions sparing pattern vision in cats. *Exp. Neurol.*, 1967, *18*, 8–25.

Glees, P. The termination of optic fibers in the lateral geniculate body of the cat. *J. Anat. (London)*, 1941, *75*, 434–440.

Glendenning, K. V., and Kofron, E. A. Projections of individual laminae of the lateral geniculate nucleus in the prosimian. *Neurosci. Abstr.*, 1974, 229.

Glickstein, M. Laminar structure of the dorsal lateral geniculate nucleus in the tree shrew *(Tupaia glis). J. Comp. Neurol.*, 1967, *131*, 93–102.

Glickstein, M. Organization of the visual pathways. *Science*, 1969, *164*, 917–926.

Glickstein, M., King, R. A., Miller, J., and Berkley, M. Cortical projections from the dorsal lateral geniculate nucleus of cats. *J. Comp. Neurol.*, 1967, *130*, 55–76.

Gouras, P. Identification of cone mechanisms in monkey ganglion cells. *J. Physiol. (London)*, 1968, *199*, 533–547.

Grafstein, B., and Laurens, R. Transport of radioactivity from eye to visual cortex in the mouse. *Exp. Neurol.*, 1973, *39*, 44–57.

Guillery, R. W. A study of Golgi preparations from the dorsal lateral geniculate nucleus of the adult cat. *J. Comp. Neurol.*, 1966, *128*, 21–50.

Guillery, R. W. The laminar distribution of retinal fibers in the dorsal lateral geniculate nucleus of the cat: A new interpretation. *J. Comp. Neurol.*, 1970, *138*, 339.

Guillery, R. W., and Kaas, J. H. A study of normal and congenitally abnormal retinogeniculate projections in cats. *J. Comp. Neurol.*, 1971, *143*, 73.

Guillery, R. W., Okoro, A. N., and Witkop, C. J., Jr. Abnormal visual pathways in the brain of a human albino. *Brain Res.*, 1975, *96*, 373–377.

Hall, W. C., and Diamond, I. T. Organization and function of the visual cortex in hedgehog. II. An ablation study of pattern discrimination. *Brain Behav. Evol.*, 1968, *1*, 215.

Harting, J. K., Diamond, I. T., and Hall, W. C. Anterograde degeneration study of the cortical projections of the lateral geniculate and pulvinar nuclei in the tree shrew *(Tupaia glis)*. *J. Comp. Neurol.*, 1973, *150*, 393–440.

Hayhow, W. R. The cytoarchitecture of the lateral geniculate body in the cat in relation to the distribution of crossed and uncrossed optic fibers. *J. Comp. Neurol.*, 1958, *110*, 1–64.

Hoffmann, K. P. Conduction velocity in pathways from retina to superior colliculus in the cat: A correlation with receptive-field properties. *J. Neurophysiol.*, 1973, *36*, 409–424.

Hoffmann, K. P., Stone, J., and Sherman, S. M. Relay of receptive-field properties in dorsal lateral geniculate nucleus of the cat. *J. Neurophysiol.*, 1972, *4*, 518–531.

Holländer, H., and Martinez-Millan, L. Short communications: Autoradiographic evidence for a topographically organized projection from the striate cortex to the lateral geniculate nucleus in the rhesus monkey *(Macaca mulatta)*. *Brain Res.*, 1975, *100*, 407–411.

Holmes, G. Disturbances of vision by cerebral lesions. *Br. J. Ophthalmol.*, 1918, *2*, 353–362.

Horel, H., Bettinger, L., Royce, G., and Meyer, D. Role of neocortex in the learning and relearning of two visual habits by the rat. *J. Comp. Physiol. Psychol.*, 1966, *61*, 66–78.

Hubel, D. H. An autoradiographic study of the retino-cortical projections in the tree shrew *(Tupaia glis)*. *Brain Res.*, 1975, *96*, 41–50.

Hubel, D. H., and Wiesel, T. N. Receptive fields of single neurons in the cat's striate cortex. *J. Physiol. (London)*, 1959, *148*, 574.

Hubel, D. H., and Wiesel, T. N. Integrative action in the cat's lateral geniculate body. *J. Physiol. (London)*, 1961, *155*, 385–398.

Hubel, D. H., and Wiesel, T. N. Receptive fields, binocular interaction and functional architecture in the cat's visual cortex. *J. Physiol. (London)*, 1962, *160*, 106–154.

Hubel, D. H., and Wiesel, T. N. Shape and arrangement of columns in cat's striate cortex. *J. Physiol. (London)*, 1963, *165*, 559–568.

Hubel, D. H., and Wiesel, T. N. Binocular interaction in striate cortex of kittens reared with artificial squint. *J. Neurophysiol.*, 1965a, *28*, 1041–1059.

Hubel, D. H., and Wiesel, T. N. Receptive fields and functional architecture in two nonstriate visual areas (18 and 19) of the cat. *J. Neurophysiol.*, 1965b, *28*, 229–289.

Hubel, D. H., and Wiesel, T. N. Receptive fields and functional architecture of monkey striate cortex. *J. Physiol. (London)*, 1968, *195*, 215.

Hubel, D. H., and Wiesel, T. N. Anatomical demonstration of columns in the monkey striate cortex. *Nature*, 1969, *221*, 747.

Hubel, D. H., and Wiesel, T. N. The period of susceptibility to the physiological effects of unilateral eye closure in kittens. *J. Physiol. (London)*, 1970a, *206*, 419.

Hubel, D. H., and Wiesel, T. N. Cells sensitive to binocular depth in area 18 of the macaque monkey cortex. *Nature*, 1970b, *225*, 41.

Hubel, D. H., and Wiesel, T. N. Laminar and columnar distribution of geniculo-cortical fibers in the macaque monkey. *J. Comp. Neurol.*, 1972, *146*, 421–450.

Hubel, D. H., and Wiesel, T. N. Uniformity of monkey striate cortex: A parallel relationship between field size, scatter, and magnification factor. *J. Comp. Neurol.*, 1974a, *158*, 295–306.

Hubel, D. H., and Wiesel, T. N. Sequence regularity and geometry of orientation columns in the monkey striate cortex. *J. Comp. Neurol.*, 1974b, *158*, 267–294.

Humphrey, N., and Weiskrantz, L. Vision in monkeys after removal of the striate cortex. *Nature*, 1967, *215*, 595–597.

Ikeda, H., and Wright, M. J. Receptive field organization of "sustained" and "transient" retinal ganglion cells which subserve different functional roles. *J. Physiol. (London)*, 1972, *227*, 769–800.

Ikeda, H., and Wright, M. J. The relationship between the "sustained-transient" and the "simple-complex" classifications of neurones in area 17 of the cat. *J. Physiol. (London)*, 1974, *244*, 59–60.

Ikeda, H., and Wright, M. J. Spatial and temporal properties of "sustained" and "transient" neurones in area 17 of the cat's visual cortex. *Exp. Brain Res.*, 1975a, *22*, 363–383.

Ikeda, H., and Wright, M. J. Retinotopic distribution, visual latency and orientation tuning of "sustained" and "transient" cortical neurones in area 17 of the cat. *Exp. Brain Res.*, 1975b, *22*, 385–398.

Ikeda, H., and Wright, M. J. The latency of visual cortical neurones in area 17 in the cat to visual stimuli with reference to the sustained (X) and transient (Y) and "simple" and "complex" cell classification. *J. Physiol. (London)*, 1975c, *245*, 114P.

Ikeda, H., and Wright, M. J. Properties of sustained-X, transient-Y, and transient-X cells in the cat's lateral geniculate nucleus. *J. Physiol. (London)*, 1976, *254*, 1, 65P.

Jacobson, M. The representation of the retina on the optic tectum of the frog. Correlation between retinotectal magnification factor and retinal ganglion cell count. *Q. J. Exp. Physiol.*, 1962, *47*, 170–178.

Jones, A. E. The lateral geniculate complex of the owl monkey *(Aotus trivirgatus)*. *J. Comp. Neurol.*, 1966, *126*, 171–180.

Joshua, D. E., and Bishop, P. O. Binocular single vision and depth discrimination. Receptive field disparities for central and peripheral vision and binocular interaction on peripheral single units in cat striate cortex. *Exp. Brain Res.*, 1970, *10*, 389–416.

Jung, R. Visual perception and neurophysiology. In Jung, R. (ed.) Central Processing of Visual Information Part A. Springer-Verlag: Berlin, 1973, pp 1–152.

Kaas, J. H., Hall, W. C., and Diamond, I. T. Cortical visual areas I and II in the Hedgehog: Relation Between evoked potential maps and architectonic subdivisions. *J. Neurophysiol.*, 1970, *33*, 595.

Kaas, J. H., Guillery, R. W., and Allman, J. M. Some principles of organization in the dorsal lateral geniculate nucleus. *Brain, Behav. Evol.*, 1972a, *6*, 253–299.

Kaas, J. H., Hall, W. C., and Diamond, I. T. Visual cortex of the grey squirrel (Sciurus carolinensis): architectonic subdivisions and connections from the visual thalamus. *J. Comp. Neurol.*, 1972b, *145*, 273–306.

Kaas, J. H., Hall, W. C., Killackey, H., and Diamond, I. T. Visual cortex of the tree shrew *(Tupaia glis)*: Architectonic subdivisions and representations of the visual field. *Brain Res.*, 1972c, *42*, 491–496.

Kaas, J. H., Guillery, R. W., and Allman, J. M. Discontinuities in the dorsal lateral geniculate nucleus corresponding to the optic disc: A comparative study. *J. Comp. Neurol.*, 1973, *147*, 163–180.

Kanagasuntheram, R., Krishnamurti, A., and Wong, W. C. Observations on the lamination of the lateral geniculate body in some primates. *Brain Res.*, 1969, *14*, 623–631.

Keating, E. G., and Horel, J. A. Cortical blindness after overlapping retinal-striate lesions: A limit to plasticity in the central visual system. *Brain Res.*, 1976, *101*, 327–339.

Kelly, D. H. Adaptation effects on spatio-temporal sine-wave thresholds. *Vision Res.*, 1972, *12*, 89.

Kennedy, J. L. The nature and physiological basis of visual movement discrimination in animals. *Psychol. Rev.*, 1936a, *43*, 494–521.

Kennedy, J. L. The effect of complete and partial bilateral extirpation of the area striata on visual movement discrimination in the cat. *Psychol. Bull.*, 1936b, *33*, 754.

Kennedy, J. L. The effects of complete and partial occipital lobectomy upon thresholds of visual real movement discrimination in the cat. *J. Genet. Psychol.*, 1939, *54*, 119–149.

Kicliter, E., Loop, M., and Jane, J. Luminous flux, wavelength and stripe orientation discrimination in ground squirrels *(Citellus tridecemlineatus)* after posterior neocortical lesions. *Soc. Neurosci. Abstr.*, 1974, 281.

Killackey, H., and Diamond, I. T. Visual attention in the tree shrew: An ablation study of the striate and extrastriate visual cortex. *Science*, 1971, *171*, 696–699.

Killackey, H., Snyder, M., and Diamond, I. T. Function of striate and temporal cortex in the tree shrew. *J. Comp. Physiol. Monogr.*, 1971, *74*, 1–29.

Killackey, H., Wilson, M., and Diamond, I. T. Further studies of the striate and extrastriate visual cortex in the tree shrew. *J. Comp. Physiol. Psychol.*, 1972, *81*, 45–63.

Kinston, W. J., Vadas, M. A., and Bishop, P. O. Multiple projection of the visual field to the medial portion of the dorsal lateral geniculate nucleus and the adjacent nuclei of the thalamus of the cat. *J. Comp. Neurol.*, 1969, *136*, 295–316.

Klüver, H. Visual functions after removal of the occipital lobes. *J. Psychol. (London)*, 1941, *11*, 23–45.

Koerner, F., and Teuber, H. L. Visual field defects after missile injuries to the geniculo-striate pathway in man. *Exp. Brain Res.*, 1973, *18*, 88–113.

Kuffler, S. W. Discharge patterns and functional organization of mammalian retina. *J. Neurophysiol.*, 1953, *16*, 37–68.

Kupfer, C. The laminar pattern and distribution of cell size in the lateral geniculate nucleus of man. *J. Neurophathol. Exp. Neurol.*, 1965, *24*, 643–652.

Lashley, K. S. The mechanism of vision. IV. The cerebral areas necessary for pattern vision in the rat. *J. Comp. Neurol.*, 1931, *53*, 419–478.

Lashley, K. S., and Frank, M. The mechanism of vision. X. Postoperative disturbances of habits based on detail vision in the rat after lesions in the cerebral visual areas. Comp. Psychol., 1934, *17*, 355–391.

Laties, A. M., and Sprague, J. M. The projection of optic fibers to the visual centers in the cat. *J. Comp. Neurol.,* 1966, *127*, 35–70.

Leicester, J., and Stone, J. Ganglion, amacrine and horizontal cells of the cat's retina. *Vision Res.,* 1967, *7*, 695.

LeGros Clark, W. E. The laminar organization and cell content of the lateral geniculate body in the monkey. *J. Anat. (London),* 1941, *75*, 419–431.

LeGros Clark, W. The laminar pattern of the lateral geniculate nucleus considered in relation to color vision. *Doc. Ophthalmol.,* 1949, *3*, 57.

LeGros Clark, W. E., and Penman, C. G. The projection of the retina in the lateral geniculate body. *Proc. Roy. Soc. London Ser. B,* 1934, *114*, 291–313.

Lepore, F., Cardu, B., Rasmussen, T., and Malmo, R. B. Rod and cone sensitivity in destriate monkeys. *Brain Res.,* 1975, *93*, 203–221.

LeVay, S., and Gilbert, C. D. Laminar patterns of geniculocortical projection in the cat. *Brain Res.,* 1976, *113*, 1–19.

LeVay, S., Hubel, D. H., and Wiesel, T. N. The pattern of ocular dominance columns in macaque visual cortex revealed by a reduced silver stain. *J. Comp. Neurol.,* 1975, *159*, 559–576.

Levick, W. R., and Cleland, B. G. Receptive fields of cat retinal ganglion cells having slowly conducting axons. *Brain Res.,* 1974a, *74*, 156–160.

Levick, W. R., and Cleland, B. G. Selectivity of microelectrodes in recordings from cat retinal ganglion cells. *J. Neurophysiol.,* 1974b, *37*, 1387–1393.

Lewellyn, D., Lowes, G., and Isaacson, R. Visually mediated behavior following neocortical destruction in the rat. *J. Comp. Physiol. Psychol.,* 1969, *69*, 25–32.

Lindsley, D., Chow, K. L., and Gollender, M. Dichoptic interactions of lateral geniculate neurons of cats to contralateral and ipsilateral eye stimulation. *J. Neurophysiol.,* 1967, *30*, 628–644.

Loop, M. S., and Berkley, M. A. Temporal modulation sensitivity of the cat. I. Behavioral measures. *Vision Res.,* 1975, *15*, 555–561.

Lopes da Silva, F. H. Dynamic characteristics of visual evoked potentials: A quantitiative study of cortical and subcortical potentials evoked in dog by sinewave modulated light and their relation to flicker fusion. Report 1.5.63-3, Institute of Medical Physics Utrecht, The Netherlands, March 25, 1970.

Maffei, L., and Fiorentini, A. Retino-geniculate convergence and the analysis of contrast. *Brain Res.,* 1971, *31*, 371–372.

Maffei, L., and Fiorentini, A. Retinogeniculate convergence and analysis of contrast. *J. Neurophysiol.,* 1972, *35*, 65–72.

Maffei, L., and Fiorentini, A. The visual cortex as a spatial frequency analyser. *Vision Res.,* 1973, *13*, 1255–1267.

Maffei, L., and Rizzolatti, G. Transfer properties of the lateral geniculate body. *J. Neurophysiol.,* 1967, *30*, 333–340.

Maffei, L., Cervetto, L., and Fiorentini, A. Transfer characteristics of excitation and inhibition in cat retinal ganglion cells. *J. Neurophysiol.,* 1970, *33*, 276–284.

Malmo, R. Effects of striate cortex ablation on intensity discrimination and spectral intensity distribution in the rhesus monkey. *Neuropsychologia (Berlin),* 1966, *4*, 9–26.

Malpeli, J. G., and Baker, F. H. The representation of the visual field in the lateral geniculate nucleus of *Macaca mulatta. J. Comp. Neurol.,* 1975, *161*, 569–594.

Marg, E., Adams, J., and Rutkin, B. Receptive fields of cells in the human visual cortex. *Experientia,* 1968, *24*, 348–350.

Marrocco, R. T., and Brown, J. B. Correlation of receptive field properties of monkey LGN cells with the conduction velocity of retinal afferent input. *Brain Res.,* 1975, *92*, 137–144.

Marshall, W., Talbot, S., and Ades, H. Cortical response of anesthetized cat to gross photic and electrical stimulation. *J. Neurophysiol.,* 1943, *6*, 1–15.

Matthews, M. R., Cowan, W. M., and Powell, T. P. S. Transneuronal cell degeneration in the lateral geniculate nucleus of the macaque monkey. *J. Anat. (London),* 1960, *94*, 145–169.

McIlwain, J. T. Receptive fields of optic tract axons and lateral geniculate cells: Peripheral extent and barbiturate sensitivity. *J. Neurophysiol.,* 1964, *27*, 1154–1173.

McIlwain, J. T. Some evidence concerning the physiological basis of the periphery effect in the cat's retina. *Exp. Brain Res.,* 1966, *1*, 265–271.

Mead. L. C. The curve of visual intensity discrimination in the cat before and after removal of the striate area of the cortex. Dissertation, 1939, University of Rochester.

Meyer, P. M. Analysis of visual behavior in cats with extensive neocortical ablations. *J. Comp. Physiol. Psychol.,* 1963, *56*, 397–401.

Meyer, P. M., Anderson, R. A., and Braun, M. G. Visual cliff preferences following lesions of the visual neocortex in cats and rats. *Psychon. Sci.*, 1966, *4*, 269–270.

Michael, C. R. Visual receptive fields of single neurons in superior colliculus of the ground squirrel. *J. Neurophysiol.*, 1972, *35*, 815–832.

Michael, C. R. Opponent-color and opponent-contrast cells in lateral geniculate nucleus of the ground squirrel. *J. Neurophysiol.*, 1973, *36*, 536–550.

Minkowski, M. Über den Verlauf, die Endigung und die Zentrale Repräsentation von gebreutzten und ungekreuzen Sehnerven fasern bei einigen Säugetieren und bei Menchen. *Schweiz. Arch. Neurol. Psychiat.*, 1920, *6*, 201–268.

Mishkin, M., and Weiskrantz, L. Effects of cortical lesions in monkeys on critical flicker frequency. *J. Comp. Physiol. Psychol.*, 1959, *52*, 660.

Mize, R. R., Wetzel, A. B., and Thompson, V. E. Contour discrimination in the rat following removal of posterior cortex. *Physiol. Behav.*, 1971, *6*, 241–246.

Movshon, J. A. The velocity tuning of single units in cat striate cortex. *J. Physiol. (London)*, 1975, *249*, 445–468.

Murphy, E. H., and Chow, K. L. Effects of striate and occipital cortical lesions on visual discrimination in the rabbit. *Exp. Neurol.*, 1974, *42*, 78–88.

Murphy, E. H., and Stewart, D. L. Effects of neonatal and adult striate lesions on visual discrimination in the rabbit. *Exp. Neurol.*, 1974, *42*, 89–96.

Murphy, E. H., Mize, R. R., and Schechter, P. B. Visual discrimination following infant and adult ablation of cortical areas 17, 18, and 19 in the cat. *Exp. Neurol.*, 1975, *49*, 386–405.

Niimi, K., and Sprague, J. M. Thalamo-cortical organization of the visual system in the cat. *J. Comp. Neurol.*, 1970, *138*, 29–250.

Noda, H., Tamaki, Y., and Iwama, K. Binocular units in the lateral geniculate nucleus of chronic cats. *Brain Res.*, 1972, *41*, 81–99.

Norton, A. C., and Clark, G. Effects of cortical and collicular lesions on brightness and flicker discrimination in the cat. *Vision Res.*, 1963a, *3*, 29–44.

Norton, A. C., and Clark, G. Acquisition of a flicker discrimination in the cortically blind cat. *Vision Res.*, 1963b, *3*, 75–79.

Norton, T. T., Galambos, R., and Frommer, G. P. Optic tract lesions destroying pattern vision in cats. *Exp. Neurol.*, 1967, *18*, 26–37.

O'Leary, J. L. Structure of the area striata of the cat. *J. Comp. Neurol.*, 1941, *75*, 131–164.

Otsuka, R., and Hassler, R. Über Aufbau und Gliederung der corticalen Sehsphare bei der Katze. *Arch. Psychiat. Ztsch. Neurol.*, 1962, *203*, 212–234.

Packwood, J., and Gordon, B. Stereopsis in normal domestic cat, Siamese cat, and cat raised with alternating monocular occlusion. *J. Neurophysiol.*, 1975, *38*, 1485–1499.

Pasik, P., Pasik, T., and Krieger, H. The effects of cerebral lesions upon optokinetic nystagmus in monkeys. *J. Neurophysiol.*, 1959, *22*, 297–304.

Pasik, T., and Pasik, P. The visual world of monkeys deprived of striate cortex and the importance of accessory optic system in its perception. Abstract of paper given at International Symposium on Visual Processes in Vertebrates, Santiago, Chile, 1970.

Pasik, P., Pasik, T., and Schilder, P. Extrageniculostriate vision in the monkey: Discrimination of luminous flux-equated figures. *Exp. Neurol.*, 1969, *24*, 421–437.

Pearlman, A. L., and Daw, N. W. Opponent color cells in the cat lateral geniculate nucleus. *Science*, 1970, *167*, 84–86.

Peters, Alan, and Palay, S. L. The morphology of laminae A and A_1 of the dorsal nucleus of the lateral geniculate body of the cat. *J. Anat.*, 1966, *100*, 451–486.

Pettigrew, J. D., Nikara, T., and Bishop, P. O. Responses to moving slits by single units in cat striate cortex. *Exp. Brain Res.*, 1968, *6*, 373.

Pitts, W., and McCulloch, W. How we know universals: The perception of auditory and visual forms. *Bull. Math. Biophys.*, 1947, *9*, 127–147.

Pollen, D. A., and Ronner, S. F. Periodic excitability changes across the receptive fields of complex cells in the striate and parastriate cortex of the cat. *J. Physiol.*, 1975, *245*, 667–697.

Pollen, D. A., Lee, J. R., and Taylor, J. H. How does the striate cortex begin the reconstruction of the visual world? *Science*, 1971, *173*, 74–77.

Polyak, S. *The Retina.* University of Chicago Press, Chicago, 1948.

Polyak, S. *The Vertebrate Visual System.* University of Chicago Press, Chicago, 1957.

Poppel, E., Held, R., and Frost, D. Residual visual function after brain wounds involving the central visual pathways in man. *Nature*, 1973, *243*, 295–296.

Poppel, E., von Cramon, D., and Backmund, H. Eccentricity-specific dissociation of visual functions in patients with lesions of the central visual pathways. *Nature,* 1975, *256,* 489–490.

Ramon y Cajal, S. *Die Retina der Wirbelthiere.* (Wiesbaden, 1892, Bergman's trans.) In S. A. Thorpe and M. Glickstein, (eds.), *The Structure of the Retina.* Thomas, Springfield, Ill., 1972.

Richards, W. Visual processing in scotomata. *Exp. Brain Res.,* 1973, *17,* 333–347.

Riddoch, G. Dissociation of visual perceptions due to occipital injuries, with especial reference to appreciation of movement. *Brain,* 1917, *40,* 15–57.

Rodieck, R. W. Quantitative analysis of cat retinal ganglion cell response to visual stimuli. *Vision Res.,* 1965, *5,* 583–601.

Rodieck, R. Receptive fields in the cat retina: A new type. *Science,* 1967, *157,* 90–92.

Rodieck, R. W. *The Vertebrate Retina: Principles of Structure and Function.* Freeman, San Francisco, 1973.

Rolls, E. T., and Cowey, A. Topography of the retina and striate cortex and its relationship to visual acuity in rhesus monkeys and squirrel monkeys. *Exp. Brain Res.,* 1970, *10,* 298–310.

Rosenquist, A. C., Edwards, S. B., and Palmer, L. A. An autoradiographic study of the projections of the dorsal lateral geniculate nucleus and the posterior nucleus in the cat. *Brain Res.,* 1974, *80,* 71–93.

Sanderson, K. J. Visual field projection columns and magnification factors in the lateral geniculate nucleus of the cat. *Exp. Brain Res.,* 1971*a, 13,* 159–177.

Sanderson, K. J. The projection of the visual field to the lateral geniculate and medial interlaminar nuclei in the cat. *J. Comp. Neurol.,* 1971*b, 143(1),* 101–117.

Sanderson, K. J. Lamination of the dorsal lateral geniculate nucleus in carnivores of the weasel *(Mustelidae),* raccoon *(Procyonidae)* and fox *(Canidae)* families. *J. Comp. Neurol.,* 1974, *153,* 239–266.

Sanderson, K. J., Darian-Smith, I., and Bishop, P. O. Binocular corresponding receptive fields of single units in the cat dorsal lateral geniculate nucleus. *Vision Res.,* 1969, *9,* 1927.

Sanderson, K., Bishop, P., and Darian-Smith, I. The properties of the binocular receptive fields of lateral geniculate neurons. *Exp. Brain Res.,* 1971, *13,* 178–207.

Sanides, F., and Hoffmann, J. Cyto- and myeloarchitecture of the visual cortex of the cat and of the surrounding integration cortices. *J. Hirnforsch.,* 1969, *11(1/2),* 79–104.

Sarmiento, R. F. The stereoacuity of macaque monkey. *Vision Res.,* 1975, *15,* 493–498.

Schilder, P. Loss of a brightness discrimination in the cat following removal of the striate area. *J. Neurophysiol.,* 1966, *29,* 888.

Schilder, P., Pasik, T., and Pasik, P. Extrageniculostriate vision in the monkey. II. Demonstration of brightness discrimination. *Brain Res.,* 1971, *32,* 383–398.

Schilder, P., Pasik, P., and Pasik, T. Extrageniculostriate vision in the monkey. III. Circle vs. triangle and "red vs. green" discrimination. *Exp. Brain Res.,* 1972, *14,* 436–448.

Schwartz, A. S., and Cheney, C. Neural mechanisms involved in the critical flicker frequency of the cat. *Brain Res.,* 1966, *1,* 369–380.

Schwartz, A., and Clark, G. Discrimination of intermittent photic stimulation in the cat without its striate cortex. *J. Comp. Physiol. Psychol.,* 1957, *50,* 468–474.

Sefton, A. J., and Bruce, I. S. Properties of cells in the lateral geniculate nucleus. *Vision Res. Suppl. No. 3,* 1971, 239–252.

Shatz, C., Lindstrom, S., and Wiesel, T. Ocular dominance columns in the cat's visual cortex. *Neurosci. Abstr.,* 1975, 56.

Sherman, S. M., Norton, T., and Casagrande, V. X- and Y-cells in the dorsal lateral geniculate nucleus of the tree shrew. *Brain Res.,* 1975, *93,* 152–157.

Shkolnik-Yarros, E. G. Neurons of the cat's retina. *Vision Res.,* 1971*a, 11,* 7–26.

Shkol'nick-Yarros, E. G. Asymmetrical dendritic fields of retinal ganglion cells. *Neurofiziologiya,* 1971*b, 3,* 301–306.

Singer, W., and Bedworth, N. Inhibitory interaction between X and Y units in the cat lateral geniculate nucuelus. *Brain Res.,* 1973, *49,* 291–307.

Singer, W., and Creutzfeldt, O. D. Reciprocal lateral inhibition of on- and off-center neurons in the lateral geniculate body of the cat. *Exp. Brain Res.,* 1970, *10,* 311.

Smith, K. U. The acuity of the cat's discrimination of visual form. *Psychol. Bull.,* 1934*a, 31,* 618–619.

Smith, K. U. Visual discrimination in the cat. I. The capacity of the cat for visual figure discrimination. *J. Genet. Psychol.,* 1934*b, 44,* 301–320.

Smith, K. U. Visual discrimination in the cat. II. A further study of the capacity of the cat for visual figure discrimination. *J. Genet. Psychol.,* 1935, *45,* 336–357.

Smith, K. U. The effect of extirpation of the striate cortex upon visually controlled palpebral reactions, compensatory eye-movements, and placing reactions of the forelimbs in the cat. *Psychol. Bull.,* 1936*a*, *33*, 606–607.

Smith, K. U. The postoperative effects of removal of the occipital cortex upon visual intensity discrimination in the cat. *Am. J. Physiol.,* 1936*b*, *116*, 145–146.

Smith, K. U. The effect of removal of the occipital cortex upon visual acuity in the cat, as measured by oculo-cephalo-gyric responses. *Psychol. Bull.,* 1936*c*, *33*, 754–773.

Smith, K. U. Visual discrimination in the cat. VI. The relation between pattern vision and visual acuity and the optic projection centers and the nervous system. *J. Genet. Psychol.,* 1938, *53*, 251–272.

Smith, K. U., and Warkentin, J. The central neural organization of optic functions related to minimum visible acuity. *J. Genet. Psychol.,* 1939, *55*, 177–195.

Snyder, M., and Diamond, I. T. The organization and function of the visual cortex in the tree shrew. *Brain Behav. Evol.,* 1968, *1*, 244–288.

Snyder, M., Hall, W. C., and Diamond, I. T. Vision in tree shrews *(Tupaia glis)* after removal of striate cortex. *Psychon. Sci.,* 1966, *6*, 243.

Snyder, M., Killackey, H., and Diamond, I. T. Color vision in the tree shrew after removal of posterior neocortex. *J. Neurophysiol.,* 1969, *32(4)*, 554–563.

Spear, P. D., and Barbas, H. Recovery of pattern discrimination ability in rats receiving serial or one-stage visual cortex lesions. *Brain Res.,* 1975, *94*, 337–346.

Spear, P. D., and Braun, J. J. Pattern discrimination following removal of visual neocortex in the cat. *Exp. Neurol.,* 1969*a*, *25*, 331–348.

Spear, P. D., and Braun, J. J. Nonequivalence of normal and posteriorly neodecorticated rats on two brightness discrimination problems. *J. Comp. Physiol. Psychol.,* 1969*b*, *67*, 235–239.

Spekreijse, H., Van Norren, D. and Van den Berg, T. J. T. P. Flicker responses in monkey lateral geniculate nucleus and human perception of flicker. *Proc. Natl. Acad. Sci. (USA),* 1971, *68*, 2802.

Spence, K., and Fulton, J. The effects of occipital lobectomy on vision in chimpanzee. *Brain,* 1936, *59*, 35.

Steinberg, R. H., Reid, M., and Lacy, P. L. The distribution of rods and cones in the retina of the cat. *J. Comp. Neurol.* 1973, *148*, 229–248.

Stewart, D. L., and Riesen, A. H. Adult versus infant brain damage: Behavioral and electrophysiological effects of striatectomy in adult and neonatal rabbits. *Adv. Psychobiol.,* 1972, *1*, 171–211.

Stone, J. Sampling properties of microelectrodes assessed in the cat's retina. *J. Neurophysiol.,* 1973, *36*, 1071–1079.

Stone, J. The naso-temporal division of the cat's retina. *J. Comp. Neurol.,* 1966, *126*, 585–600.

Stone, J., and Dreher, B. Projection of X- and Y-cells of the cat's lateral geniculate nucleus to area 17 and 18 of visual cortex. *J. Neurophysiol.,* 1973, *36*, 551–567.

Stone, J., and Fabian, M. Specialized receptive fields of the cat's retina. *Science,* 1966, *152*, 1277–1279.

Stone, J., and Fukuda, Y. Properties of cat retinal ganglion cells: A comparison of W-cells with X- and Y-cells. *J. Neurophysiol.,* 1974*a*, *37*, 722–748.

Stone, J., and Fukuda, Y. The naso-temporal division of the cat's retina re-examined in terms of Y-, X- and W-cells. *J. Comp. Neurol.,* 1974*b*, *155*, 377–394.

Stone, J., and Hansen, S. M. The projection of the cat's retina on the lateral geniculate nucleus. *J. Comp. Neurol.,* 1966, *126*, 601–624.

Stone, J., and Hoffmann, P. Conduction velocity as a parameter in the organization of the afferent relay in the cat's lateral geniculate nucleus. *Brain Res.,* 1971, *32(2)*, 454–459.

Stone, J., and Hoffmann, P. Very slow-conducting ganglion cells in the cat's retina: A major, new functional type? *Brain Res.,* 1972, *43*, 610–616.

Stone, J., and Holländer, H. Optic nerve axon diameters measured in the cat retina: Some functional considerations. *Exp. Brain Res.,* 1971, *13*, 498.

Suzuki, H., and Kato, E. Binocular interaction at cat's lateral geniculate body. *J. Neurophysiol.,* 1966, *29*, 909.

Szentagothai, J. Neuronal and synaptic architecture of the lateral geniculate nucleus. In R. Jung (ed.), *Handbook of Sensory Physiology,* Vol. VII/3: *Central Processing of Visual Information,* Part B: *Visual Centers in the Brain.* Springer-Verlag, New York, 1973, pp. 141–176.

Talbot, S. A., and Marshall, W. H. Physiological studies on neural mechanisms of visual location and discrimination. *Am. J. Ophthalmol.,* 1941, *24*, 1255–1264.

Tansley, K. *Vision in Vertebrates.* Chapman & Hall, London, 1965.

Taravella, C. L., and Clark, G. Discrimination of intermittent photic stimulation in normal and brain-damaged cats. *Exp. Neurol.,* 1963, *7,* 282–293.

TerBraak, J., and Van Vliet, A. Subcortical optokinetic nystagmus in the monkey. *Psychiat. Neurol. Neurochirurg. (Amsterdam),* 1963, *66,* 277–283.

TerBraak, J. W. G., Schenk, V. W. D., and Van Vliet, A. G. M. Visual reactions in a case of long-lasting and cortical blindness. *J. Neurol. Neurosurg. Psychiatr.,* 1971, *34,* 140.

Teuber, H. L., Battersby, W., and Bender, M. *Visual Field Defects after Penetrating Missile Wounds of the Brain.* Harvard University Press, Cambridge, Mass., 1960.

Thompson, R. Retention of a brightness discrimination following neocortical damage in the rat. *J. Comp. Physiol. Psychol.,* 1960, *53,* 212–215.

Thuma, B. D. Studies on the diencephalon of the cat. 1. The cyto-architecture of the corpus geniculatum laterale. *J. Comp. Neurol.,* 1928, *46,* 173–198.

Tucker, T. J., Kling, A., and Scharlock, D. P. Sparing of photic frequency and brightness discrimination after striatectomy in neonatal cats. *J. Neurophysiol.,* 1968, *31,* 818–832.

Tusa, R. The retinotopic organization of V1, V2 and V3 in the cat. *Anat. Rec.,* 1975, *181,* 497.

Updyke, B. V. The patterns of projection of cortical areas 17, 18, and 19 onto the laminae of the dorsal lateral geniculate nucleus in the cat. *J. Comp. Neurol.,* 1975, *163,* 377–396.

Urbaitis, J. C., and Meikle, T. H., Jr. Relearning a dark-light discrimination by cats after cortical and collicular lesions. *Exp. Neurol.,* 1968, *20,* 295.

von Freund, H. J., Lauff, D., and Grunewald, G. Binoculare Interabtion in Corpus geniculatum laterale der Katze. *Pfluegers Arch. Ges. Physiol.,* 1967, *297,* 85.

Walls, G. *The Vertebrate Eye and its Adaptive Radiation.* Cranbrook Institute Scientific Bulletin 19, Cranbrook Press, Bloomfield Hills, N.J., 1942.

Walls, G. L. *The Lateral Geniculate Nucleus and Visual Histophysiology.* University of California Publication in Physiology, Vol. 9, University of California Press, Berkeley, 1953.

Ward, J. P., and Masterton, B. Encephalization and visual cortex in the tree shrew *Brain Behav. Evol.,* 1970, *3,* 421–469.

Ware, C. B., Casagrande, V. A., and Diamond, I. T. Does the acuity of the tree shrew suffer from removal of striate cortex? *Brain Behav. Evol.,* 1972, *5,* 18–29.

Ware, C. B., Diamond, I. T., and Casagrande, V. A. Effects of ablating the striate cortex on a successive pattern discrimination: Further study of the visual system in the tree shrew *(Tupaia glis). Brain Behav. Evol.,* 1974, *9,* 264–279.

Wässle, H., Levick, W. R., and Cleland, B. G. The distribution of the alpha-type of ganglion cells in the cat's retina. *J. Comp. Neurol.,* 1975, *159,* 419–438.

Watkins, D. W., and Berkley, M. A. The orientation selectivity of single neurons in cat striate cortex. *Exp. Brain Res.,* 1974, *19,* 433–446.

Weiskrantz, L. Contour discrimination in a young monkey with striate cortex ablation. *Neuropsychologia,* 1963, *1,* 145–164.

Weiskrantz, L., and Cowey, A. Striate cortex lesions and visual acuity of the rhesus monkey. *J. Comp. Physiol. Psychol.,* 1963, *56,* 225–231.

Weiskrantz, L., and Cowey, A. Comparison of the effects of striate cortex and retinal lesions on visual acuity in the monkey. *Science,* 1967, *155,* 104–106.

Weiskrantz, L., and Cowey, A. Filling in the scotoma: A study of residual vision after striate cortex lesions in monkeys. *Progr. Physiol. Psychol.,* 1970, *3,* 237–260.

Weiskrantz, L., and Cowey, A. Effects of striate cortex removals on visual discrimination. *Brain Res.,* 1971, *31,* 376.

Weiskrantz, L., Warrington, E. K., Sanders, M. D., and Marshall, J. Visual capacity in the hemianopic field following a restricted occipital ablation. *Brain,* 1974, *97,* 709–728.

Wetzel, A. B. Visual cortical lesions in the cat: A study of depth and pattern discrimination. *J. Comp. Physiol. Psychol.,* 1969, *68,* 580–588.

Wiesel, T. N., and Hubel, D. H. Spatial and chromatic interactions in the lateral geniculate body of the rhesus monkey. *J. Neurophysiol.,* 1966, *29,* 1115–1156.

Wiesel, T. N., Hubel, D. H., and Lam, D. M. K. Autoradiographic demonstration of ocular-dominance columns in the monkey striate cortex by means of transneuronal transport. *Brain Res.,* 1974, *79,* 273–279.

Wiesenfeld, Z., and Kornel, E. E. Receptive fields of single cells in the visual cortex of the hooded rat. *Brain Res.,* 1975, *94,* 401–412.

Wilson, M. E., and Cragg, B. G. Projections from the lateral geniculate nucleus in the cat and monkey. *J. Anat. (London),* 1967.

Wilson, M. E., and Toyne, M. J. Retino-tectal and cortico-tectal projections in *Macaca mulatta. Anat. Rec.,* 1969, *163*, 286.

Wilson, P. D., and Stone, J. Evidence of W-cell input to the cat's visual cortex via the laminae of the lateral geniculate nucleus. *Brain Res.,* 1975, *92*, 472–478.

Winans, S. A. Visual form discrimination after removal of the visual cortex in cats. *Science,* 1967, *158*, 944.

Winans, S. S. Visual cues used by normal and visual-decorticate cats to discriminate figures of equal luminous flux. *J. Comp. Physiol. Psychol.,* 1971, *74*, 167–178.

Winkler, C., and Potter, A. *An Anatomical Guide to Experimental Researches on the Cat's Brain.* W. Versluys, Amsterdam, 1914.

Wong-Riley, M. T. T. Changes in the dorsal lateral geniculate nucleus of the squirrel monkey after unilateral ablation of the visual cortex. *J. Comp. Neurol.,* 1972, *146*, 519–547.

Wood, C. C., Spear, P. D., and Braun, J. J. Effects of sequential lesions of suprasylvian gyri and visual cortex on pattern discrimination in the cat. *Brain Res.,* 1974, *66*, 443–466.

Wurtz, R. H. Visual receptive fields of striate cortex neurons in awake monkeys. *J. Neurophysiol.,* 1969, *32(5)*, 727–742.

7

Visual System: Pulvinar-Extrastriate Cortex

Martha Wilson

Introduction

Until a few decades ago, it was commonly believed that there is one primary projection from each peripheral receptor system to the cortex. Cortex which was not accounted for by these sensory areas, and which was not identifiable as motor cortex, was defined as association cortex. This view of cortical organization was agreeable for a number of reasons. It accounted for the minimal effects on sensory function of removing various portions of association cortex, it was consistent with the Empiricists' notions of how percepts are achieved by combination of elements of experience, and it fit equally well with the Behaviorists' insistence that learning consists of associations between stimuli and responses.

Thus these physiological ideas were put to several kinds of use in psychological theory. On the one hand, association cortex was asked to bind sensations into perceptions, and, on the other hand, to provide connections between stimuli and motor acts. However, neuropsychologists could treat these issues as empirical problems, and in the 1950s the functions of these presumed nonsensory areas were actively investigated in a number of laboratories.

It became clear that association cortex in the posterior part of the brain is, first, modality specific, and, second, critical for the performance of many kinds of tasks, involving many kinds of presumed psychological processes. More and more refined behavioral tasks were devised and pressed into service in order to discover

Martha Wilson   Department of Psychology, University of Connecticut, Storrs, Connecticut 06268. The writing of this chapter was supported by Grant BMS 74-09745 from the National Science Foundation.

which aspects of function could be assigned to cortical sensory processes and which could be assigned to cortical association processes.

However, during these years of experimental activity, little attention was given to cortex adjoining striate cortex. Several early studies seemed to confirm Lashley's (1948) conclusion that if there were visual engrams they did not reside in these cortical areas. Interest was centered instead on the inferior convexity of the temporal lobe, an area which was clearly critical for the performance of tasks based on visual information. Thus visual association cortex came to be functionally identified with inferotemporal cortex and extrastriate, nontemporal areas remained even more of a mystery (Klüver and Bucy, 1938).

By 1970, ideas of how the visual system is organized, structurally and functionally, had changed dramatically. The visual system now was thought to include no less than five projections from the retina to midbrain and diencephalic structures. In addition to the well-studied geniculostriate pathways, projections to the pretectum, superior colliculus, accessory optic systems, and ventral lateral geniculate had been identified in one or more primate species. In addition, new cortico-cortical connections of some complexity had emerged, with many more to follow. Areas of extrastriate cortex, to which no obvious functions could be assigned previously, were found to play a necessary role in both the processing and relaying of visual information. Multiple, topographic representations of the visual hemifield were encountered anterior to striate cortex, and new subcortical-cortical relationships were discovered which cast fresh doubt on the serial model of sensory and association areas which had prevailed for so long.

Thus several decades of investigation have served to expand our conception of sensory cortex at the expense of association cortex. Even more recently, the proliferation of new techniques has opened the way for more sophisticated analyses of the structural and functional characteristics of the remaining association cortex, as well as former association cortex. In what follows, what is known at present about the functional organization of primate extrastriate visual pathways will be summarized. It will be seen that new complexities have superseded the appealing simplicity of the old doctrines.

However, it is possible to impose some order on the vast number of new experimental findings by conceptualizing the visual pathways as a system made up of three subsystems, each with its own functional specialization. These subsystems involve both horizontal and vertical circuits, and thus cut across distinctions based on anatomical and physiological data. The problem of describing extrastriate cortical function is equivalent to the problem of explaining visual perception, and thus the first issues to be discussed must be psychological.

We will take as a starting point the assumption that visual perception does not consist solely of the encoding of stimulus features which are extracted from the visual array and combined through convergent mechanisms to produce a given percept. It is clear that visual perception involves more than a passive recognition of stimulus location and quality. Rather, it is an event achieved through active looking, which requires spatial integrating mechanisms to bring selected parts of the visual field into central gaze. However, even if the importance of acquiring information, as well as identifying information, is granted, it must also be emphasized that perceptual events are influenced by ongoing activity in the nervous system. Such activity represents the residual effects of previous stimulation and acts as a referent which determines the effects of current stimulation. Stimulus categorization, perceptual schemata, and, ultimately, object recognition depend on such processes.

If we turn our attention to the vertical organization of the visual system, at least three ascending thalamocortical pathways can be identified in a model primate. Two of these, the tectal-pulvinar-prestriate and the geniculostrate pathways, can be described as "lemniscal" (Benevento and Rezak, 1976). That is, they convey direct, "labeled line" afferent input from receptor to cortex, rapidly, reliably, and faithfully (Semmes, 1970). Experimental evidence shows that locating and identifying stimulus inputs depend critically on these two systems. The third ascending thalamocorticical pathway, the lateral pulvinar-prestriate and inferotemporal system, is "extralemniscal" in that afferent sensory input is indirect, and dependent on corticothalamocortical pathways. This system appears to be critical for categorization and recognition of visual input, although information from the lemniscal systems is clearly indispensable for its function.

A model of cerebral mechanisms in vision must take into account the interdependence of these functional systems. In order to locate potentially useful information, it is necessary to identify stimulus attributes to some extent. And in order to identify an object, critical stimulus features must be located. And both locating and identifying particular kinds of information will be determined in part by categorization, based on experience with similar inputs. Such schemata will, in turn, be continuously affected by information from locating and identifying mechanisms.

Horizontal circuits at all levels of the visual system link the vertical circuits and provide for integration of perceptual function. The elaboration and extension of lemniscal pathways cross-cortically provide for further convergence of foveal and extrafoveal information. In addition, large areas of extrastriate cortex receive input from all three functional systems, providing the anatomical capability for integration of past and present stimulation. It is clear that a simple model of IN-UP-OVER- and OUT does not do justice either to the brain or to visual perception.

FUNCTIONAL UNITS IN EXTRASTRIATE CORTEX

Lateral (a) and medial (b) views of the macaque brain are shown in Fig. 1 with the boundaries of extrastriate cortex indicated. It can be seen that extrastriate visual cortex composes a large part of the cortex as a whole, attesting to the importance of visual function in primates. Since we cannot assume that visual cortex is a homogeneous structure with unitary function, a first step in understanding its organization more fully is to arrive at units of analysis which will reveal meaningful relationships between structure and function.

Architectonically defined areas, corticocortical connections, thalamocortical projections, and functional properties have all been used as bases for identifying

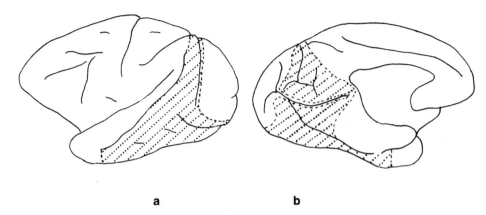

Fig. 1. Lateral (a) and medial (b) views of the macaque brain. Slashed areas represent extent of extrastriate visual cortex. Based on drawings in von Bonin and Bailey (1947).

units within extrastriate cortex, as well as areas over the whole cortex. At the very least, cortical maps are necessary in order for an investigator to have some means of reporting locations on the cortex.

CYTOARCHITECTURAL AREAS

Differences in the size, characteristics, and arrangements of neurons in various areas of cortex can be used to define these areas. Von Bonin and Bailey (1947) provided a standard map for the macaque brain, making use of the lettering system devised by von Economo (1929) for his map of the human brain.

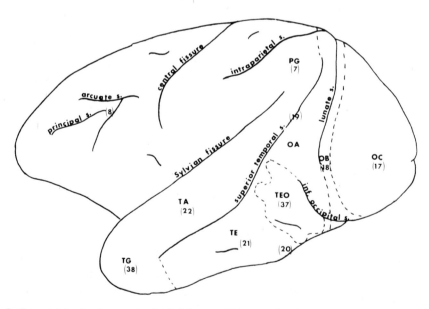

Fig. 2. Extrastriate visual cortex and adjoining cortical areas, labeled according to von Bonin and Bailey (1947) and Brodmann (1905) in terms of cytoarchitectural areas. Extent of area TEO is also shown as defined by von Bonin and Bailey (1950).

The areas so defined in extrastriate cortex are similar to Brodmann's (1905) map of numbered areas. Figure 2 shows a lateral view of the macaque brain with von Bonin and Bailey's parcellation of extrastriate cortex and neighboring areas, together with Brodmann's numerical labels for approximately similar areas.

Prestriate or parastriate cortex, OB, lies adjacent to striate cortex, OC. Peristriate cortex, OA, lies adjacent to OB. Together they make up the circumstriate belt, Brodmann's areas 18 and 19. The posterior inferotemporal area, TEO, and the anterior inferotemporal area, TE, are located on the inferior convexity and lateral surface of the temporal lobe. The temporal pole, TG, is not part of extrastriate visual cortex, either cytoarchitecturally or functionally, and appears to be more closely related to other limbic structures. Anterior to the extrastriate region lie auditory (TA) and somatosensory (PG) areas of cortex.

Von Bonin and Bailey questioned the distinctiveness of the boundary between Brodmann's areas 18 and 19, and this distinction is still under discussion (Tigges *et al.*, 1973*a*; Zeki, 1969*b*). Von Bonin and Bailey were also puzzled about the line of demarcation between OA and TE. Originally, they assigned a question mark rather than a letter designation to the cortex at the temporal-occipital junction. This latter point subsequently aroused the interest of Mishkin and his collaborators, since it raised the question of what cortical extent should be functionally defined as inferotemporal association cortex (Ettlinger *et al.*, 1968; Iwai and Mishkin, 1969). As described below, a series of behavioral experiments led them to accept von Bonin and Bailey's (1950) relabeling of this area as TEO and to pursue the investigation of functional differences between TEO and anterior inferotemporal cortex, TE. However, this matter is still also under discussion (Gross, 1972, 1973). It is clear that useful definitions of functional units will be based on electrophysiological, anatomical and behavioral criteria, as well as differences in architectonics.

CORTICAL VISUAL REPRESENTATIONS

Exploration of extrastriate cortex by anatomical and electrophysiological techniques leads to further parcellation of these cortical areas. Beyond area 17, many more areas can be distinguished than those based on cytoarchitectural criteria. At present, no less than six representations of the visual hemifield in Brodmann's areas 18 and 19 are identifiable in rhesus and owl monkeys, and work on these and other species suggests that this list may be just the beginning of the roster of cortical areas concerned with visual function.

Figure 3 represents a composite of findings in the rhesus monkey based on both anatomical and electrophysiological methods (Cragg, 1969; Zeki, 1969*a,b*, 1971*a,b*). Visualization of these subdivisions of extrastriate cortex is extremely difficult since much of the cortex is located in the banks and depths of sulci and is therefore not revealed in a view of the lateral surface of the brain. In addition, boundaries between areas do not often coincide with convenient landmarks so that their extent involves somewhat tortuous specification. Worse yet, several visual areas are interdigitated in a complex fashion. In order to show the locations of these areas in terms of cortical geography, the extrastriate visual areas are

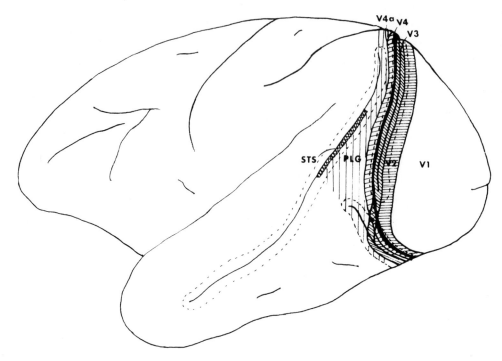

Fig. 3. Lateral surface of the brain, showing multiple visual representations as determined by Zeki (1969a,b, 1971a,b) and Cragg (1969). Heavy lines represent the depths of sulci, and dashed lines represent the banks of sulci, drawn as if they were laid open. See text for description of the boundaries of these areas. PLG, Prelunate gyrus; STS, superior temporal sulcus.

depicted on the lateral surface of the hemisphere, with the banks and depths of the lunate, inferior occipital, and superior temporal sulci drawn as if they were laid open.

Anterior to the primary visual projection in striate cortex lies a second visual area, V2. The boundary between V1 and V2 represents points in the visual field lying on the vertical meridian. This striate-prestriate border runs dorsoventrally on the lateral surface of the cortex. It is met in the area representing foveal vision by the primary projection of the horizontal meridian, which extends from this junction to the occipital pole and on to the medial surface. In V2, as well as V1, the upper quadrant of the contralateral visual hemifield is represented ventrally, while the lower quadrant is represented dorsally. Cells with receptive fields in the temporal periphery are thus found in the medial wall of the hemisphere, dorsally in the upper arm of the calcarine fissure, and ventrally in the lower bank of the calcarine fissure, as is also true in V1. This second visual area extends from the striate-prestriate border to the middle of the posterior bank of the lunate sulcus, dorsally, and to the depths of the inferior occipital sulcus, ventrally. The anterior boundary of V2 represents points lying on the horizontal meridian, such that the entire contralateral visual hemifield is represented visuotopically between these two boundaries. However, in visualizing this representation of the cortex, the situation is complicated, ventrally, by the intrusion of two other visual areas, V4 and V4a, into the posterior bank of the inferior occipital sulcus.

Two more visual representations (the V_3 complex) extend from the anterior boundary of V_2 dorsally to the middle of the anterior bank of the lunate sulcus, and ventrally to the middle of the inferior occipital sulcus. Again, the lower quadrant of the visual field is represented dorsally, while the upper quadrant is represented ventrally. The anterior border of the V_3 complex represents the vertical meridian. Proceeding anteriorly, the V_4 complex, which may contain two or more representations, lies adjacent to the V_3 complex dorsally, and is intercalated ventrally into V_2 in the posterior bank of the inferior occipital sulcus. The fourth visual complex may extend over the prelunate gyrus to the posterior bank of the superior temporal sulcus. From data now available, it appears that the V_4 complex represents only central vision. Finally, two additional visual areas are located in the medial and lateral portions of the posterior bank of the superior temporal sulcus, with the horizontal and vertical meridians again represented (Zeki, 1969a,b; 1971a, 1974a,b, 1977).

These six or more visual representations are included in Brodmann's areas 18 and 19 and part of TEO. Portions of the circumstriate belt which include cortex in parts of the lunate, inferior occipital, and superior temporal sulci, and cortex lying between, make up the foveal representations in prestriate cortex (Zeki, 1969a), 1977). This area is shown diagrammatically, and in tems of cortical landmarks, in Fig. 4. However, it is not clear how these representations are organized in the more anterior regions of the circumstriate belt area (Zeki, 1969b). The quadrantic organization found in V1, V2, and V3 appears to break down, although some topographic organization is discernible in the representation in the superior

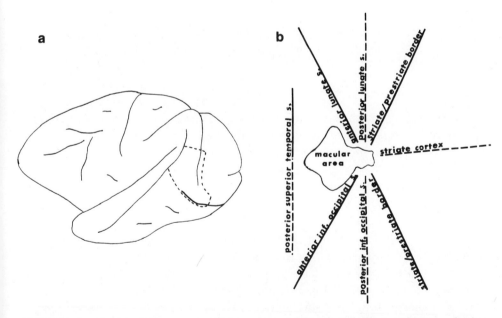

Fig. 4. (a) Area in circumstriate cortex which receives a projection from the macular area of striate cortex. Projections in the banks and depths of sulci are not shown. (b) Arrangement of representations of the horizontal (dotted lines) and vertical (uninterrupted lines) meridians in terms of location on the cortex. Redrawn from Zeki (1969b).

temporal sulcus (Zeki, 1974a). The extent and number of the visual areas located on the anterior prelunate gyrus remain a puzzle. Nevertheless, these findings provide the first hints of the way in which extrastriate cortex is organized in rhesus monkey.

Before turning to the questions that immediately arise from these data, we may ask if this organization is a general feature of the primate extrastriate visual system. While detailed mapping has not yet been accomplished for a large number of species, the evidence that is available suggests that multiple, visuotopic representations are found in all primate species.

Area 18 is a visually responsive area in the squirrel monkey, organized in a distorted mirror-image fashion with respect to area 17 (Cowey, 1964). There is also a visual area in the superior temporal gyrus in the squirrel monkey (Doty *et al.*, 1964) which is visuotopically organized (Martinez-Millán and Holländer, 1975). Further, it appears that a visual area can be identified in a number of primate species, lying in the dorsal part of the middle of the temporal lobe, labeled the "middle temporal area" (Allman and Kaas, 1971). Thus the bushbaby (Allman *et al.*, 1973), the marmoset (Woolsey, 1971), and the owl monkey (Allman and Kaas, 1971), as well as the rhesus and squirrel monkeys, possess an area representing the visual hemifield which is distant from striate cortex, and which is identified as the middle temporal area in all of these species by some, if not all, investigators (Martinez-Millán and Holländer, 1975; Spatz and Tigges, 1972).

Adjacent points on the cortex lying between area 17 and the middle temporal area, in the owl monkey and bushbaby, exhibit the same progression of receptive fields toward and away from the vertical meridian that is characteristic of extrastriate areas in the rhesus monkey (Allman and Kaas, 1971; Allman *et al.*, 1973). This fact suggests that a number of representations of the visual hemifield exist, and a recent series of studies in the owl monkey demonstrates just such a set of visuotopically organized areas anterior to striate cortex (Allman, 1976; Allman and Kaas, 1971, 1974a,b, 1975).

Studies of extrastriate cortex in the owl monkey reveal that not one but at least five distinct cortical visual areas lie adjacent to area 18. Most likely this is true of the bushbaby as well. Four of these areas have been extensively studied and appear to be organized around representations of the horizontal and vertical meridians. Figure 5 shows the primary visual projection, V1, with V2 adjoining. The striate-prestriate border represents the vertical meridian except for a small extent devoted to the temporal periphery on the medial wall of the hemisphere. Anterior and adjacent to V2 lie a medial area, on the medial wall, a dorsomedial area, a dorsointermediate area, a dorsolateral area, and an unspecified visual area ventral to the dorsolateral area. The common border of each of these areas with V2 represents the horizontal meridian. These areas, lying in Brodmann's area 19, are labeled "third tier" areas since V1 and V2 are denoted as the "first tier" and "second tier," respectively (Allman and Kaas, 1974a). Anterior to the dorsolateral area, and almost completely surrounded by it, lies the middle temporal area. As shown in Fig. 5, the current state of mapping does not exhaust the known visual areas anterior to striate cortex.

Within each of the third tier areas and the middle temporal area, the upper quadrant is represented ventrally, and the lower quadrant dorsally, with the horizontal meridian bisecting the area. Each of these areas can be further characterized in terms of the proportion of the total area which is devoted to central vision. The middle temporal area and all of the third tier areas with the exception of the medial area represent the central area of the visual field in large part with little of their areas concerned with the periphery. The medial area, in owl monkey, differs strikingly in that most of its area (96%) is concerned with the peripheral portions of the visual hemifield (Allman, 1976). This finding provides another example of the amazing specificity exhibited by functional areas outside of striate cortex.

Examining Fig. 5, in the light of what is known about the rhesus monkey, leads to the conclusion that multiple representations of visual fields are a common feature of extrastriate organization in primates. This fact is incompatible with

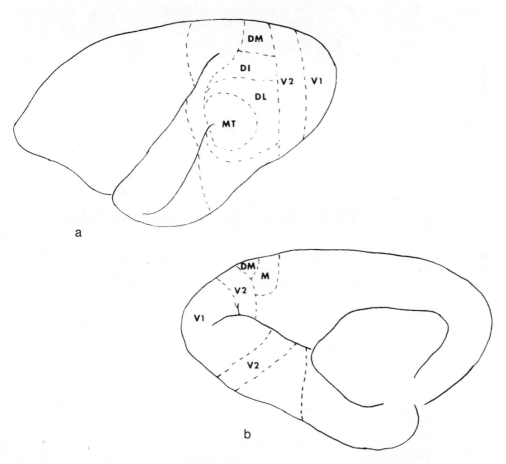

Fig. 5. Extent of visual representations in striate and extrastriate cortex in the owl monkey on lateral (a) and medial (b) surfaces of cortex. Shown are the medial (M), dorsomedial (DM), dorsointermediate (DI), dorsolateral (DL), and middle temporal (MT) areas. Unlabeled areas represent additional, unmapped visual areas. Based on Allman and Kaas (1974a,b) and Wagor et al. (1975).

early descriptions of the cortical visual system as consisting of striate cortex, or V1, belt areas, V2 and V3, and temporal cortex association areas. Rather, there appears to be a mosaic of visual areas anterior to striate cortex. Another similarity that can be noted is that the common border between V1 and V2 represents the vertical meridian, a feature of the visual system which has been found in many mammals (Glendenning *et al.*, 1975). Furthermore, in both rhesus monkey and owl monkey, the border between V2 and the third tier, or V3, represents the horizontal meridian.

Beyond this, the questions about organization become more compelling than the similarities, at this stage in our knowledge. Area 19 is divided into a number of visuotopically organized subareas in the owl monkey and bushbaby, while topographic organization may become progressively degraded in visual areas anterior to V3 in the rhesus monkey. It is possible, however, that complete mapping of extrafoveal areas in the rhesus monkey will reveal a visuotopic organization similar to that seen clearly in the more easily accessible cortex of the owl monkey and bushbaby. The problem remains of adducing the relationships between the third tier areas in owl monkey and the visual areas intercalated between the striate cortex and the superior temporal sulcus in the rhesus monkey.

CORTICOCORTICAL CONNECTIONS

Given that there are multiple visual representations in the extrastriate visual system, one obvious first step in elucidating their function is to discover the afferent and efferent connections of each area. In primates, the most complete description of corticocortical projections now available comes from work on the rhesus monkey. But even without complete descriptions of other primates, a number of common relationships can be discerned.

Figure 6 shows a composite of the corticocortical projections found in rhesus monkey (Cragg, 1969; Jones and Powell, 1970; Kuypers *et al.*, 1965; Zeki, 1969*a,b*, 1971*b*, 1977). There are a number of interlocking and overlapping projections from striate cortex to multiple areas in prestriate and circumstriate cortex, and from these areas to inferotemporal cortex. These findings are in substantial agreement where they overlap, but the precise pattern of projections from various subdivisions of the circumstriate cortex to inferotemporal cortex, and from inferotemporal cortex to prestriate cortex, is still unclear.

It is certain, however, that area 17 (V1) sends direct projections to V2 and V3, the V4 complex, to the fundus of the intraparietal sulcus, and medial cortex in the superior temporal sulcus. There is also a sparse projection to the frontal eye fields (area 8) from V1. These connections apparently exhaust the direct corticocortical projections from striate cortex.

V2 and V3 project independently to V4, V4a, the anterior prelunate gyrus, and the superior temporal sulcus. The precise relationship of points in the visual hemifield found in V1 and V2 may no longer obtain in these areas. One reason may lie in the fact that points in the lower and upper quadrants, represented in dorsal and ventral V3, appear to be connected. This would, in itself, produce a breakdown in visuotopic organization in the areas to which V3 projects (Zeki,

1971*b*). As noted previously, though, the superior temporal sulcus exhibits a crude, topographic organization: this area receives multiple inputs, some topographical and some convergent (Zeki, 1971*a*). Reciprocal connections from the superior temporal sulcus to V1 have not been demonstrated, but this area projects back to V2 and V3 (McLoon *et al.*, 1975). And there is a reciprocal projection from V2 to V1 in both the rhesus monkey (Kuypers *et al.*, 1965) and the squirrel monkey (Tigges *et al.*, 1973*a*).

The circumstriate belt area projects to inferotemporal cortex (area 20), to the frontal eye fields (area 8), and to the intraparietal sulcus (Kuypers *et al.*, 1965). Area 20 projects to area 21, part of the amygdala, and area 8 (Jones and Powell, 1970). Area 21, in turn, sends projections to the superior temporal sulcus, the temporal pole, the frontal lobe, and the amygdala (Jones and Powell, 1970; Kuypers *et al.*, 1965; Jones and Mishkin, 1972; Whitlock and Nauta, 1956; Van Hoesen and Pandya, 1975). Reciprocal projections from inferotemporal cortex to prestriate areas are in doubt (Jones and Powell, 1970), although they have been reported (cf. Gross, 1973). The superior temporal sulcus also receives fibers from the posterior parietal area, 7.

Data from other primate species also point to a complex set of interconnections between cortical visual areas. In squirrel monkey, V1 projects directly to V2, V3, and the middle temporal area (Cowey, 1964; Martinez-Millán and Holländer, 1975; Spatz *et al.*, 1970). Similarly, in the marmoset, efferent fibers from V1 travel

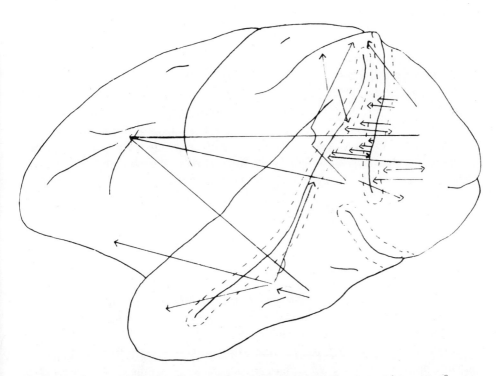

Fig. 6. Corticocortical projections from striate and prestriate cortical areas to other areas of cortex. Areas within dashed lines indicate banks of sulci. Arrows represent projections from one area to another but do not indicate topographic or density variables.

to the middle temporal area (Spatz, 1975), which in turn projects to areas 8, 22, medial 17 and 19, and what Allman and Kaas would describe as the dorsolateral and dorsomedial areas (Spatz and Tigges, 1972). The bushbaby is similar in terms of direct projections from V1 to V2 and the middle temporal area (Tigges *et al.,* 1973*b*) but apparently differs from monkeys in that no projections are known from V1 to third tier areas. Less information is available for the owl monkey: connections are reported from the dorsomedial area to the dorsolateral area, the superior tip of the Sylvian fissure, and the temporal cortex. There are also reciprocal connections between the middle temporal area and area 7 (Wagor *et al.,* 1975).

In all primate species, interhemispheric connections also link visual areas beyond striate cortex. In prestriate cortex, only midline portions of the visual field appear to be so connected in rhesus monkey. That is, areas representing the vertical meridian and/or the foveal representation are joined interhemispherically via the caudal third of the corpus callosum (Pandya *et al.,* 1971; Zeki, 1970). In V4 and V4a, callosal connections may represent all parts of the visual field, since precise visuotopic representation is no longer present. Inferotemporal areas are linked by fibers traveling in the anterior commissure, and, as discussed below, the information transferred is also not limited to the foveal area.

Interhemispheric connections in other primate species are also prominent in the third tier and middle temporal areas. There are connections between the middle temporal area in one hemisphere and contralateral middle temporal, dorsolateral, and posterior parietal areas in the marmoset (Spatz and Tigges, 1972). In the owl monkey, the dorsomedial area projects to contralateral dorsomedial, middle temporal, and posterior parietal areas (Wagor *et al.,* 1975). In these projections topographic information from all parts of the visual hemifield appears to be transferred interhemispherically (Spatz and Tigges, 1972).

The picture that emerges from these studies of corticocortical connections in extrastriate cortex is one of multiple, overlapping, and often reciprocal relationships between subdivisions of this visual cortex. Thus, even at this level, the notion of simple, serial processing of visual input is difficult to envisage. And the picture is hardly complete since another major source of cortical visual information arises from direct, thalamocortical projections to extrastriate cortex from the pulvinar nucleus. This information may be of a different sort than that transmitted through the lateral geniculate-striate-extrastriate system, and we will next consider how the tectal-pulvinar-extrastriate system is organized.

AFFERENT CONNECTIONS OF THE PULVINAR

Before turning to the organization of the pulvinar-extrastriate component of the cortical visual system, it is necessary to consider the connections of the pulvinar itself. Drawings of the pulvinar in the tree shrew, an insectivore, and in four representative primate species are shown in Figs. 7 and 8. In the tree shrew, the pulvinar appears to be a single homogeneous structure. In the other four of these species, the bushbaby, owl monkey, squirrel monkey, and rhesus monkey, various subdivisions of the pulvinar have been identified, in terms both of cytoarchitectural differences and of afferent and efferent connections. While the labels used to distinguish these subdivisions may represent premature homologizing, the similar arrangement of the labels in the four species suggests that this may be a useful first step in understanding the functional organization of the pulvinar.

The tree shrew pulvinar, as shown in Fig. 7, displays no obvious boundaries within its limits, as discussed in a number of studies by Diamond and his collaborators (Harting *et al.*, 1972, 1973). The lack of cytoarchitectonic subdivisions implies a corresponding lack of differential, functional connections, and, indeed, this seems to be the case. The entire pulvinar in the tree shrew is the target of fibers from the superior colliculus. Since similar results hold for a number of mammals, this arrangement may be representative of a common mammalian plan.

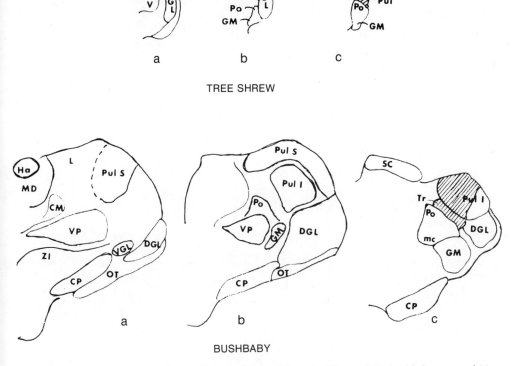

Fig. 7. Frontal sections through the pulvinar nucleus of the tree shrew and the bushbaby at rostral (a), intermediate (b), and caudal (c) levels. In the tree shrew, slashed areas, representing tectorecipient portions, include the whole extent of the pulvinar. Shown are the lateral nucleus (L), ventral group (V), pulvinar (Pul), dorsal lateral geniculate nucleus (DGL), posterior nucleus (Po), and superior colliculus (SC). Based on Harting *et al.* (1973). Tectorecipient portion (slashed area) in the bushbaby is limited to part of the caudal sector of the inferior pulvinar and to the transition zone lying between the inferior pulvinar and the posterior nucleus. Shown are the superior pulvinar (Pul S), inferior pulvinar (Pul I), transition area (Tr), ventral lateral geniculate nucleus (VGL), optic tract (OT), medial geniculate nucleus (GM), ventral posterior nucleus (VP), habenula (Ha), nucleus medialis dorsalis (MD), centre median (CM), cerebral peduncle (CP), and other structures, labeled as above. From Glendenning *et al.* (1975).

In the bushbaby (Fig. 7), a superior portion of the pulvinar appears to differentiate out of the posterior portion of the lateral nucleus. This sector has, at present, no known direct sensory input from subcortical structures. In contrast, part of the inferior portion, which lies more caudally in the thalamus, receives a projection from the superficial layers of the superior colliculus, as does the transition area, a small mass of cells lying between the inferior pulvinar and the posterior nucleus (Glendenning *et al.*, 1975). On purely geographic grounds, one might speculate that the transition zone is homologous to the intergeniculate portion of the inferior pulvinar in monkey, thus bringing the prosimian and simian pulvinars together in a common organization. However, evolutionary processes may not have provided such an outcome, no matter how attractively simple it is.

The pulvinar nucleus in the owl monkey (Fig. 8) is also divided into inferior and superior subdivisions. These are distinguished on the basis of their cytoarchi-

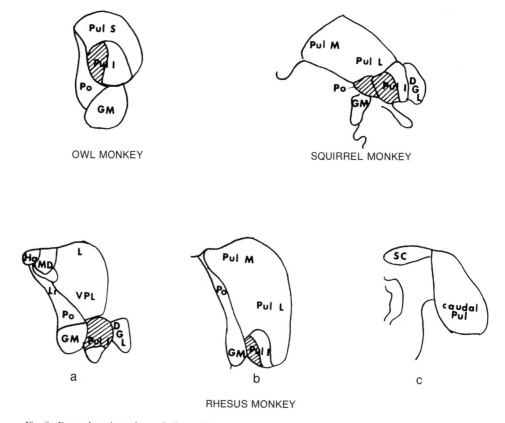

Fig. 8. Frontal sections through the pulvinar nucleus of the owl monkey, squirrel monkey, and rhesus monkey. The tectorecipient area (slashed area) in owl monkey is assumed to be in the medial part of the inferior pulvinar, adjacent to the posterior nucleus, as in the bushbaby. From Lin *et al.* (1974). In squirrel monkey, the inferior pulvinar (Pul I), lateral pulvinar (Pul L), medial pulvinar (Pul M), and other structures, labeled as in Fig. 7, are shown. From Mathers (1971). The pulvinar nucleus of the rhesus monkey is shown at rostral (a), intermediate (b), and caudal (c) levels. Shown are the inferior pulvinar (Pul I), lateral pulvinar (Pul L), medial pulvinar (Pul M), caudal pole of pulvinar (caudal Pul), nucleus limitans (Li), and ventral posterior nucleus, lateral division (VPL). Other structures labeled as in Fig. 7. Based on Benevento and Fallon (1975).

tectonic features and anatomical connections (Allman *et al.,* 1972). In this species, the two sectors lie in approximately the same plane on the rostral-caudal axis of the thalamus, caudal to the lateral geniculate nucleus.

Three subdivisions are apparent in the pulvinar of the squirrel monkey and the rhesus monkey (*cf.* Fig. 8). In squirrel monkey, fibers from the superior colliculus project to the ventromedial two-thirds of the inferior pulvinar, as well as to a portion of the posterior nucleus (Mathers, 1971). In the rhesus monkey, the inferior pulvinar is made up of an intergeniculate portion, lying between the medial and lateral geniculate nuclei, and a more caudal portion which is inferior and adjacent to the lateral subdivision. Fibers from the superficial layers of the superior colliculus terminate in the dorsomedial and lateral portions of the inferior pulvinar, adjacent to the lateral geniculate. There is also tectal input to the medial portion of the inferior pulvinar, which lies between the medial geniculate nucleus and the lateral subdivision of the pulvinar (Benevento and Fallon, 1975). Thus, in both the squirrel monkey and the rhesus monkey, there is a tectorecipient portion of the inferior pulvinar and, by implication, a nontectorecipient portion of the inferior pulvinar. The lateral pulvinar is not tectorecipient: its sole input appears to come from occipital cortex. The medial pulvinar receives projections from the deep layers of the superior colliculus but not from the superficial layers or from the cortex (Benevento and Fallon, 1975).

Thus it is known that in the prosimian bushbaby, and in at least two simian species, the pulvinar is divided into those portions which receive afferent input from the ascending visual system via the superficial layers of the superior colliculus and those portions which do not receive any tectal input but may receive cortical input. Since at one time it was believed that none of the pulvinar received extrathalamic input, these results force us to reconsider the functional role of the inferior pulvinar, as dictated by its direct sensory input from the superior colliculus. In addition, the inferior pulvinar is visuotopically organized in owl monkey and rhesus monkey (Allman *et al.,* 1972), which suggests a functional specificity not previously attributed to it. These findings suggest that there are two thalamic lemniscal systems and put the inferior pulvinar on an equal footing with the dorsal lateral geniculate as a sensory gateway to the cortex.

Two further points related to the question of afferent input to the pulvinar can be made. First, while part of the pulvinar has been shown to receive input from the superior colliculus, this area is by no means the only target of ascending tectothalamic fibers. There are projections from the superficial layers of the superior colliculus to a number of thalamic nuclei, including the dorsal and ventral lateral geniculates, medialis dorsalis, and the midline and intralaminar nuclei (Benevento and Fallon, 1975; Myers, 1963). Thus, whatever its role in vision, the inferior pulvinar does not play a unique role in relaying visual information from the superior colliculus to the cortex unless various projections represent different kinds of information about the visual world.

Second, the inferior pulvinar is not only tectorecipient. It is also the target of corticofugal fibers, as are other sectors of the pulvinar (Benevento and Rezak, 1976). Striate cortex sends descending projections to the lateral and inferior divisions of the pulvinar in rhesus monkey (Campos-Ortega *et al.,* 1970*b*), bushbaby (Campos-Ortega, 1968), and tree shrew (Harting and Casagrande, 1974).

The superior temporal sulcus or middle temporal area projects to the lateral and inferior pulvinars in rhesus monkey (McLoon *et al.*, 1975), marmoset (Spatz and Tigges, 1972), and owl monkey (Lin and Kaas, 1975). Similarly, in the squirrel monkey, fibers from prestriate and inferotemporal cortex terminate in the inferior pulvinar (Mathers, 1972).

There is still a question about whether the inferior pulvinar receives direct input from the retina. Both positive (Campos-Ortega *et al.*, 1970*a*) and negative (Trojanowski and Jacobson, 1975) findings are available. However, the pulvinar does receive afferent input from the lateral geniculate nucleus, the claustrum, and the reticular nucleus, as well as from the superior colliculus (Trojanowski and Jacobson, 1975).

Thus the pulvinar nucleus in primates consists of lemniscal portions, receiving input from the retina, as well as from cortical visual areas, and extralemniscal portions, which are apparently entirely dependent on corticofugal input.

PULVINAR-EXTRASTRIATE CONNECTIONS

Early anatomical studies using retrograde methods provided evidence of projections from the pulvinar to prestriate and temporal areas of cortex in the rhesus monkey (Chow, 1950; Walker, 1938). Additional sources of information can be found in behavioral studies which report sites of retrograde thalamic degeneration after restricted lesions of extrastriate visual cortex.

A notable beginning in understanding the pulvinar-extrastriate system in the bushbaby has been provided by Diamond and his collaborators. This system can now be compared with that of the less hominoid tree shrew and the more hominoid rhesus monkey, as defined by the pulvinar differentiation in these species described above. Figure 9 shows those areas of extrastriate cortex which receive projections from subdivisions of the pulvinar (Glendenning *et al.*, 1975).

Portions of the caudal pulvinar, described as lemniscal by virtue of their connections with the superior colliculus, project to a circumscribed area in the middle of the dorsal part of the temporal lobe. This area, as noted above, is labeled the "middle temporal area" and can be identified in a number of species. Retrograde degeneration which is restricted to the caudal pulvinar after middle temporal lesions confirms this pathway in the bushbaby (Harting *et al.*, 1972; Wilson *et al.*, 1975). A similar pulvinar–middle temporal projection is found in the owl monkey (Lin *et al.*, 1974).

The superior pulvinar in the bushbaby, the input to which is not known, is, in any case, nontectorecipient, and this sector of the pulvinar projects to more ventral and inferior portions of the temporal lobe, as well as to areas 18 and 19. These two thalamocortical projections are nonoverlapping, so that two systems with different input can be identified for further study.

The rhesus monkey demonstrates more complexity in pulvinar-extrastriate connections. Consistent with earlier data, autoradiographic methods show that the inferior pulvinar projects widely to extrastriate cortical areas in a topographic manner (Benevento and Rezak, 1976). This projection includes parts of areas 18,

19, 20, and 21. The intergeniculate portion, adjacent to the caudal pole of the lateral geniculate, projects to medial and dorsolateral prestriate cortex and the floor of the intraparietal sulcus. This projection, which includes cortex in the lunate and inferior occipital sulci, is associated with both corticorecipient and tectorecipient portions of the pulvinar. The more caudal portions of the inferior pulvinar, receiving tectal but not cortical input, send fibers to cortex in the superior temporal sulcus and the ventrolateral prestriate and posterior inferotemporal areas.

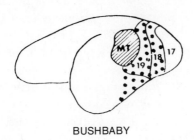

BUSHBABY

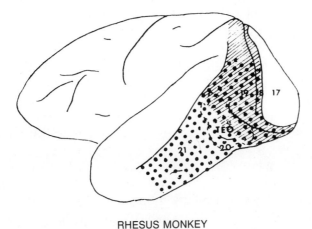

RHESUS MONKEY

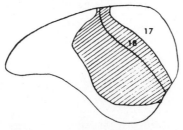

TREE SHREW

Fig. 9. Tectorecipient (slashed area) and nontectorecipient (dotted area) cortical projections in the bushbaby (based on Glendenning *et al.*, 1975), the rhesus monkey (based on Benevento and Rezak, 1976), and the tree shrew (based on Harting *et al.*, 1973).

From early anatomical retrograde degeneration studies and a host of behavioral experiments in which inferotemporal cortex was ablated, it is known that the lateral pulvinar projects to large sectors of occipital and temporal cortex. Some of these projections in the occipital lobe overlap with the projection field of the inferior pulvinar (Benevento and Rezak, 1976). The rostral corticorecipient part projects topographically to medial and dorsolateral prestriate cortex, as does the rostral portion of the inferior pulvinar. However, the caudal portions of the lateral pulvinar, also corticorecipient, project to area TE so this area of inferotemporal cortex is served only by nontectorecipient parts of the pulvinar complex.

A puzzling aspect of the pulvinar-extrastriate systems in various species has been brought into focus by Diamond (1976). Figure 7 shows the pulvinar projection in the tree shrew. All of the pulvinar, it will be remembered, is tectorecipient and it projects in a topographic manner to extrastriate cortex from the striate-prestriate border, where the vertical meridian is represented, to almost all of the temporal lobe. The adjacent cortical projection fields of the lateral geniculate and the pulvinar are elegant, although not surprising, in view of the fact that the pulvinar and lateral geniculate nuclei adjoin in the thalamus, with the vertical meridian represented on their common boundary.

Although the tectorecipient portion of the inferior pulvinar in the bushbaby also adjoins the vertical meridian representation at the border of the lateral geniculate, its cortical projection is *not* adjacent to V1. It is separated from striate cortex by prestriate cortex and lies in the middle of the temporal lobe. The problem has two aspects. First, areas defined as 18 and 19 in the tree shrew and bushbaby receive very different kinds of thalamic input. Second, the tectal-pulvinar system in the bushbaby projects to a cortical target which is not adjacent to the lateral geniculate-striate cortex projection.

One alternative in facing this issue is to assume that the bushbaby is an aberrant species in terms of primate evolution. The fact that a similar tectal-pulvinar-middle temporal organization is apparent in the owl monkey argues against this possibility. Another alternative is that the pulvinar projections in the rhesus monkey may combine features of both tree shrew and bushbaby organization, in that both lateral and inferior pulvinar projections adjoin striate cortex. Thus, it can be cautiously pointed out, both tectorecipient (tree shrew plan) and nontectorecipient (bushbaby plan) systems send information to areas adjacent to striate cortex in the rhesus monkey. If nontectorecipient pulvinar cortical projections represent a newer development in the primate visual system, this cortically modulated projection system may have interdigitated itself between the two older, primary routes to the cortex.

Summary

In the search for functional subdivisions in extrastriate cortex, it is clear that it is no longer tenable to hold to a distinction between primary visual cortex receiving direct sensory input and visual association areas receiving indirect sensory input from primary sensory cortex. Rather, we are faced with the prospect of finding functional correlates for a number of structurally related areas, some of which receive direct afferent input and some of which receive indirect corticocortical and corticothalamocortical information.

The geniculostriate system can be identified as one lemniscal component. A second lemniscal component, the tectal-pulvinar-extrastriate system, projects to cortical areas which are also the targets of geniculostriate projections. The portions of the pulvinar complex which are corticorecipient but not tectorecipient form another component of the visual system, defined as extralemniscal. This system projects to circumstriate cortex, where it overlaps with lemniscal projections, and to anterior temporal cortex, where it does not.

These extrastriate areas can be defined in terms of their anatomical connections, but they are interrelated at many levels. Each is linked to the others by corticocortical connections, subcortical connections, and corticothalamic connections such that all of these areas can potentially influence the activity of any or all of the others. Ultimately, the visual system must be thought of in terms of one integrated system, a view dictated by our visual experience as well as by our anatomy.

Response Properties of Extrastriate Areas

With some notion of the arrangement and anatomical connections of extrastriate visual areas, it is now possible to ask what these areas are contributing to visual function. One approach, which has been successful in the geniculostriate system, is to find out what characteristics of visual stimulation are encoded by neural units at various levels of the system, and to infer from this what each level is contributing to the processing of visual input. This enterprise has not proceeded very far in the extrastriate cortical visual system, but from what is already known it is clear that the cortical visual areas described above do not simply represent redundant versions of the same information. Rather, they appear to be organized in such a way as to specify particular aspects of the potential information in a visual stimulus.

Circumstriate Cortex

The elucidation of the functional characteristics of cells in striate cortex and prestriate areas in the monkey by Hubel and Wiesel (1968, 1970) is widely known. This work shows how the visuotopic organization of striate cortex is well suited for analysis of spatial attributes, orientation, eye preference, and directionality of movement, in terms of where these stimulus events occur in the visual field. Anterior to striate cortex, other attributes of visual stimuli become important in determining response. In V2 and V3, some cells in the banks and depths of the lunate sulcus respond to simultaneous stimulation of both eyes, as well as to stimulation of either eye. Other cells respond only to stimulation of both eyes. Since many of these cells exhibit disparity in the receptive fields of the two eyes, it is hypothesized that they may subserve stereoscopic depth perception.

More of these binocular depth cells are found as points on the cortex lying farther away from striate cortex are sampled. Neighboring cells respond to the same degree of horizontal disparity in the receptive fields of the two eyes, suggesting a columnar organization for stereoscopic depth receptors similar to the organization previously found for orientation detectors in striate cortex. Columns specific for orientation are also found in V2 and V3.

More anteriorly, cells in the V4 complex respond in a variety of ways to specific color information (Zeki, 1973). The properties of these cells contrast with those of the "color cells" in striate cortex, which do not display very complicated response characteristics. In what appears to be more and more typical an organization, cells preferring a specific color are found together in a column through the cortex.

Charting other subdivisions of circumstriate cortex has not demonstrated unique response properties until the areas in the superior temporal sulcus (one of which may be homologous to the middle temporal area) are reached. A series of studies by Zeki (Dubner and Zeki, 1971; Zeki, 1974a,b) indicates that a medial area may be involved in the analysis of moving stimuli. Cells located here are responsive either to movement in a specific direction (usually away from the center of gaze) or to movement in any direction, provided that the movement is rapid. Again, the data suggest a columnar organization in that cells preferring a specific directionality of movement are clustered together. A small subset of cells can also be identified which require edges moving toward or away from each other, in order to trigger a response. Even more rarely, units are encountered which fire when opposed, changing inputs to the two eyes are presented, such as would obtain if a stimulus moved toward or away from the organism. These cells are obviously binocularly driven.

A lateral area in the posterior bank of the superior temporal sulcus contains a high percentage of cells responsive to color. Specificity to either short or long wavelengths can be shown, as well as responses based on opponent processes.

The size of receptive fields in the superior temporal sulcus movement area shows wide variation (Zeki, 1974b). Some cells include the area of central vision, and these cells typically exhibit smaller receptive fields than those cells whose fields lie outside the center of gaze. A number of cells have fields which extend into the ipsilateral visual hemifield, a feature even more pronounced for units in inferotemporal cortex, which are described next.

INFEROTEMPORAL CORTEX

One of the historical definitions of association cortex was that such areas are "electrically silent" in contrast to sensory areas from which evoked potentials could be recorded after peripheral stimulation. Nevertheless, gross changes in electrical activity in inferotemporal cortex do occur during visual discrimination by monkeys (Chow, 1961; Gerstein et al., 1968). Responses from individual neurons in temporal cortex (area TE) can also be demonstrated (Gross et al., 1967). Such units have very large receptive fields that invariably include the fovea and are often bilateral. Stimuli moving in a direction orthogonal to the longer axis are preferred as are complex, colored, patterned stimuli. These facts suggest that rather specific inputs are coded by inferotemporal neurons, and Gross *et al.* (1972) summarize their findings by proposing that the function of inferotemporal cells can be described as providing increasingly specific information about wider areas of the visual field.

A combined lesion-electrophysiological study (Rocha-Miranda *et al.*, 1975) supports the anatomical possibility that visual information is routed from striate cortex to inferotemporal cortex through circumstriate cortex and the forebrain commissures, and that response characteristics of inferotemporal cells can be attributed to input from the striate-circumstriate pathway. As noted above, a majority of these cells have bilateral receptive fields. Abolishing the input from one striate cortex eliminates inferotemporal response to the hemifield represented by that hemisphere. This manipulation also changes the response characteristics of inferotemporal receptive fields in the remaining hemifield. Thus both ipsilateral and contralateral inputs from striate cortex are important for inferotemporal function.

In contrast to the effects of eliminating striate input, inferotemporal responsiveness to visual stimuli is not abolished by pulvinar lesions (Gross *et al.*, 1973). But a striking effect is noted after pulvinar lesions: cells in inferotemporal cortex display no receptive field. This is one of the rare examples of a demonstrated pulvinar effect on visual function.

Cortical evoked potentials also provide evidence for striate influence on inferotemporal function (Vaughan and Gross, 1969). Lesions of striate cortex affect the variability and, to some extent, the amplitude of late components of responses to flashes of light. However, there is no reciprocal effect of inferotemporal lesions on striate evoked potentials, nor do lesions alter the excitability characteristics of evoked striate responses (Schwartzkroin *et al.*, 1969). These results are compelling evidence for a serial processing model of inferotemporal function. But other facts argue that striate input to inferotemporal cortex via the circumstriate pathways may not be the whole story. Some response latencies in inferotemporal cortex are shorter than the latencies of striate response, or of single-unit responses in inferotemporal cortex. In addition, section of the optic tract severely reduces inferotemporal response on the same side, suggesting a subcortical input rather than a convergent, corticocortical input.

PULVINAR

The nature of visual input to which the pulvinar is responsive is not well understood at this time. Only small, dark bars or slits of light were used in mapping receptive fields in the pulvinar of owl monkey since the main concern was to establish the nature of the visual representation (Allman *et al.*, 1972). Some specificity of response is indicated by the facts that stationary stimuli as opposed to moving stimuli do not evoke responses and that responses are minimal to onset or offset of stimuli. And pulvinar and prestriate, but not lateral geniculate or striate, responses are affected by changes in contour density and contrast (Perryman and Lindsley, 1974). This effect appears to depend on eye movements since immobilizing the eye attenuates the response. Thus the importance of stimulus movement or eye movement in eliciting pulvinar response supports a description of its role in vision in terms of locating information in the visual field.

It is difficult to ascribe response properties in the pulvinar to any specific inputs, cortical or subcortical, at this time. Since the pulvinar receives input from striate, prestriate, and temporal cortex, as well as the superior colliculus, and since the superior colliculus receives input from these areas as well as from the retina, the task is as formidable as anywhere else in the visual system.

SUMMARY

Zeki (1974*a*) has summarized the response properties of the multiple visual areas found in monkey extrastriate visual areas, and he points to two generalizations that hold for these areas. First, there is a "division of labor" within circumstriate cortex such that different areas emphasize different functional attributes of visual stimulation. Second, this specificity is ordered within a given area so that cells which show the same preferences for particular values on a stimulus dimension are grouped together in a columnar arrangement.

Thus, beyond area 17, and its topographic analysis of orientation, length, width, eye laterality, color and direction of movement, the two visual hemifields are joined across the midline in area 18, and stereoscopic depth mechanisms are elaborated. In area 19, one region, the fourth visual complex, is specialized for the appreciation of color, and another area in the superior temporal sulcus also codes spectral characteristics of stimuli, and yet another area analyzes movement. In addition, large areas of the two hemifields converge upon single cells in inferotemporal cortex and respond to particular patterns of visual input.

These features of visual organization in the extrastriate cortex are consistent with the anatomical connections known to be present. Additional and different kinds of information about how extrastriate cortex contributes to visual function can be obtained from behavioral studies, to which we turn next.

EXTRASTRIATE CORTEX AND BEHAVIOR

Unlike the anatomical and electrophysiological studies summarized above, behavioral experiments have usually addressed themselves to the problem of evaluating one or another model of cortical functioning in behavior. Historically, this approach has taken the form of investigating cortical localization of function, on the assumption that behavioral functions are (more or less) definable, and the remaining problem is simply to understand how the brain mediates between stimulus input and behavioral response.

This can be understood if it is appreciated that neuropsychology has its roots in psychology, and to the extent that other neuroscientists involved themselves with behavioral questions, they accepted the classical psychological categories given to them. Thus if a taxonomy of behavioral processes defined a process called perception, for example, the neuropsychologist saw it as his task to discover how and where in the central nervous system the patterns of activity correlated with appreciation of objects in the real world are represented.

This tendency to work back from behavior, or experience, to the brain led to a plethora of experiments in which the investigator devised a task which was presumed to tap a particular behavioral process, such as "attention" or "discrimination" or "memory," and then noted the effect of one or more lesions of biological interest on this presumed function. This point has been made by a number of writers, usually accompanied by the observation that our understanding of brain-behavior relationships has not been advanced very quickly by this approach (Gross, 1972, 1973; Mishkin, 1966; Pribram, 1971; Wilson, 1968). However, the results of these studies were valuable when the investigator operationally defined the processes under investigation, and were less valuable only when arbitrary labels were attached to tasks which may intrude into many categories of behavior. Comprehensive reviews of studies relating extrastriate cortex and visual behavior have been provided by Gross (1972; 1973) and by Weiskrantz (1974), and the history of these investigations will not be repeated here. In what follows, an attempt will be made to describe the effects of disrupting the functions of circumscribed areas of extrastriate cortex in terms of the three functional systems described above.

Visual Function in the Tree Shrew

The tree shrew is a useful animal with which to begin behavioral studies of extrastriate cortex because of the striking development of the pulvinar-extrastriate system (Masterton *et al.*, 1974). In addition, as shown in Figs. 7 and 9, the whole pulvinar receives input from the superior colliculus and projects to most of the temporal lobe. This species thus affords the opportunity to study well-developed, parallel thalamocortical projection systems, the geniculostriate and the pulvinar-extrastriate, in relative isolation. We can approach the results of behavioral studies in two ways: after ablation of one or the other of these cortical areas, we can ask what visual functions the animal is still capable of, using the remaining system, or we can ask what functions are impaired after loss of either system.

A series of studies on the tree shrew shows that animals with complete removal of striate cortex can catch moving bait, avoid obstacles, and relearn form, pattern, and color discrimination without great difficulty (Killackey *et al.*, 1971; Snyder and Diamond, 1968; Snyder *et al.*, 1969; Ware *et al.*, 1972). Furthermore, without striate cortex, tree shrews show unimpaired depth discrimination and simple stimulus equivalence (Jane *et al.*, 1972). Once a discrimination is learned, tree shrews with striate lesions are able to shift responses to a previously unrewarded cue (Killackey *et al.*, 1971) or learn to ignore cues that had served as a signal for reward, and attend to cues that were previously irrelevant (Killackey *et al.*, 1972).

These findings, taken alone, might suggest that visual functions can proceed perfectly adequately in the absence of striate cortex. However, parametric studies reveal acuity deficits after striate lesions (Ward *et al.*, 1975; Ward and Masterton, 1970), suggesting that striate cortex in the tree shrew does play an important role in visual processes. And the addition of constant or variable extraneous information to a simple pattern discrimination produces a striking deficit. Destriated tree shrews which are able to discriminate between two patterns are unable to do so if the patterns are surrounded by an annulus (Killackey *et al.,* 1971). Similarly, if a form discrimination is complicated by the addition of uncorrelated color cues, striate lesions have a profound effect on performance (Killackey *et al.,* 1972).

Temporal cortical lesions, in contrast, produce different effects on residual function compared to striate lesions. While temporal lesions retard initial learning and relearning, with or without extraneous cues, animals with temporal lesions are able to succeed on these kinds of tasks. However, if the task demands the adoption of a new strategy, as when reward contingencies are reversed, or different cues are made relevant, temporal lesions produce severe deficits.

Thus, while both striate and temporal cortex are necessary for visually guided behavior of a complex nature, the functions served by each area in the tree shrew appear to be different. Striate cortex, in addition to its role in stimulus-analyzing mechanisms, is implicated in the selection of relevant stimulus information in the spatial domain. Temporal cortex, in contrast, appears to be important in the selection of relevant stimulus information over time. We must conclude that the lemniscal systems in the tree shrew cortex subserve both "sensory" and "higher-order" functions, perhaps because all of the visual cortex is accounted for in terms of these direct sensory projections.

VISUAL FUNCTION IN THE BUSHBABY

Striate lesions in the bushbaby produce a sensory loss which appears to be more profound than that in the tree shrew (Atencio *et al.,* 1975). Indeed, it is difficult to catalogue functions that remain unaffected by striate lesions since so much of visually guided behavior is altered. It is possible with stepwise procedures and remedial training to demonstrate pattern discrimination learning in bushbabies with partial striate lesions, but total striate lesions have a devastating effect on such tasks. Furthermore, bushbabies with striate cortex removed display faulty depth perception and difficulty in localizing stationary as well as moving objects.

Visual function is also impaired by lesions of temporal cortex. While animals with ventral temporal lesions are capable of visual localization and visual following, and demonstrate no gross impairment in object and pattern vision, they show a deficit on a variety of tasks which involve visual learning.

Since temporal cortex in the bushbaby can be divided into projections from lemniscal and extralemniscal systems, an obvious next step is to ask if there are differences in the functions of these cortical areas. It appears that there are (Wilson *et al.,* 1975). Different types of impairment are seen following ablation of ventral temporal cortex and the middle temporal area. Bushbabies with ventral temporal lesions are impaired on visual discrimination learning either with or without extraneous, irrelevant information. In addition, such animals have difficulty in shifting responses from one set of cues to a previously irrelevant set of cues, when the reward contingencies are changed. These impairments are reminiscent of those seen in tree shrews with temporal cortex lesions. The middle temporal lesions, on the other hand, produce difficulty in utilizing a visual cue which is separated from the response site, and which varies in location from trial to trial. It is not going far beyond the data to suggest that some kind of visuospatial function is implicated here. The sensory status of animals with the two kinds of lesions of extrastriate cortex does not appear to differ, as measured by size discrimination thresholds.

Thus ventral temporal and middle temporal areas appear to be involved in different behavioral functions in the bushbaby, both of which differ from the role of striate cortex. The middle temporal and striate areas, representing the projections of direct, sensory channels to the cortex, can be characterized as critical for location and analysis of stimulus information. Visual processes which depend on the appropriate utilization of past inputs, such as learning and shifting responses, depend on ventral temporal cortex which is not the recipient of direct, sensory input. However, in neither of the studies described was circumstriate cortex as well as ventral temporal cortex ablated, so the total cortical projection area of the nontectorecipient pulvinar has not yet been investigated.

VISUAL FUNCTION IN THE RHESUS MONKEY

A vast literature has now accumulated on the effects of disrupting various extrastriate visual areas in the rhesus monkey. There are no studies comparable, though, to Humphrey's 8-year series of experiments on the effect of total striate removal, which examined the course of a wide range of visual functions (1975). Nevertheless, from that study, some general conclusions about residual visual capacity, based on what remained of the extrastriate systems, can be reached. It appears that Helen, the rhesus monkey with striate cortex removed (except for a miniscule portion remaining in the depths of the calcarine fissure), was capable of figure-ground differentiation, visual localization, ambient vision, and little else.

From the data summarized above, it can be appreciated that all of the major input to circumstriate cortex is affected by striate lesions, so that removal of striate cortex will functionally deafferent circumstriate cortex to a large extent (Atencio *et al.*, 1975; Benevento and Rezak, 1976). Furthermore, efferents from circumstriate cortex to other areas in the parietal, temporal, and frontal lobes will be similarly altered through disruption of corticocortical and, to a greater or lesser degree, thalamocortical input, following striate lesions.

Granted that it is impossible to infer the functions of the geniculostriate system in isolation from the rest of the brain, it is still valuable to see what are the contributions of this system to the total visual function of the organism. It is clear from Humphrey's study that the visual capacities of rhesus monkey, while greater than previously thought (Pasik *et al.*, 1969; Schilder *et al.*, 1972, 1971), are nevertheless minimal when cortical visual function is dependent on the striate-deficient contributions of the tectal-pulvinar-extrastriate visual system. With these facts in mind, we can next ask what visual functions are lost when portions of the extrastriate system are removed, rather than what functions remain in the presence of these areas.

Modern history, in the investigation of behavioral functions of extrastriate cortex, begins with two series of investigations by Mishkin. The first emphasized the importance of prestriate cortical areas for visual functions, and the second emphasized differences in visual functions in two regions of inferotemporal cortex.

In the first set of experiments, Mishkin (1966) showed that the visual impairment characteristic of inferotemporal lesions such as deficits in pattern discrimination learning could be produced by eliminating input from striate cortex to inferotemporal cortex. This result was presaged in an experiment by Ettlinger (1959): monkeys with a unilateral lesion in inferotemporal cortex, contralateral section of the optic tract, and section of the corpus callosum were impaired on visual discrimination tasks. Mishkin accomplished the effect by removing striate cortex in one hemisphere and inferotemporal cortex in the contralateral hemisphere, and then sectioning the single, crossed pathway in the corpus callosum that remained as a functional connection between the intact striate and inferotemporal areas. This manipulation produces a severe deficit in pattern discrimination as does a unilateral prestriate lesion in the same hemisphere as a striate lesion, provided that all of circumstriate cortex which receives projections from striate cortex is removed (Mishkin, 1972). Any spared portion of the prestriate area seems to be sufficient for providing input to the inferotemporal area, which may explain the lack of disruption after prestriate manipulations found in other studies (Pribram *et al.*, 1966, 1969; Reitz, 1969). Thus, whether or not the striate-circumstriate-inferotemporal pathway is the only critical set of connections, the importance of the demonstrated prestriate relay, for maintaining both response properties of inferotemporal cells and visual discriminative processes, is well established.

Given that circumstriate cortex plays an important part in relaying visual information from striate cortex to more anterior areas, the question remains as to whether this area is also involved in stimulus processing. Or, to ask the question in a different way, does the prestriate area contribute to behavioral functions in and of itself? The fact that cells in circumstriate areas demonstrate complex response requirements is one reason for believing that it does, and behavioral data point to the same conclusion. Early lesion studies of posterior parietal cortex in rhesus monkeys (Bates and Ettlinger, 1960; Wilson, 1957) included cortex lying between the intraparietal sulcus and the lunate sulcus, an area which is the target of striate and prestriate projections from extrafoveal, lower quadrant portions of the visuotopic representations in these areas. A common finding is that monkeys with such a lesion are prone to misreaching and spatial disorientation. Moreover, this may occur only when the response is under visual control (Wilson, 1957). An impairment in visuospatial function is also suggested by the fact that monkeys with posterior parietal lesions have difficulty in learning a task when the cue and response sites are separated in space (Bates and Ettlinger, 1960; Pohl, 1973). Since this cortical area represents part of the tectorecipient pulvinar projection, these results are consistent with the behavioral effects of middle temporal lesions in the bushbaby. Localization of, or orientation to, events in the visual field which are significant appears to be at least one of the functions of this system.

Results of a second series of studies by Iwai and Mishkin (1968, 1969) led to the conclusion that the inferotemporal area can be subdivided into two areas with different functional specializations. In a search for the posterior boundary of inferotemporal cortex, Iwai and Mishkin discovered that ablation of cortex at the juncture of the occipital and temporal lobes is sufficient to produce the deficit in visual pattern discrimination learning that is seen after the classical inferotemporal lesion. The expanded area extends the inferotemporal area to cortex labeled TEO, and to an area dorsal to and including both banks of the inferior occipital sulcus; lesions in either of these restricted areas as well as lesions in more anterior inferotemporal cortex are sufficient to interfere with visual discrimination learning. Figure 10 shows the extent of each of the subtotal lesions, O–IV, which are effective.

If several of these strip lesions are combined into larger lesions, O + I, I + II, III + IV, a double dissociation of function emerges. The more posterior lesions produce a greater deficit on pattern discrimination than on concurrent learning of object discriminations, while the reverse is true of the anterior lesion (Mishkin, 1972). A number of experiments on the effects of ablating posterior and anterior inferotemporal areas have led to the suggestion that the posterior lesion may be tapping "attentional-perceptual" mechanisms and the anterior area may be involved in "associative-mnemonic" functions (Cowey and Gross, 1970; Gross *et al.*, 1971; Manning, 1971*a,b*; Manning *et al.*, 1971).

However, many problems arise in drawing conclusions from these data, together with data from other studies. The first difficulty lies in attempting to relate the locus of various lesions, which has varied from experiment to experiment, to what is known about the anatomical and physiological organization of

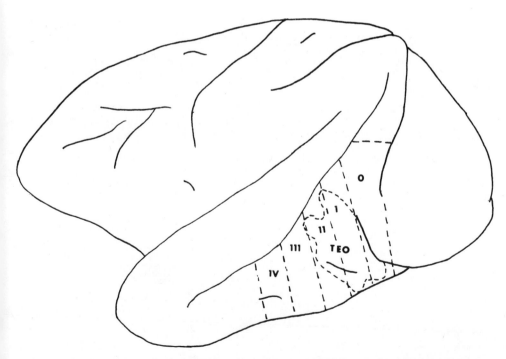

Fig. 10. Lateral view of the macaque cortex showing areas labeled O–IV in inferotemporal cortex, which, when removed singly, impair pattern discrimination learning. From Iwai and Mishkin (1969).

these areas. Cowey and Gross (1970) define a foveal prestriate area which is contrasted with the anterior inferotemporal area. The minimal common foveal prestriate lesion includes the posterior portion of TEO and the ventral portion of the foveal prestriate projection (Zeki, 1969*b*) while the maximal extent of foveal prestriate lesions includes all of TEO, the foveal prestriate area, and some extrafoveal areas. The O + I posterior inferotemporal lesion is coextensive with the minimal foveal prestriate lesion, but the I + II posterior lesion includes very little of the foveal prestriate area. Moreover, the latter lesion extends into inferotemporal cortex which receives different thalamic input (compare Figs. 9 and 11). Yet both of the posterior lesions produce greater impairment on pattern discrimination, a "perceptual" task, than on concurrent learning, an "associative" task. Furthermore, none of the lesions includes all of the prestriate areas which are critical for producing pattern discrimination deficits (Mishkin, 1972). These ambiguities make it difficult to relate lesion effects to known corticocortical and thalamocortical systems.

A second difficulty in interpreting what is known about the behavioral effects of circumscribed extrastriate lesions lies in the fact that the obtained effects imply

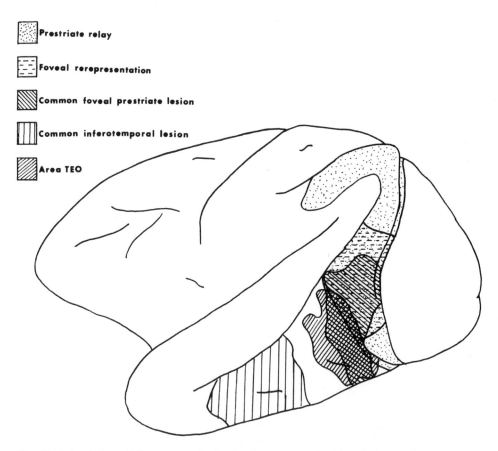

Fig. 11. Lateral view of the macaque brain showing extents of various lesions and cortical areas included within them. Shown are the prestriate relay (Mishkin, 1972), the macular rerepresentation (Zeki, 1969*b*), the common foveal prestriate and inferotemporal lesions from Cowey and Gross (1970), and area TEO (von Bonin and Bailey, 1950).

quantitative differences which do not lend themselves easily to an understanding of the cortical substrates involved. That is, both posterior and anterior inferotemporal lesions produce impairments relative to normal control animals on pattern discrimination and concurrent learning, even though the degree of deficit can be doubly dissociated in the two operated groups. In other studies, both posterior and anterior inferotemporal groups are impaired on pattern discrimination learning relative to a control group, but the operated groups do not differ among themselves (Bender, 1973; Oscar-Berman and Butters, 1976). In still other studies, one lesion group behaves like a normal control group while the other lesion group does not. For example, monkeys with anterior inferotemporal lesions and normal control animals are sensitive to reinforcement schedule while monkeys with posterior inferotemporal lesions are not (Manning *et al.*, 1971).

More perplexing are data that are simply not in agreement. In some studies, monkeys with posterior inferotemporal lesions but not anterior inferotemporal lesions perform more poorly when extraneous information is added to a discrimination (Gross *et al.*, 1971) and are facilitated by the addition of additional information when such information is relevant (Manning, 1971*b*). In other studies, monkeys with anterior but not posterior inferotemporal lesions perform more poorly when extraneous cues are added (Rothblat, 1968) while monkeys with posterior but not anterior lesions fail to make use of redundant information (Wilson *et al.*, 1972). And monkeys with posterior but not anterior inferotemporal lesions may be impaired on color discrimination learning tasks (Butter, 1974*a*) while monkeys with anterior but not posterior lesions show poor performance on matching-to-sample problems with color cues (Wilson *et al.*, 1972). In the face of all the difficulties in interpretation noted above, it appears that solution of the problem of extrastriate function still eludes us.

Since Iwai and Mishkin's functional dissociation of inferotemporal cortex into anterior and posterior areas left the classical inferotemporal area largely undisturbed, the previous behavioral findings relevant to this area remain of interest. However, since most of these studies were directed to testing one or another hypothesis about function, discussion of these and more recent behavioral results will be presented in that context. It is agreed that inferotemporal cortex is concerned exclusively with visual processes, and no changes basic to visual function such as impairments in acuity have been detected. It can be further stated that monkeys with inferotemporal lesions behave inappropriately when faced with any task demanding the utilization of visual input in a choice situation (cf. reviews by Gross, 1972, 1973). Beyond these areas of agreement, interpretation of inferotemporal function has taken a number of directions.

THEORIES OF INFEROTEMPORAL FUNCTION

As noted above, most of the hypotheses relating visual cortex and visual function have made use of taxonomic categories derived from observations of behavior. Thus the inferotemporal involvement in visual discrimination learning was usually explained by pointing to either the discriminative aspects or the learning aspects of the tasks. As a greater variety of situations has been employed, this dichotomy has been broadened into "perceptual" and "memory" hypotheses of inferotemporal function, which, we have seen, reached an apparent resolution in the functional dissociation of inferotemporal cortex. The answer appeared to lie in the fact that the classical inferotemporal lesion invades both the posterior sector, presumably responsible for perceptual processes, and the anterior sector, presumably responsible for memory processes (Iversen, 1970, 1973). However, this solution is not well supported by the location of lesions in many studies, even given a belief in perception and memory as sequential processes. And before the extension of inferotemporal cortex to include more posterior areas, and the distinction between anterior and posterior inferotemporal cortex, theories of inferotemporal function based on more anterior removals included both "perceptual" and "memory" hypotheses. The perceptual hypotheses can be further broken down into those which stress a particular feature of the perceptual process: visual sampling, selective attention, stimulus equivalence, stimulus categorization, or pattern recognition. The memory hypotheses can be fractionated into those stressing consolidation, storage, or retrieval of visual input.

The memory hypotheses have been easier to attack experimentally. Both monkeys and baboons show 15-min and 24-hr retention deficits following inferotemporal lesions, although it is not clear whether such deficits result from a failure of consolidation, storage, or retrieval mechanisms (Iversen, 1970; Iversen and Weiskrantz, 1964, 1970). And, although the details vary, there is ample evidence that monkeys with inferotemporal lesions are subject to proactive and retroactive interference during learning and performance of visual tasks (Cowey and Gross, 1970; Iversen, 1970; Wilson et al., 1972). Still, the possibility must again be considered that such deficits are due to inadequately perceived stimulus traces.

Both electrophysiological and lesion studies speak to this point, although not unambiguously. Results of several studies of short-term memory point to adequate appreciation of stimulus characteristics but difficulty in establishing and/or retrieving information about cue-reward relationships (Kovner and Stamm, 1972; Wilson et al., 1968b). Other studies stress that impairment of short-term memory processes following inferotemporal lesions is the result of a difficulty in establishing appropriate associations, rather than in retrieval processes. The fact that the perceptual difficulty of the tasks may be a factor in the amount of impairment observed argues against a pure memory hypothesis, however (Goldrich et al., 1970; Levine et al., 1970). Nevertheless, there is evidence that monkeys with inferotemporal lesions are able to establish, maintain, and retrieve information about cue-reward relationships, although they remember different kinds of information than do normal controls (Wilson et al., 1968a). We seem to be left with the conclusion that we started with: monkeys lacking inferotemporal cortex behave stupidly in situations in which they must make appropriate choices based on past experiences.

The memory hypotheses are less popular than they once were (Iversen, 1973; Weiskrantz, 1974). Turning to a consideration of how inferotemporal cortex might be implicated in perceptual processes, broadly defined, leads to a number of hypotheses. We are also led back to theories which include all of extrastriate cortex, in view of the great, if not complete, dependence of inferotemporal cortex on striate and prestriate input.

The model of inferotemporal cortex which is easiest to grasp holds that this area is the end point in a chain of stimulus-analyzing mechanisms which begin in the geniculostriate system. Convergent mechanisms such as have been hypothesized to account for the response properties of complex and hypercomplex cells in prestriate areas are assumed to be further elaborated in inferotemporal cortex. In such a scheme, inferotemporal cortex is the grandest feature detector of them all. However, it is difficult even theoretically to account for the perception of the visual world, with its constancies and its flux, on this basis. Nor do present experimental data support an "elaboration" hypothesis, if we accept performance on an orientation discrimination as a measure of the activity of stimulus-analyzing mechanisms. Foveal striate lesions affect thresholds of angular discrimination to a greater extent than either anterior or posterior inferotemporal lesions (Blake *et al.*, 1974), whereas the serial elaboration model predicts that the anterior inferotemporal area should provide the best feature analysis.

Effective object and pattern discrimination involves a number of processes, however. It is assumed, for example, that visual stimuli are normally brought into focus in central vision so that detailed analysis of stimulus attributes can be carried out by foveal mechanisms. Gross (1973) has suggested that inferotemporal cortex may serve to integrate information from the tectal-pulvinar system about the position of the head and eyes, relative to a stimulus, with information from the geniculostriate system about various stimulus features. This "input-combining" hypothesis can be tested by employing combined striate-collicular lesions and comparing the effect of such lesions with those of posterior inferotemporal lesions, considered the better candidates for integrative functions of this type (Butter, 1974*b*). The results indicate that both striate-collicular lesions and inferotemporal lesions impair acquisition of a pattern discrimination task, which supports the hypothesis. However, as Butter points out, an interaction between the geniculostriate system and the tectal-pulvinar system might take place subcortically rather than cortically. This is certainly consistent with the anatomical facts. That is, the interaction might consist of striate input to the superior colliculus, which in turn determines orientation and eye movements, which in turn affect the input to striate cortex. But this is clearly a different hypothesis than one which states that object or pattern recognition depends on two kinds of information which are integrated in inferotemporal cortex: the position of stimulus features in space as determined by gaze and orientation factors, and the actual stimulus features as determined by attributes of the stimulus. Furthermore, the "input-combining" hypothesis is weakened by the finding that posterior inferotemporal but not striate-collicular lesions affect retention, as opposed to learning, of a pattern discrimination task. This finding argues that inferotemporal cortex serves other functions than combining striate and tectal input.

The elaboration hypothesis, as described above, stresses inferotemporal cortex as the end stage in a hierarchical feature extraction mechanism. The hypothesis can be construed in another way if different aspects of the model are emphasized. Let us assume that pattern recognition involves detecting invariances in stimulation over a wide set of changing retinal inputs. If convergence of information from central and peripheral portions of the visual field is emphasized, rather than convergence of elements leading to specificity of stimulus features, the elaboration hypothesis suggests that the inferotemporal area provides a mechanism for enlarging receptive field size so that a stimulus can be recognized regardless of its locus in the visual field (Rocha-Miranda *et al.*, 1975). In the absence of such a mechanism, pattern discrimination would involve an incredible number of separate habits producing highly inefficient learning. [Interestingly, this multiplicity of habits, which neuropsychological theory ascribes only to brain-damaged animals, is postulated in theories of normal human learning such as those of Guthrie and Estes (cf. Hilgard and Bower, 1975).]

Visual perception is also thought to involve sampling processes, a necessary activity if potentially interesting extrafoveal information is to be brought into central vision. There are several lines of evidence that suggest that inferotemporal cortex is critical for this function. Monkeys with inferotemporal lesions pick fewer novel objects in search of reward (Pribram, 1960), do not utilize cues which are less salient (Butter, 1968; Butter *et al.*, 1965), and do not exploit redundant cues that are spatially separated from the response site (Butter and Hirtzel, 1970).

But restricting visual input is also thought to be important in visual function, and it has been found that monkeys with inferotemporal lesions show more responses to altered stimuli (Butter and Doehrman, 1968) and are distracted by extraneous stimulus features (Butter, 1969, 1972). Such impairments have been interpreted as reflecting deficits in selective attention, and have sometimes been attributed to invasion of the posterior inferotemporal cortex, in line with the perceptual-memory distinction (Butter, 1969).

Rothblat and Pribram (1972) also stress the role of inferotemporal cortex in selecting information. This view gains support from the demonstration of differences in electrical activity in inferotemporal cortex which precede response selection of one or another aspect of a compound stimulus and which are correlated with the dimension of the stimulus that is appropriate in terms of reinforcement. Since, with overtraining, striate activity also reflects such activity, the authors conclude that attentional mechanisms are not solely response linked but can, with experience, serve as filters on incoming information. The importance of inferotemporal cortex, however, is thought to lie in its responsiveness to various aspects of stimulation which guide behavior selectively (Bagshaw *et al.*, 1972).

Pribram's model of inferotemporal function as a mechanism for selective attention implies an efferent control of stimulus input, and Pribram has pointed to the known projections from inferotemporal cortex to subcortical structures as support for his views. The issue has also been addressed experimentally a number of times with both positive and negative results (Pribram, 1971; Schwartzkroin *et al.*, 1969). In his model, Pribram (1974) distinguishes between stable, preprogrammed feature detectors, around which a relatively unmodifiable primary sensory system is organized, and a labile, experience-sensitive mechanism, depending on inferotemporal cortex function, which selects and controls responses to afferent input in terms of its own activity. Thus recognizing a particular pattern or object requires processes which are independent of specific stimulus input, yet can be modified by specific input. Although not directly relevant to tests of the efferent model, Turvey (1973) has arrived at a similar distinction, on the basis of behavioral data, between visual features which are "context independent," and are appreciated by feature-detecting systems, and visual features which are "context dependent," and arise from more global representations and more central decisions. And Weiskrantz (1972) also points to inferotemporal cortex as necessary for "the construction of a stable visual world of solid things out of the literal and constantly changing response to stimulus features carried out by striate cortex."

Thus both elaboration and gating hypotheses of inferotemporal function postulate mechanisms for providing perceptual invariances, although the nature and importance of the neural connections postulated vary. An elaboration model emphasizes convergent, afferent input as providing a stable representation of the visual world. Gross's interaction notion could be included here if information from ambient vision (Trevarthen, 1968; Held, 1970) contributes to such a representation. A gating model, on the other hand, emphasizes efferent control over afferent input as providing a representation of the visual world. The problem now becomes one of stating how and where visual configurations are abstracted from the stimulus array, in neuropsychological terms.

However, stimuli are not only extracted from a visual array. Input is also categorized and assigned meaning on the basis of relevant past experience with similar input. The problem of how stimuli are categorized leads directly back to the hypothesis that inferotemporal cortex is implicated in memory processes, unsatisfactory as that hypothesis proved at first test. But if stimulus categorization is conceived broadly as a process including features of what we call memory and perception (cf. Helson, 1964), a great deal of conflicting data about inferotemporal function can be reconciled. Iversen (1973) has pointed out that, in addition to the processes of cue extraction, contextual effects and "strategies of looking" contribute to what is perceived. In a similar vein, Wilson has argued that utilization of visual input involves the processing of stimulus information over both time and space, and has hypothesized a tradeoff between attention to present and past, focal and peripheral, information in visual stimuli (Wilson, 1968; Mason and Wilson, 1974; Wilson et al., 1972; Soper et al., 1975). Thus the participation of all three cortical visual systems will be involved in any perceptual event. Whether stimulus categorization, which involves the organization of stimulus input, demands efferent as well as afferent processes is still open to question.

It should also be noted that any model of how the visual system functions must account for the lability as well as the stability of the perceptual world (Pribram, 1974; Soper et al., 1975). While organisms respond to changing stimuli as coherent configurations, it is also true that organisms respond differently to stimulus input with the same physical attributes, when reinforcement contingencies change or when stimuli display different relationships to stored information (Wilson, 1971, 1972). Thus any model of cortical function in vision must account for the flexibility and adaptability of perception, as well as for the constancies which characterize the visual world.

CONCLUDING COMMENTS

How can extrastriate function in vision be understood in relation to variables that have been discussed? Consideration of the response properties of neurons, organization of visual representations, corticocortical and thalamocortical connections, species differences, and behavioral correlates may provide some grounds for speculation if taken in conjunction.

The dichotomy between sensory and association areas and functions can be replaced with a new dichotomy between a world of visual features and a world of visual things. The complexities of anatomical and functional organization in the visual system, as now understood, do not lead to a parallel distinction between peripheral and central processes, or between striate and extrastriate cortex. Vertical and horizontal circuits integrate central and peripheral, striate and extrastriate, components at every level of the visual system, and it appears that the search for a "central processor" can be safely abandoned.

Two ways of seeing, which have been labeled "locating and identifying" (Schneider, 1969), "noticing and examining" (Weiskrantz, 1972), or "ambient and focal" (Trevarthen, 1968), can perhaps be identified with the lemniscal components of both extrastriate and striate cortex. But the spatial mode is insufficient to account for the perception of the visual world, and a temporal dimension must also be invoked. To the extent that previous stimulus inputs are stored over time, and act as a referent for categorizing present stimuli, we can look to the contributions of the extralemniscal system and expect to find even greater independence from the particular form of physical energy that constitutes the stimulus than that provided by the elaboration of the lemniscal systems.

Thus the world of features might be thought of as being exemplified by the specificity of response properties found in visual cortex, while the world of things, depending on both past and present input, is relatively independent of specific stimulus input. The development of extrastriate cortex, reaching its apex in primate evolution, can be conceived as providing for the elaboration of both spatial and temporal processing, integrating direct-line and reverberating circuits, and continuing the process of trading off information which is seen at every level of the visual system beginning with the duplex retina. We might attribute the flexibility of primate function to this ability to sacrifice appreciation of some events in space or time, in order to better appreciate other events in space and time, and to change priorities when appropriate.

In conclusion, while the distinction between visual features and the visual world appears to be consistent with both our present knowledge about the organization of visual cortex and current perceptual theory, it must be remembered that the same could be said of the sensory-association model which preceded it.

Acknowledgments

I am grateful to Doris Walters for expert secretarial help during the preparation of this chapter.

REFERENCES

Allman, J. M. Representation of the visual field on the medial wall of occipital-parietal cortex in the owl monkey. *Science*, 1976, *191*, 572–575.

Allman, J. M., and Kaas, J. H. A representation of the visual field in the caudal third of the middle temporal gyrus of the owl monkey (*Aotus trivirgatus*). *Brain Res.*, 1971, *31*, 85–105.

Allman, J. M., and Kaas, J. H. The organization of the second visual area (V 11) in the owl monkey: A second order transformation of the visual hemifield. *Brain Res.*, 1974a, *76*, 247–265.

Allman, J. M., and Kaas, J. H. A cresent-shaped cortical visual area surrounding the middle temporal area (MT) of association cortex in the owl monkey, *Aotus* trivirgatus. *Brain Res.*, 1974b, *81*, 199–213.

Allman, J. M., and Kaas, J. H. The dorsomedial cortical visual area: A third tier area in the occipital lobe of the owl monkey (*Aotus trivirgatus*). *Brain Res.*, 1975, *100*, 473–487.

Allman, J. M., Kaas, J. H., Lane, R. H., and Miezin, F. M. A representation of the visual field in the inferior pulvinar nucleus in the owl monkey (*Aotus trivirgatus*). *Brain Res.*, 1972, *40*, 291–302.

Allman, J. M., Kaas, J. H., and Lane, R. H. The middle temporal visual area (MT) in the bushbaby, *Galago senegalensis*. *Brain Res.*, 1973, *57*, 197–202.

Atencio, F. W., Diamond, I. T., and Ward, J. P. Behavioral study of the visual cortex of *Galago senegalensis*. *J. Comp. Physiol. Psychol.*, 1975, *89*, 1109–1135.

Bagshaw, M. H., Mackworth, N. H., and Pribram, K. H. The effect of resections of the inferotemporal cortex or the amygdala on visual orienting and habituation. *Neuropsychologia*, 1972, *10*, 153–162.

Bates, J. A. V., and Ettlinger, G. Posterior biparietal ablations in the monkey. *AMA Arch. Neurol.*, 1960, *3*, 177–192.

Bender, D. B. Visual sensitivity following inferotemporal and foveal prestriate lesions in the rhesus monkey. *J. Comp. Physiol. Psychol.*, 1973, *84*, 613–621.

Benevento, L. A., and Fallon, J. H. The ascending projections of the superior colliculus in the rhesus monkey. *J. Comp. Neurol.*, 1975, *160*, 339–362.

Benevento, L. A., and Rezak, M. The cortical projections of the inferior pulvinar and adjacent lateral pulvinar in the rhesus monkey (*Macaca mulatta*): An autoradiographic study. *Brain Res.*, 1976, *108*, 1–24.

Blake, L., Jarvis, C., and Mishkin, M. Pattern discrimination deficits after partial inferior temporal or striate lesions in monkeys. *Brain Res.*, 1977, *120*, 209–220.

Bonin, G. von, and Bailey, P. *The Neocortex of Macaca Mulatta*. University of Illinois Press, Urbana, Ill., 1947.

Bonin, G. von, and Bailey, P. *The Isocortex of the Chimpanzee*. University of Illinois Press, Urbana, Ill., 1950.

Brodmann, K. Beitrage zur histologischen Lokalisation der Grosshirnrinde IIIte Mitteilung: Die Rindenfelder der neideren Affen. *J. Psychol. Neurol.*, 1905, *4*, 177–226.

Butter, C. M. The effect of discrimination training on pattern equivalence in monkeys with inferotemporal and lateral striate lesions. *Neuropsychologia*, 1968, *6*, 27–40.

Butter, C. M. Impairments in selective attention to visual stimuli in monkeys with inferotemporal and lateral striate lesions. *Brain Res.*, 1969, *12*, 374–383.

Butter, C. M. Detection of masked patterns in monkeys with inferotemporal, striate or dorsolateral frontal lesions. *Neuropsychologia*, 1972, *10*, 241–243.

Butter, C. M. Effect of superior colliculus, striate, and prestriate lesions on visual sampling in rhesus monkeys. *J. Comp. Physiol. Psychol.*, 1974a, *87*, 905–917.

Butter, C. M. Visual discrimination impairments in rhesus monkeys with combined lesions of superior colliculus and striate cortex. *J. Comp. Physiol. Psychol.*, 1974b, *87*, 918–929.

Butter, C. M., and Doehrman, S. R. Size discrimination and transposition in monkeys with striate and temporal lesions. *Cortex*, 1968, *4*, 35–46.

Butter, C. M., and Hirtzel, M. Impairment in sampling visual stimuli in monkeys with inferotemporal lesions. *Physiol. Behav.*, 1970, *5*, 369–370.

Butter, C. M., Mishkin, M., and Rosvold, H. E. Stimulus generalization following inferotemporal and lateral striate lesions in monkeys. In D. Mostofsky (ed.), *Stimulus Generalization*. Stanford University Press, Stanford, Calif., 1965, pp. 119–133.

Campos-Ortega, J. A. Descending subcortical projections from the occipital lobe of *Galago crassicaudatus*. *Exp. Neurol.*, 1968, *21*, 440–454.

Campos-Ortega, J. A., Hayhow, W. R., and Clüver, P. F. deV. A note on the problem of retinal projections to the inferior pulvinar nucleus of primates. *Brain Res.*, 1970a, *22*, 126–130.

Campos-Ortega, J. A., Haybow, W. R., and Clüver, P. F. deV. The descending projections from the cortical visual fields of *Macaca mulatta* with particular reference to the question of a cortico-lateral geniculate pathway. *Brain Behav. Evol.*, 1970b, *3*, 368–414.

Chow, K. L. A retrograde degeneration study of the cortical projection field of the pulvinar in the monkey. *J. Comp. Neurol.*, 1950, *93*, 313–340.

Chow, K. L. Anatomical and electrographical analysis of temporal neocortex in relation to visual discrimination learning in monkey. In J. F. Delafresnaye (ed.), *Brain Mechanisms and Learning.* Thomas, Springfield, Ill., 1961, pp. 507–525.

Cowey, A. Projection of the retina on the striate and prestriate cortex in the squirrel monkey, *Saimiri sciureus. J. Neurophysiol.,* 1964, *27,* 366–393.

Cowey, A., and Gross, C. G. Effects of foveal prestriate and inferotemporal lesions on visual discriminations by rhesus monkeys. *Exp. Brain Res.,* 1970, *11,* 128–144.

Cragg, B. G. The topography of the afferent projections in the circumstriate visual cortex of the monkey studied by the Nauta method. *Vision Res.,* 1969, *9,* 733–757.

Diamond, I. T. Organization of the visual cortex: Comparative anatomical and behavioral studies. *Fed. Proc.,* 1976, *35,* 60–67.

Doty, R. W., Kimura, D. S., and Mogenson, G. J. Photically and electrically elicited responses in the central visual system of the squirrel monkey. *Exp. Neurol.,* 1964, *10,* 19-51.

Dubner, R., and Zeki, S. M. Response properties and receptive fields of cells in an anatomically defined region of the superior temporal sulcus in the monkey. *Brain Res.,* 1971, *35,* 528–532.

Ettlinger, G., Iwai, E., Mishkin, M., and Rosvold, H. E. Visual discrimination in the monkey following serial ablation of inferotemporal and preoccipital cortex. *J. Comp. Physiol. Psychol.,* 1968, *65,* 110–117.

Ettlinger, G. Visual discrimination following successive temporal ablations in monkeys. *Brain,* 1959, *82,* 232–250.

Gerstein, G. L., Gross, C. G., and Weinstein, M. Inferotemporal evoked potentials during discrimination performance by monkeys. *J. Comp. Physiol. Psychol.,* 1968, *65,* 526–528.

Glendenning, K. K., Hall, J. A., Diamond, I. T., and Hall, W. C. The pulvinar nucleus of *Galago senegalensis. J. Comp. Neurol.,* 1975, *161,* 419–458.

Goldrich, S. G., Pond, F. J., Livesey, P., and Schwartzbaum, J. S. Electrically-induced afterdischarges in the inferotemporal cortex of monkeys: Effects on visual discrimination and discrimination-reversal performance. *Neuropsychologia,* 1970, *8,* 417–430.

Gross, C. G. Visual functions of inferotemporal cortex. In R. Jung (ed.), *Handbook of Sensory Physiology,* Vol. 7, Part 3. Springer-Verlag, Berlin, 1972, pp. 451–482.

Gross, C. G. Inferotemporal cortex and vision. In E. Stellar and J. M. Sprague (eds.), *Progress in Physiological Psychology,* Vol. 5. Academic Press, New York, 1973, pp. 77–123.

Gross, C. G., Schiller, P. H., Wells, C., and Gerstein, G. L. Single unit activity in temporal association cortex of the monkey. *J. Neurophysiol.,* 1967, *30,* 833–843.

Gross, C. G., Rocha-Miranda, C. E., and Bender, D. B. Visual properties of neurons in inferotemporal cortex of the macaque. *J. Neurophysiol.,* 1972, *35,* 96–111.

Gross, C. G., Cowey, A., and Manning, F. J. Further analysis of visual discrimination deficits following foveal prestriate and inferotemporal lesions in rhesus monkeys. *J. Comp. Physiol. Psychol,* 1971, *76,* 1–7.

Gross, C. G., Bender, D. B., and Rocha-Miranda, C. E. Inferotemporal cortex: A single unit analysis. In F. O. Schmitt and F. G. Worden (eds.), *The Neurosciences: A Third Study Program.* MIT Press, Cambridge, Mass., 1973, pp. 229–238.

Harting, J. K., and Casagrande, V. A. Afferent connections of the pulvinar nucleus in the tree shrew. *Neurosci. Abstr.,* 1974, 248.

Harting, J. K., Hall, W. C., and Diamond, I. T. Evolution of the pulvinar. *Brain Behav. Evol.,* 1972, *6,* 424–452.

Harting, J. K., Diamond, I. T., and Hall, W. C. Anterograde degeneration study of the cortical projections of the lateral geniculate and pulvinar nuclei in the tree shrew (*Tupaia glis*). *J. Comp. Neurol.,* 1973, *150,* 393–440.

Held, R. Two modes of processing spatially distributed information. In F. O. Schmitt (ed.), *The Neurosciences: Second Study Program.* Rockefeller University Press, New York, 1970, pp. 317–324.

Helson, H. Adaptation-level theory. Harper and Row, New York, 1964.

Hilgard, E. R., and Bower, G. H. *Theories of Learning,* 4th ed. Prentice-Hall, Englewood Cliffs, N.J., 1975.

Hubel, D. H., and Wiesel, T. N. Receptive fields and functional architecture of monkey striate cortex. *J. Physiol., (London),* 1968, *195,* 215–243.

Hubel, D. H., and Wiesel, T. N. Cells sensitive to binocular depth in area 18 of the macaque monkey cortex. *Nature,* 1970, *225,* 41–42.

Humphrey, N. K. Vision in a monkey without striate cortex: A case study. *Perception,* 1974, *3,* 241–255.

Iversen, S. D. Interference and inferotemporal memory deficits. *Brain Res.,* 1970, *19,* 277–289.

Iversen, S. D. Visual discrimination deficits associated with posterior inferotemporal lesions in the monkey. *Brain Res.,* 1973, *62,* 89–101.

Iversen, S. D., and Weiskrantz, L. Temporal lobe lesions and memory in the monkey. *Nature*, 1964, *201*, 740–742.

Iversen, S. D., and Weiskrantz, L. An investigation of a possible memory defect produced by inferotemporal lesions in the baboon. *Neuropsychologia*, 1970, *8*, 21–36.

Iwai, E., and Mishkin, M. Two visual foci in the temporal lobe of monkeys. In N. Yoshii and N. A. Buchwald (eds.), *Neurophysiological Basis of Learning and Behavior*. Osaka University Press, Osaka, Japan, 1968.

Iwai, E., and Mishkin, M. Further evidence on the locus of the visual area in the temporal lobe of the monkey. *Exp. Neurol.*, 1969, *25*, 585–594.

Jane, J. A., Levey, N., and Carlson, N. J. Tectal and cortical function in vision. *Exp. Neurol.*, 1972, *35*, 61–77.

Jones, B., and Mishkin, M. Limbic lesions and the problem of stimulus-reinforcement association. *Exp. Neurol.*, 1972, *36*, 362–377.

Jones, E. G., and Powell, T. P. S. An anatomical study of converging sensory pathways within the cerebral cortex of the monkey. *Brain*, 1970, *93*, 793–820.

Killackey, H., Snyder, M., and Diamond, I. T. Function of striate and temporal cortex in the tree shrew. *J. Comp. Physiol. Psychol.*, 1971, *74*, 1–29.

Killackey, H., Wilson, M., and Diamond, I. T. Further studies of the striate and extrastriate visual cortex in the tree shrew. *J. Comp. Physiol. Psychol.*, 1972, *81*, 45–63.

Klüver, H., and Bucy, P. C. A analysis of certain effects of bilateral temporal lobectomy in the rhesus monkey with special reference to "psychic blindness." *J. Psychol.*, 1938, *5*, 33–54.

Kovner, R., and Stamm, J. S. Disruption of short-term visual memory by electrical stimulation of inferotemporal cortex in the monkey. *J. Comp. Physiol. Psychol.*, 1972, *81*, 163–172.

Kuypers, H. G. J. M., Szcwarcbart, M. K., Mishkin, M., and Rosvold, H. E. Occipitotemporal corticocortical connections in the rhesus monkey. *Exp. Neurol.*, 1965, *11*, 245–262.

Lashley, K. S. The mechanism of vision. XVIII. Effects of destroying the visual "associative areas" of the monkey. *Genet. Psychol. Monogr.*, 1948, *37*, 107–166.

Levine, M. S., Goldrich, S. G., Pond, F. J., Livesey, P., and Schwartzbaum, J. S. Retrograde amnestic effects of inferotemporal and amygdaloid seizures upon conditioned suppression of lever-pressing monkeys. *Neuropsychologia*, 1970, *8*, 431–442.

Lin, C. S., and Kaas, J. H. Some efferent and afferent connections of a medial division of the inferior pulvinar nucleus in the owl monkey (*Aotus trivirgatus*). *Neurosci. Abstr.*, 1975, 44.

Lin, C. S., Wagor, E., and Kaas, J. H. Projections from the pulvinar to the middle temporal visual area (MT) in the owl monkey, *Aotus trivirgatus*. *Brain Res.*, 1974, *76*, 145–149.

Manning, F. J. Punishment for errors and visual discrimination learning by monkeys with inferotemporal cortex lesions. *J. Comp. Physiol. Psychol.*, 1971*a*, *75*, 146–152.

Manning, F. J. The selective attention "deficit" of monkeys with ablations of foveal prestriate cortex. *Psychon. Sci.*, 1971*b*, *25*, 291–292.

Manning, F. J., Gross, C. G., and Cowey, A. Partial reinforcement: Effects on visual learning after foveal prestriate and inferotemporal lesions. *Physiol. Behav.*, 1971, *6*, 61–64.

Martinez-Millán, L., and Holländer, H. Cortico-cortical projections from striate cortex of the squirrel monkey (*Saimiri sciureus*): A radioautographic study. *Brain Res.*, 1975, *83*, 405–417.

Mason, M., and Wilson, M. Temporal differentiation and recognition memory for visual stimuli in rhesus monkeys. *J. Exp. Psychol.*, 1974, *103*, 383–390.

Masterton, M., Skeen, L. C., and RoBards, M. J. Origins of anthropoid intelligence II. Pulvinar-extrastriate system and visual reversal learning. *Brain Behav. Evol.*, 1974, *10*, 322–353.

Mathers, L. H. Tectal projection to the posterior thalamus of the squirrel monkey. *Brain Res.*, 1971, *35*, 295–298.

Mathers, L. H. The synaptic organization of the cortical projection to the pulvinar of the squirrel monkey. *J. Comp. Neurol.*, 1972, *146*, 43–60.

McLoon, S. C., Santos-Anderson, R., and Benevento, L. A. Some projections of the posterior bank and floor of the superior temporal sulcus in the rhesus monkey. *Neurosci. Abstr.*, 1975, 64.

Mishkin, M. Visual mechanisms beyond the striate cortex. In R. Russell (ed.), *Frontiers of Physiological Psychology*. Academic Press, New York, 1966, pp. 93–119.

Mishkin, M. Cortical visual areas and their interaction. In A. G. Karczmar and J. C. Eccles (eds.), *Brain and Human Behavior*. Springer-Verlag, New York, 1972, pp. 187–208.

Myers, R. E. Projections of the superior colliculus in the monkey. *Anat. Rec.*, 1963, *145*, 264.

Oscar-Berman, M., and Butters, N. Sequential and single-stage lesions of posterior association cortex in rhesus monkeys. *Physiol. Behav.*, 1976, *17*, 287–296.

Pandya, D. N., Karol, E. A., and Heilbron, D. The topographical distribution of the interhemispheric projections in the corpus callosum of the rhesus monkey. *Brain Res.*, 1971, *32*, 31–43.

Pasik, P., Pasik, T., and Schilder, P. Extrageniculostriate vision in the monkey: Discrimination of luminous flux-equated figures. *Exp. Neurol.,* 1969, *23,* 421–437.

Perryman, K. M., and Lindsley, D. B. Visually evoked responses in pulvinar, lateral geniculate, and visual cortex to patterned and unpatterned stimuli in squirrel monkey. *Neurosci. Abstr.,* 1974, 371.

Pohl, W. Dissociation of spatial discrimination deficits following frontal and parietal lesions in monkeys. *J. Comp. Physiol. Psychol.,* 1973, *82,* 227–239.

Pribram, K. H. The intrinsic systems of the forebrain. In J. Field (ed.), *Handbook of Physiology,* Vol. 2. American Physiological Society, Washington, D.C., 1960.

Pribram, K. H. *Languages of the Brain: Experimental Paradoxes and Principles in Neuropsychology.* Prentice-Hall, Englewood Cliffs, N.J., 1971.

Pribram, K. H. How is it that sensing so much we can do so little? In F. O. Schmitt and F. G. Worden (eds.), *The Neurosciences: Third Study Program.* MIT Press, Cambridge, Mass., 1974, pp. 249–261.

Pribram, K. H., Blehert, S. R., and Spinelli, D. N. Effects on visual discrimination of crosshatching and undercutting the inferotemporal cortex of monkeys. *J. Comp. Physiol. Psychol.,* 1966, *62,* 358–264.

Pribram, K. H., Spinelli, D. N., and Reitz, S. L. The effects of radical disconnection of occipital and temporal cortex on visual behavior of monkeys. *Brain,* 1969, *92,* 301–312.

Reitz, S. L. Effects of serial disconnection of striate and temporal cortex on visual discrimination performance in monkeys. *J. Comp. Physiol. Psychol.,* 1969, *68,* 139–146.

Rocha-Miranda, C. E., Bender, D. B., Gross, C. G., and Mishkin, M. Visual activation of neurons in inferotemporal cortex depends upon striate cortex and forebrain commissures. *J. Neurophysiol.,* 1975, *38,* 475–491.

Rothblat, L. Functions of the temporal lobe in selective attention: A behavioral analysis. Unpublished Ph.D. thesis, University of Connecticut, 1968.

Rothblat, L., and Pribram, K. H. Selective attention: Input filter or response selection? An electrophysiological analysis. *Brain Res.,* 1972, *39,* 427–436.

Schilder, P., Pasik, T., and Pasik, P. Extrageniculostriate vision in the monkey. II. Demonstration of brightness discrimination. *Brain Res.,* 1971, *32,* 383–398.

Schilder, P., Pasik, P., and Pasik, T. Extrageniculostriate vision in the monkey: III. Circle vs. triangle and "red vs. green" discrimination. *Exp. Brain Res.,* 1972, *14,* 436–448.

Schneider, G. E. Two visual systems. *Science,* 1969, *163,* 895–902.

Schwartzkroin, P. A., Cowey, A., and Gross, C. G. A test of an "efferent model" of the function of inferotemporal cortex in visual discrimination. *Electroencephalogr. Clin. Neurophysiol.,* 1969, *27,* 594–600.

Semmes, J. Protopathic and epicritic sensation: A reappraisal. In A. L. Benton (ed.), *Contributions to Clinical Neuropsychology.* Aldine, Chicago, 1970.

Snyder, M., and Diamond, I. T. The organization and function of the visual cortex in the tree shrew. *Brain Behav. Evol.,* 1968, *1,* 244–288.

Snyder, M., Killackey, H., and Diamond, I. T. Color vision in the tree shrew after removal of posterior neocortex. *J. Neurophysiol.,* 1969, *32,* 554–563.

Soper, H. V., Diamond, I. T., and Wilson, M. Visual attention and inferotemporal cortex in rhesus monkeys. *Neuropsychologia,* 1975, *13,* 409–419.

Spatz, W. B. An efferent connection of the solitary cells of Meynert: A study with horseradish peroxidase in the marmoset *Callithrix. Brain Res.,* 1975, *92,* 450–455.

Spatz, W. B., and Tigges, J. Experimental-anatomical studies on the "middle temporal visual area (MT)" in primates. *J. Comp. Neurol.,* 1972, *146,* 451–464.

Spatz, W. B., Tigges, J., and Tigges, M. Subcortical projections, cortical associations and some intrinsic intralaminar connections of the striate cortex in the squirrel monkey (*Saimiri*). *J. Comp. Neurol.,* 1970, *140,* 155–174.

Tigges, J., Spatz, W. B., and Tigges, M. Reciprocal point-to-point connections between parastriate and striate cortex in the squirrel monkey (*Saimiri*). *J. Comp. Neurol.,* 1973a, *148,* 481–490.

Tigges, J., Tigges, M., and Kalaha, C. S. Efferent connections of area 17 in *Galago. Am. J. Phys. Anthropol.,* 1973b, *38,* 393–398.

Trevarthen, C. B. Two mechanisms of vision in primates. *Psychol. Forsch.,* 1968, *31,* 299–337.

Trojanowski, J. Q., and Jacobson, S. Peroxidase labeled subcortical afferents to pulvinar in rhesus monkey. *Brain Res.,* 1975, *97,* 144–50.

Turvey, M. T. On peripheral and central processes in vision: Inferences from an information-processing analysis of masking with patterned stimuli. *Psychol. Rev.,* 1973, *80,* 1–52.

Van Hoesen, G. W., and Pandya, D. N. Some connections of the enterhinal (area 28) and perirhinal (area 35) cortices of the rhesus monkey. I. Temporal lobe afferents. *Brain Res.,* 1975, *95,* 1–24.

Vaughan, H. G., Jr., and Gross, C. G. Cortical responses to light in unanaesthetized monkeys and their alteration by visual system lesions. *Exp. Brain Res.,* 1969, *8,* 19–36.

von Economo, C. *The Cytoarchitectonics of the Human Cerebral Cortex.* Oxford University Press, London, 1929.

Wagor, E., Lin, C. S., and Kaas, J. H. Some cortical projections of the dorso-medial visual area (DM) of association cortex in the owl monkey, *Aotus trivirgatus. J. Comp. Neurol.,* 1975, *163,* 227–250.

Walker, A. E. *The Primate Thalamus.* University of Chicago Press, Chicago, 1938.

Ward, J. P., and Masterton, R. B. Encephalization and visual cortex in the tree shrew (*Tupaia glis*). *Brain Behav. Evol.,* 1970, *3,* 421–469.

Ward, J. P., Frank J., and Moss, M. Visual acuity deficits in destriate tree shrews as a function of stimulus area and stripe separation. *Neurosci. Abstr.,* 1975, 71.

Ware, C. B. Casagrande, V. A., and Diamond, I. T. Does the acuity of the tree shrew suffer from removal of striate cortex? *Brain Behav. Evol.,* 1972, *5,* 18–29.

Weiskrantz, L. Review lecture: Behavioral analysis of the monkey's visual nervous system. *Proc. Roy. Soc. London Ser. B.,* 1972, *182,* 427–455.

Weiskrantz, L. The interaction between occipital and temporal cortex in vision: An overview. In F. O. Schmitt and F. G. Worden (eds.), *The Neurosciences: A Third Study Program.* MIT Press, Cambridge, Mass., 1974, pp. 189–204.

Whitlock, D. G., and Nauta, W. J. H. Subcortical projections from the temporal neocortex. *J. Comp. Neurol.,* 1956, *106,* 183–212.

Wilson, M. Effects of circumscribed cortical lesions upon somesthetic and visual discrimination in the monkey. *J. Comp. Physiol. Psychol.,* 1957, *50,* 630–635.

Wilson, M. Inferotemporal cortex and the processing of visual information in monkeys. *Neuropsychologia,* 1968, *6,* 135–140.

Wilson, M. Shifts in categorization and identifiability of visual stimuli by rhesus monkeys. *Percept. Psychophy.,* 1971, *10,* 271–272.

Wilson, M. Assimilation and contrast effects in visual discrimination by rhesus monkeys. *J. Exp. Psychol.,* 1972, *93,* 279–282.

Wilson, M., Rothblat, L., and Kirstein, E. Frequency and recency of reward and inferotemporal lesions. *Psychon. Sci.,* 1968a, *11,* 237–238.

Wilson, M., Wilson, W. A., Jr., and Sunenshine, H. S. Perception, learning and retention of visual stimuli by monkeys with inferotemporal lesions. *J. Comp. Physiol. Psychol.,* 1968b, *65,* 404–412.

Wilson, M., Kaufman, H. M., Zieler, R. E., and Lieb, J. P. Visual identification and memory in monkeys with inferotemporal lesions. *J. Comp. Physiol. Psychol.,* 1972, *78,* 173–183.

Wilson, M., Diamond, I. T., Ravizza, R. J., and Glendenning, K. K. A behavioral analysis of middle temporal and ventral temporal cortex in the bushbaby (*Galago senegalensis*). *Neurosci. Abstr.,* 1975, 73.

Woolsey, C. N. Comparative studies on cortical representation of vision. *Vision Res. Suppl.,* No. 3, 1971, 365–382.

Zeki, S. M. The secondary visual areas of the monkey. *Brain Res.,* 1969a, *13,* 197–226.

Zeki, S. M. Representation of central visual fields in prestriate cortex of monkey. *Brain Res.,* 1969b, *14,* 271–291.

Zeki, S. M. Interhemispheric connections of prestriate cortex of monkey. *Brain Res.,* 1970, *19,* 63–75.

Zeki, S. M. Convergent input from the striate cortex (area 17) to the cortex of the superior temporal sulcus in the rhesus monkey. *Brain Res.,* 1971a, *28,* 338–340.

Zeki, S M. Cortical projections from two prestriate areas in the monkey. *Brain Res.,* 1971b, *34,* 19–35.

Zeki, S. M. Colour coding in rhesus monkey prestriate cortex. *Brain Res.,* 1973, *53,* 422–427.

Zeki, S. M. Functional organization of a visual area in the posterior bank of the superior temporal sulcus of the rhesus monkey. *J. Physiol. (London),* 1974a, *236,* 549–573.

Zeki, S. M. Cells responding to changing image size and disparity in the cortex of the rhesus monkey. *J. Physiol. (London),* 1974b, *242,* 827–841.

Zeki, S. M. Colour coding in the superior temporal sulcus of rhesus monkey visual cortex. *Proc. R. Soc. London Ser. B.,* 1977, *197,* 195–223

8

Somatosensory System

C. Vierck

Introduction

The intent of this chapter is to describe research which provides correlations of neural events in the somatosensory system with their sensory accompaniments. The first part outlines the anatomical and physiological organization of the system at the early stages of processing (i.e., the periphery and spinal cord), because all subsequent coding operations of the CNS depend fundamentally on this information. The later sections of the chapter examine the system from a behavioral viewpoint; there, neural coding is discussed in relation to several sensory qualities that in the past have been studied as submodalities of somesthesis.

Receptors and Peripheral Fibers

Many of the earliest studies of somesthetic receptors used anatomical techniques in an attempt to reveal whether a given type of receptor was consistently present under skin areas (or spots) that when stimulated evoked a particular sensation (e.g., Weddell *et al.*, 1954). This method did not yield clear answers, and it has been replaced with a more open-ended physiological approach that is not so dependent on the hypothesis that all receptive fields consist of discrete spots or that the skin is a mosaic of mutually exclusive receptive fields, each with one and only one receptor. As will become apparent, modern techniques of recording from single peripheral nerve fibers have been successful in generating a number of fiber categories that express relatively unique sets of response properties, and

C. VIERCK   Department of Neuroscience, University of Florida College of Medicine, Gainesville, Florida 32601.

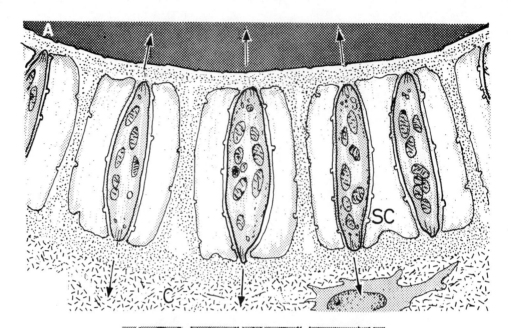

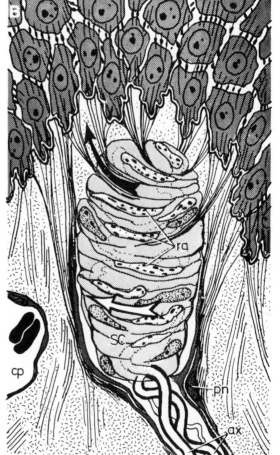

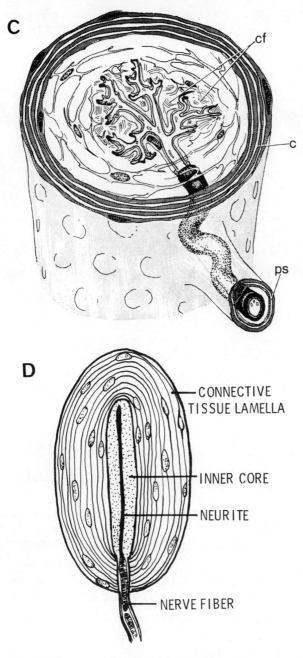

Fig. 1. A: Lanceolate guard and down hair receptors. The dark shaded area represents the hair shaft, and the arrows indicate the direction of effective mechanical stimuli. SC, Schwann cells; C, corium of hair follicle. B: A Meissner's corpuscle, showing tonofibrils of epithelial cells, some of which enter the corpuscle or are continuous with its endoneural sheath. The black arrow indicates movement of the receptor that could be produced via the tonofibrils. ra, Coiled receptor axon; pn, perineural sheath; ax, myelinated axons; cp, capillary. C: Cross section of a tubular Ruffini corpuscle containing a corpusle space between the capsule and the nerve terminal. cf, Collagen fibers of the inner core; c, capsule, formed from the perineural sheath, ps. (A, B, and C from Andres and von Düring (1973). D: A Pacinian corpuscle showing the neurite within a gelatinous inner core, which is surrounded by concentric lamellae.

many of these fiber categories can be linked to a specific receptor type (Iggo, 1974; Andres and Von Düring, 1973; Munger, 1971; Lynn, 1975; Burgess and Perl, 1973). A class of peripheral fibers that responds to a unique set of adequate stimuli, has distinctive physiological characteristics, and is (or is presumed to be) associated with a certain receptor specialization has been termed an "afferent unit" (Iggo, 1966b). In the discussion that follows, several of the more prevalent afferent units will be described.

Hair Receptors

Hair receptors are located in hair follicles and are exquisitely sensitive to the bending of the hair (see Fig. 1). Since they do not exhibit a maintained discharge with continued stimulation, they are also classified as transient detectors or even velocity detectors, because their rate of response is proportional to the velocity of hair distortion. Hair receptors and their afferent fibers can be subdivided into at least two main groups and several subgroups, each with distinctive morphological and physiological properties.

Guard Hairs. Guard hairs are the largest of the pelage hairs and are innervated by a longitudinally oriented pallisade of lanceolate endings within the follicles. The lanceolate endings are composed of nerve terminals that are sandwiched between Schwann cell processes and are oriented so that one edge of each protruding terminal faces the hair shaft. Four classes of guard hairs are supplied by large (A-alpha) myelinated fibers, and these have been designated T (tylotrich), G_1, intermediate, and G_2 (Burgess et al., 1968; Brown and Iggo, 1967; Merzenich and Harrington, 1969; Perl, 1968). The tylotrich endings are more abundant in rabbits than in cats, and they are not present in primates (Burgess and Perl, 1973; Straile, 1960). They are located adjacent to touch domes (see below). Among the more common guard receptors, the G_1 fibers produce the most transient response to hair bending, requiring a high-velocity stimulus, showing no preference for the direction of hair bending, and fatiguing rapidly to repeated stimulations. The G_2 fibers respond to lower velocities of stimulation, adapt more slowly with maintained hair deflection, show a slight preference for hair bending away from the rest position as opposed to release toward the rest position (linear directionality, Burgess and Perl, 1973), and may discharge more vigorously in one radial direction (spatial directionality, Burgess and Perl, 1973). The properties of intermediate fibers fall generally between those of G_1 and G_2 fibers. Each type of guard hair fiber can be excited by stimulation of a single hair in its receptive field, but the receptive fields involve more than one hair and can be large (up to 6 cm² in the cat, Iggo, 1974).

Down Hairs. Down hairs are thinner and shorter than guard hairs, and their follicles are supplied by a whorl of endings from small myelinated (A-delta) peripheral fibers. These D fibers are distinguished from G fibers by their responsivity to deflection of the down hairs, but the D hairs also respond to guard hair stimulation (Burgess et al., 1968; Brown and Iggo, 1967; Merzenich and Harrington, 1969; Perl, 1968). The D fibers show little linear or spatial directionality and supply a number of hairs in fairly large receptive fields; hence they do not provide precise information about the locus or direction of a stimulus. However, they have very low thresholds for excitation and are readily excited by movement of a stimulus (e.g., air) across the skin.

Touch Receptors

Touch receptors (see Figs. 1 and 2) are quite varied in their response properties, the morphology of their receptor specializations, and the spectrum of afferent fiber diameters supplying them. Although the response properties of a given receptor differ when located in hairy vs. glabrous skin because the receptivity of the ending is influenced by the characteristics of the surrounding tissue, these differences have not been identified in detail and will not be emphasized here. A large (and likely important) species difference must be taken into account, however. It is estimated that 75% of the tactile receptors in humans are slowly adapting, while the percentages appear to be nearly reversed in monkeys, with 80% rapidly adapting receptors (Knibestöl and Vallbo, 1970).

PACINIAN CORPUSCLES. Pacinian corpuscles are supplied by the largest myelinated fibers in cutaneous nerves, and they display a remarkable capability for detection of transient stimuli (Merzenich and Harrington, 1969; Hunt and McIntyre, 1960; Hunt, 1961, 1974; Lynn, 1969; Talbot et al., 1968). The Pacinian corpuscle is a distinct, laminated capsule that provides exquisite sensitivity for brief mechanical distortion of the outer lamellae and effectively filters out the effects of slow displacements. Thus the receptor responds at minimum threshold (is tuned) to sinusoidal stimulation in the range of 50–400 Hz, and at these frequencies the Pacinian fibers will follow the vibratory stimulus faithfully. The discharge of the fibers is limited to one or a few impulses per stimulus (fast adapting with no position response), and there is no linear directionality. Because the receptor can respond to indentations as small as 1 μm, the Pacinian corpuscle is sensitive to remote vibrations that are transmitted through the tissue (particularly by bone conduction). The most superficial Pacinian corpuscles are located deep in the subcutaneous tissue and are concentrated in the hands and feet. They are also distributed in a number of deep regions, including periosteum, connective tissue of the abdominal cavity, and near large blood vessels. Small, modified "Paciniform" corpuscles are found within muscles and joints.

FIELD RECEPTORS. Field receptors in hairy skin can be excited by hair stimulation, but they respond to direct indentation of the skin as well. They are supplied by large myelinated (A-alpha) fibers that are characterized as velocity detectors (as distinct from transient detectors such as Pacinian corpuscles or G_1 hair receptors). The morphology of the field receptors in hairy skin has not been determined, but there are at least two types of fibers (F_1 and F_2) that have response properties similar to and yet distinct from those of the intermediate and G_2 hair receptors (Burgess et al., 1968; Perl, 1968). As velocity detectors with intermediate adaptation rates and minimal (F_1) to intermediate (F_2) position responsivity and linear directionality, the field receptors have characteristics that are transitional between those of the transient detectors and those of the type I and type II position detectors (see below).

A

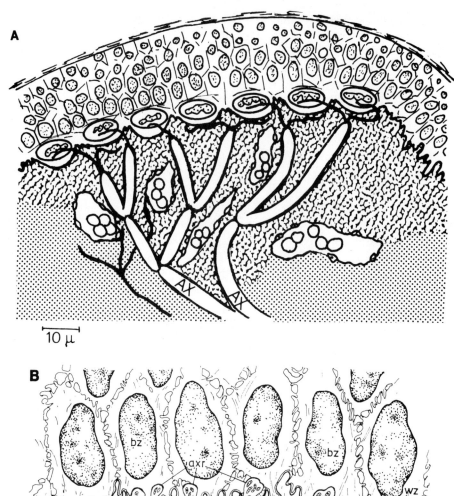

10 μ

B

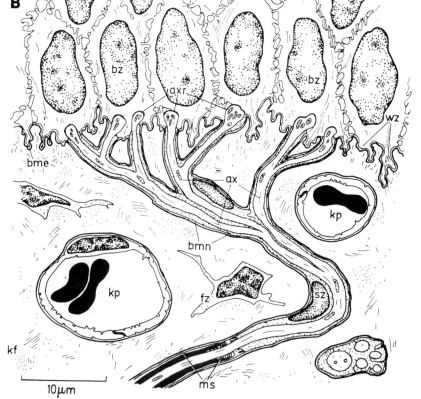

10μm

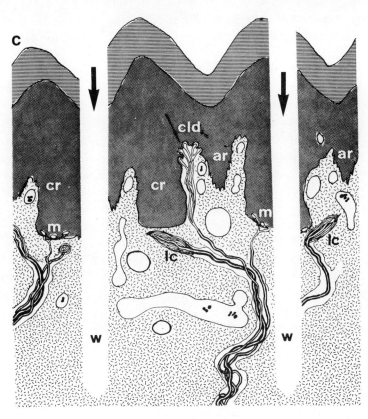

Fig. 2. A: A type I, slowly adapting touch corpuscle in hairy skin, showing the innervation of Merkel's disks within a dome of skin. From Iggo and Muir (1969). B: A cold receptor in hairy skin. ms, Myelin sheath; sz, Schwann cell; ax, axon; axr, receptive endings with mitochondria; bz, basal epidermal cells; bmn, basal membrane of nerve terminals: bme, basal membrane of epidermis. From Hensel (1973). C: Locations of cold receptors (cld) and Merkel cell–neurite complexes (m) in glabrous skin. The cold receptor is situated at the top of a dermal papilla, with its terminals penetrating into the basal epidermis. The Merkel cell–neurite complexes are located in the epithelium of columnar ridges (cr). w, Wire holes to locate cold receptor; le, lamellated Paciniform receptors. From Hensel *et al.* (1974).

MEISSNER'S CORPUSCLES. Meissner's corpuscles are plentiful in the glabrous skin of primates, and a similar form is present in the hairless skin of cats (Lynn, 1969; Cauna, 1962; Malinovsky, 1966; Jänig, 1971). The oval corpuscle is found in the papillary ridges and consists of flattened laminar cells that encompass many nerve endings. Large myelinated fibers (A-alpha) with field receptor properties innervate glabrous skin and are probably associated with Meissner's corpuscles, although some investigators refer to them only as "rapidly adapting glabrous units" (Talbot *et al.*, 1968; Jänig, 1971; Knibestöl and Vallbo, 1970; Lindblom, 1965; Hagbarth *et al.*, 1970).

MERKEL CELL–NEURITE COMPLEXES. Merkel cell–neurite complexes are receptor specializations that do not involve encapsulation of the nerve endings in the manner of Pacinian or Meissner's corpuscles. Myelinated A-alpha fibers divide into a number of terminal branches that have disk-shaped endings associated with specialized tactile cells within the basal layer of the epidermis (Cauna, 1962; Iggo and Muir, 1969; Munger, 1965). In hairy skin, the Merkel–neurite complexes are associated with domes or "touch spots," and in glabrous skin they are located at the tips of columnar epidermal ridges that have been termed "rete pegs." Merkel–neurite complexes are supplied by type I or slowly adapting fibers that display both velocity and position sensitivities (Iggo and Muir, 1969; Brown and Iggo, 1967; Perl, 1968; Knibestöl and Vallbo, 1970; Iggo, 1966b; Harrington and Merzenich, 1970; Tapper, 1964). When a tactile dome is directly compressed, the initial, dynamic discharge is proportional to the rate of stimulus movement; if contact is maintained, a static discharge rate develops which is proportional to the amount of pressure exerted on the skin over a long period of time. The receptive fields are small and punctate, including only a few domes on hairy skin. Linear directionality is prominent, with excitation only on compression of the receptors.

RUFFINI ENDINGS. Ruffini endings are complex, lamellated receptors that are thought to be situated in the dermis, beneath points on hairy and glabrous skin that are innervated by type II slowly adapting fibers (Burgess and Perl, 1973; Iggo, 1966b; Chambers et al., 1972). Type II units show both velocity and position responses, with accentuation of the latter, in comparison with type I fibers. Type II fibers are distinguished by their regular discharge rates and particularly by the fact that they are excited by stretch of the skin (often in one direction only—spatial directionality). In comparison, type I receptors do not respond at all to skin stretch, but require direct deformation of the skin overlying the receptor. Both type I and type II receptors respond to rapid cooling of the skin, and extreme heat or cold will suppress responsivity to tactile stimulation.

C MECHANORECEPTORS. C mechanoreceptors compose about half of the cutaneous unmyelinated afferent fibers from the hairy skin of cats (Conrad et al., 1974), but they are less abundant in monkeys (Burgess and Perl, 1973) and may be absent in man (Torebjörk and Hallin, 1974). The discovery that unmyelinated fibers respond to light mechanical indentation of the skin over small receptive fields is surprising in the context of classical notions that C fibers are given over to reception of noxious stimulation of large receptive fields (Heinbecker et al., 1933; Zotterman, 1939; Douglass and Ritchie, 1957; Iggo, 1960; Bessou et al., 1971). The C mechanoreceptors have been classified as velocity detectors, because they respond to slowly moving stimuli; they require at least 150 msec of skin contact, in contrast to only a few milliseconds for myelinated touch fibers. The C fibers fatigue readily to repeated stimulation of one portion of their receptive fields, without affecting responses from the remainder of the field. A prominent feature of the C mechanoreceptors is an afterdischarge that continues for several seconds after slow stroking of the skin. In addition to the "dynamic" response to slow velocities of stimulus movement, the C touch fibers exhibit a position response that adapts in 20–30 sec, as compared with time constants of many minutes for type I and type II fibers. Both the velocity and position responses are more pronounced with indentation than with release of a stimulus (linear directionality), but the afterdischarge is apparently symmetrical. The terminals of the unmyelinated cutaneous fibers are present in the superficial dermis and the epidermis. Although several functional groupings have been identified for the unmyelinated afferents (see below), no distinctive specializations of the endings or their surrounding tissues have been discerned.

TEMPERATURE RECEPTORS

Temperature receptors have been identified as clearly distinct from the touch fibers that respond to rapid temperature changes (type I, type II, and C mechanoreceptors) and from the thermal nociceptors (see below). The thermoreceptor fibers are more sensitive to temperature change, show a static discharge that is more reliably related to skin temperature, do not respond to mechanical distortion, and display threshold sensitivities that are comparable to human thresholds for thermal sensation (Hensel *et al.*, 1960; Iggo, 1959; Iggo and Young, 1975; Hensel, 1973; Sumino *et al.*, 1973).

COLD RECEPTORS. Cold receptors show a dynamic discharge in response to decreases in skin temperature when the initial skin temperature ranges from approximately 15°C to 40°C, and the frequency of the impulses is related to the rate of temperature change. Warming of the skin from the same range of initial temperatures produces a transient off-response unless the heat is extreme (approximately 53°C), producing a "paradoxical" response (Long, 1973). Regardless of whether the skin temperature is increased or decreased to a new level, if that level is maintained within a cold fiber's sensitivity range there is a static discharge rate that can be related to the imposed temperature. The sensitivity functions of individual fibers are in the form of an inverted U, with maxima between 20°C and 35°C. That is, a given discharge rate can be produced by skin temperatures on either side of the maximum (e.g., 18°C and 34°C). Recent evidence indicates that cold-fiber terminals end in a characteristic pattern in relation to basal epidermal cells of hairy skin (Hensel *et al.*, 1974). Cold fibers are both myelinated (A-delta) and unmyelinated (C).

WARM RECEPTORS. Warm receptors have not been characterized morphologically, but there are unmyelinated fibers that respond selectively to warming of the skin in the approximate range of 30–48°C. The dynamic discharge of warm fibers is opposite to that of cold fibers, as would be expected. Warming the skin produces a burst of impulses, and cooling decreases the rate of discharge. Warm receptors also discharge statically when skin temperature is maintained at levels from approximately 35°C to 48°C, and the activity peak occurs at 40–45°C. Temperatures above 42°C activate thermal nociceptors (see below).

NOCICEPTORS

Nociceptors are defined as high-threshold units that have sensitivity ranges for mechanical or thermal stimuli that begin near levels which damage the tissue. In addition, some of these fibers respond to chemical stimuli that have been shown to produce pain responses in human subjects. The substances that produce or potentiate pain reactions and have been suggested as possible "intermediaries" for the enduring pain that accompanies tissue damage are histamine (Rosenthal, 1968), potassium (Benjamin, 1968), bradykinin and other polypeptides (Hunt and McIntyre, 1960), acetylcholine (Keele and Armstrong, 1964), serotonin (Sicuteri *et al.*, 1974), acidity (Lindahl, 1974), and a substance P (Lewis, 1942). It is only recently that technique has permitted isolated recordings from small pain fibers, and the major attention has been directed to classification of responses of cutaneous receptors to mechanical and thermal stimuli (Hunt and McIntyre, 1960; Perl, 1968; Burgess and Perl, 1967; Iggo, 1959, 1960; Bessou and Perl, 1969; Iggo and Ogawa, 1971; Iniuchijima and Zotterman, 1960). The endings of pain fibers are unencapsulated and have been termed "free nerve endings," but some specializations must account for the different response properties that have been described.

MECHANICAL NOCICEPTORS. Mechanical nociceptors have been identified in both the A-delta and C fiber classes. Both types require high-intensity mechanical stimulation of the skin for excitation, are weakly stimulated or unaffected by thermal stimuli, and are unresponsive to chemical stimulation if the skin is not broken. The small myelinated fibers are velocity detectors, and most do not discharge statically with maintained stimulation (even puncture) of the skin. The receptive fields consist of a number of spots in hairy and glabrous skin that fatigue independently with repeated stimulation. The terminals of unmyelinated mechanical nociceptors appear to be located in subcutaneous fatty tissue, and they adapt more slowly to continued stimulation than do the myelinated fibers. They are best stimulated by skin puncture within uniform receptive fields (i.e., not containing discrete receptive spots).

MECHANICAL AND THERMAL NOCICEPTORS. Mechanical and thermal nociceptors supply the skin in several distinguishable forms: A-delta fibers that respond to intense mechanical stimulation and heat over 45°C; C fibers that respond selectively to strong mechanical and noxious cold stimulation; and a group of C fibers that have been termed "polymodal nociceptors." The polymodal nociceptors respond to noxious mechanical and heat stimulation, and they are excited by application of irritant chemicals (e.g., dilute acids) to the skin. The receptive fields consist of one small area. A characteristic feature is sensitization with repeated heat stimulation, so that successive thresholds are decreased and response magnitudes to replications of a given temperature are increased. Heat stimulation also sensitizes the fibers to subsequent mechanical stimulation. Sensitization does not appear to result from repeated mechanical stimulation, but a low-frequency background activity often follows a sequence of mechanical insults. The velocity response resembles that of low-threshold mechanical C fibers; the most effective stimuli are slow scratching, rubbing, and prodding with a sharp object. Adaptation to maintained stimulation occurs within several seconds.

DEEP PRESSURE-PAIN RECEPTORS. Deep pressure-pain receptors have not been characterized in detail but have been observed in muscles (Paintal, 1960). They are supplied primarily by A-delta and C fibers and are not associated with corpuscular endings. These "free nerve endings" are clearly distinct from muscle spindle receptors and do not respond vigorously to muscle stretch or twitch. They respond to compression or puncture of the muscle. The unmyelinated fibers appear also to be excited by muscle ischemia (Iggo, 1966*a*).

VISCERAL AFFERENTS. Many visceral afferents are unmyelinated and respond to manipulations of the viscera that can be associated with pain (Iggo, 1957). For example, some fibers are stimulated by either distention or contraction of the hollow viscera, and thus they are stretch or tension receptors. Other afferents have been excited by chemical stimulation such as lowering the pH of the stomach contents to 3.0 or less.

JOINT RECEPTORS

Joint receptors have been considered for some time to be the exclusive peripheral agents for position sense (the conscious appreciation of limb position with exclusion of visual cues, Rose and Mountcastle, 1959). Although this view seems entirely reasonable, recent studies have uncovered a number of problems associated with identification of the code(s) (see below). Also, there are suggestions that other somatic afferents may play a major role in the determination of limb position. Despite these difficulties in interpretation, it is clear that several distinctive receptor varieties are present in the vicinity of joints, and that each of these supplies different information concerning the movements and positions of the limbs (Andrew, 1954; Skoglund, 1956; Burgess and Clark, 1969*b*; Boyd and Roberts, 1953). Nearly all the information on joint receptors has been obtained from the knee joints of cats.

RUFFINI ENDINGS. Ruffini endings are "spray-type" terminals located in the connective tissue of joint capsules. Their large myelinated fibers exhibit a phasic discharge that is specific for a given direction of joint movement and is proportional to the speed of movement in the preferred direction. Movement in the opposite direction decreases a fiber's discharge rate below the normal spontaneous rate, and this attenuation is also sensitive to rate of movement. Within a limited range of end positions, the Ruffini endings provide a tonic level of discharge. Because tension of the muscles acting at a joint affects the capsule and these receptors, the Ruffini discharge is different with active vs. passive movement of a limb or with active movement under different conditions of resistance. Thus the information provided by these fibers appears to reflect the direction and speed of movement, the resistance to movement, and static limb position, when the joint is held within a certain portion of its movement field.

PACINIFORM ENDINGS. Paciniform endings are also present in joint capsules, and are supplied by large myelinated fibers. These endings are smaller, with fewer laminations, than the cutaneous Pacinian corpuscles. These receptors are rapidly adapting velocity detectors that respond to all movements at the relevant joint regardless of start position, or direction of movement. These movement detectors do not give a static discharge when the joint position is maintained.

GOLGI RECEPTORS. Golgi receptors are present in the ligaments and otherwise are not distinguishable from Golgi tendon organs. These spray-type endings are supplied by large myelinated fibers, and their response properties are similar to but distinguishable from those of the capsular Ruffini endings. The Golgi endings are phasically sensitive to the velocity and direction of movement but not to the degree seen in the Ruffini endings. The static position responses of Golgi endings are not influenced by muscle tension, and therefore they more accurately signal true limb position. The maximum discharge of Golgi endings commonly occurs at the extremes of flexion or extension. This pattern is termed a "single-ended code" for position, as compared with many of the Ruffini endings that discharge maximally at an intermediate position, with a double-ended decrement at positions in both directions from the "best" position.

Muscle and Tendon Receptors

Muscle and tendon receptors have been extensively studied with respect to their sensitivities, spinal reflex actions, and CNS connections (Granit, 1970; Mathews, 1972), but little attention can be directed to the detailed literature in this brief overview.

Muscle Spindle Receptors. Muscle spindle receptors are located on intrafusal muscle fibers within spindle organs that are situated in parallel with extrafusal muscle fibers. This arrangement causes the spindle endings to be excited by stretch of the muscle, and contraction of the extrafusal fibers decreases the spindle discharge. Recently, it has been shown that there are two kinds of intrafusal muscle fibers, usually called "nuclear bag" and "nuclear chain" fibers. Also, there is evidence that each type of fiber can be independently excited by separate classes of small (gamma) motoneurons. When the intrafusal fibers contract, the associated spindle endings discharge. Thus the spindle receptor activity is dictated by a combination of gamma motoneuron input to the intrafusal fibers and large alpha motoneuron input to the extrafusal fibers of the same muscle and/or its antagonist.

The primary or annulospiral receptors of muscle spindles end on the central or polar region of both nuclear bag and nuclear chain intrafusal fibers. Also, there are secondary or flower-spray receptors that end off-center, predominantly on the nuclear chain fibers. Although both kinds of fibers are within the A-alpha range, the primary fibers are distinctive as the largest myelinated fibers (designated group Ia). The secondary fiber diameters are within the range of large cutaneous afferents (A-alpha group II). The primary endings are more sensitive to the velocity of phasic muscle stretch, but primary and secondary endings display similar tonic position responses. Because of their greater dynamic sensitivity, the primary endings are more responsive to brief tendon taps, and they are more easily driven by vibration of the muscle.

Golgi Tendon Organs. Golgi tendon organs are said to be situated in series with the muscle, because either passive stretch or active contraction of the muscle will exert tension on the tendon. In fact, passive stretch of a muscle excites tendon receptors only when extreme, while active contraction is a potent activator of these spray-type receptors at the musculotendinous junction.

The preceding outline of peripheral somatosensory receptor properties depicts an unexpected variety of potential codes for discrimination of the nature of stimuli that impinge on the body surface or result from activity of the organism. On the one hand, the precision or "purity" of the peripheral inputs appears remarkable in that each major category (hair, touch, temperature, pain, joint, and muscle) contains distinctive component populations of fibers. On the other hand, when the response properties of each of these components are analyzed, it is apparent that there is a good deal of confounding of information concerning different aspects of an adequate stimulus for each fiber. For example, many peripheral fibers combine velocity sensitivity with position responses, so that accurate interpretation of the latter will not occur until the former is fully adapted, and this can be a matter of seconds. Furthermore, it seems strange that these functions would be combined in several component populations that are differentiated by the presence of other response characteristics (e.g., type I and II touch fibers, Ruffini and Golgi joint afferents). This apparent confounding of potential codes provides a distinct challenge to the neurobiologist who wishes to match the behavior of the organism with the biology of the system. One of the major avenues of solution to the problem must be to chart the fate of these potential codes from the periphery as they ascend the central nervous system. It is inevitable that the physiological properties of the system components will change with repeated divergence and convergence of the units within and between a number of central relays. As this analysis progresses, it becomes increasingly apparent that peripheral input characteristics are combined and altered repeatedly, so that the degrees of freedom of the system are expanded considerably; and there is also a sorting process that provides intriguing opportunities for revealing the functions of certain groupings of response properties. For example, at the spinal cord level, the ascending somatosensory pathways are divided cleanly into separate channels that are independently dissectable and possess fiber populations with different spectra of physiological properties (see Fig. 3).

DORSAL COLUMN SYSTEM

The dorsal column system of the spinal cord was viewed for some time as a straight-through pathway for all of the large primary afferents necessary for so-called discriminative somesthesis. Recent anatomical, physiological, and behavioral studies have combined to reveal important exceptions and contradictions to this view: (1) Only a small percentage (25%) of the primary afferents that enter the dorsal columns from lower segmental levels remain there at cervical levels (Whitsel et al., 1967b; Petit and Burgess, 1968). (2) Some fibers relay into the dorsal columns from the dorsal horn (Angaut-Petit, 1975; Uddenberg, 1968). (3) Cells contributing ascending fibers to the lateral columns receive major inputs from large peripheral afferents that should support fine tactile and proprioceptive discriminations (Willis *et al.*, 1974, 1975; Brown and Franz, 1969; Bryan *et al.*, 1974). (4) In fact, a number of somatosensory discriminations have been shown to be intact after interruption of the dorsal columns (Vierck, 1966, 1974, 1975; Norrsell, 1966; DeVito *et al.*, 1964; Diamond *et al.*, 1964; Mettler and Liss, 1959; Reynolds *et al.*, 1972; Schwartzman and Bogdonoff, 1968, 1969).

Most of the physiological studies defining the response properties of primary afferent fibers that ascend directly to the dorsal column nuclei have described the projection from hindlimbs (Burgess and Clark, 1969*b*; Brown, 1968; Petit and Burgess, 1968; Whitsel *et al.*, 1969*a*). In primates, all the long projection fibers without a spinal synapse are in the A-alpha range of conduction velocities and are fast adapting. Thus guard hairs, Pacinian afferents, field receptors, and Paciniform joint fibers are represented, while down hairs, types I and II slowly adapting receptors, C mechanoreceptors, thermoreceptors, nociceptors, deep pressure-pain receptors, visceral afferents, Ruffini and Golgi joint afferents, spindle recep-

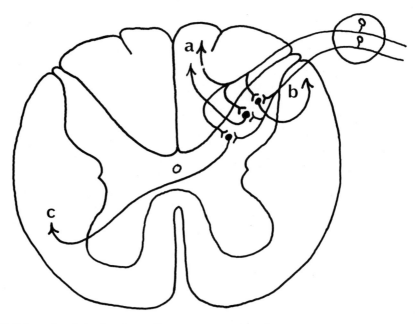

Fig. 3. Schematic of the long ascending somatosensory pathways considered in this chapter. a, Collaterals of large dorsal root afferents and secondary fibers from the dorsal horn contribute to the dorsal columns. b, Dorsal horn cells send axons into the ipsilateral dorsolateral column as two ascending pathways: the spinocervicothalamic tract and the aberrant dorsal column tract. Fibers of the dorsal columns and the aberrant dorsal column tract synapse in the dorsal column nuclei (gracilis and cuneatus) in the lower medulla. Projection cells of the dorsal column nuclei cross the midline in the medulla and ascend (as the medial lemniscus) to synapse in the thalamus (primarily nucleus ventralis posterolateralis). Fibers of the spinocervicothalamic tract synapse in the lateral cervical nucleus, which is situated at the dorsolateral edge of the dorsal horn at levels C1–C3. Axons of projection cells from the lateral cervical nucleus cross in the upper cervical cord and ascend to join the medial lemniscus in the medulla. c, Some dorsal horn cells send axons across the spinal cord to ascend in the contralateral anterolateral column. Some of these fibers ascend all the way to the thalamus as the spinothalamic tract, while other spinoreticular fibers terminate in the brain stem reticular formation.

tors, and Golgi tendon organs are excluded. The situation is slightly different in the cat, with primary fiber projections from type II tactile units and slowly adapting mechanoreceptors at the base of the claws. Group I muscle afferents from the cat's forelimbs ascend the cervical dorsal columns directly to the external cuneate nuclei.

Although the qualitative features of the primary dorsal column afferents are preserved in large part through their bulbar relay, some convergent features have been seen among cells of the dorsal column nuclei. Receptive fields become larger than those of primary afferents (Norton and Kruger, 1973), but many remain small compared to the other spinal pathways. In experiments using chloralose anesthesia in cats, wide-field neurons have been seen that respond to contralateral as well as ipsilateral input (Blum and Whitehorn, 1973). Convergences between receptor types have also been noted. For example, some nuclear cells respond to stimulation of hairs and to light, moving touch of the skin (Angaut-Petit, 1975); other cells can be driven by either cutaneous or proprioceptive stimulation (Kostyuk and Skibo, 1969; Rosen, 1967); and there is even a class of polymodal cells that increase their discharge rate with noxious stimulation (Angaut-Petit, 1975) (see below). At present, it is difficult to interpret the functions of these "atypical" dorsal column cells—in part, because it is likely that many of them are interneurons that do not project directly with the medial lemniscus to the somatosensory thalamus and cortex. Presence of a cell in the central nest region of the nuclei is somewhat predictive that the unit projects to the thalamus in cat (Gordon and Horrobin, 1967) but not in monkeys (Albe-Fessard *et al.*, 1975). The central nest region of cats contains a large portion of the modality-pure neurons with small receptive fields (Gordon and Seed, 1961).

Recent studies have shown that a significant proportion (10%) of the fibers in fasciculi gracilis and cuneatus have their cells of origin in the dorsal horn rather than in the dorsal root ganglion (Uddenberg, 1968; Angaut-Petit, 1975; Rustioni, 1973, 1974). Approximately 20% of these postsynaptic fibers (DCPS) respond to stimulation of hairs and are similar to primary DC fibers. The majority of the relayed DC fibers are distinct from primary afferents in that they are sensitive to noxious stimulation. A few DCPS fibers respond selectively to painful stimuli, but most are polymodal—i.e., they are activated by hair bending and maintained skin contact, and noxious pinch produces the highest and most regular discharge rate. In addition, these units respond to both cold and noxious heat. Since the polymodal fibers do not project to the cell nest region of the feline dorsal column nuclei, which contains cells that project to the thalamus, it has been suggested that DCPS cells exert a modulating influence on DC-lemniscal transmission (Angaut-Petit, 1975).

SPINOCERVICOTHALAMIC TRACT

The functional significance of the ascending dorsolateral tracts of the spinal cord has been a subject of considerable debate since discovery of the spinocervicothalamic tract (SCTT) in the 1950s (Morin, 1955). Although this pathway is prominent and has been studied extensively in cats (Brown, 1971, 1973; Brown and Franz, 1969; Boivie, 1970; Horrobin, 1966), its existence has been questioned for primates, particularly man. However, the lateral cervical nucleus is present in monkeys and man (Truex *et al.*, 1970), and its connections have begun to be described anatomically and physiologically in monkeys (Ha, 1971; Bryan *et al.*, 1974). Still, there is physiological evidence that the "importance" of this tract may be greater in cats than in primates (e.g., Morin, 1955). Although behavioral studies have indicated that the dorsolateral tracts of monkeys contribute information that is utilized for a variety of somesthetic discriminations, these studies do not implicate the spinocervicothalamic tract as distinct from other sensory fibers in the ipsilateral dorsolateral column (Levitt and Schwartzman, 1966; Vierck, 1966, 1973*a,b*) (see below).

Cells of origin of the spinocervicothalamic tract have been identified by extracellular recording of cells in the dorsal horn that are (1) backfired by dorsolateral tract stimulation below the level of the lateral cervical nucleus (C1–C3) and (2) not backfired by similar stimulation at C1. These cells are characterized by distinct patterns of convergence from different categories of primary afferent fibers. In the cat, four types of cells have been distinguished on this basis (Brown, 1973). Types I, II, and III receive prominent inputs from the major classes of hair receptors plus different combinations of heat, cold, joint, muscle, and high-threshold mechanical receptors, while type IV receives only the high-threshold inputs. The high dynamic range of these neurons suggests that coding of stimulus attributes is conveyed primarily by the discharge patterns of SCTT cells. The somatotopic organization of the SCTT apparently is not precise, as it is for the dorsal columns, suggesting that spatial coding is not well developed within the SCTT. Also, different forms of natural stimulation evoke distinguishable patterns of discharge in individual SCTT neurons. The spinocervicothalamic tract resembles the dorsal columns in the reception of fast-adapting hair input and in the lack of representation of slowly adapting touch afferents. Unlike the dorsal columns, the SCTT receives little or no input from low-threshold touch or joint afferents, and the distal extremities are poorly represented. Conversely, although both pathways contain a large number of hair afferents, only the SCTT conveys input from the exquisitely sensitive down hairs. The DC and SCTT pathways also are distinctive with regard to inhibitory influences that play upon them (see below).

Recent investigations of the projection pattern of primary afferents that ascend the dorsal columns have shown that a large number of them leave the DC to synapse in the dorsal horn (Burgess and Clark, 1969*b*; Petit and Burgess, 1968; Whitsel *et al.*, 1969*a*). Some portion of the secondary neurons then send axons into the ipsilateral dorsolateral column, and these fibers appear to synapse within the DC nuclei (Dart and Gordon, 1973). Because this pathway begins and ends with the dorsal column system but ascends the cord in the DL columns, it will be referred to as the "aberrant DC system." The physiological properties of this system have not been elucidated in detail, but a large proportion of the cells in cats respond to low-threshold cutaneous stimulation (usually hair, Dart and Gordon,

1973). Since type I and II slowly adapting touch receptors and Ruffini and Golgi joint afferents are not represented by fibers of the spinocervicothalamic tract or the direct component of the dorsal column system (Whitsel *et al.,* 1969*a*; Petit and Burgess, 1968; Brown and Franz, 1969; Angaut-Petit, 1975), it will be interesting to see if slowly adapting afferents relay through the aberrant DC system. Type I slowly adapting input is conducted rostrally via postsynaptic DC fibers (Angaut-Petit, 1975), but this input converges onto polymodal cells that may not project directly onto DC–lemniscal relay cells. A spinal route for type II input has not been established, but slowly adapting touch-pressure cells have been observed in the dorsal column nuclei (Brown *et al.,* 1970; Perl *et al.,* 1962; Yamamoto and Miyajima, 1961; Kruger *et al.,* 1961). The importance of type II receptors for cutaneous pressure sensation has been emphasized (Harrington and Merzenich, 1970).

SPINOTHALAMIC TRACTS

The classical view of the crossed anterolateral or spinothalamic tracts is that they are the exclusive spinal routes for pain and temperature senses and that they convey minimal tactile and proprioceptive information. This reputation has arisen primarily from clinical experience that anterolateral chordotomy in humans produces profound losses of pain and temperature sensation, with little impairment of touch or proprioception. However, it is now apparent that thermal and mechanical nociceptors project on SCT and relayed DC cells. Although the functional significance of these connections has not been determined, it is well known that pain sensitivity eventually returns following chordotomy (White and Sweet, 1969). Furthermore, the input to spinothalamic cells from touch fibers is considerable, and some tactile discriminations are not affected (Vierck, 1977, 1974) or deteriorate only partially (Levitt and Schwartzman, 1966; Vierck, 1977) following section of the ipsilateral spinal tracts.

Several anterior spinal pathways can be implicated as participants in the direct rostral conduction of somatosensory input to the brain stem and diencephalon (e.g., Mehler, 1966; Mehler *et al.,* 1960; Boivie, 1971; Kerr, 1975; Kerr and Lippman, 1974; Lundberg and Oscarsson, 1962): (1) the lateral spinothalamic or neospinothalamic tract, (2) the spinoreticular or paleospinothalamic tract, (3) the ventral spinothalamic tract, and (4) the contralateral ventral flexor reflex tract. The present discussion will focus on recent descriptions of spinal cord cells that can be backfired by contralateral stimulation in the caudal diencephalon of primates (Willis, 1975; Albe-Fessard *et al.,* 1974; Applebaum *et al.,* 1975). These cells will be referred to simply as "spinothalamic tract cells," in the absence of functional distinctions between separate crossed anterolateral pathways. It is important to recognize that the spinothalamic tract is better developed in primates than in cats (Morin, 1955; Andersson *et al.,* 1975; Mehler, 1957).

Spinothalamic tract cells of the monkey uniformly show convergent responses from noxious mechanical and thermal input, in keeping with their presumed role in pain conduction. Additional convergent inputs are more selective, and four groups of cells have been discerned, based on receptivities to nonnoxious mechanical or proprioceptive stimulation: (1) Displacement and release of down hairs or guard hairs produces rapidly adapting on- and off-responses of spinothalamic hair units. (2) Gentle mechanical stimulation produces a rapidly adapting response, while sustained, *firm* pressure elicits a tonic discharge from low-threshold touch units. (3) Another group of high-threshold touch units exhibits the slowly adapting response to substantial skin pressure, but a low-threshold, phasic component is not seen. (4) Slowly adapting deep units are sensitive to manipulations of muscles or joints.

There are several other types of input which have been shown to converge on a portion of the spinothalamic cells without a discernable preference for any of the above groups. Nonnoxious thermal stimulation has been shown to evoke activity in some of the hair, low-threshold, and high-threshold touch cells, but no units respond exclusively to thermal stimuli (Martin *et al.*, 1975). It is of course possible that more "pure" temperature information projects directly to regions other than the ventrobasal thalamus, and this presumed projection pattern could be related to the dual role of temperature input for sensation and for body temperature regulation. High-threshold visceral afferents have also been shown to project onto both low- and high-threshold mechanoreceptive spinothalamic projection cells (Hancock *et al.*, 1975; Selzer and Spencer, 1969; Fields *et al.*, 1970). This finding supports the notion that referred pain can be explained by convergence of visceral pain onto cells with a somatic local sign (Ruch, 1961). The categories of peripheral afferents that appear not to project onto spinothalamic units are Pacinian corpuscles, type I and II slowly adapting receptors, and possibly C mechanoreceptors.

The spinothalamic tract is somatotopically organized, and the individual units have well-defined but large receptive fields, ranging from an average of 18 cm² for high-threshold cells to around 40 cm² for low-threshold touch and hair cells. Superficially, these values suggest that the spinothalamic tract can support reasonably good localization of painful stimuli but less accurate localization of light skin contact. It is not clear, however, that small receptive fields are necessarily optimal for tactile localization (to be elaborated on later).

Inhibitory Influences

Before attempting to interpret the bewildering complexity of input sorting among the long somatosensory pathways, it is necessary to complicate the picture with a cursory examination of the nature of afferent and descending inhibitory influences on them. This is particularly apparent for the spinocervicothalamic tract, which is subject to a powerful and curious modality masking by descending influences. In the preceding account of physiological categories for SCTT fibers, the profiles of convergence onto groups I–IV were not detailed, because they differ dramatically in the decerebrate and spinal states (Brown, 1971, 1973). In the presence of descending inhibition (decerebrate cats), SCTT group I units respond only to tylotrich hair stimulation, group II only to guard hair stimulation, group III to all types of hair input, and group IV units are unresponsive. With the inhibition removed (spinal cats), high-threshold input is added to all groups so that (with a few "minor" exceptions) groups I–III look alike and respond to all types of hair stimulation, extreme heat and cold, high-threshold touch, muscle and joint input, and mechanoreceptive C fiber activation. Group IV cells respond to touch, temperature, and joint and muscle influences but not to manipulation of hair receptors. In addition to this imposition of receptor selectivity by inhibition from above, the SCTT is subject to afferent, spatial inhibition such that stimulation of large contralateral or ipsilateral body areas can attenuate the responsivity of SCTT cells of all types (groups I–IV).

Some spinothalamic tract cells are subject to similar afferent inhibitory influences from contralateral or bilateral stimulation of the skin or hair (Willis *et al.,* 1974), and the effect is exerted in part on cells that respond only to noxious stimuli. Conversely, activation of descending inhibition by stimulation of the somatosensory or primary motor cortex selectively depresses the responsivity of low-threshold spinothalamic units (Coultier *et al.,* 1974). Thus it appears that afferent and descending inhibitory influences exert complementary effects on spinothalamic conduction.

Lemniscal projection cells of the dorsal column nuclei maintain the qualitative purity of inputs from the long collaterals of primary afferents. Thus inhibitory influences cannot switch modality for a given lemniscal neuron. However, there is evidence from cats that stimulation of the somatosensory cortex inhibits lemniscal conduction of hair units but not touch or pressure cells (Towe, 1973). Thus modality switching appears to operate over the population of lemniscal cells in cats. This is not apparent for monkeys, in which small numbers of both hair and touch units are inhibited (Towe, 1973). A more distinctive inhibitory feature within the dorsal column–lemniscal system has previously been described as a spatial, surround inhibition (Gordon and Jukes, 1964; Gordon and Manson, 1967; Poggio and Mountcastle, 1963). Although it is generally assumed that this afferent inhibition increases spatial resolution (von Békésy, 1967), the functional significance of an inhibitory surround has been questioned because it has been demonstrated for only a small percentage of lemniscal units in some experiments (e.g., 5% in awake monkeys, Whitsel *et al.,* 1973). However, Laskin (1969) has clarified the situation considerably by showing that the inhibitory field is not limited to the borders of the excitatory field. Using a conditioning-test paradigm, he showed that the test responses of nearly all cortical SI units studied were diminished when the conditioning stimulus occurred up to 70 msec before the test stimulus. The suppression was maximal when the conditioning stimulus was strong and when it was applied near the *center* of the excitatory receptive field of the unit. The magnitude of the inhibition decreased as the conditioning stimulus moved away from the receptive field center, and only occasionally did the inhibitory field extend beyond the confines of the excitatory field (giving the appearance of surround inhibition). Apparently, the inhibitory fields of dorsal column nuclear cells are often larger than the excitatory fields, giving a high yield of apparent surround inhibition, but the relative field sizes change with successive synapses until they are quite similar at the SI cortex. Thus temporal as well as spatial effects of afferent inhibition in the dorsal column–lemniscal system must be considered.

Stimuli that are applied within the receptive field of a cell in this system will produce an excitation that is followed by a period of diminished responsivity for successive stimulation. To complete the present picture of inhibitory influences, it must be mentioned that the output of the cuneate nucleus can be decreased by stimulation of vagoaortic afferent fibers (Gahery and Vigier, 1974), and even visual or auditory stimulation can depress cuneate conduction in chloralose-anesthetized animals (Jabbur and Atweh, 1975).

AFFERENT INTERACTIONS

Throughout the history of somatosensory research, vigorous debate has centered on the degree to which somesthetic qualities are determined by selective activity from identifiable forms of peripheral receptors. The classical argument is exemplified by the positions of von Frey and of Weddell *et al.* (1954), who have promoted an "either/or" approach to the question of somatosensory coding. That is, there has been an attempt to settle on one principle of coding such that somesthetic qualities are specified either by activity *per se* from independent populations of receptors or by different patterns of activity that originate from one or a few receptor varieties. The preceding account of afferent units with complex adequate stimuli and complicated discharge properties that are variously sorted at the first stage of processing in the central nervous system brings several points to bear on this oversimplistic dichotomy of specificity vs. patterning: (1) Since nearly any form of stimulation of the body surface excites a large number of complex receptor categories, it is risky to attempt to match a given receptor or discharge pattern with a category of somatic sensation. (2) When consideration is given to the numerous discriminative somatosensory capacities that have been revealed by psychophysical investigations (e.g., see Lindahl, 1974; Gibson, 1962; Weinstein, 1968; Burgess, 1974), it becomes exceedingly difficult to define elemental somesthetic qualities to be linked with peripheral entities. (3) It is reasonable to expect that all available mechanisms of information transfer are utilized by the somesthetic systems, and it is now apparent that spatial and temporal representations of peripheral events repeatedly interact within the nervous system.

In some cases, an apparent sensory code changes with conduction through the nervous system, with little obvious alteration of information. This may increase the efficiency of information transfer (see section on position sense) or it may occur when the initial code cannot be maintained through successive synapses (see vibration). In circumstances of stimulus interaction, there may be modification of some parametric value of a code (and its associated sensory attribute) without a change in the fundamental quality of the sensation. This type of interaction has been termed "nonsynthetic" (Burgess, 1974) and often involves additive or subtractive changes in intensity. Also, there are synthetic interactions that produce emergent sensory experiences that cannot be related directly to the elemental afferent units. Some examples of the latter might be itch, tickle, heaviness, wetness, and texture.

Predictions and cautions that each spinal pathway cannot be considered alone but must be investigated as part of an integrated functional system (Melzack and Wall, 1962) have been abundantly reaffirmed. For example: (1) Stimulation of the dorsal columns or dorsal column nuclei has been shown to inhibit transmission along the spinocervical tract (Brown and Martin, 1972) and to affect pain conduction that is accomplished in large part through the anterolateral columns (White and Sweet, 1969; Sheally, 1974). (2) After a dorsal column lesion creates a void of "lemniscal" neurons within areas 3b and 1 of the postcentral gyrus (Dreyer *et al.,* 1974), a subsequent lesion of the contralateral anterolateral column releases the cells from some masking influence, so that 96% of them display lemniscal properties (Levitt and Levitt, 1974*a,b*). These and other related findings remind us that any effect that is observed to follow ablation of part of the somatosensory system must be considered in terms of the capabilities of a residual system that is likely to be disrupted. This situation leads to the prediction that such a system of interdependent conduction channels should be extremely susceptible to loss of any of its components. Indeed, some unexpected deficits have been observed to follow restricted lesions of the spinal cord (e.g., Vierck *et al.,* 1971; Kruger and Mosso, 1974), but much more common and impressive is the finding that expected deficits do not occur at all or do not endure after lesion of a single cord sector (i.e., ipsilateral dorsal column, ipsilateral dorsolateral column, or contralateral anterolateral column) (Levitt and Schwartzman, 1966; Vierck, 1966, 1973*a,b*, 1974, 1975; Norrsell, 1966; DeVito *et al.,* 1964; Diamond *et al.,* 1964; Dobry and Casey, 1972*a*; Mettler and Liss, 1959; Liu *et al.,* 1975; Reynolds *et al.,* 1972; Schwartzman and Bogdonoff, 1968, 1969; Kitai and Weinberg, 1968; Schwartz *et al.,* 1972). Also, several of these investigations have shown that transection of two pathways produces significant alterations of sensory capacity that are not seen with lesions isolated to one of the cord sectors (Levitt and Schwartzman, 1966; Vierck, 1966, 1973*a*; DeVito *et al.,* 1964; Liu *et al.,* 1975; Kitai and Weinberg, 1968; Tapper, 1970; Norrsell, 1966; Sjoqvist and Weinstein, 1942). It is apparent, then, that there is a great deal of redundancy of elemental information transfer by the different spinal pathways, and if each tract has unique functions these will most often be revealed as specialized transformations or interactions of the same or similar inputs that are utilized for different means by other pathways. Certainly the neat functional dichotomy of epicritic and protopathic pathways (i.e., a discriminative dorsal column–lemniscal system vs. a crudely organized spinothalamic system, respectively) has lost the experimental foundation that once seemed powerful (Head, 1920; Mountcastle, 1961).

Because extensive progress has not been made in cleanly differentiating the functional somatosensory categories that are meaningful to the nervous system, the remaining sections will review research that has focused on principles of coding that apply to certain arbitrary and general sensory qualities. The complex projections of the somatosensory system from the spinal cord to the brain stem and thalamus will largely be ignored in favor of concentrating on the spinal cord and cerebral cortex. It is at these extremes of the neuraxis that our present knowledge is best developed.

Receptive field size has been thought for some time to be the most fundamental determinant of spatiotactile localization and discrimination. This concept is based in large part on the fact that the distal extremities and the tongue of most animals are supplied by numerous peripheral units with small excitatory fields, and low thresholds for tactile resolution have been obtained from these regions (Weinstein, 1968). The most popular method for clinical and experimental testing of tactile resolution has been the two-point or compass test, which has been viewed as a definitive indicator of the integrity of the dorsal column–medial lemniscal system. Receptive fields of lemniscal projection cells in the dorsal column nuclei are smaller than those of either the spinocervicothalamic tract or the spinothalamic tract (Gordon, 1973), giving support to this classical view. Hence it is unsettling to discover that precise surgical lesions of the dorsal columns do not elevate two-point thresholds in monkeys (Levitt and Schwartzman, 1966) or man (Cook and Browder, 1965). Apparently, the clinical usefulness of the test is in detecting involvement of the ipsilateral dorsal *and* dorsolateral columns, as indicated by the finding that lesions of the dorsal quadrant of the monkey cord produce deficits that are not seen with isolated interruption of either the dorsal or the dorsolateral columns (Levitt and Schwartzman, 1966). However, even the spinothalamic tract cannot be neglected as a significant contributor to spatiotactile resolution, since it has been shown recently that surgical section of the contralateral anterolateral column (chordotomy) in humans can lead to elevation of the two-point threshold (Kruger and Mosso, 1974). These studies point out the need to reevaluate the role of receptive field size *per se* in spatial coding. This topic has been analyzed cogently by Erickson (1968), who concludes that broadly tuned neurons (in this case, having large receptive fields) can perform some localizing functions as effectively as narrowly tuned neurons (Vierck and Jones, 1969). This works out because there is a tradeoff between field size and amount of overlap of the receptive fields of the neuron population "representing" a skin area. Thus small receptive fields would be a disadvantage in many respects for spatial resolution if they were not dense enough to overlap extensively. Accordingly, the small fields supplying the distal extremities come at the price of high innervation density, as reflected by the area of somatosensory cortex that is given over to the distal extremities, in approximate proportion to innervation density (rather than skin area).

At this point, in order to appreciate spatial coding mechanisms of the somatosensory system, it is important to consider the cortical representation of tactile space, because it represents the furthest development of somatotopy—another feature that has been thought to be critical to spatial discrimination. Classically, the dorsal column–medial lemniscal relay through thalamic nucleus VPL has been considered the primary source of input to the primary somatosensory area (SI), and the SI cortical area appears to display the finest-grained somatotopic organization of the cortical somesthetic areas. Several single-unit recording studies have sought to confirm the importance of the dorsal column projection to SI but have revealed only subtle changes in the "map" following dorsal column lesions in either cats or monkeys (Eidelberg and Woodbury, 1972; Eidelberg *et al.*, 1975; Levitt and Levitt, 1968; Dobry and Casey, 1972*b*).

On the other hand, when attention is carefully directed toward cytoarchitectural areas within SI (areas 3 b, 2, or 1) and the mediolateral position of the electrode within the postcentral cortex, Dreyer *et al.* (1974) have shown that some portions of the SI map are dramatically altered by dorsal column section. In addition to a general reduction in units responding to cutaneous tactile stimulation (as opposed to stimulation of "deep" muscle, joint, and other receptors), the percentage of "lemniscal" units is greatly reduced in the central core of the somatosensory strip (area 3b and the anterior portion of area 1). This loss of lemniscal representation is, in addition, more widespread in the regions of SI that receive input from the distal extremities, where all cytoarchitectural zones are affected. The "nonlemniscal" neurons encountered in this preparation are often unresponsive to mechanical stimulation of the skin, will not respond to repeated stimulations, or are responsive to stimulation over unusually large areas of skin. This study represents a satisfying confirmation of the classical notion of dorsal column input to SI cortex, but it increases puzzlement over the lack of a two-point tactile deficit following dorsal column lesions. We are confronted with normal performance despite a major reduction in innervation density by elimination of large numbers of fast-conducting, small-field afferents and a severe disruption of the primary somatotopic map.

One view of the role of somatotopy in spatiotactile discrimination is exemplified by von Békésy's (1967) geometrical neural unit theory. A basic assumption of the theory is that spatial attributes of somatosensory stimuli can be given by the profile of activity that exists across the population of neurons in a somatotopic map (e.g., SI cortex). In the case of two-point stimulation, each point stimulus would elicit activity in an approximately disk-shaped area of the SI cortex, with maximum discharge rates for neurons near the center of the disk area (and possibly a surrounding ring of inhibited cells). If it is possible for the organism to scan over the "map" and "perceive" these activity profiles, then separation of the two points could be given by some minimal separation of the areas of activity. This is an appealing logic that nicely "explains" tactile perception of stimulus location and handles certain interactive phenomena, such as funneling (Gardner and Spencer, 1972) and masking (Laskin, 1975).

If direct mapping functions do support sensory discrimination, it is likely that they do so on a limited basis, and a variety of other mechanisms underlying somesthetic perception must be sought. This becomes more and more evident as complexities of somesthetic cortical topography are revealed by anatomical and physiological studies. Within the SI map, there are differences in the distribution of superficial and deep receptor categories that correlate roughly with cytoarchitectural zones (Paul *et al.*, 1972; Powell and Mountcastle, 1959; Dreyer *et al.*, 1974). The density of touch units decreases gradually from area 3b (approximately 90%) to area 2 (approximately 20% distal extremity and 60% proximal extremity). There are gross geometrical distortions of the map that reflect innervation density, and the dorsal column–lemniscal system predominantly supplies the core zone (primarily areas 3b and 1), while the dorsolateral tracts supply the fringes (areas 3a and 2). Also, the "map" is organized to preserve point-to-point connections along the dermatomal innervation pattern, but this results in each point on the body surface being "represented" or localized within several disjoint areas on the SI cortex (Werner and Whitsel, 1968; Paul *et al.*, 1972). Thus a map-scanning process within SI would apparently encounter multiple peaks of activity in response to a single-point stimulus on the skin. It seems likely, then, that the cortical activity profiles from two-point stimulation could be confused with the redundant profiles from a single stimulus. The question of the functional signifi-cance of somatosensory cortical mapping increases considerably in scope with demonstration of additional somatotopic representations beyond the confines of SI (Werner and Whitsel, 1973). Posterior and lateral to SI is the second somato-sensory area (SII), which can be further subdivided into an anterior part that is similar in organization to SI and a posterior region containing cells with large receptive fields for touch that also receive nociceptive auditory and visual input (Carreras and Andersson, 1963; Whitsel *et al.*, 1969*b*). Furthermore, a third somatotopic area has been described within area 5 of the parietal lobe (Darian-Smith *et al.*, 1966; Blomquist and Lorenzini, 1965).

The above data show that redundant organizations of somatosensory input exist for different cerebral cortical areas as well as for the ascending spinal pathways. However, as pointed out earlier, spinal pathways or cortical regions that redundantly transfer or code certain functions (such as spatial discrimination) can be expected not to function equipotentially for all aspects of those generalized functions. With this in mind, it is useful to evaluate further lesion studies at cord and cortical levels that have utilized behavioral tasks of spatial discrimination other than the two-point test. One interpretational difficulty that we face with apparent demonstrations of redundancy is the possibility that different pathways (or areas) permit the same end point of behavioral discrimination through quite different coding mechanisms. This is suggested by an experiment using a spatiotactile task requiring that monkeys discriminate the size of an object placed on the glabrous skin of the foot (Vierck, 1973*a*). Dorsal column lesions elevate tactile size thresh-olds, but the thresholds return to normal values after several months of postopera-tive testing. Subsequent section of the ipsilateral dorsalateral column reinstates a deficit that does not disappear with extended training. One interpretation of this finding is that the initial deficit results from removal of one of several spatial codes, so that the stimuli feel to the animal as if they have been altered. The postoperative training could then permit relearning on the basis of new cues that are as effective as those utilized preoperatively. In this case, the redundancy would be only apparent and the task could be considered as inadequate to differentiate the nature of any spatial "information" exclusively supplied by each pathway. An alternate possibility is that, over the 2-month period, the input normally con-ducted over the dorsal columns is distributed more potently to the spinal cells of origin of the intact ascending pathways.

Following the logic presented above, it is likely that each spinal pathway is (1) sufficient but not necessary for certain functions and (2) necessary and sufficient for other functions. Several examples of the latter can be given. In the context of spatiotactile discrimination, several experiments have indicated that dorsal column input becomes critical when a temporal (or sequential spatial) factor is added to the task. If monkeys are required to detect the direction of movement of a brush across the skin (Vierck, 1974) or identify the form of a stimulus by moving the skin along an edge contour (Azulay and Schwartz, 1975), then dorsal column lesions produce enduring deficits. These deficits can possibly be related to interruption of afferent conduction of quickly adapting units with small receptive fields and afferent inhibition. This type of unit predominates in the dorsal column–lemniscal system, which should provide a sharply limited burst of activity among cells with receptive fields centered at the location of an edge contour moving across the skin. Thus we return to somatotopy and the question of cortical map scanning.

Recent physiological studies suggest that directional sensitivity is abstracted at the cortex and fed onto individual cells (Whitsel et al., 1973). It may be that the major "purpose" of a somatotopic map is to provide an orderly source of inputs for the derivation of specific detection capabilities (such as direction) among certain cells. However, the finding of specific directionally sensitive cells does not circumvent the problem of whether spatial discrimination can be subserved by processes that do not depend on a map-scanning process. It seems as if it would be necessary for the nervous system to identify which directionally sensitive cells are firing at a given point in time, and this would be efficiently given by the geometrical position of the neurons. It is not known whether the directionally sensitive cells are located in an arrangement that generates a cortical map for stimulus direction. Directionally sensitive units have been observed in SI, SII, and cytoarchitectural areas 5 and 7 (Whitsel et al., 1973; Mountcastle et al., 1975). Cortical lesion studies in cats and dogs have revealed a deficit in directionality tasks following SII or SI plus SII lesions, but not after lesions of SI alone (Allen, 1947; Glassman, 1970). Thus it might be fruitful to explore thoroughly the second somatosensory area in terms of the representation and organization of cells with directional specificity.

In general, the history of investigations using the ablation method to seek exclusive functional roles for each cortical somatosensory area has paralleled the spinal lesion studies in revealing apparent redundancies. Lesions confined to the primary or secondary areas have failed to produce enduring performance deficits in roughness discrimination (Ruch and Fulton, 1935; Zubeck, 1952) (monkeys, cats), absolute touch thresholds (Schwartzman and Semmes, 1971; Norrsell, 1967) (dogs, monkeys), tactual localization (Diamond et al., 1964) (cats), or a variety of shape and texture discriminations (Cole and Glees, 1954; Teitelbaum et al., 1968; Orbach and Chow, 1959) (monkeys, cats). In some studies, combined ablation of areas SI and SII has been ineffective (Orbach and Chow, 1959; Teitelbaum et al., 1968; Diamond et al., 1964; Norrsell, 1967), while other investigators have obtained significant impairment with the more extensive lesions (Allen, 1947; Zubeck, 1952). Depending on the studies chosen, then, either of the following conclusions could be entertained: (1) that discriminative somesthesis is handled equally well by either the primary or the secondary area but depends on one of these being intact or (2) that discriminative somesthesis, while it may be served in part by areas SI and SII, is critically dependent on some other cortical area. The first conclusion, coupled with the atypical studies on directional sensitivity, contradicts the classical notion (implied by the SI and SII labels) that the primary area is the major lemniscal receiving zone and should be fundamental to all further cortical processing of precise somatosensory cues. The second conclusion represents an extreme and heretical extension of this refutation of classical dictum, because anatomical data have shown that the SI and SII areas receive nearly all of the thalamocortical projections from the specific somatosensory thalamic nuclei (primarily from the ventrobasal complex, receiving input from all three cord sectors) (Bowsher, 1965; Jones and Powell, 1973). Several recent experiments, however, have taken the bite out of these conclusions. First, it has been demonstrated that sensory motor cortical lesions, involving cytoarchitectural area 4 in addition to areas 3, 1, and 2, render monkeys unable to perform on a stereognostic form task (Kruger and Porter, 1958). Because the task involved active palpation of the stimuli by the monkeys, it is difficult to be sure that the impairment is not related to a motoric ataxia rather than a difficulty with sensory decoding. Thus, in subsequent studies, Semmes and Porter (1972) and Semmes *et al.* (1974) have restricted lesions to portions of the sensorimotor strip and found the following: (1) lesions of the motor cortex are without effect on a battery of active form discriminations, indicating that the monkeys can compensate for clumsy tactile exploration; (2) lesions of the posterior portion of the postcentral SI region produce deficits on the most difficult form discriminations (e.g., square vs. diamond and convex vs. concave cylinders), indicating that proper design of the behavioral task can reveal specialized functions for the SI cortex; and (3) anterior lesions of the postcentral area, including the posterior bank of the central sulcus (area 3b), produce severe deficits on nearly all the discrimination tasks tested. The last finding fits with anatomical evidence that area 3b receives most of the thalamo-cortical afferents from the ventrobasal complex in the monkey (Jones and Powell, 1970) and area 3b contains the preponderance of SI units responding to tactile (as opposed to deep) stimulation. The Semmes and Porter finding brings the monkey data more in line with the human deficits that follow damage to the postcentral gyrus (Corkin *et al.*, 1964), and it can explain some of the negative results of primate lesions if area 3b has been spared in these studies. It does not explain the results of lesions in carnivores, because areas 3b, 1, and 2 of the cat receive comparable thalamocortical projections (Jones and Powell, 1969*b*). Also, it seems that lesions of cytoarchitectural areas 1 and 2 would often isolate the thalamic input to area 3b in the monkey, preventing communication with other important parietal cortical areas (see below).

If the above findings are summarized in terms of major questions left unanswered, it is apparent that we are still far from understanding the fundamentals of cortical somatosensory processing. In the monkey, the area 3b lesions could be effective by interruption of a major input channel rather than disruption of the SI "map." Also, it should be noted that area 3b is nearly contiguous with the motor cortex, and the Semmes and Porter tasks involved active palpation; discrimination of passively received stimuli might yield different results. In the cat, there is a suggestion that SII lesions produce deficits in passive discriminations, while the most obvious SI impairments are motor related (Glassman, 1970). There are insufficient data to generate a guess as to the functions of SII in monkeys.

Whatever the resolutions to these questions turn out to be, it is clear that elucidation of cortical somatosensory functions will depend heavily on investigations focusing on areas beyond the confines of SI and SII. In fact, Diamond (1967) has developed the idea that "association" cortex is more primitive than the sensory koniocortex—reinforcing the notion that the precise organization of the somatotopic maps has developed in response to imposed requirements for orderly input systems more than as areas providing new, intrinsic functional capabilities. The cortical regions receiving the heaviest direct projections from SI are the motor area (and supplementary motor area) of the frontal lobe and area 5 of the parietal lobe (projecting in turn to area 7, Jones and Powell, 1969a). SII joins in the projection to the motor areas. Since the functions of parietal areas as well as the motor areas have been linked to somatomotor control operations, it is necessary to return to the periphery and consider proprioception.

PROPRIOCEPTION

In 1959, Rose and Mountcastle reviewed what seemed like compelling evidence that receptors in joint capsules and ligaments are responsible for sensations of limb position. They excluded muscle and tendon receptors as contributors to position sense on the grounds that the discharge of neither is linearly related to muscle length or joint angle. The gamma motor innervation of muscle spindles introduces a potent driving source other than muscle stretch, and the tendon organs will respond to contraction force under isometric conditions. Furthermore, muscle and tendon afferents were thought to project heavily to the cerebellum, but not the cerebral cortex, and cerebellar lesions have been claimed (on the basis of crude evidence) not to produce sensory defects of limb position sense (Holmes, 1922). Early psychophysical studies reported that anesthetization of joints (and not the relevant muscles) produced anesthesia for position of the joint (Browne *et al.,* 1954), and the muscle spindles in the extraocular muscles were said not to indicate the position of the eyes (Brindley and Merton, 1960). The clinching bit of evidence seemed to be provided by the observation that stimulation of the group I fibers in a muscle nerve could not be detected by cats (Swett and Bourassa, 1967).

Despite the weight of the preceding evidence, the issue has been reopened by reversals of some of the earlier observations, particularly by a comprehensive set of studies by Goodman *et al.* (1972). Muscle projections to area 3a of the cerebral cortex have been demonstrated (Oscarsson and Rosen, 1963; Phillips *et al.,* 1971). Extraocular muscles and muscles supplying anesthetized joints or limbs with artificial joints may support position sense (Skavenski, 1971; Clark *et al.,* 1975; Goodman *et al.,* 1972; Cross and McCloskey, 1973). Lesions of cerebellocortical projections in the brachium conjunctivum have been shown to produce an impairment of weight discrimination when combined with lesions of the medial lemniscus, but isolated lemniscal section produces little deficit (Sjoqvist and Weinstein, 1942). And Goodwin *et al.* (1972) have shown that vibration, which effectively activates spindle receptors, can produce illusions of limb movement. Although the vibration also appears to activate joint receptors (Millar, 1973), the illusions are consistently in the direction that corresponds to stretch of the muscle receiving the vibration, and it is not clear whether joint receptors are appropriately stimulated selectively by vibration of different muscles. Thus it is now necessary to consider both the muscle and the joint receptors as possible contributors to the sensations of limb movement and limb position.

The slowly adapting Golgi and Ruffini endings, situated in ligaments or joint capsules, respectively, have been considered as likely contributors to the sense of limb position, and they compose a large portion of fibers that have been isolated in nerves supplying joints (Skoglund, 1973) (Fig. 4). However, the physiological properties of these fibers are quite complex and would appear not to support position sense without extraction of certain specific features by central neurons. The first problem, one that has been studied in some detail, concerns the receptive angles of slowly adapting joint receptors. Although some peripheral fibers have been shown to respond, with fairly narrow "tuning," to intermediate positions of a joint, the majority respond maximally at the extremes of flexion or extension (Skoglund, 1956; Burgess and Clark, 1969a). Thus, if limb position is coded by detection of which neurons are active in the relevant population, it appears that the intermediate angles are underrepresented. Furthermore, a large percentage of the peripheral neurons may respond both to flexion and extension (Burgess and Clark, 1969a). These difficulties appear to have been resolved by the demonstration that slowly adapting joint neurons in the ventrobasal thalamus of monkeys are of two types; they respond maximally only to full flexion or full extension, and their receptive angles are large, overlapping the intermediate joint positions (Mountcastle et al., 1963). Thus joint angle could be determined by the relative intensities of discharge in these two populations of neurons receiving convergent input from peripheral fibers. The density of peripheral receptors with particular ranges of sensitivity appears to be correlated with the discharge rate imposed on a thalamic cell by different joint positions.

Unfortunately, several major questions remain unanswered. Both types of peripheral fibers and the thalamic joint units display a phasic (onset transient) response that is extremely sensitive to the rate of movement of a limb to a given end point (Skoglund, 1973). In the case of the thalamic units, the steady-state discharge rate that accurately signals end position is not evident until approximately 5 sec has elapsed after the limb reaches an end position (Mountcastle et al., 1963). This means that if position sense were determined by activity of these units, one of the following situations would be required: (1) The observer would have to wait at least 5 sec after each movement to discriminate position independent of rate of movement to that position. Psychophysical experiments have not demonstrated such inordinately long response latencies (e.g., Vierck, 1975; Lloyd and Caldwell, 1965). (2) Cortical (or other) neurons may be capable of responding to either the phasic or the tonic component of an input system, as indicated for feline cortical cells sensitive to stimulation of slowly adapting sinus hairs (Galbraith et al., 1974). However, this has not been demonstrated for the proprioceptive system, and it is difficult to imagine a synaptic process that could extract one of two discharge components that are confounded in single primary afferents without

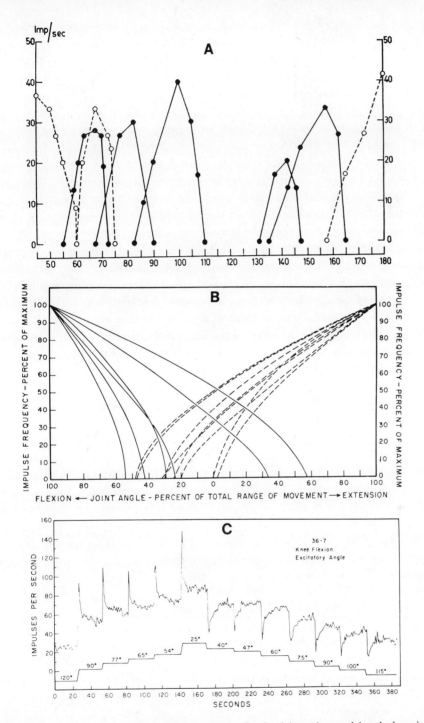

Fig. 4. A: Impulse frequency for eight *peripheral,* slowly adapting joint units supplying the knee joint of the cat. Note the restricted ranges of sensitivity for each fiber. From Skoglund (1956). B: Sensitivity ranges for slowly adapting joint units in the ventrobasal thalamus. The curves cover a wide range of joint angles, are single ended, and have their maxima only at the extremes of flexion and extension. From Mountcastle *et al.* (1963). C: A sequence of stimulations of a ventrobasal joint neuron showing the onset transient response (or inhibition) and the steady-state discharge that is related to the amount of flexion. From Mountcastle *et al.* (1963).

retaining the 5-sec latency to onset of the static response. (3) It is possible that initial judgments of a newly attained limb position are made by comparing the discharges of fast-adapting neurons responding only to rate with the discharge of slowly adapting neurons responding to rate and position. The properties of central neurons detecting velocity of limb movement have not been worked out in detail.

In addition to the superimposition of velocity and position sensitivities onto slowly adapting joint afferents, it has been suggested that twisting the limb can alter the discharge to flexion or extension (Burgess and Clark, 1969a); this factor has not been adequately explored, either peripherally or centrally. Also, it has been shown that the Ruffini endings are sensitive to muscular tension at the joint (Skoglund, 1956). The importance of this influence for the discharge of central, proprioceptive neurons is not known.

The contributions of the major ascending spinal pathways to proprioceptive functions are not well understood. Position sense can be severely disturbed in humans and monkeys following ipsilateral cord lesions (Lashley, 1917; Vierck, 1966), but, contrary to classical notions, surgical interruption of the dorsal columns does not impair discrimination of limb position (Vierck, 1966; Cook and Browder, 1965). Recent physiological results explain this finding on the basis that slowly adapting joint afferents and muscle afferents leave the dorsal columns to synapse in the dorsal horn (Burgess and Clark, 1969b; Williams et al., 1973). It would be valuable to know whether the fast-adapting joint afferents that remain in the dorsal columns must be intact for an animal to discriminate rate of joint movement, but little attention has been directed to aspects of proprioceptive sensation other than static position. Since joint input has not been described for the spinocervicothalamic tract (Brown, 1973), it is possible that a major source of slowly adapting joint information travels via the aberrant dorsal column tract to the dorsal column nuclei (Dart and Gordon, 1973; Korner and Landgren, 1969). However, contradictory results leave unresolved the question of slowly adapting joint representation in the gracile nucleus (Williams et al., 1973; Kruger et al., 1961). The spinocerebellar tracts, receiving input from both muscle and joint receptors, cannot be ruled out entirely as contributors to proprioceptive sensation, and joint receptors contribute input to the spinothalamic tract (Willis et al., 1975).

Proprioceptive input from muscles and joints has been thought to be of major importance for the coordination of muscular activity, and the neural pathways that are critical for this function may overlap or be independent of those responsible for the rostral conduction of proprioceptive sensations. Classically, a distinction between conscious proprioception (position sense) and unconscious proprioception (direct feedback to motor systems for coordination) has been applied to functions of the dorsal column–lemniscal and the spinocerebellar systems, respectively. However, the disorders of movement that follow dorsal column section do not necessarily support this distinction. Neurological testing of reflex and spontaneous movements has described lesioned animals as ataxic and lacking in ability or inclination to tactually explore and manipulate objects in "extrapersonal space" (Ferraro and Barrera, 1934; Gilman and Denny-Brown, 1966). When monkeys or cats are trained in a variety of tasks requiring complicated motor sequences to acquire reinforcement, they exhibit a variety of impairments (Dubrovsky *et al.,* 1971; Melzack and Bridges, 1971; Melzack and Southmayd, 1974; Dubrovsky and Garcia-Rill, 1973) that are difficult to characterize precisely, but in different circumstances the animals are slow to initiate motor acts that are often inaccurately directed. It has been suggested that the problem concerns proper sequencing of individual motor acts or an attentional deficiency rather than being related to a loss of position sense. These experiments, coupled with the frequent finding that dorsal column lesions do not impair sensory discriminations, have fostered the idea that the dorsal columns provide a special form of information that is directly linked to motor activity—i.e., that they do not participate in the detection of passively received somesthetic stimuli but are involved with the initiation, programming, and evaluation of the consequences of motor activities (Semmes, 1969; Wall, 1970; Melzack and Bridges, 1971). An observation that has frequently been cited as a particularly telling argument in favor of this notion is that human subjects can identify two-dimensional shapes by active palpation but not after passive impression of the object on the skin (Gibson, 1962). A similar formulation has been reviewed in terms of the importance of efferent eye movement commands for the acquisition of visual information (Festinger, 1971). In the case of object recognition by somesthesis, however, Schwartz *et al.* (1973) have shown that there is no advantage to active palpation in comparison with similar movement of the objects passively over the skin.

As reviewed earlier, dorsal column lesioned animals are impaired on some passive discrimination tasks (Vierck, 1973*a,b,* 1974), and, contrary to early indications in rats (Wall, 1970), cats with isolated dorsal columns (all other spinal pathways cut) can detect the presence of passively received stimuli (Frommer *et al.,* 1975; Myers *et al.,* 1974). Thus dorsal column functions are not entirely motor related. Also, when tested for execution of simple motor tasks, monkeys show little or no impairment in latency, speed, or accuracy of directing an arm or leg to a target (Vierck, 1975). These animals are impaired, however, in coordination of the actions of their distal extremities—particularly the fractionation of finger movements. The dorsal column–lemniscal system has evolved in approximate pace with the pyramidal motor system; the primary somatosensory and motor areas are directly linked; and the pyramidal tract exerts direct effects on conduction through the dorsal column nuclei (Jones and Powell, 1973; Towe, 1973). It is not surprising, then, that lesions of the motor cortex or the pyramidal tract produce impairments of distal extremity movement that are quite similar to those following dorsal column lesions (Beck and Chambers, 1970; Bucy *et al.,* 1966; Ridley and Ettlinger, 1975). The importance of the fast-adapting and fast-conducting dorsal column input for finely regulated manipulative activities is emphasized, without claiming that all dorsal column functions serve manipulation.

It remains to be determined whether incoordination of the distal extremities can account for the impairments on tasks requiring complex motor sequencing, or whether the problem shows up in distal movements because they involve complex and precisely timed sequences of muscular action. That is, are the distal impairments a special case of sequencing errors, or are individual movements of distal muscles impaired to the extent that they serve as critical interrupters of complex, whole-body activities? What will be required is to build up a sequence of movements so that each component can be observed in isolation and as a part of the integrated activity. Several other problems that need to be resolved are as follows: (1) The motor deficits are more severe for the hands than for the feet (Gilman and Denny-Brown, 1966; Ferraro and Barrera, 1934; Vierck, 1975). Lesions of fasciculus cuneatus involve all forelimb fibers of the dorsal column–lemniscal system, muscle afferent projections to motor cortex, and fibers destined for the cerebellum (Oscarsson and Rosen, 1963; Landgren *et al.*, 1967), while lesions of fasciculus gracilis spare the aberrant dorsal column tract (including muscle afferents to motor cortex) and spinocerebellar fibers. Thus cord lesions should be compared with dorsal column nuclear and medial lemniscal lesions and various cerebellar lesions. At the present time, it is not possible to differentiate clearly motor impairments resulting from interruption of pathways to the somatosensory cortex, the motor cortex, or the cerebellum. (2) It would be instructive to see if dorsal column lesions affect passive discriminations of limb movement and position at the distal extremities more than at the proximal joints.

A number of experiments using monkeys with section of all the dorsal roots supplying one or more limbs have revealed a remarkable capacity for motor performance (Allen *et al.*, 1975; Knapp *et al.*, 1963; Bossom and Ommaya, 1966; Vierck, 1975). After extensive training, these animals are able to accurately direct a limb toward a target, grasp a reward, bring it to the mouth, and retrieve the food from the hand. This can be accomplished without visual guidance and from a variable start position, requiring that different movements be executed on each trial. This is not to say that the animals are unimpaired motorically; they have great difficulty immediately after surgery, even with visual guidance. The movements are jerky, and very few attempts at directed movement are successful. Although these early deficits in gross reaching contrast sharply with the initial performance of dorsal column lesioned animals, the point of interest for the present discussion is that the deafferented monkeys can eventually program and regulate certain aspects of motor performance with little or no proprioceptive feedback. The reason for the qualifying statement about the availability of proprioceptive feedback is that afferent fibers have been shown to enter the central nervous system via the ventral roots (Clifton *et al.*, 1974; Vance *et al.*, 1975; Ryall and Piercey, 1970).However, nearly all of the ventral root afferents that have been characterized so far are nociceptors, and most of these innervate the viscera. The few proprioceptors present would provide extremely meager input for estimating the position and rate of movement of the joints.

A variety of evidence from sources other than the deafferented preparation has led to the conclusion that there is a class of movements, termed "ballistic," that are not dependent on proprioceptive feedback (e.g., Kornhuber, 1971). Because these movements are of too short a duration to effectively utilize information from peripheral receptors, they are programmed and run off from a "packaged" command. In the execution of a ballistic movement by a normal animal, there most likely is an assessment of all relevant sensory information before and at the termination of a movement, but evidence is building that somesthetic input from the active limb is inhibited during movement (Coultier, 1974; Ghez and Pisa,

1972; Dyhre-Poulsen, 1975). If an effective feedback system is operative during ballistic movements, it probably involves return loops within the motor systems, permitting regulation of the force of muscular contractions. The effectiveness of motor preprogramming and/or motoric reafference is indicated by demonstrations that human subjects can actively move a limb to a target more accurately than they can discriminate passive excursions of the same limb (Paillard and Brouchon, 1968). Also, Lashley (1917) reported that a patient with spinal cord damage and a complete loss of the senses of limb movement and position could accurately guide the affected limb to a target, without visual control, and accuracy was directly related to the speed of the motion. With the above considerations in mind, it is not surprising that dorsal column lesions leave a good deal of motor capacity intact, and the importance of sequencing becomes apparent. These animals would be expected to have difficulty in stringing together a rapid progression of fast movements that are improvised on the basis of their sensory consequences (e.g., object manipulation).

At the cortical level, lesions within the parietal lobe have effects that are not dissimilar to those following dorsal column section. Deficits of position sense or weight discrimination are not evident following lesions of SI in cats or monkeys (Glassman, 1971; Ruch and Fulton, 1935; Levitt and Levitt, 1969), but mild disturbances of motor control, affecting primarily the distal extremities, have been noted frequently to result from removal of SI or posterior parietal cortex (Zubeck, 1952; Glassman, 1970; Bates and Ettlinger, 1960; Kennard and Kessler, 1940; Lamotte and Acuna, 1975; Denny-Brown and Chambers, 1958). Sufficient data are not available to be sure of which aspects of motor behavior depend on somatosensory projections anterior to the motor cortex or posterior to parietal "association" regions, but it is likely that the projection to motor cortex is important for making adjustments to perturbations of a limb (Tatton *et al.*, 1975; Evarts and Tanji, 1974; Conrad *et al.*, 1974), while the parietal areas have been implicated in the initiation or monitoring of consciously directed activity (Mountcastle *et al.*, 1975). The latter is supported by recent studies of single-unit activity in parietal areas 5 and 7 of monkeys, revealing several classes of cells that either require motor activity for activation (Hyvarinen and Poranen, 1974; Mountcastle *et al.*, 1975) or require combinations of sensory input that would ordinarily occur only during motor activity (Sakata *et al.*, 1973; Duffy and Burchfiel, 1971).

Brodmann's area 5 of the monkey contains a large proportion of cells that are classified as joint receptive but that may include responsivity to muscle receptors (Duffy and Burchfiel, 1971; Sakata *et al.*, 1973; Mountcastle *et al.*, 1975). Although investigators disagree on the proportion of units responding to movement at a single joint, all agree that area 5 contains proprioceptive neurons with convergent properties not observed for the joint neurons of adjacent area 2. Some respond only to stimulation at more than one joint, or movement of both limbs, and many discharge more vigorously to active movement than to passive rotation. Other cells require specific interactions of tactile and proprioceptive cues. For example, stroking in one direction over a field restricted to a portion of the arm can cause a cell to discharge if the shoulder is adducted, but similar stroking with the shoulder abducted and stroking in other directions with the shoulder adducted are not effective stimuli (Sakata *et al.*, 1973). A wide variety of these interactions have been described. Area 5 neurons that respond to passively received tactile stimuli usually are sensitive only to moving stimuli, and directional selectivity is the rule.

Several types of neurons present in both areas 5 and 7 appear to respond only during active movements. One class of neurons does not respond to passive manipulation of the limbs, but a projection of a limb by the animal toward a "desired" object produces vigorous discharge. Some of these cells require any goal-directed movement of one arm (usually contralateral), while others respond with movement of either arm in a specific direction. Hand manipulation neurons of areas 5 and 7 also are not excited by passive stimulation, but manipulation of an object by the animal is a very effective stimulus. While area 5 is distinguished by a large number of neurons with complex proprioceptive receptivities, area 7 contains cells that may be uniquely characterized by complex adequate stimuli with strong visual components. For example, visual fixation cells respond only when the animal focuses on objects of interest that are located within reach (although it is not necessary that a reach occur). "Interest" can be defined by the object's novelty or by its reward value. Visual tracking neurons respond not to visual fixation on an object but to smooth visual pursuit of an interesting item. These cells usually display a directional preference. A small number of neurons require visual tracking and projection of the arm toward the tracked cue.

The physiological properties of parietal neurons are intuitively consonant with some of the concepts of parietal functions that have arisen from observations following lesions of posterior parietal cortex. Although it is difficult to imagine a topographic arrangement of units that would coherently organize the diverse combinations of specific somatosensory, visual, and motor "fields," it has been suggested that the parietal cortex provides awareness of the location of the body parts within the immediate extrapersonal space (Hyvarinen and Poranen, 1974). This notion of a three-dimensional map of the immediate environment is reinforced by the dramatic instances of unilateral neglect of the body and external objects located contralateral to the side of a parietal lesion in humans (Critchley, 1969). Although it must be cautioned that human lesions producing the most prominent neglect involve areas that may be unique to the human (Brodmann's areas 39 and 40), lesioned monkeys display perceptual rivalry (extinction), where bilateral stimulation of the body is intepreted as stimulation only of the side ipsilateral to the lesion (Eidelberg and Schwartz, 1971; Heilman *et al.*, 1970). Thus it is predicted that animals with parietal lesions will be severely impaired on behavioral tasks that require perception of the spatial relationships of objects to the animal.

A related formulation proposes that parietal neurons provide command signals to direct manual and visual exploration of near objects (Mountcastle *et al.*, 1975). Unfortunately, it is difficult experimentally to distinguish between deficits that would relate directly to disruption of a command apparatus and disruption of a mapping function on which the motor commands would depend. For example, parietal lesions induce a reluctance of animals to move and errors of reaching when a movement does occur (Denny-Brown and Chambers, 1958; Critchley, 1969); this appears to indicate disruption of a motor comand apparatus but could also result from deficient recognition of significant stimuli or a disordered perception of the position of the stimuli in relation to the animal. Conversely, neglect and extinction could logically result from an absence of certain directed motor commands as well as from a perceptual deficit. Although the large number of parietal neurons that respond only with active movement seems to demand a unifying principle of organization that includes motor functions, the artificial distinction between sensory and motor operations and the tendency to ascribe one global function to this region of diverse inputs, cells, and outputs will probably give way to a description of multiple functions that cannot be described as exclusively sensory or motor. One possibility in this regard is that many parietal neurons participate in evaluation of whether an ongoing movement is on target. That is, their neuronal discharges might depend on a match-up (convergence or gating) of specific corollary discharges from motor areas (e.g., motor cortex) and certain sensory signals.

Early behavioral studies of animals with posterior parietal lesions utilized tests of stereognosis, on the assumption that recognition of an object's form by touch and proprioception would require spatial and temporal integration of information beyond that which is evident at the level of SI cortex. Although lesioned animals often are slow to learn these tasks, even difficult form discriminations can be learned with extensive training (e.g., Pribram and Barry, 1956; Semmes, 1973; Ridley and Ettlinger, 1975; Munger, 1965). This is surprising, because any of a number of expected deficits should interfere with these tasks: (1) clumsy palpation, (2) disruption of feedback from palpation (as provided by hand manipulation neurons?), (3) impaired appreciation of spatial relationships, or (4) difficulty in recognition of the rewarded cues in the environment as "significant." Furthermore, it should be noted that the extinction phenomenon and errors of reaching also recover in monkeys after parietal lesions (Mountcastle *et al.*, 1975; Heilman *et al.*, 1970). Recovery on these tasks could occur for any or all of the following reasons: because the animals adopt performance strategies that permit compensation for and masking of deficits that are actually enduring; because the lesions have spared some critical area of tissue (e.g., temporal "association" cortex, Wilson *et al.*, 1975); or because the behavioral significance of the parietal areas has yet to be revealed. Pursuit of the last alternative should be most fruitful, and it is likely that properly designed behavioral experiments will reveal striking and enduring deficits with restricted lesions (e.g., to areas 5 and 7). Recent analyses of spatial discriminations serve as a demonstration of the way in which behavioral experiments will change our conceptualization of parietal functions.

For many parietal cells, the animal's body appears to serve as the spatial referent for neural discharge triggered by activity directed at an external object. That is, the cells respond with movement of a limb toward or focusing the eyes on an object in a given position (or moving in a given direction) relative to the central body axis. This implies that a parietal-lesioned animal should have difficulty with tasks testing egocentric spatial localization—i.e., the relation of objects to the body. However, frontal lesions but not parietal lesions impair learning of tasks such as position reversal or delayed response, where the animal must remember that one of two identical objects is significant because of its position relative to the animal's body (Pohl, 1973). Conversely, the landmark test of allocentric spatial localization has revealed deficits from parietal but not frontal lesions. Allocentric discriminations are made on the basis of the spatial relationships of external objects to each other and do not depend on the animal's position as a referent. In the landmark task, two foodwells are covered with identical objects, and food is placed under the object nearest a landmark cue. This task appears to indicate that allocentric relationships are coded by the parietal areas, but the landmark task can be learned, with extra training (Pohl, 1973). Also, Mendoza and Thomas (1975) have pointed out that the landmark task confounds allocentric cues with spatial separation of the cue and the reinforcement (see Fig. 5). When these factors are dissociated by placing the reinforcement under the significant (cueing) element of a spatial pattern, parietal-lesioned animals have little difficulty making an allocentric spatial pattern discrimination. However, when the reinforcement is placed under an element other than the significant cue, the task is not learned with extensive training, following parietal damage. The message from these experiments is not entirely clear, but the following is suggested: parietal-lesioned animals can appreciate the location of significant objects and their relationship to the body and to external referents, and a motor response can be directed accurately to a significant object; but the transfer of significance from one object to another is impaired under certain as yet undefined circumstances. Possibly these relationships will be clarified by experiments that determine the pathways and conditions responsible for establishment of the significance features of parietal cellular responses.

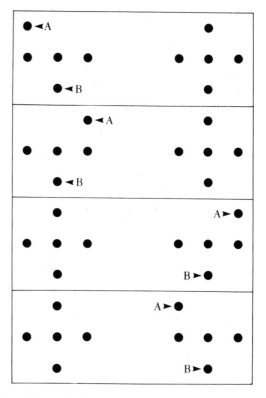

Fig. 5. An example of an allocentric discrimination task without separation of cue and reward. The reward is placed under the sphere that is located out of place in one of the two patterns (reward locus indicated by the A arrows). Parietal-lesioned animals solve this problem. An allocentric discrimination with separation of cue (out-of-place sphere) and reward (indicated by the B arrows; always located at the bottom of the disrupted pattern). Parietal-lesioned animals have difficulty with this task. Adapted from Mendoza and Thomas (1975).

Consideration of the locus of interactions that interject significance as a determinant of neural discharge to environmental stimulation can usefully begin by deciding whether this attentional factor appears *de novo* at the parietal cortex by convergence of sensory inputs with other projections. An alternative possibility is offered by the presence of descending inhibitory inputs onto cells of origin and relay cells of each of the major somatosensory pathways, suggesting that filtering for stimulus significance might be present at all stages of somesthetic conduction. Although there is no evidence that cells of the primary somesthetic relays (dorsal horn, dorsal column nuclei, ventrobasal thalamus, SI and SII cortex) respond selectively to significant stimuli, unit activity in these regions has not been extensively sampled in awake-behaving animals. Clearly, attentional processes that determine significance are multifaceted, and different aspects of attention may be contributed by each of the major pathways. For example, it has been reported that monkeys or humans with dorsal column lesions have lapses of attention during somesthetic sensory testing (Wall, 1970; Schwartzman and Bogdonoff, 1969), and deficient orientation to significant stimuli can occur during execution of a complex motor sequence (Dubrovsky and Garcia-Rill, 1973). In the latter case, the investigators believe that high cervical lesions interrupt proprioceptive feedback that is critical for proper coordination of head and eye movements, making it difficult for the animals to track moving stimuli. Thus dorsal column lesions appear to produce effects that interfere with attention under certain circumstances, but defects that might be expected to result from disruption of a precise topographic system are not seen (e.g., neglect or perceptual rivalry or gross errors of reaching) (Eidelberg and Schwartz, 1971; Vierck, 1975). The spinocervicothalamic tract has been implicated as especially important for attentional processes, because somatosensory conduction to the cerebral cortex is quickest over this pathway (Taub, 1964), and the SCTT sends a projection to an area of the subthalamus which participates in the maintenance of behavioral wakefulness and an activated EEG (Denavit and Korsinski, 1968; Naquet *et al.*, 1966). However, lesions of the spinal dorsolateral columns have not been reported to produce deficient orientation to environmental stimulation.

The functions of arousal and attention often have been thought to be linked together as attributes of the reticular formation, which exerts a powerful ascending drive of sleep-wakefulness rhythms and extensive modulation of sensory conduction and motor activity (Jasper *et al.*, 1958). Thus it has been instructive to compare the results of section of the long ascending pathways with lesions of the reticular formation. If convergence of both systems is necessary for attention, then either type of lesion should leave the animal unable to select and orient to significant stimuli, while selective contributions of each system that do not depend on the integrity of the other should be revealed by medial vs. lateral lesions of the brain stem. Lateral midbrain lesions involve the dorsal column–lemniscal, spinocervical, and spinothalamic tracts and spare most of the reticular core above the level of direct somesthetic input and collateral input from the lateral pathways (primarily from the spinothalamic tracts; see Pompeiano, 1973). Lateral tract lesions have been shown to produce a profound and enduring inattention to somesthetic stimulation, even though the animals are fully aroused and active

(Sprague *et al.*, 1963). Conversely, lesions of the reticular core induce a transient somnolence and inattention that recover to the point that the animals (cats) can be aroused and are then described as hyperdistractable, implying a release of the tendency to orient to any novel or salient stimulus, regardless of the consequences for ongoing behavior. These data suggest that (1) input over at least one of the somatosensory pathways in the lateral brain stem is crucial for localizing somesthetic stimuli and orienting to them, even though the reticular system is theoretically capable of such actions (Bowsher, 1975) and may direct them in primitive organisms, and (2) in mammalian systems the nonspecific reticular systems may function to hold attention, once "focused." Thus it may be that the filtering of sensory conduction by reticular connections with the specific sensory systems comes into play after a stimulus has been localized and labeled as significant by the specific systems.

If the scanning, localizing, and reinforcement (significance) aspects of attention are dependent on conduction by the specific somatosensory pathways, with considerable redundancy among them, the question can still be asked whether these functions are elaborated before or at the cerebral cortex. This is particularly the case since inattention resulting from lateral midbrain lesions was not confined to somatosensory stimuli, and the lesions were not strictly limited to involvement of the lateral tracts (Sprague, 1963). It is most likely that involvement or deafferentation of the tectum contributed to the deficit of attention because the colliculi have long been thought to be important for orienting reactions, and neglect and errors of localization are seen with tectal lesions (Sprague and Meikle, 1965; Keating, 1974). Furthermore, recordings from single tectal units in awake, behaving monkeys have revealed responsivities for visual stimuli within a receptive field only when they are fixated for reward (Goldberg and Wurtz, 1972). Although the colliculi have generally been considered to be visual and auditory relays, recent investigations have revealed tactile units in the superior colliculus that are arranged topographically and in a systematic relationship with visual fields (Dräger *et al.*, 1975; Stein *et al.*, 1974).

It is difficult to define the unique functions of the tectum, as distinct from those of the posterior parietal cortex, with regard to attentional processes. In addition to organizing certain reflex orienting reactions, the colliculi appear to contribute input to the parietotemporooccipital association cortex. For example, in a prosimian (bushbaby), the superior colliculus projects through the inferior pulvinar nucleus to several temporal lobe regions (Glenndenning *et al.*, 1975). In this regard, it is interesting to note that tactile discrimination of edible from nonedible objects is disrupted by disconnection of the parietal and temporal lobes in monkeys (Keating and Horel, 1971).

Vibration

Geldard (1940) has argued that vibration should be referred to as a sense or submodality within somesthesis. The case is based primarily on evidence that vibration enjoys a private peripheral line of conduction. This point has been solidly confirmed by a number of elegant investigations that have identified the Pacinian corpuscle and associated large myelinated fibers as the peripheral transmitting elements (Verrillo, 1966; Lamotte and Mountcastle, 1975; Mountcastle *et al.*, 1969; Merzenich and Harrington, 1969). Pacinian afferents are entrained by high frequencies of stimulation (to at least 400 Hz) and respond to parametric manipulations in a manner that closely matches psychophysical estimations by monkey and human observers of the same continua. Thus, at the periphery, there is receptor specificity for vibration sensitivity and interval coding of vibration frequency. One of the intriguing puzzles that has come out of this research relates to the fate of the interval code with transmission across successive CNS synapses that eliminate the occurrence of entrainment at frequencies which can be discriminated by the psychophysical observers. Indeed, the temporal code fades and cannot be detected at the cerebral cortex (Mountcastle *et al.*, 1969). At the present, it must be concluded that some forms of detailed perceptual awareness do not require participation of cerebral cortical regions or that the temporal code for vibration frequency is transformed dramatically. Occurrence of either would not be unique within the somatosensory system.

Regardless of the outcome of the vibration-coding problem, the "purpose" of exquisite vibratory sensitivity on the skin is not apparent for the many organisms equipped with remarkable auditory acuity. There are few meaningful stimuli in the environments of most mammals that would appear to exclusively excite Pacinian corpuscles. The match of psychophysical discrimination capabilities with activity and entrainment of Pacinian afferents indicates that this input can be selectively attended to, but synthetic interactions with other afferents may provide the most useful information to organisms in their natural environment. For example, it is possible that accurate discrimination of the frequency components of a stimulus is important to the appreciation of texture, which appears to be perceived most accurately with movement of the skin over an object, often producing a series of sharp transient stimuli to a given skin spot. Consistent with this notion, Pacinian corpuscles are particularly plentiful in the hands and the tongue, where texture discrimination is especially acuitive. However, the fact that Pacinian corpuscles are widely distributed and are often located deep to the skin must be taken into account in ascribing functions to these afferent units. Other afferent interactions that have been observed to involve vibratory stimulation are as follows: (1) Pain threshold is elevated by concurrent vibration of a nearby locus (Sullivan, 1968), but when intense stimuli are perceived as painful in the presence of vibration, the pain reaction may be intensified over control trials without vibration (Melzack and Wall, 1963). (2) Although it is not clear whether the following effects result from direct action to vibration on skin receptors other than Pacinian corpuscles or from interactions of these inputs with Pacinian afferents, vibration appears to reduce the perceived area of a stimulus and increase the separability of individual stimuli, but it impairs localization of skin contact (von Békésy, 1967; Vierck and Jones, 1970). (3) Focal vibratory stimulation sets up traveling waves that should effectively excite Pacinian corpuscles over a wide area of the body because of the extraordinary sensitivity of these receptors. However, the vibratory stimulus is perceived as focal rather than generalized, indicating that the effective excitatory area is reduced centrally. (4) In addition to the brief discharge of fast and slowly adapting touch units that will occur with initial contact of a vibrating stimulus on the skin, it has been shown that sustained vibration quite effectively excites muscle receptors (Goodman *et al.*, 1972).

It is evident from the above that mechanical stimulation of the skin by brief sinusoids sets off complicated patterns of activity that would not be expected to be contained within a single afferent conduction channel within the CNS. Nevertheless, physiological data indicate that Pacinian afferents project via the dorsal columns but not the spinocervical or spinothalamic tracts (Brown, 1973). This indicates that the sensation of vibration is carried exclusively by the DC pathway, and that modulating effects are exerted through collateral axons to the dorsal horn, without a one-to-one transference of Pacinian activity to dorsal horn cells. It is surprising to find, however, that neither vibratory detection nor roughness (texture) discrimination is permanently lost following dorsal column lesions (Cook and Browder, 1965; Schwartzman and Bogdonoff, 1969; Dobry and Casy, 1972*a;* Kitai and Weinberg, 1968). It is possible that Pacinian afferents ascend the dorsolateral columns as aberrant dorsal column fibers, but the general rule is that it is the slowly adapting fibers that exit the dorsal columns in this fashion. Before concluding that the dorsal columns are not necessary for normal vibratory discrimination, it will be necessary to test lesioned animals for awareness of vibratory frequency and intensity, rather than the mere presence of stimulus oscillation. It has been noted, for example, that some elements of the brain stem reticular formation are especially sensitive to sharp, transient stimulation (tap, Bowsher *et al.*, 1968). Conduction through this or other systems might be sufficient to identify stimulus oscillation, but temporal resolution should not be great (Pompeiano, 1973). Consistent with the inability to detect a cortical code for vibratory frequency, deficits of vibratory detection have not been seen following lesions of areas SI and SII (Schwartzman, 1972), but here, too, more demanding discriminations should be evaluated.

Pain

In 1965, Melzack and Wall presented their gate control theory of pain, which offered a physiological explanation for an observation that had appeared frequently in the clinical literature (Livingston, 1943)—that pain conduction, initiated in small myelinated and unmyelinated fibers, is opposed by central interactions with input from large myelinated fibers. Several propositions that were offered by the gate control theory have met difficulty: (1) The inhibition from large fibers was thought to occur presynaptically on small fiber terminals synapsing with pain transmission cells of the spinal cord. However, subsequent physiological investigations have shown neither that inhibitory effects are exclusively presynaptic nor that they arise only from large fiber activity (Franz and Iggo, 1968; Vyklicky *et al.*, 1969; Wagman and Price, 1969; Zimmerman, 1968). (2) The pain transmission cells were thought to be those dorsal horn cells with a wide dynamic range, such that pain would be coded by intense activity in these cells rather than by the discharge of a group of units responding exclusively to noxious stimulation. Recent studies have determined that there are both peripheral afferent units and central cells that respond only to stimuli that can be regarded as noxious (Burgess and Perl, 1967; Bessou and Perl, 1969; Christensen and Perl, 1970). (3) The small cells within substantia gelatinosa (laminae II and III) were implicated as the inhibitory interneurons on the basis of indirect evidence from gross recording techniques, and subsequent research has not produced definitive evidence on this question. Because the substantia gelatinosa cells are too small to isolate by microelectrode recording, their inputs have not been determined. Anatomical evidence can be interpreted to support an inhibitory action of substantia gelatinosa neurons on pain transmission via cells in laminae I or IV (Rethelyi and Szentogothai, 1973), but the spinothalamic tract cells that originate in deeper laminae of the spinal gray matter (Willis *et al.*, 1974) apparently would escape this influence.

Although it has been difficult to pin down the circuitry responsible for afferent inhibition of pain, the phenomenon of afferent modulation has continued to receive empirical support and has generated the clinical technique of primary afferent stimulation for control of pain (Fields *et al.*, 1974; Shealy, 1974). At the level of behavioral analyses of clinical pain or experimentally induced pain, the evidence is inconclusive as to the optimum form of conditioning stimulation, and therefore these data resemble those from the physiological studies in not delineating a singular mechanism of inhibition. Either nonpainful stimulation of large fibers or noxious input is effective (Fields *et al.*, 1974; Melzack, 1975; Vierck *et al.*, 1974); not all types of clinical pain are affected (Fields *et al.*, 1974; Melzack, 1975); there is conflicting evidence as to whether the stimulation must be delivered to certain points on the body surface, whether superficial or deep stimulation is more effective, and whether certain waveforms and frequencies of stimulation are optimal; and the effect is quite variable, even for a given subject under what appear to be constant conditions (Melzack, 1975; Vierck *et al.*, 1974). At this point, it is clear only that the level of pain conduction is not determined solely by the intensity of a noxious stimulus. In addition to the importance of afferent interactions, there are supraspinal sources of powerful inhibition that act in part on pain conduction at the spinal cord level. For example, stimulation of a portion of the midbrain central gray has been reported to obliterate overt responses to noxious levels of stimulation that otherwise elicit obvious signs of discomfort (Mayer and Liebeskind, 1974).

The lateral spinothalamic tract has been regarded as the principal spinal pathway for conduction of pain sensations in primates, as evidenced by a decrease of pain sensitivity below the level of an anterolateral chordotomy (White and Sweet, 1969). However, this lesion does not completely obliterate pain sensitivity, and after a postoperative period in excess of several months pain sensations typically recur (King, 1957; White and Sweet, 1969). There is little indication at present as to which pathway(s) is critically involved with the "secondary" conduction of pain or why the recovery process is slow. The period of several months is suggestive of the occurrence of axonal sprouting, which could increase the density and potency of existing connections and/or bring small fiber inputs to influence a population of spinal cells not normally contacted. Considering the former alternative, a number of pathways other than the crossed spinothalamic have been linked with pain conduction: (1) The possibility of uncrossed spinothalamic fibers has been mentioned frequently, but this cannot account for the recovery that occurs following bilateral chordotomies (White and Sweet, 1969). (2) Although the existence of an anterior spinothalamic tract has been frequently mentioned in medical textbooks, the evidence for it was shaky until a recent anatomical demonstration of the presence of such a pathway in the anterior column of the monkey cord (Kerr, 1975; Kerr and Lippman, 1974). There have been no studies which would establish the functional role of this pathway, but its rostral connections are similar to those of the lateral spinothalamic tract, and it is not likely to conduct only touch information, as suggested in numerous texts. (3) The spinocervical tract contains units with a wide dynamic range that could signal pain by high rates of discharge. This pathway has been implicated in the transmission of pain in carnivores, where the spinothalamic tract is poorly developed (Kennard, 1954; Andersson et al., 1975). (4) Lissauer's tract has access to a prominent input from small-diameter peripheral afferents and could provide a multisynaptic ascending route for pain (Basbaum, 1973) or could be involved in the redistribution of pain input to neurons other than the injured spinothalamic cells. (5) Finally, even the dorsal columns contain relayed fibers with a nociceptive input component (Uddenberg, 1968; Angaut-Petit, 1975), and dorsal column lesions attenuate pain reactivity (Vierck et al., 1971).

Lesions of either the anterolateral spinal column or the ventral column interrupt, in addition to direct spinothalamic fibers, important inputs to the brain stem reticular formation via spinothalamic collaterals and direct spinoreticular fibers (Bowsher, 1975; Bowsher et al., 1968). Clinical evidence suggests that these reticular regions and their rostral projections (e.g., to intralaminar thalamic nuclei) overlay distinctive emotional qualities on the discriminative sensory aspects of pain. For example, stereotaxic lesions of intralaminar nuclei in human patients with intractable pain have been reported to decrease emotional reactions to pain without diminishing appreciably the sensation of pain (White and Sweet, 1969; Mark et al., 1963). Conversely, mesencephalic tractotomy, which interrupts the spinothalamic tract but spares the medial (paleospinothalamic) reticular system, produces a very disturbing accentuation of chronic pain (Pagni, 1974). Units within the spinoreticulothalamic projection system respond differentially to noxious input and connect with limbic and hypothalamic structures that participate in the evocation of emotional reactions (Casey et al., 1974).

It is important to note that most of the cells within the paleospinothalamic projection system respond to nonnoxious touch stimuli exclusively or in addition to stimuli evoking pain (Phillips et al., 1971). Hence it can be expected that this system is not entirely (or even primarily) concerned with the elaboration of intense autonomic and behavioral reactions to pain. The receptive fields of these units are typically very large, often extending bilaterally on the body surface. Contrary to early reports of single-unit recordings from "specific" somatosensory relays (e.g., thalamic nucleus VPL and SI cortex), such large-field neurons are not strictly confined to the nonspecific reticular system but are interspersed among cells with small fields in the somatotopically organized regions (Baker *et al.*, 1971; Jabbur *et al.*, 1972). These cells are more readily demonstrated following lesions of some portion of the specific system (Bava *et al.*, 1968; Dreyer *et al.*, 1974; Levitt and Levitt, 1974*a*), indicating that the activity of some of them is normally masked (inhibited) by activity of the small-field projection cells. Conversely, discharge of the small-field cells to stimulation of their receptive fields must be influenced by activity in the wide-field neurons, and it will be intriguing to learn more about the nature of the nonspecific influence as well as the optimum conditions generating it. Wide-field neurons typically habituate rapidly to repetitive stimulation, and if some of them are inhibitory interneurons they could accentuate the saliency of novel stimuli. That is, a new stimulus would excite a restricted number of small-field neurons and would exert more powerful inhibition on other cells via wide-field interneurons than would a nonnovel stimulus. Also, it is possible that the wide-field neurons selectively modulate activity in certain submodality classes of cells (e.g., pain).

It is unlikely that all large-field neurons receive their input entirely from the reticular projection system or that they all should be considered only as modulators of coding functions in other cells. For example, the neurons with large receptive fields in the posterior nuclear complex of the thalamus and SII cortex are certain to be involved with coding of various aspects of somatosensory information, in addition to a possible role in pain mediation (Curry, 1972; Poggio and Mountcastle, 1960; Berkley and Parmer, 1974), but there are few clues as to what functions should be attended to. This situation is in part related to the fact that somatosensory receptive fields have been defined consistently with punctate stimulation, which is unlikely to reveal their most important features. The recent use of a stroking stimulus has led to the suggestion that large-field neurons can be fired preferentially by certain sequences of stimulation of separate portions of their receptive fields (Whitsel *et al.*, 1973, 1978). Also, Whitsel *et al.* have shown that the variability of SII cells is related to their mean rate of discharge in such a manner that different groups of these cells (as well as those of SI) are selectively tuned to different rates and frequencies of stimulation *across* their receptive fields. Another formulation proposes that the phenomenon of stimulus constancy depends on the presence of a loosely coupled system (i.e., one with extensive interconnectedness and large fields, Glassman *et al.*, 1975). That is, the ability to transfer the recognition of a pattern of cutaneous stimulation on one portion of the body to distant patches of skin might not be possible for a system that is uniformly composed of tightly coupled input-output relations.

PRESSURE

When a physical object lightly contacts the skin surface, there is a sensation of pressure that varies with the magnitude (force and/or displacement) of the stimulus. Although both quickly and slowly adapting tactile units are affected by the initial skin contact, the sensation persists beyond the period of time in which units with only a velocity sensitivity are responding vigorously. Thus experiments on pressure sensation have attended to the type I and type II slowly adapting receptors. Only these afferent units respond differentially to pressures that span the entire range of intensities discriminated by human subjects (assuming that the code is given by impulse frequency) (Harrington and Merzenich, 1970; Werner and Mountcastle, 1965). Several sets of experiments have plotted the discharge rates of slowly adapting primary afferents in monkeys during the early steady-state period (i.e., after the onset transient response) and have compared these functions with estimates of the growth of perceived intensity in humans, using the method of magnitude estimation (Harrington and Merzenich, 1970; Mountcastle et al., 1966; Werner and Mountcastle, 1965). Using similar stimulus probes and intensity ranges, both type I and type II units and the behavioral data generate power functions with similar slopes for stimulation of comparable skin regions. The exponents of the power functions for hairy skin range from 0.4 to 0.7, and exponents for glabrous skin are near unity. These differences indicate that the transfer functions of the receptors are strongly influenced by characteristics of the tissue in which they are embedded. Also, the close correspondence of the functions derived from peripheral units and human behavioral responses has led to the proposition that estimates of stimulus intensity are based on functional properties of first-order afferents and that further CNS transformations of the peripheral code are linear. This point of view has been sdrongly criticized on a number of counts (Kruger and Kenton, 1973): e.g.; (1) power functions often are not the best fit for the data, (2) exponents are strongly influenced by threshold values and a variety of important procedural details, and (3) there is considerable variability in the functions generated by peripheral afferents.

When the relationship between stimulus intensity and its evoked sensory magnitude is plotted for different rates of stimulus onset (e.g., 3.4–33 μm/msec, Harrington and Merzenich, 1970) the curves are congruent, indicating that the subjects' judgments of the pressure sensation are not strongly influenced by the onset transient response of slowly adapting units. This conclusion follows from observations that the initial phasic response is quite sensitive to the rate of stimulus onset. Apparently contradictory results are obtained, however, if the rate of stimulus onset is much slower (less than 0.5 μm/sec, Horch et al., 1975). Under these conditions, large indentations that should provoke a static discharge in slowly adapting units do not elicit a sensation of pressure. Possibly the necessary conditions for evocation of the pressure sense include an initially abrupt increase in receptor activity, even though estimates of pressure are not based entirely on the early discharge frequency. A similar sensitivity to the rate of change of discharge occurs in reverse at the removal of a stimulus. If skin contact is terminated abruptly, the pressure sensation disappears, but an aftersensation lingers following slow removal of the probe (Horch et al., 1975).

Although the preceding account of possible neural mechanisms for pressure sensation is confusing in its particulars, it is evident that pressure sensations are not given by a simple decoding of the impulse frequency offered by slowly adapting primary afferents. Soon it should be possible to make more positive statements about the precise coding operations that act on slowly adapting tactile input, because the type I and II units can be stimulated selectively by directing a small probe to a tactile dome (type I) or to intervening skin. In the few instances in which this approach of precise stimulation has been utilized, contradictory results have been obtained. If a single tactile dome of a cat is stimulated, the animal can use that stimulus as a conditioned cue (Tapper, 1970), but similar stimulation of human skin has been reported not to elicit a sensation of pressure (Harrington and Merzenich, 1970). Possibly summation from several receptors is required for humans. It is unlikely that stimulation of the type I unit does not have sensory consequences, but it is reasonable to expect that they will differ from those resulting from type II stimulation. The probability is also high that these receptors provide crucial input for tactile discriminative capabilities that are not simply related to the static pressure exerted by an object on the skin.

The static discharge of slowly adapting peripheral units does not continue indefinitely with sustained stimulation but eventually declines to near-spontaneous levels of activity (Chambers *et al.,* 1972; Horch and Burgess, 1975). Thus it might be expected that the overall sensitivity of the receptors is depressed with adaptation, such that they would be less sensitive to superimposed, transient changes in stimulus pressure, but the opposite is the case (Horch and Burgess, 1975). This suggests that a major function of the slowly adapting receptors is to extend the range of phasic skin sensitivity to circumstances involving high levels of background pressure. In general, we are more acutely aware of changes in tactile stimulation than we are of continual pressure (e.g., as produced by clothing). The type II receptor has several features of interest in relation to other tactile capabilities. Unlike type I receptors, Ruffini endings are exquisitely sensitive to stretch of the skin, and they exhibit some specificity for the direction of stretch (Chambers *et al.,* 1972). The importance of this observation is emphasized by a recent demonstration that skin stretch is the most salient cue for directional sensitivity on the human forearm (Gould and Vierck, 1976). Type II receptors are also characterized by their extremely regular rates of discharge, which presents some interesting possibilities for interval coding of the contour profile (texture) of an object impressed on the skin. Amassian and Giblin (1974) have proposed that cuneate nucleus touch neurons driven by different periodic inputs from convergent afferents (i.e., stimulated by a rough object) put out interspike interval patterns that theoretically can be discriminated from outputs resulting from similar convergent rates of input firing (stimulation with a smooth object), even though the mean rates of discharge are similar (see Fig. 6).

Several attempts have been made to assess the importance of the different spinal pathways for sensitivity to skin contact. Because absolute thresholds for touch could depend on any of the sensitive mechanoreceptors, it seems unlikely that any one pathway would be critical for this type of task, but a classical distinction between fine, epicritic touch and gross, protopathic touch could apply (Head, 1920). The implication is that the lemniscal system is optimally organized for spatial resolution, while the crossed tactile pathways contain units with large, overlapping receptive fields (extensive convergence) that are ideally suited for pressure sensitivity. Deficits of absolute pressure sensitivity in carnivores are produced by combined section of the ipsilateral dorsal and dorsolateral columns (Tapper, 1970; Norrsell, 1966), but similar impairments are not seen with either or both of these lesions in monkeys (Vierck, 1977).

Although absolute touch thresholds probably do not reflect activity only of slowly adapting receptors, discrimination of suprathreshold pressures might be dependent on slowly adapting units because of their wide range of pressure sensitivity. When monkeys are trained to discriminate differences in stimulus pressure applied to their feet, the resulting difference thresholds are elevated by dorsal column lesions, then recover to normal, are again elevated by dorsolateral lesions, and then return to preoperative levels of discrimination (Vierck, 1977). In monkeys, both type I and II units are thought to exit the dorsal columns and travel in the aberrant dorsal column pathway (Whitsel *et al.*, 1969a). Also, the convergence of touch input onto spinocervicothalamic cells of high dynamic range implicates the dorsolateral columns as a likely transmitter of pressure differentials. Thus it is surprising that dorsal column lesions have an effect on difference thresholds for pressure and also that there appears to be complete recovery of pressure discrimination after dorsal quadrant cord lesions in monkeys. Appar-

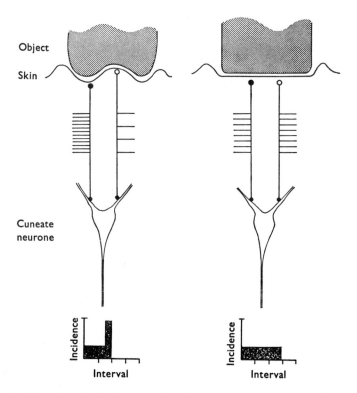

Fig. 6. Hypothetical mode of tactile discrimination of texture. In each case, several regularly discharging type II afferents are shown to project onto a single dorsal column nuclear cell. A rough stimulus (left) would cause a more marked difference in frequency of discharge in the two afferents (compared with the smooth stimulus on the right), resulting in a different pattern of postsynaptic discharge as depicted by the interspike interval histograms. From Amassian and Giblin (1974).

ently there are a variety of cues available to the animal for discrimination of punctate pressure. For example, stronger stimuli indent a wider area of skin than weaker stimuli and therefore excite a greater number of afferent units, in addition to provoking more intense discharge in those receptors near the probe.

TEMPERATURE

The sensations of cutaneous warmth and cold seem to be the easiest of the somesthetic "submodalities" to understand in terms of neural coding, because there exist singular "pure" receptor categories for each (Hensel, 1973). Thus it would be expected that the thermoneutral temperature would correspond to that point where the cold and warm fiber sensitivity curves intersect and that the intensities of cold and warmth sensations would simply be related to the relative discharge rates of cold vs. warm fibers supplying a given skin region. Several problems with this simplistic notion are presented, however, by the following relationships: assuming that warm spots are intermingled with cold receptors (which may not be valid, Poulos, 1975), the intersection of the sensitivity curves is probably higher (e.g., between 35°C and 40°C, Hensel, 1973) than the thermoneutral point (e.g., 30–35°C, Iggo and Young, 1975), which is higher than the peak of the cold-fiber sensitivity curve (less than 28°C, Gahery and Vigier, 1974; Iggo and Young, 1975; Poulos, 1975). Thus the thermoneutral point occurs at a temperature that evokes little or no activity in warm fibers and a mean rate of discharge in cold fibers that is comparable to that produced by distinctively colder stimuli (acting on the downslope of the sensitivity curve). This difficulty applies equally to sensing quick temperature changes or maintained levels, because the curves for mean rates of discharge during the dynamic or static phases of activity of cold receptors have similar forms. Since psychophysical difference thresholds for step decreases in temperature are comparable when the temperature pulses originate at adapting temperatures from 29°C to 41°C (Darian-Smith *et al.,* 1975), it appears that some factor other than mean rate of discharge contributes discriminative information. The necessity for some code other than overall discharge rate is less apparent in the warm range of temperatures, since the sensitivity curves of warm fibers are sharply truncated at high temperatures (that also evoke activity in thermal nociceptors).

Several possibilities have been offered for resolution of the dilemma presented by the sensitivity curves of cold fibers: (1) The type I and type II slowly adapting mechanoreceptors respond monotonically to decreasing temperature, below the sensitivity range of warm receptors (Poulos, 1975), and they might contribute useful thermal information if the nervous system could distinguish the activity generated in these units by mechanical and thermal stimuli (e.g., by the patterns of discharge elicited). (2) Evidence from several laboratories provides an interesting model of temporal coding in the sequencing of cold fiber action potentials (Iggo and Young, 1975; Poulos, 1975). Throughout much of their sensitivity range (e.g., below 35°C), cold fibers fire in bursts that are cleanly

C. VIERCK

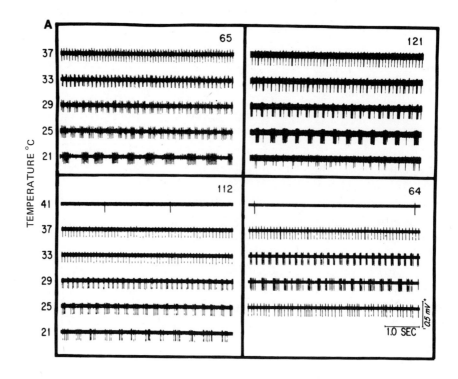

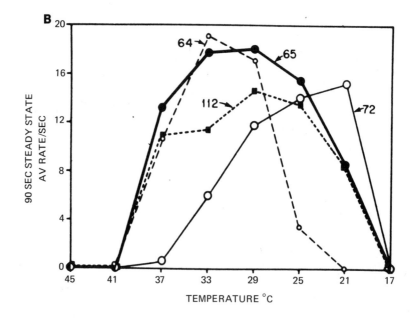

separated by silent periods, and the number of impulses per burst increases monotonically with decreasing temperature (see Fig. 7). In the trigeminal system, the bursting pattern is present at both peripheral and thalamic levels.

Beyond the observation that temperature sensation is lost following anterolateral chordotomy in humans (White and Sweet, 1969), there is a paucity of data on the participation of the different spinal pathways in transmission of information supplied by the peripheral temperature fibers. Because careful psychophysical measurements have not been made on chordotomy patients over a long recovery period, neither the severity of the initial deficit nor the possibility of recovery with pain sensitivity has been adequately evaluated, and companion studies on laboratory animals are not available. This is an important issue in light of the rarity of pure temperature units in any of the major ascending spinal pathways, including the spinothalamic tract of monkeys (Willis *et al.*, 1974; Brown, 1973).

Single-unit and lesion studies at the cerebral cortical level have similarly failed to reveal areas that are critically involved in temperature discrimination (Werner and Whitsel, 1973; Cragg and Downer, 1967). In monkeys, combined lesion of areas SI, SII, and posterior parietal areas 5 and 7 is without substantial effect on thresholds of thermal discrimination, although the number of errors is increased at small temperature differences that are difficult for normal monkeys to differentiate (1°C, Cragg and Downer, 1967). Thus it would seem as if the cerebral cortex is not involved in any way with temperature sensations, except for a fascinating

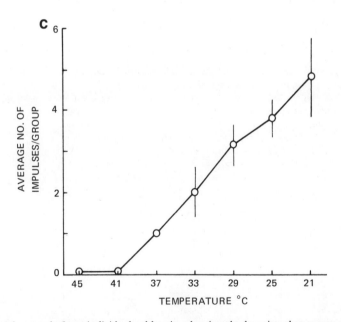

Fig. 7. A: Sample records from individual cold units, showing the bursting that occurs with increased prominence at lower temperatures. B: Curves of average steady-state response rates as functions of temperature for three of the units in A (i.e., Nos. 64, 65, and 112). C: Average number of spikes per group for the cold fibers, showing a direct relationship with temperature, rather than the curvilinear curves of B. From Poulos (1975).

contradiction that has come from studies of interhemispheric transfer of thermal discriminations. If normal monkeys are trained to recognize gross temperature differences (15°C vs. 45°C) by palpation of the stimulus objects with one hand (or foot), there is immediate transfer of the discrimination to the other hand (or foot). Other monkeys that receive a complete section of the corpus callosum (or lesion of the somatosensory areas of the "trained" hemisphere), before or after training of the first limb, show no subsequent transfer of the skill to the second limb (Cragg and Downer, 1967; Ebner and Myers, 1962). The impression gained from these results is that the critical information processed by the cortex and transferred by the corpus callosum has more to do with "strategies" of discriminative behavior than the fundamental thermal cues. This is reinforced by anatomical observations that the distal extremity regions of the SI and SII areas of the two sides do not connect through the corpus callosum (although the proximal limb regions are interconnected, Jones and Powell, 1973).

References

Albe-Fessard, D., Levante, A., and Lamour, Y. Origin of spinothalamic tract in monkeys. *Brain Res.,* 1974, *65,* 503–509.

Albe-Fessard, D., Boivie, J., Grant, G., and Levante, A. Labelling of cells in the medulla oblongata and the spinal cord of the monkey after injections of horseradish peroxidase in the thalamus. *Neurosci. Lett.,* 1975, *1,* 75–80.

Allen, G. C., Orbach, J., Berman, D., and Berman, A. J. Forelimb deafferentation in rhesus monkeys: Precise movements without visual guidance. *Neurosci. Abstr.,* 1975, *1,* 155.

Allen, W. F. Effect of partial and complete destruction of the tactile cerebral cortex on correct conditioned differential foreleg response from cutaneous stimulation. *Am. J. Physiol.,* 1947, *151,* 325–337.

Amassian, V. E., and Giblin, D. Periodic components in steady-state activity of cuneate neurones and their possible role in sensory coding. *J. Physiol. (London),* 1974, *243,* 353–385.

Andersson, S. A., Finger, S., and Norrsell, U. Cerebral units activated by tactile stimuli via a ventral spinal pathway in monkeys. *Acta Physiol. Scand.,* 1975, *93,* 119–128.

Andres, K. H., and von Düring, M. Morphology of cutaneous receptors. In *Handbook of Sensory Physiology,* Vol. II. Springer-Verlag, Berlin, 1973, pp. 3–28.

Andrew, B. L. The sensory innervation of the medial ligament of the knee joint. *J. Physiol. (London),* 1954, *123,* 241–250.

Angaut-Petit, D. The dorsal column system. II. Functional properties and bulbar relay of the post-synaptic fibers of the cat's fasciculus gracilis. *Exp. Brain Res.,* 1975, *22,* 471–493.

Applebaum, A. E., Beall, J. E., Foreman, R. D., and Willis, N. D. Organization and receptive fields of primate spinothalamic tract neurons. *J. Neurophysiol.,* 1975, *38,* 572–586.

Azulay, A., and Schwartz, A. S. The role of the dorsal funiculus of the primate in tactual discriminations. *Exp. Neurol.,* 1975, *46,* 315–332.

Baker, M. A., Tyner, C. F., and Towe, A. L. Observations on single neurons recorded in the sigmoid gyre of awake, nonparalyzed cats. *Exp. Neurol.,* 1971, *32,* 388–403.

Basbaum, A. Conduction of the effects of noxious stimulation by short-fiber multisynaptic systems in the spinal cord of the rat. *Exp. Neurol.,* 1973, *40,* 699–716.

Bates, J. A. V., and Ettlinger, G. Posterior biparietal ablations in the monkey. *Arch. Neurol. (Chicago),* 1960, *9,* 333–335.

Bava, A., Fadiga, E., and Mangoni, T. Extra lemniscal reactivity and commissural linkages in the VPL nucleus of cats with chronic cortical lesions. *Arch. Ital. Biol.,* 1968, *106,* 204–206.

Beck, C., and Chanbers, W. W. Speed, accuracy and strength of forelimb movement after unilateral pepamidotomy in rhesus monkeys. *J. Comp. Physiol. Psychol. Monoqr.,* 1970, *70,* 1–22.

Benjamin, F. G. Release of intracellular potassium as a factor in pain production. In D. R. Kenshalo (ed.), *The Skin Senses.* Thomas, Springfield, Ill., 1968, pp. 466–479.

Berkley, K. J., and Parmer, R. Somatosensory cortical involvement in response to noxious stimulation in the cat. *Exp. Brain Res.*, 1974, *20*, 363–374.

Bessou, P., and Perl, E. R. Response of cutaneous sensory units with unmyelinated fibers to noxious stimuli. *J. Neurophysiol.*, 1969, *32*, 1025–1043.

Bessou, P., Burgess, P. R., Perl, E. R., and Taylor, C. B. Dynamic properties of mechanoreceptors with unmyelinated (C) fibers. *J. Neurophysiol.*, 1971, *34*, 116–131.

Blomquist, A. J., and Lorenzini, C. A. Projection of dorsal roots and sensory nerves to cortical sensory motor regions of squirrel monkey. *J. Neurophysiol.*, 1965, *28*, 1195–1205.

Blum, P., and Whitehorn, D. Wide-field neurons in the cuneate nucleus of cat. *Fed. Proc.*, 1973, *32*, 399.

Boivie, J. The termination of the cervicothalamic tract in the cat: An experimental study with silver impregnation methods. *Brain Res.*, 1970, *19*, 333–360.

Boivie, J. The termination of the spinothalamic tract in the cat. An experimental study with silver impregnation methods. *Exp. Brain Res.*, 1971, *12*, 331–353.

Bossom, J., and Ommaya, A. K. Visuomotor adaption (to prismatic transformation of the retinal image) in monkeys with bilateral dorsal rhizotomy. *Brain*, 1966, *91*, 161–172.

Bowsher, D. The anatomophysiological basis of somatosensory discrimination. *Int. Rev. Neurobiol.*, 1965, *8*, 35–75.

Bowsher, D. Characteristics of central non-specific somatosensory systems. In H. H. Kornhuber (ed.), *The Somatosensory System.* Georg Theime, Stuttgart, 1975, pp. 68–77.

Bowsher, D., Mallart, A., Petit, D., and Albe-Fessard, D. A bulbar relay to the centre median. *J. Neurophysiol.*, 1968, *31*, 288–300.

Boyd, I. A., and Roberts, T. D. M. Proprioceptive discharges from stretch receptors in the knee joint of the cat. *J. Physiol. (London)*, 1953, *122*, 38–58.

Brindley, G. S., and Merton, P. A. The absence of position sense in the human eye. *J. Physiol. (London)*, 1960, *153*, 127–130.

Brown, A. G. Cutaneous afferent fiber collaterals in the dorsal column of the cat. *Exp. Brain Res.*, 1968, *5*, 293–305.

Brown, A. G. Effects of descending impulses on transmission through the spinocervical tract. *J. Physiol. (London)*, 1971, *219*, 103–125.

Brown, A. G. Ascending and long spinal pathways: Dorsal columns, spinocervical tract and spinothalamic tract. In *Handbook of Sensory Physiology*, Vol. II. Springer-Verlag, Berlin, 1973, pp. 315–338.

Brown, A. G., and Franz, D. N. Responses of spinocervical tract neurones to natural stimulation of identified cutaneous receptors. *Exp. Brain Res.*, 1969, *7*, 231–249.

Brown, A. G., and Iggo, A. A quantitative study of cutaneous receptors and afferent fibers in the cat and rabbit. *J. Physiol. (London)*, 1967, *193*, 707–733.

Brown, A. G., and Martin H. F., III. Effects on transmission through the spinocervical tract evoked from the dorsal columns and the dorsal column nuclei. *J. Physiol. (London)*, 1972, *224*, 34–35P.

Brown, A. G., Gordon, G., and Kay, R. H. Cutaneous receptive properties of single fibers in the cat's medial lemniscus. *J. Physiol. (London)*, 1970, *211*, 37–39P.

Browne, M. C., Lee, J., and Ring, P. A. The sensation of passive movement at the metatarso-phalangeal joint of the great toe in man. *J. Physiol. (London)*, 1954, *126*, 448–458.

Bryan, R. N., Coultier, J. D., and Willis, W. D. Cells of origin of the spinocervical tract in the monkey. *Exp. Neurol.*, 1974, *42*, 574–536.

Bucy, P. C., Ladpli, R., and Ehrlich, A. Destruction of the pyramidal tract in the monkey. *J. Neurosurg.*, 1966, *25*, 1–20.

Burgess, P. R. Patterns of discharge evoked in cutaneous nerves and their significance for sensation. *Adv. Neurol.*, 1974, *4*, 11–18.

Burgess, P. R., and Clark, F. J. Characteristics of knee joint receptors in the cat. *J. Physiol. (London)*, 1969a, *203*, 301–317.

Burgess, P. R., and Clark, F. J. Dorsal column projection of fibers from the cat knee joint. *J. Physiol. (London)*, 1969b, *203*, 281–299.

Burgess, P. R., and Perl, E. R. Myelinated afferent fibers responding specifically to noxious stimulation of the skin. *J. Physiol. (London)*, 1967, *190*, 541–562.

Burgess, P. R., and Perl, E. R. Cutaneous mechanoreceptors and nocicepto_s. In *Handbook of Sensory Physiology*, Vol. 2. Springer-Verlag, Berlin, 1973, pp. 29–78.

Burgess, P. R., Petit, D., and Warren R. M. Receptor types in cat hairy skin supplied by myelinated fibers. *J. Neurophysiol.*, 1968, *31*, 833–855.

Carreras, M., and Andersson, S. A. Functional properties of neurons of the anterior ectosylvian gyrus of the cat. *J. Neurophysiol.*, 1963, *26*, 100–126.

Casey, K. L., Keene, J. J., and Morrow, T. Bulboreticular and medial thalamic unit activity in relation to aversive behavior and pain. *Adv. Neurol.*, 1974, *4*, 197–206.

Cauna, N. Functional significance of the submicroscopical, histochemical and microscopical organization of the cutaneous receptor organs. *Anat. Anz.*, 1962, *3*, Suppl. 2, 181–197.

Cauna, N. Fine structure of the receptor organs and its probable functional significance. In A. V. S. de Reuk and J. Knight (eds.), *Touch, Heat and Pain.* Churchill, London, 1966, pp. 117–127.

Chambers, M. F., Andres, K. H., Duering, M. V., and Iggo, A. The structure and function of the slowly adaptive type II receptor in hairy skin. *A. J. Exp. Physiol.*, 1972, *57*, 417–445.

Christensen, B. N., and Perl, E. R. Spinal neurons specifically excited by noxious or thermal stimuli: Marginal zone of the dorsal horn. *J. Neurophysiol.*, 1970, *33*, 293–307.

Clark, F. J., Horch, K. W., Burgess, P. R., and Bach, S. M. Static awareness of knee joint angle is not affected by local anesthetic block of knee joint receptors. *Neurosci. Abstr.*, 1975, *1*, 132.

Clifton, G. L., Vance, W. H., Applebaum, M. L., Coggeshall, R. F., and Willis, W. D., Jr. Responses of unmyelinated afferents in the mammalian ventral root. *Brain Res.*, 1974, *32*, 163–167.

Cole, J., and Glees, P. Effects of small lesions in sensory cortex in trained monkeys. *J. Neurophysiol.*, 1954, *17*, 1–13.

Conrad, B., Matsunami, K., Meger-Lohmann, J., Wiesendanger, N., and Brooks, V. B. Cortical load compensation during voluntary elbow movements. *Brain Res.*, 1974, *71*, 507–514.

Cook, A. W., and Browder, E. J. Function of posterior columns in man. *Arch. Neurol. (Chicago)*, 1965, *12*, 72–79.

Corkin, S., Milner, B., and Rasmussen, T. Effects of different cortical excisions on sensory thresholds in man. *Trans. Am. Neurol. Assoc.*, 1964, 112–116.

Coultier, J. D. Sensory transmission through lemniscal pathway during voluntary movement in the cat. *J. Neurophysiol.*, 1974, *37*, 831–845.

Coultier, J. D., Maunz, R. A., and Willis, W. D. Effects of stimulation of sensorimotor cortex on primate spinothalamic neurons. *Brain Res.*, 1974, *65*, 351–356.

Cragg, B. G., and Downer, J. de C. Behavioral evidence for cortical involvement in manual temperature discrimination in the monkey. *Exp. Neurol.*, 1967, *19*, 433–442.

Critchley, J. *The Parietal Lobes.* Hafner, New York, 1969.

Cross, M. J., and McCloskey, D. I. Position sense following surgical removal of joints. *Brain Res.*, 1973, *55*, 443–445.

Curry, M. J. The exteroceptive properties of neurones in the somatic part of the posterior groups (PO). *Brain Res.*, 1972, *44*, 439–462.

Darian-Smith, I., Isbister, J., Mok, H., and Yokota, T. Somatic sensory cortical projection areas excited by tactile stimulation of the cat: A triple representation. *J. Physiol. (London)*, 1966, *182*, 671–689.

Darian-Smith, I., Johnson, K. O., and LaMotte, C. Peripheral neural determinants in the sensing of changes in skin temperature. In H. H. Kornhuber (ed.), *The Somatosensory System.* Georg Thieme, Stuttgart, 1975, 23–37.

Dart, A. M., and Gordon, G. Some properties of spinal connections of the cat's dorsal column nuclei which do not involve the dorsal columns. *Brain Res.*, 1973, *58*, 61–68.

Denavit, M., and Korsinski, E. E. Somatic afferents to the cat subthalamus. *Arch. Ital. Biol.*, 1968, *106*, 391–411.

Denny-Brown, D., and Chambers, R. A. The parietal lobe and behavior. *Assoc. Res. Nerv. Ment. Dis.*, 1958, *36*, 35–117.

DeVito, J. L., Ruch, T. C., and Patton, H. D. Analysis of residual weight discriminatory ability and evoked potentials following section of dorsal columns in monkeys. *Indian J. Physiol. Pharmacol.*, 1964, *8*, 117–126.

Diamond, I. T. The sensory neocortex. *Contrib. Sensory Physiol.* 1967, *2*, 51.

Diamond, I. T., Randall, W., and Springer. L. Tactual localization in cats deprived of cortical areas SI and SII and the dorsal columns. *Psychon. Sci.*, 1964, *1*, 261–262.

Dobry, P. J. K., and Casey, K. L. Roughness discrimination in cats with dorsal column lesions. *Brain Res.*, 1972*a*, *44*, 385–397.

Dobry, P. J. K., and Casey, K. L. Coronal somatosensory unit responses in cats with dorsal column lesions. *Brain Res.*, 1972*b*, *44*, 399–416.

Douglass, W. W., and Ritchie, J. M. Non-medullated fibers in the saphenous nerve which signal touch. *J. Physiol. (London)*, 1957, *139*, 385–399.

Dräger, V. C., and Hubel, D. H. Responses to visual stimulation and relationship between visual, auditory and somatosensory inputs in mouse superior colliculus. *J. Neurophysiol.*, 1975, *36*, 690–713.

Dreyer, D. A., Schneider, R. J., Metz, C. B., and Whitsel, B. L. Differential contributions of spinal pathways to body representation in postcentral gyrus of *Macaca mulatta. J. Neurophysiol.,* 1974, *37,* 119–145.

Dubrovsky, B., and Garcia-Rill, E. Role of dorsal columns in sequential motor acts requiring precise forelimb projection. *Exp. Brain Res.,* 1973, *18,* 165–177.

Dubrovsky, B., Davelaar, F., and Garcia-Rill, E. The role of dorsal columns in serial order acts. *Exp. Neurol.,* 1971, *33,* 93–102.

Duffy, F. H., and Burchfiel, J. L. Somatosensory system: Organizational hierarchy from single units in monkey area 5. *Science,* 1971, *172,* 273–275.

Dyhre-Poulsen, P. Increased vibration threshold before movements in human subjects. *Exp. Neurol.,* 1975, *47,* 516–522.

Ebner, F. F., and Myers, R. F. Corpus callosum and the interhemispheric transfer of tactual learning. *J. Neurophysiol.,* 1962, *25,* 380–391.

Eidelberg, E., and Schwartz, A. S. Experimental analysis of the extinction phenomenon in monkeys. *Brain,* 1971, *94,* 91–108.

Eidelberg, E., and Woodbury, C. M. Apparent redundancy in the somatosensory system in monkeys. *Exp. Neurol.,* 1972, *37,* 573–581.

Eidelberg, E., Kreinick, C. J., and Langescheid, C. On the possible functional role of afferent pathways in skin sensation. *Exp. Neurol.,* 1975, *47,* 419–432.

Erickson, R. P. Stimulus coding in topographic and non-topographic modalities: On the significance of the activity of individual sensory neurons. *Psychol. Rev.,* 1968, *75,* 447–465.

Evarts, E. V., and Tanji, J. Gating of motor cortex reflexes by prior instruction. *Brain Res.,* 1974, *71,* 479–494.

Ferraro, A., and Barrera, S. E. Effects of experimental lesions of the posterior columns in *Macacus rhesus* monkeys. *Brain,* 1934, *57,* 307–332.

Festinger, L. Eye movements and perception. In P. Bach-Y-Rita *et al.* (eds.), *The Control of Eye Movements.* Academic Press, New York, 1971, pp. 259–273.

Fields, H. L., Partridge, L. D., and Winter, D. L. Somatic and visual receptive field properties of fibers in ventral quadrant white matter of the cat spinal cord. *J. Neurophysiol.,* 1970, *33,* 827–837.

Fields, H. L., Adams, J. E., and Hosobuchi, Y. Peripheral nerve and cutaneous electrohypalgesia. *Adv. Neurol.,* 1974, *4,* 749–754.

Franz, D. N., and Iggo, A. Dorsal root potentials and ventral root reflexes evoked by non myelinated fibers. *Science,* 1968, *162,* 1140–1142.

Frommer, G. P., Trefz, B. R., and Casey, K. L. Somatosensory function and cortical unit activity in cats with only dorsal column fibers. *Neurosci. Abstr.,* 1975, *1,* 120.

Gahery, Y., and Vigier, D. Inhibitory effects in the cuneate nucleus produced by vago-aortic afferent fibers. *Brain Res.,* 1974, *75,* 241–246.

Galbraith, G. C., Gottschaldt, K.-M., and Schultz, W. Unit activity in the somatosensory cortex of the cat and its relation to discharge in primary afferent fibers from the sinus hair follicles. *Proc. Physiol. Soc.,* 1974, *244,* 73–74P.

Gardner, E. P., and Spencer, W. A. Sensory funneling. II. Cortical neuronal representation of patterned cutaneous stimuli. *J. Neurophysiol.,* 1972, *35,* 954–977.

Geldard, F. The perception of mechanical vibration. I. History of a controversy. *J. Gen. Psychol.,* 1940, *22,* 243–269.

Ghez, C., and Pisa, M. Inhibition of afferent transmission in cuneate nucleus during voluntary movement in the cat. *Brain Res.,* 1972, *40,* 145–151.

Gibson, J. J. Observations on active touch. *Psychol. Rev.,* 1962, *69,* 477–491.

Gilman, S., and Denny-Brown, D. Disorders of movement and behavior following dorsal column lesions. *Brain,* 1966, *89,* 397–418.

Glassman, R. B. Cutaneous discrimination and motor control following somatosensory cortical ablations. *Physiol. Behav.,* 1970, *5,* 1009–1019.

Glassman, R. B. Discrimination of passively received kinesthetic stimuli following sensorimotor cortical ablations in cats. *Physiol. Behav.,* 1971, *7,* 239–243.

Glassman, R. B., Forgus, M. W., Goodman, J. E., and Glassman, H. N. Somesthetic effects of damage of cat's ventrobasal complex, medial lemniscus or posterior group. *Exp. Neurol.,* 1975, *48,* 460–492.

Glenndenning, K. K., Hall, J. A., Diamond, I. T., and Hall, W. C. The pulvinar nucleus of *Galago senegalensis. J. Comp. Neurol.,* 1975, *161,* 419–458.

Goldberg, M. E., and Wurtz, R. H. Activity of superior colliculus in behaving monkey. II. Effect of attention on neuronal responses. *J. Neurophysiol.,* 1972, *35,* 560–574.

Goodwin, G. M., McCloskey, D. I., and Mathews, P. B. C. The contribution of muscle afferents to kinesthesia shown by vibration induced illusions of movement and by the effects of paralysing joint afferents. *Brain,* 1972, *95*, 705–748.

Gordon, G. The concept of relay nuclei. In *Handbook of Sensory Physiology,* Vol. II. Springer-Verlag, Berlin, 1973, pp. 137–150.

Gordon, G., and Horrobin, D. Antidromic and synaptic responses in the cat's gracile nucleus to cerebellar stimulation. *Brain Res.,* 1967, *5*, 419–421.

Gordon, G., and Jukes, M. G. M. Dual organization of the exteroceptive component of the cat's gracile nucleus. *J. Physiol. (London),* 1964, *173*, 263–290.

Gordon, G., and Manson, J. R. Cutaneous receptive fields of single nerve cells in the thalamus of the cat. *Nature (London),* 1967, *215*, 597–599.

Gordon, G., and Seed, W. A. An investigation of nucleus gracilis of the cat by antidromic stimulation. *J. Physiol.,* 1961, *155*, 589–601.

Gould, W. R. and Vierck, C. T., Jr. Cues supporting recognition orientation of tactile stimuli. *Neuroscience Abst.* 1976, *2*, 936.

Granit, R. *The Basis of Motor Control.* Academic Press, New York, 1970.

Ha, H. Cervicothalamic tract in the rhesus monkey. *Exp. Neurol.,* 1971, *33*, 205–212.

Hagbarth, K.-E., Hongell, A., Hallin, R. G., and Torebjörk, H. E. Afferent impulses in median nerve fascicles evoked by tactile stimuli of the human hand. *Brain Res.,* 1970, *24*, 423–442.

Hancock, M. B., Foreman, R. D., and Willis, W. D. Convergence of visceral and cutaneous input onto spinothalamic tract cells in the thoracic spinal cord of the cat. *Exp. Neurol.,* 1975, *47*, 240–248.

Hardy, J. D., and Oppel, T. W. Studies in temperature sensation. III. the sensitivity of the body to heat and the spatial summation of the end organ response. *J. Clin. Invest.,* 1937, *16*, 533–540.

Harrington, T., and Merzenich, M. M. Neural coding of the sense of touch: Human sensations of skin indentation compared with the responses of slowly adapting mechanoreceptive afferents innervating the hairy skin of monkeys. *Exp. Brain Res.,* 1970, *10*, 251–264.

Head, H. *Studies in Neurology.* Oxford, London, 1920.

Heilman, K., Pandya, D. N., and Geschwind, N. Trimodal inattention following parietal lobe ablations. *Trans. Am. Neurol. Assoc.,* 1970, *95*, 259–261.

Heinbecker, P., Bishop, G. H., and O'Leary, J. Pain and touch fibers in peripheral nerves. *Arch. Neurol. Psychiat.,* 1933, *29*, 771–789.

Hensel, H. Cutaneous thermoreceptors. In *Handbook of Sensory Physiology, Vol.* II. Springer-Verlag, New York, 1973, pp. 79–110.

Hensel, H., Iggo, A., and Witt, I. A quantitative study of sensitive thermoreceptors with C afferent fibers. *J. Physiol.,* 1960, *153*, 113–126.

Hensel, H. Andres, K. H., and During, M. V. Structure and function of cold receptors. *Pflügers Arch.,* 1974, *352*, 1–10.

Holmes, G. Cronnian lectures on the clinical symptoms of cerebellar disease. Lecture IV. *Lancet,* 1922, *2*, 111–115.

Horch, K. W., and Burgess, P. R. Effect of activation and adaptation on the sensitivity of slowly adapting cutaneous mechanoreceptors. *Brain Res.,* 1975, *98*, 109–118.

Horch, K. W., Burgess, P. R., and Poulos, D. A. Temporal effects on magnitude sensations produced by skin indentation in humans. *Neurosci. Abstr.,* 1975, *1*, 122.

Horrobin, D. F. The lateral cervical nucleus of the cat; an electrophysiological study. *Q. J. Exp. Physiol.,* 1966, *51*, 351–371.

Hunt, C. C. On the nature of vibration receptors in the hind limb of the cat. *J. Physiol. (London)* 1961, *155*, 175.

Hunt, C. C. The Pacinian corpuscle. In J. I. Hubbard (ed.), *The Peripheral Nervous System.* Plenum, New York, 1974, pp. 405–420.

Hunt, C. C., and McIntyre, A. K. An analysis of fibre diameter and receptor characteristics of myelinated cutaneous afferent fibres in cat. *J. Physiol. (London),* 1960, *153*, 99–112.

Hyvarinen, J., and Poranen, A. Function of the parietal associative area 7 as revealed from cellular discharges in alert monkeys. *Brain,* 1974, *97*, 673–692.

Iggo, A. Gastric mucosal receptors with vagal afferent fibres in the cat. *Q. J. Exp. Physiol.,* 1957, *42*, 398–409.

Iggo, A. Cutaneous heat and cold receptors with slowly conducting (C) afferent fibres. *Q. J. Exp. Physiol.,* 1959, *44*, 362–370.

Iggo, A. Cutaneous mechanoreceptors with afferent C fibres. *J. Physiol. (London),* 1960, *152*, 337–353.

Iggo, A. Pain and pain receptors. In A. V. S. de Reuck and J. Knight (eds.), *Touch, Heat and Pain.* Little, Brown, Boston, 1966*a*, pp. 360–366.

Iggo, A. Cutaneous receptors with a high sensitivity to mechanical displacement. In A. V. S. de Reuck and J. Knight (eds.), *Touch, Heat and Pain.* Little, Brown, Boston, 1966*b*, pp. 237–256.

Iggo, A. Cutaneous receptors. In J. I. Hubbard (ed.), *The Peripheral Nervous System.* Plenum, New York, 1974, pp. 347–404.

Iggo, A., and Muir, A. R. The structure and function of a slowly adapting touch corpuscle in hairy skin. *J. Physiol. (London),* 1969, *200,* 763–796.

Iggo, A., and Ogawa, H. Primate cutaneous thermal nociceptors. *J. Physiol. (London),* 1971, *216,* 77–78P.

Iggo, A., and Young, D. W. Cutaneous thermoreceptors and thermal nociceptors. In H. H. Kornhuber (ed.), *The Somatosensory System.* Georg Thieme, Stuttgart, 1975, pp. 5–22.

Iniuchijima, J., and Zotterman, Y. The specificity of afferent cutaneous C fibres in mammals. *Acta Physiol. Scand.,* 1960, *49,* 267–273.

Jabbur, S. J., and Atweh, S. I. Visual, auditory and somatic interactions in the cuneate nucleus. In H. H. Kornhuber (ed.), *The Somatosensory System.* Georg Thieme, Stuttgart, 1975, pp. 115–122.

Jabbur, S. J., Baker, M. A., and Towe, A. L. Wide-field neurons in thalamic nucleus ventralis posterolateralis of the cat. *Exp. Neurol.,* 1972, *36,* 213–238.

Jänig, W. Morphology of rapidly and slowly adapting mechanoreceptors in the hairless skin of the cat's hind foot. *Brain Res.,* 1971, *28,* 217–232.

Jasper, H. H. *et al.* (eds.). *The Reticular Formation of the Brain.* Little, Brown, Boston, 1958.

Jones, E. G., and Powell, T. P. S. Connections of the somatic sensory cortex of the rhesus monkey. I. Ipsilateral cortical connections. *Brain,* 1969*a,* *92,* 504–531.

Jones, E. G., and Powell, T. P. S. The cortical projection of the ventroposterior nucleus of the thalamus in the cat. *Brain Res.,* 1969*b,* *13,* 298–318.

Jones, E. G., and Powell, T. P. S. Connections of the somatic sensory cortex of the rhesus monkey. III. Thalamic connections. *Brain,* 1970, *93,* 37–56.

Jones, E. G., and Powell, T. P. S. Anatomical organization of the somatosensory cortex. In *Handbook of Sensory Physiology,* Vol. 2. Springer-Verlag, Berlin, 1973, pp. 579–620.

Keating, E. G. Impaired orientation after primate tectal lesions. *Brain Res.,* 1974, *67,* 533–541.

Keating, E. G., and Horel, J. A. Somatosensory deficit produced by parietal-temporal cortical disconnection in the monkey. *Exp. Neurol.,* 1971, *33,* 547–565.

Keele, C. A., and Armstrong, D. *Substances Producing Pain and Itch.* Arnold, London, 1964.

Kennard, M. A. The course of ascending fibers in the spinal cord of the cat essential to the recognition of painful stimuli. *J. Comp. Neurol.,* 1954, *100,* 511–524.

Kennard, M. A., and Kessler, M. M. Studies of motor performance after parietal ablations in monkeys. *J. Neurophysiol.,* 1940, *3,* 248–257.

Kerr, F. W. L. The ventral spinothalamic tract and other ascending systems of the ventral funiculus of the spinal cord. *J. Comp. Neurol.,* 1975, *159,* 335–356.

Kerr, F. W. L., and Lippman, H. H. The primate spinothalamic tract as demonstrated by anterolateral cordotomy and commissural myelotomy. *Adv. Neurol.,* 1974, *4,* 147–156.

King, R. B. Postchordotomy studies of pain threshold. *Neurology,* 1957, *7,* 610–669.

Kitai, S. T., and Weinberg, J. Tactile discrimination study of the dorsal column–medial lemniscal system and spino-cervico-thalamic tract in cat. *Exp. Brain Res.,* 1968, *6,* 234–246.

Knapp, H. D., Taub, E., and Berman, A. J. Movements in monkeys with deafferented limbs. *Exp. Neurol.,* 1963, *7,* 305–315.

Knibestöl, M., and Vallbo, A. B. Single unit analysis of mechanoreceptor activity from the human glabrous skin. *Acta Physiol. Scand.,* 1970, *80,* 178–195.

Korner, L., and Landgren, S. Projections of low threshold joint afferents to the cerebral cortex of the cat. *Acta Physiol. Scand.,* 1969, *76,* 5A–7A.

Kornhuber, H. H. Motor functions of cerebellum and basal ganglia: The cerebellocortical saccadic (ballistic) clock, the cerebellonuclear hold regulator, and the basal ganglia ramp (voluntary speed smooth movement) generator. *Kybernetik,* 1971, *8,* 157–162.

Kostyuk, P. G., and Skibo, G. G. Synaptic transmission of proprioceptive and cutaneous volleys through the Burdach nucleus. *Neurosci. Transl.,* 1969, *6,* 623–630.

Kruger, L., and Kenton, B. Quantitative neural and psychophysical data for cutaneous mechanoreceptor function. *Brain Res.,* 1973, *49,* 1–24.

Kruger, L., and Mosso, J. A. An evaluation of duality in the trigeminal afferent system. *Adv. Neurol.,* 1974, *4,* 73–82.

Kruger, L., and Porter, P. A behavioral study of the functions of the rolandic cortex in the monkey. *J. Comp. Neurol.,* 1958, *109,* 439–469.

Kruger, L., Siminoff, R., and Witkovsky, P. Single neuron analysis of dorsal column nuclei and spinal nucleus of trigeminal in cat. *J. Neurophysiol.*, 1961, *24*, 333–349.

Lamotte, R. H., and Acuna, C. Defects in accurate projection of the contralateral arm into extrapersonal space in monkeys after removal of the posterior parietal association cortex. *Neurosci. Abstr.*, 1975, *1*, 131.

Lamotte, R. H., and Mountcastle, V. B. Capacities of humans and monkeys to discriminate between vibratory stimuli of different frequency and amplitude. *J. Neurophysiol.*, 1975, *38*, 539–559.

Landgren, S., Silfvenius, H., and Wolsk, D. Somato-sensory paths to the second cortical projection areas of the group I muscle afferents. *J. Physiol. (London)*, 1967, *191*, 543–559.

Lashley, K. S. The accuracy of movement in the absence of excitation from the moving organ. *Am. J. Physiol.*, 1917, *43*, 169–194.

Laskin, S. E. Cortical correlates of cutaneous masking: A comparison of psychophysical and electrophysiological inhibitory functions. Doctoral dissertation, New York University, 1975.

Lawrence, D. G., and Kuypers, H. G. J. M. The functional organization of the motor system in the monkey. I. The effects of bilateral pyramidal lesions. *Brain*, 1968, *91*, 1–14.

Levitt, M., and Levitt, J. Sensory hind limb representation of Sm I cortex of the cat after spinal tractotomies. *Exp. Neurol.*, 1968, *22*, 276–302.

Levitt, M., and Levitt, J. Limb position sense after Rolandic cortex ablations. *Anat. Rec.*, 1969, *163*, 218.

Levitt, J., and Levitt, M. Post central somatic mechanoreception. I. Dorsal column and anterolateral lesions. *Proc. Soc. Neurosci.*, 1974*a*, *4*, 306.

Levitt, M., and Levitt, J. Post central somatic mechanoreception. II. Dorsal quadrant, hemisection and anterolateral lesions. *Proc. Soc. Neurosci.*, 1974, *4*, 307.

Levitt, M., and Schwartzman, R. J. Spinal sensory tracts and two-point tactile sensitivity. *Anat. Rec.*, 1966, *154*, 377.

Lewis, T. *Pain.* Macmillan, New York, 1942.

Lim, R. K. S. Pain. *Annu. Rev. Physiol.*, 1970, *32*, 269–288.

Lindahl, O. Pain—a general chemical explanation. *Adv. Neurol.*, 1974, *4*, 45–48.

Lindblom, V. Properties of touch receptors in distal glabrous skin of the monkey. *J. Neurophysiol.*, 1965, *28*, 966–985.

Liu, C. N., Yu, J., Chambers, W. W., and Ha, H. The role of the medial lemniscal and spinocervicothalamic pathways on tactile reactions in cats. *Acta Neurobiol. Exp.* 1975, *35*, 149–157.

Livingston, W. K. *Pain Mechanisms: A Physiologic Interpretation of Causalgia and Its Related States.* Macmillan, New York 1943.

Lloyd, A., and Caldwell, L. S. Accuracy of active and passive positioning of the leg on the basis of kinesthetic cues. *J. Comp. Physiol. Psychol.*, 1965, *60*, 102–106.

Long, R. R. Cold fiber heat sensitivity: Dependency of "paradoxical" discharge on body temperature. *Brain Res.*, 1973, *63*, 389–392.

Lundberg, A., and Oscarsson, O. Two ascending spinal pathways in the ventral part of the cord. *Acta. Physiol. Scand.*, 1962, *51*, 270–286.

Lynn, B. The nature and location of certain phasic mechanoreceptors in the cat's foot. *J. Physiol. (London)*, 1969, *201*, 765–773.

Lynn, B. Somatosensory receptors and their CNS connections. *Annu. Rev. Physiol.*, 1975, *37*, 105–127.

Malinovsky, L. Variability of sensory nerve endings in foot pads of a domestic cat. *Acta. Anat.*, 1966, *64*, 82–106.

Mark, V. H., Ervin, F. R., and Yakolw, P. I. Stereotaxic thalamotomy. III. The verification of anatomical lesion sites in the human thalamus. *Arch. Neurol.*, 1963, *8*, 528–538.

Martin, R. F., Applebaum, A. E., Forman, R. D., Beall, J. E., and Willis, W. D. Responses to cutaneous thermal stimulation of spinothalamic tract neurons in the monkey. *Neurosci. Abstr.*, 1975, *1*, 147.

Mathews, P. B. *Mammalian Muscle Receptors and Their Central Actions.* Williams and Wilkins, Baltimore, 1972.

Mayer, D. J., and Liebeskind, J. C. Pain reduction by focal electrical stimulation of the brain: An anatomical and behavioral analysis. *Brain Res.*, 1974, *68*, 73–93.

Mehler, W. R. The mammalian "pain" tract in phylogeny. *Anat. Rec.*, 1957, *127*, 332.

Mehler, W. R. Some observations on secondary ascending afferent systems in the central nervous system. In R. S. Knighton and P. R. Dumke (eds.), *Pain.* Little, Brown, Boston, 1966, pp. 11–32.

Mehler, W. R., Feferman, M. E., and Nauta, W. J. H. Ascending axon degeneration following anterolateral cordotomy: An experimental study in the monkey. *Brain*, 1960, *83*, 718–750.

Melzack, R. Prolonged relief of pain by brief, intense transcutaneous somatic stimulation. *Pain*, 1975, *1*, 357–374.

Melzack, R., and Bridges, J. A. Dorsal column contributions to motor behavior. *Exp. Neurol.*, 1971, *33*, 53–68.

Melzack, R., and Southmayd, S. E. Dorsal column contributions to anticipatory motor behavior. *Exp. Neurol.,* 1974, *42*, 274–281.

Melzack, R., and Torgerson, W. S. On the language of pain. *Anesthesiology,* 1971, *34*, 50.

Melzack, R., and Wall, P. D. On the nature of cutaneous sensory mechanisms. *Brcin,* 1962, *85*, 331–356.

Melzack, R., and Wall, P. D. Masking and metacontrast phenomena in the skin sensory system. *Exp. Neurol.,* 1963, *8*, 35–46.

Melzack, R., and Wall, P. D. Pain mechanisms: A new theory. *Science,* 1965, *150*, 971–979.

Mendoza, J. E., and Thomas, R. K. Effects of posterior parietal and frontal neocrotical lesions in the squirrel monkey. *J. Comp. Physiol Psychol.,* 1975, *89*, 170–182.

Merzenich, N. M., and Harrington, T. H. The sense of flutter-vibration evoked by stimulation of the hairy skin of primates: Comparison of human sensory capacity with the responses of mechanoreceptive afferents innervating the hairy skin of the monkeys. *Exp. Brain Res.,* 1969, *9*, 236.

Mettler, F. A., and Liss, H. Functional recovery in primates after large subtotal spinal cord lesion. *J. Neuropathol. Exp. Neurol.,* 1959, *18*, 509–516.

Millar, J. Joint afferent fibre responding to muscle stretch, vibration and contraction. *Brain Res.,* 1973, *63*, 380–383.

Morin, F. A new spinal pathway for tactile impulses. *Am. J. Physiol.,* 1955, *183*, 245–252.

Mountcastle, V. B. Some functional properties of the somatic afferent system. In W. A. Rosenblith (ed.), *Sensory Communication.* Wiley, New York, 1961.

Mountcastle, V. B., Poggio, G. F., and Werner, G. The relation of thalamic cell response to peripheral stimuli varied over an intensive continuum. *J. Neurophysiol.,* 1963, *26*, 807–834.

Mountcastle, V. B., Talbot, W. H., and Kornhuber, H. H. The neural transformation of mechanical stimuli delivered to the monkey's hand. In A. de Reuck and J. Knight (eds), *Touch, Heat and Pain.* Little, Brown, Boston, 1966, pp. 325–345.

Mountcastle, V. B., Talbot, W. H., Sakata, H., and Hyvarinen, J. Cortical neuronal mechanisms in flutter-vibration studied in unanesthetized monkeys. Neuronal periodicity and frequency discrimination. *J. Neurophysiol.,* 1969, *32*, 452–484.

Mountcastle, V. B., Lynch, J. C., Georgopoulos, A., Sakata, H., and Acuna, C. Posterior parietal association cortex of the monkey: Command functions for operations within extrapersonal space. *J. Neurophysiol.,* 1975, *38*, 871–908.

Munger, B. L. The intraepidermal innervation of the snout skin of the opposum: A light and electron microscope study, with observations on the nature of Merkel's Tastzellen. *J. Cell Biol.,* 1965, *26*, 79.

Munger, B. L. Patterns of organization of peripheral sensory receptors. In *Handbook of Sensory Physiology,* Vol. I. Springer-Verlag, New York, 1971, pp. 524–553.

Myers, D. A., Hostetter, G., Bourassa, C. M., and Swett, J. E. Dorsal columns in sensory detection. *Brain Res.,* 1974, *70*, 350–355.

Naquet, R., Denevit, M., and Albe-Fessard, D. Comparaison entre le rôle du subthalamus et celui des afférents structures bulbomésencéphaliques dans le maintien de la vigilance. *Electroencephalogr. Clin. Neurophysiol.,* 1966, *20*, 149–164.

Norrsell, U. The spinal afferent pathways of conditioned reflexes to cutaneous stimuli in the dog. *Exp. Brain Res.,* 1966, *2*, 269–282.

Norrsell, V. A conditioned reflex study of sensory defects caused by cortical somatosensory ablations. *Physiol. Behav.,* 1967, *2*, 73–81.

Norton, A. C., and Kruger, L. *The Dorsal Column System of the Spinal Cord: An Updated Review..* Brain Information Service, Los Angeles, Calif., 1973.

Orbach, J., and Chow, K. L. Differential effects of resections of somatic areas I and II in monkeys. *J. Neurophysiol.,* 1959, *22*, 195–203.

Oscarsson, O., and Rosen, I. Projection to cerebral cortex of large muscle spindle afferents in forelimb nerves of the cat. *J. Physiol. (London),* 1963, *169*, 924–945.

Pagni, C. A. Pain due to central nervous system lesions: Physiopathological considerations and therapeutical implications. *Adv. Neurol.,* 1974, *4*, 339–348.

Paillard, J., and Brouchon, M. Active and passive movements in the calibration of position sense. In S. J. Freedman (ed.), *The Neuropsychology of Spatially Oriented Behavior.* Dorsey Press, Honeward, Ill., 1968.

Paintal, A. S. Functional analysis of group III afferent fibres of mammalian muscles. *J. Physiol.,* 1960, *152*, 250–270.

Paul, R. L., Merzenich, M., and Goodman, H. Representation of slowly and rapidly adapting cutaneous mechanoreceptors of the hand in Brodman's areas 3 and 1 of *Macaca mulatta. Brain Res.,* 1572, *36*, 229–249.

Perl, E. R. Myelinated afferent fibers innervating the primate skin and their response to noxious stimuli. *J. Physiol. (London)*, 1968, *197*, 593.

Perl, E. R., Whitlock, D. G., and Gentry, J. R. Cutaneous projection to second-order neurons of the dorsal column system. *J. Neurophysiol.*, 1962, *25*, 337–358.

Petit, D., and Burgess, P. R. Dorsal column projection of receptors in cat hairy skin supplied by myelinated fibers. *J. Neurophysiol.*, 1968, *31*, 849–855.

Phillips, C. G., Powell, T. P. S., and Wiesendanger, M. Projection from low-threshold muscle afferents of hand and forearm to area 3a of baboon's cortex. *J. Physiol. (London)*, 1971, *217*, 419–446.

Poggio, G. F., and Mountcastle, V. B. A study of the functional contributions of the lemniscal and spinothalamic systems to somatic sensibility: Central nervous mechanisms in pain. *Bull. Johns Hopkins Hosp.*, 1960, *25*, 337–358.

Poggio, G. F., and Mountcastle, V. B. The functional properties of ventrobasal thalamic neurons studied in unanesthetized monkeys. *J. Neurophysiol.*, 1963, *26*, 775–806.

Pohl, W. Dissociation of spatial discrimination deficits following frontal and parietal lesions in monkeys. *J. Comp. Physiol. Psychol.*, 1973, *82*, 227–239.

Pompeiano, O. Reticular formation. In *Handbook of Sensory Physiology*, Vol. II. Springer-Verlag, New York, 1973, pp. 381–488.

Poulos, D. A. Central processing of peripheral temperature information. In H. H. Kornhuber (ed.), *The Somatosensory System*. Georg Thieme, Stuttgart, 1975, pp. 78–93.

Powell, T. P. S., and Mountcastle, V. B. Some aspects of the functional organization of the cortex of the post central gyrus of the monkey: A correlation of findings obtained in a single unit analysis with cytoarchitecture. *Bull. Johns Hopkins Hosp.*, 1959, *105*, 133–162.

Pribram, H. B., and Barry, J. Further behavioral analysis of parieto-temporo-preoccipital cortex. *J. Neurophysiol.*, 1956, *19*, 99–106.

Rethelyi, M., and Szentagothai, J. Distribution and connections of afferent fibres in the spinal cord. In *Handbook of Sensory Physiology*, Vol. 2. Springer-Verlag, New York, 1973, pp. 207–253.

Reynolds, P. J., Talbot, R. E., and Brookhart, J. M. Control of postural reactions in the dog: The role of the dorsal column feedback pathway. *Brain Res.*, 1972, *40*, 159–164.

Ridley, R. M., and Ettlinger, G. Tactile and visuo-spatial discrimination performance in the monkey: The effects of total and partial posterior parietal removals. *Neuropsychologia*, 1975, *13*, 191–206.

Rose, J. E., and Mountcastle, V. B. Touch and kinesthesis. In *Handbook of Physiology*, Section I: *Neurophysiology*. 1959, 387–429.

Rosen, I. Functional organization of group I activated neurons in the cuneate nucleus of the cat. *Brain Res.*, 1967, *6*, 770–772.

Rosenthal, S. R. Histamine as the chemical mediator for referred pain. In D. R. Kenshalo (ed.), *The Skin Senses*. Thomas, Springfield, Ill., 1968, pp. 480–498.

Ruch, T. C., Pathophysiology of pain. In T. C. Ruch, H. D. Patton, J. W. Woodbuury, and A. L. Towe (eds.), *Neurophysiology*. Saunders, Philadelphia, 1961, 350–368.

Ruch, T. C., and Fulton, J. F. Cortical localization of somatic sensibility; the effect of precentral, postcentral and posterior parietal lesions upon the performance of monkeys trained to discriminate weights. *Res. Publ. Assoc. Nerv. Ment. Dis.*, 1935, *15*, 289–330.

Rustioni, A. Non-primary afferents to the nucleus gracilis from the lumbar cord of the cat. *Brain Res.*, 1973, *51*, 81–95.

Rustioni, A. Non-primary afferents to the cuneate nucleus in the brachial dorsal funiculus of the cat. *Brain Res.*, 1974, *75*, 247–259.

Ryall, R. W., and Piercey, M. F. Visceral afferent and efferent fibers in sacral ventral roots in cats. *Brain Res.*, 1970, *23*, 57–65.

Sakata, H., Takaoka, Y., Kawarasaki, A., and Shibutani, H. Somatosensory properties of neurons in the superior parietal cortex (area 5) of the rhesus monkey. *Brain Res.*, 1973, *64*, 85–102.

Sanwald, J. C., and Vierck, C. J., Jr. The afferent spinal pathways mediating light tactile sensation. *Proc. Int. Un. Physiol. Sci.*, 1968, *7*, 385.

Schwartz, A. S., Eidelberg, E., Marchok, P., and Azulay, A. Tactile discrimination in the monkey after section of the dorsal funiculus and lateral lemniscus. *Exp. Neurol.*, 1972, *37*, 582–596.

Schwartz, A. S., Perey, A. J., and Azulay, A. Further analysis of active and passive touch in pattern discrimination. In preparation, 1977.

Schwartzman, R. J. Somatesthetic recovery following primary somatosensory cortex ablations. *Arch. Neurol.*, 1972, *27*, 340–349.

Schwartzman, R. J., and Bogdonoff, M. D. Behavioral and anatomical analysis of vibration sensitivity. *Exp. Neurol.*, 1968, *20*, 43–51.

Schwartzman, R. J., and Bogdonoff, M. D. Proprioception and vibration sensibility discrimination in the absence of the posterior columns. *Arch. Neurol.*, 1969, *20*, 349–353.

Schwartzman, R. J., and Semmes, J. The sensory cortex and tactile sensitivity. *Exp. Neurol.*, 1971, *33*, 147–158.

Selzer, M., and Spencer, W. A. Convergence of visceral and cutaneous afferent pathways in the lumbar spinal cord. *Brain Res.*, 1969, *14*, 331–348.

Semmes, J. Protopathic and epicritic sensation: A reappraisal. In A. L. Benton (ed.), *Contributions to Clinical Neuropsychology*. Aldine, Chicago, 1969, pp. 142–171.

Semmes, J. Somesthetic effects of damage to the central nervous system. In *Handbook of Sensory Physiology*, Vol. 2. Springer-Verlag, New York, 1973, pp. 719–742.

Semmes, J., and Porter, L. A comparison of precentral and postcentral cortical lesions on somatosensory discrimination in the monkey. *Cortex*, 1972, *8*, 249–264.

Semmes, J., Porter, L., and Randolph, M. C. Further studies of anterior postcentral lesions in monkeys. *Cortex*, 1974, *10*, 55–68.

Sheally, C. N. Six year's experience with electrical stimulation for control of pain. *Adv. Neurol.*, 1974, *4*, 775–782.

Sicuteri, F., Franchi, G., and Michelacci, S. Biochemical mechanisms of ischemic pain. *Adv. Neurol.*, 1974, *4*, 39–44.

Sjoqvist, O., and Weinstein, E. A. The effect of section of the medial lemniscus on proprioceptive functions in chimpanzees and monkeys. *J. Neurophysiol.*, 1942, *5*, 69–74.

Skavenski, A. A. Inflow as a source of extraretinal eye position information. *Vision Res.*, 1971, *12*, 221–229.

Skoglund, S. Anatomical and physiological studies of knee joint innervation in the cat. *Acta Physiol. Scand.*, 1956, *36*, Suppl. 124.

Skoglund, S. Joint receptors and kinesthesis. In *Handbook of Sensory Physiology*, Vol. 2. Springer-Verlag, New York, 1973, pp. 111–136.

Sprague, J. M., and Meikle, T. H. The role of the superior colliculus in visually guided behavior. *Exp. Neurol.*, 1965, *11*, 115–146.

Sprague, J. M., Levitt, M., Robson, K., Liu, C. N., Stellar, E., and Chambers, W. W. A neuroanatomical and behavioral analysis of the syndromes resulting from midbrain lemniscal and reticular lesions in the cat. *Arch. Ital. Biol.*, 1963, *101*, 225–295.

Stein, B. E., Magalhaes-Castro, B., and Kruger, L. Relation between visual and somatic organization in the cat superior colliculus. *Soc. Neurosci. Abstr.* 1974, *4*, 436.

Straile, W. E. Sensory hair follicles in mammalian skin: The tylotrich follicle. *Am. J. Anat.*, 1960, *106*, 133–147.

Sullivan, R. Effect of different frequencies of virbation on pain threshold detection. *Exp. Neurol.*, 1968, *20*, 135–142.

Sumino, R., Dubner, R., and Starkman, S. Responses of small myelinated "warm" fibers to noxious heat stimuli applied to the monkey's face. *Brain Res.*, 1973, *62*, 260–263.

Swett, J. E., and Bourassa, C. M. Comparison of sensory discrimination thresholds with muscle and cutaneous nerve volleys in the cat. *J. Neurophysiol.*, 1967, *30*, 530–545.

Talbot, W. H., Darian-Smith, I., Kornhuber, H. H., and Mountcastle, V. B. The sense of flutter-vibration: Comparison of the human capacity with response patterns of mechanoreceptive afferents from the monkey hand. *J. Neurophysiol.*, 1968, *31*, 301–334.

Tapper, D. M. Cutaneous slowly adapting mechanoreceptors in the cat. *Science*, 1964, *143*, 53–54.

Tapper, D. M. Behavioral evaluation of the tactile pad receptor system in hairy skin of the cat. *Exp. Neurol.*, 1970, *26*, 447–459.

Tatton, W. G., Forner, S. D., Gerstein, G. L., Chambers, W. W., and Liu, C. N. The effect of post central cortical lesions on motor responses to sudden limb displacements in monkeys. *Brain Res.*, 1975, *96*, 108–113.

Taub, A. Local, Segmental and supraspinal interactions with a dorsolateral spinal cutaneous afferent system. *Exp. Neurol.*, 1964, *10*, 357–374.

Teitelbaum, H., Sharphos, S. K., and Byck, R. Role of somatosensory cortex on interhemispheric transfer of tactile habits. *J. Comp. Physiol. Psychol.*, 1968, *66*, 623–632.

Thach, W. T. Timing of activity in cerebellar dentate nucleus and cerebral motor cortex during prompt volitional movement. *Brain Res.*, 1975, *88*, 233–241.

Torebjörk, H. E., and Hallin, R. G. Identification of afferent C fibers in intact skin nerves. *Brain Res.*, 1974, *67*, 387–403.

Towe, A. L. Somatosensory cortex: Descending influences on ascending systems. In *Handbook of Sensory Physiology*, Vol. 2. Springer-Verlag, New York, 1973, pp. 315–338.

Truex, R. C., Taylor, M. J., Smythe, M. Q., and Gildenberg, P. L. The lateral cervical nucleus of cat, dog, and man. *J. Comp. Neurol.*, 1970, *139*, 93–104.

Uddenberg, N. Functional organization of long, second order afferents in the dorsal funiculus. *Exp. Brain Res.*, 1968, *4*, 377–382.

Vance, W. H., Clifton, G. L., Coggeshall, R. E., and Willis, W. D., Jr. Receptive field properties of unmyelinated ventral root afferents. *Fed. Proc.*, 1975, *34*, 388.

Verrillo, R. T. Vebrotactile sensitivity and the frequency response of the Pacinian corpuscle. *Psychon. Sci.*, 1966, *4*, 135–136.

Vierck, C. J., Jr. Spinal pathways mediating limb position sense. *Anat. Rec.*, 1966, *154*, 437.

Vierck, C. J., Jr. Alterations of spatio-tactile discrimination after lesions of primate spinal cord. *Brain Res.*, 1973, *58*, 69–79.

Vierck, C. J., Jr. Tactile movement detection and discriminating following dorsal column lesions in monkeys. *Exp. Brain Res.*, 1974, *20*, 331–346.

Vierck, C. J., Jr. Proprioceptive deficits after dorsal column lesions in monkeys. In H. H. Kornhuber (ed.), *The Somatosensory System*. Georg Thieme, Stuttgart, 1975, pp. 311–318.

Vierck, C. J., Jr. Absolute and differential sensitivities to touch stimuli after spinal cord lesions in monkeys. *Brain Res.*, 1977, *134*, 529–539.

Vierck, C. J., Jr., and Jones, M. B. Size discrimination on the skin. *Science*, 1969, *158*, 488–489.

Vierck, C. J., Jr., and Jones, M. B. Influences of low and high frequency oscillation upon spatio-tactile resolution. *Physiol. Behav.*, 1970, *5*, 1431–1435.

Vierck, C. J., Jr., Hamilton, D. M., and Thornby, J. I. Pain reactivity of monkeys after lesions to the dorsal and lateral columns of the spinal cord. *Exp. Brain Res.*, 1971, *13*, 140–158.

Vierck, C. J., Jr., Lineberry, C. G., Lee, P. K., and Calderwood, H. W. Prolonged hypalgesia following "acupuncture" in monkeys. *Life Sci.*, 1974, 1277–1289.

von Békésy, G. *Sensory Inhibition*. Princeton University Press, Princeton, N.J., 1967.

Vyklicky, L., Rudomin, P., Zajac, F. E., III, and Burke, R. E. Primary afferent depolarization evoked by a painful stimulus. *Science*, 1969, *165*, 184–186.

Wagman, I. H., and Price, D. D. Responses of dorsal horn cells of *M. mulatta* to cutaneous and sural nerve A and C fiber stimuli. *J. Neurophysiol.*, 1969, *32*, 803–817.

Wall, P. D. The origin of a spinal cord slow potential. *J. Physiol. (London)*, 1962, *164*, 508–526.

Wall, P. D. The sensory and motor role of impulses traveling in the dorsal columns towards cerebral cortex. *Brain*, 1970, *93*, 505–524.

Weddell, G., Palmer, E., and Pallie, W. Nerve endings in mammalian skin. *Biol. Rev.*, 1954, *30*, 159–193.

Weinstein, S. Intensive and extensive aspects of tactile sensitivity as a function of body part, sex and laterality. In D. Kenshalo (ed.), *The Skin Senses*. Thomas, Springfield, Ill., 1968, pp. 195–222.

Werner, G., and Mountcastle, V. B. Neural activity in mechanoreceptive cutaneous afferents: Stimulus-response relations, Weber functions, and information transmission. *J. Neurophysiol.*, 1965, *28*, 359–397.

Werner, G., and Whitsel, B. L. Topology of the body representation in somatosensory area I of primates. *J. Neurophysiol.*, 1968, *31*, 856–869.

Werner, G., and Whitsel, B. L. Functional organization of the somatosensory cortex. In *Handbook of Sensory Physiology*, Vol. 2. Springer-Verlag, New York, 1973, pp. 579–620.

White, J. C., and Sweet, W. H. *Pain and the Neurosurgeon*. Thomas, Springfield, Ill., 1969.

Whitsel, B. L., Petrucelli, L. M., and Sapiro, G. Modality representation in the lumbar and cervical fasciculus gracilis of squirrel monkey. *Brain Res.*, 1969a, *15*, 67–78.

Whitsel, B. L., Petrucelli, L. M., and Werner, G. Symmetry and connectivity in the map of the body surface in somatosensory area II of primates. *J. Neurophysiol.*, 1969b, *32*, 170–183.

Whitsel, B. L., Roppolo, J. R., and Werner, G. Cortical information processing of stimulus motion on the skin. *J. Neurophysiol.*, 1973, *35*, 691–717.

Whitsel, B. L., Schreiner, R. C., and Essick, G. K. Analysis of variability in somatosensory cortical neuron discharge. In preparation, 1978.

Williams, W. J., BeMent, S. L., Yim, T. C. T., and McCall, W. D., Jr. Nucleus gracilis responses to knee joint motion; a frequency response study. *Brain Res.*, 1973, *64*, 123–140.

Willis, W. D., Maunz, R. A., Foreman, R. D., and Coultier, J. D. Static and dynamic responses of spinothalamic tract neurons to mechanical stimuli. *J. Neurophysiol.*, 1975, *38*, 587–600.

Willis, W. W., Trevino, D. L., Coultier, J. D., and Maunz, R. A. Responses of primate spinothalamic tract neurons to natural stimulation of hindlimb. *J. Neurophysiol.*, 1974, *37*, 358–372.

Wilson, M. Tactual discrimination learning in monkeys. *Neuropsychologia*, 1965, *3*, 353–361.

Wilson, M., Diamond, I. T., Ravissa, R. J., and Glendenning, K. K. A behavioral analysis of middle temporal and ventral temporal cortex in the bushbaby *(Galago senegaleusis) Neursci. Abstr.*, 1975, *1*, 73.

Yamamoto, S., and Miyajima, M. Unit discharges recorded from dorsal portion of medulla responding to adequate exteroreceptive and proprioceptive stimulation in cats. *Jap. J. Physiol.*, 1961, *11*, 619–626.

Zimmerman, M. Drosal root potentials after C-fiber stimulation. *Science,* 1968, *160*, 896–898.

Zotterman, Y. Touch, pain and tickling: An electrophysiological investigation on cutaneous sensory nerves. *J. Physiol. (London),* 1939, *95*, 1–28.

Zubeck, J. P. Studies in somesthesis. II. Role of somatic sensory areas I and II in roughness discrimination in cat. *J. Neurophysiol.,* 1952, *15*, 401–408.

9

The Vestibular System: Basic Biophysical and Physiological Mechanisms

MANNING J. CORREIA AND FRED E. GUEDRY, JR.

INTRODUCTION

The vestibular sense organs behave analogously to an inertial guidance system. They respond to angular and linear accelerations of the head. The linear acceleration to which they respond may result from translational head motion or change in orientation of the head relative to gravity. Like certain proprioceptors and unlike certain exteroceptors, the vestibular sense organs not only detect energies in the environment but also provide feedback to the organism concerning the current state of motion and orientation of the head (and whole body) relative to the Earth's or some other force field. Skillful control of whole body movement usually involves integration of vestibular information with that supplied by other senses to produce appropriate, smooth, and coordinated motor responses. The extent of this integration is reflected by the neural pathways which exist between the vestibular sensory end organs and structures such as the cerebellum, the extraocular muscles, and the flexor and extensor muscles of the neck, torso, and limbs. This association is illustrated in general in Fig. 1.

A more specific block diagram of the structures related to the vestibular sensory-motor system is presented in Fig. 2, which illustrates some of the diverse

MANNING J. CORREIA Departments of Otolaryngology, Physiology, and Biophysics, University of Texas Medical Branch, Galveston, Texas 77550. FRED E. GUEDRY, JR. Naval Aerospace Medical Research Laboratory, Naval Air Station, Pensacola, Florida 32504. Some of the results reported in this chapter were supported by a NASA Contract, NAS 9–14641, to M. J. Correia.

MANNING J. CORREIA
AND
FRED E. GUEDRY, JR.

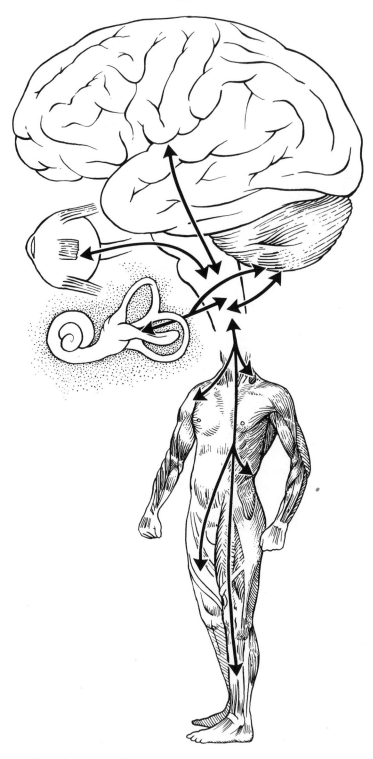

Fig. 1. General illustration of the diffuse interrelations of the vestibular apparatus and other neural systems.

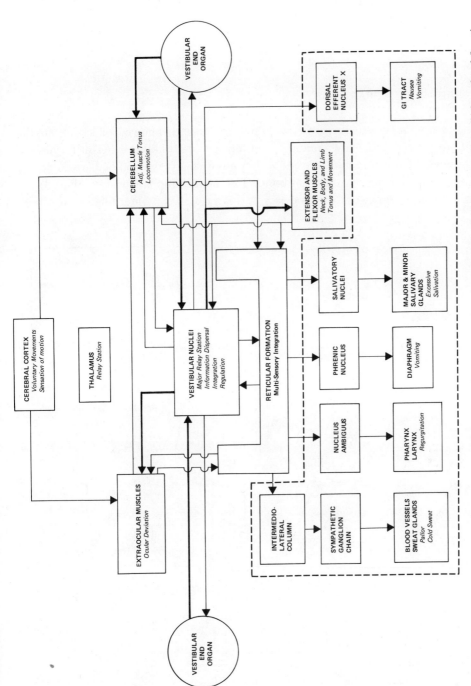

Fig. 2. Interrelations of various neural structures associated with the vestibular system. The role of each structure's vestibular-related function is indicated in its box. Interrelations of structures which play major roles in purposive and reflexive behavior in response to physiological vestibular stimulation are indicated by heavy dark arrows. The structures associated with vegetative effects of excessive nonphysiological vestibular stimulation are bounded by a dashed line. Modified from McCabe et al. (1972).

interrelations of this system and others. While it is beyond the scope of this chapter to summarize the massive literature which has accumulated on these various interrelations, the reader is asked to bear them in mind as some basic neurobiological principles of the vestibular system are presented in relation to their behavioral implications.

VESTIBULAR APPARATUS

The sensory structures of the vestibular system, known collectively as the vestibular apparatus, are contained within a membranous labyrinth which is supported by fibrous strands inside a contoured cavity, the bony labyrinth, in the petrous portion of the temporal bone. The membranous labyrinth (Fig. 3), an interconnected series of tubes and sacs, forms a closed container filled with a fluid,

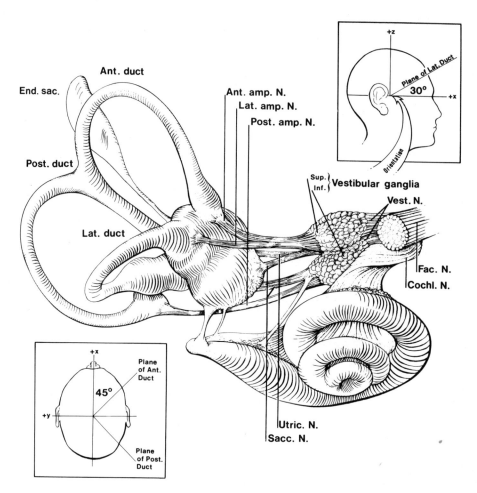

Fig. 3. Orientation and gross morphology of the semicircular ducts and otolith organs, as well as their innervation. Modified from Hardy (1934). The major planes of the semicircular ducts relative to the cardinal head axes (cf. Hixson *et al.*, 1966) are shown in the insets.

endolymph. This extracellular fluid is remarkable in that it has a high potassium and low sodium content (144 mmol/liter K^+, 16 mmol/liter Na^+) (Smith *et al.*, 1954). The space outside the membranous labyrinth, between it and the bony labyrinth, is filled with perilymph, which, like cerebrospinal fluid, has a high sodium (150 mmol/liter) and low potassium (5 mmol/liter) content (e.g., Rauch and Koestlin, 1958). The membranous labyrinth contains two types of sensory organs: the semicircular ducts, whose sensory receptors are primarily sensitive to angular acceleration, and the otolith organs, the utricle and saccule, whose sensory receptors are primarily sensitive to linear acceleration and change in linear acceleration.

SEMICIRCULAR DUCTS[1]

Three semicircular ducts, the anterior, the posterior, and the lateral, form part of the membranous labyrinth in each inner ear (Fig. 3). In man, each duct is roughly in a single plane and approximately at right angles to the other two. The lateral duct is in a plane inclined about 30° from the horizontal head plane, while the anterior and posterior ducts are approximately in vertical head planes (Fig. 3). The anterior semicircular duct of the labyrinth in one ear is coplanar with the posterior semicircular duct of the labyrinth in the contralateral ear. This plane is approximately 45° from the sagittal head plane (see Fig. 3).

The ends of each semicircular duct connect with the lumen of the utricle (Fig. 3) to form a closed loop, but there are only five entranceways to the utricle because the anterior and posterior ducts merge to form a common crus which enters the ceiling of the utricle (Fig. 3). In man, the average cross-sectional diameter of the arm of each of the semicircular ducts is approximately 0.25 mm (Igarashi, 1966), whereas the diameter of a cross-section of the utricle is between 2 and 4 mm.

Each semicircular duct widens at one point before it joins the utricle. This dilation, the ampulla, which is approximately 2.0 mm in diameter (Igarashi, 1966), contains the neuroepithelium of the semicircular duct. This neuroepithelium as well as supporting cells, connective tissue, blood vessels, and nerve fibers form the crista ampullaris (Fig. 4). The crista ampullaris is a saddle-shaped ridge which extends across the floor of the ampulla at right angles to the long axis of the ampulla (see, e.g., posterior crista, Fig. 4). The shape of the crista ampullaris is a minimum surface of revolution, i.e., a revolved catenary, and as such it facilitates maximum packing of neuroepithelial cells in a small area (Landolt *et al.*, 1975). Sensory neuroepithelium (see below) covers the major part of the crista ampullaris. This neuroepithelium consists of specialized mechanoreceptor sensory cells (hair cells). From the apical end of these hair cells, cilia extend upward into the cupula, a gelatinous mass (mucopolysaccharides within a keratin meshwork, e.g., Dohlman, 1971), which forms a fluid-tight partition or flap across the ampulla by

---

[1]In this chapter when describing the morphology of the vestibular apparatus and related neural structures, descriptive terms are used in accordance with *Nomina Anatomica* (1968). Customarily, in the areas of environmental and clinical medicine more global equivalent terms are used. In those areas, for example, semicircular canal as compared to semicircular duct is used to describe the sensory end organ which detects angular acceleration of the head.

MANNING J. CORREIA
AND
FRED E. GUEDRY, JR.

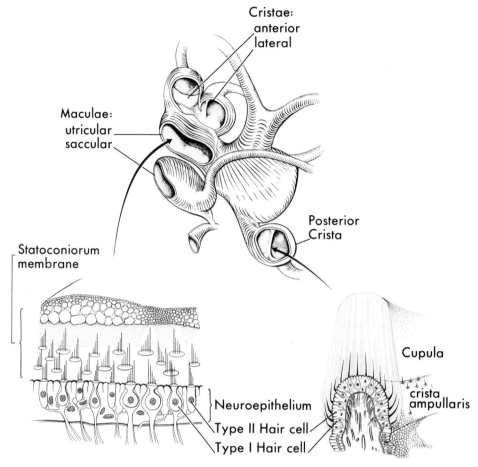

Fig. 4. Contents of the utricle, saccule, and ampullae. Enlarged cross-section through the utricular macula and the crista ampullaris of the posterior ampulla illustrate the covering of the macula, the statoconiorum membrane, and the covering of the crista, the cupula, as well as hair cells (type I and type II) whose cilia are embedded in the statoconiorum membrane and the cupula. In this figure, the tallest of the cilia for each hair cell represents the kinocilium. This figure is a composite of figures redrawn from Anson *et al.* (1967), Lindeman (1969), and Wersall (1956).

virtue of the fact that the fan-shaped cupula extends from the crista to the roof of the ampulla with its peripheral edge contacting the membranous wall all the way around the ampullary chamber above the crista.

OTOLITH ORGANS

The anterior part of the utricle widens into a recess in which a spade-shaped sensory area, the macula utriculi, is located (Fig. 4). The surface area of the utricular macula is of a complex shape; however, its major plane is nearly horizontal when the head is erect. The saccular macula is hook-shaped, and its major plane is perpendicular to the plane of the utricular macula (cf. Lindeman,

1969, Fig. 4, p. 18). Like the cristae ampullares, the maculae of the utricle and saccule consist of neuroepithelium, supporting cells, vessels and a nerve fiber complex. Cilia extend from the apical ends of the macular mechanoreceptor hair cells into a gelatinous membrane (mucopolysaccharides, e.g., Young *et al.*, 1974), the statoconiorum membrane, containing the otoliths or statoconia, like the "frost- ing" on a gelatinous cake (Fig. 4). The statoconia, which in mammals are calcite crystals (Carlstrom *et al.*, 1953), make the "frosting" on the superstructure of this sensory detector more dense than the surrounding endolymphatic fluid. Within the statoconiorum membrane there is a central curved area, the striola (Werner, 1933), which is structurally distinctive and physiologically important, as discussed below (see Lindeman, 1969, Fig. 44, p. 89). In the statoconiorum membrane of the utricle it is identifiable as a groove (Fig. 4) and in the saccular statoconiorum membrane it appears as a ridge.

FUNCTIONAL PRINCIPLES BASED ON MORPHOLOGY

The specific gravity of the calcite crystals, which are the statoconia in mam- mals, is 2.71, whereas that of the endolymph, perilymph, and the cupula is approximately 1.00 (Money *et al.*, 1971). The equivalence of the specific gravity of the cupula and surrounding endolymph and the fact that the semicircular ducts form circular closed loops as they communicate via the utricle are physical features which suggest that this sensory system normally detects angular acceleration (and not linear acceleration) of the head. The difference in specific gravity between the statoconia and the surrounding endolymph in the utricle and saccule is a feature which suggests that these structures operate like inertial mass linear accelerometers.

NEUROEPITHELIA OF THE VESTIBULAR APPARATUS

MORPHOLOGY AND INNERVATION. The basic features of the sensory cells of the maculae and cristae are the same and hence they will not be discussed separately. The vestibular neuroepithelia consist of sensory cells partitioned from subepithelial tissue by a basement membrane. Each sensory cell is surrounded by six or seven supporting cells.

There are fundamentally two types of sensory hair cells (Wersall, 1956), type I cells, which are amphora shaped (Fig. 4) with the nucleus in the rounded bottom, and type II cells, which are roughly cylindrical in shape (Fig. 4). Type I and type II cells are innervated in different ways. The peripheral axons of the bipolar ganglion cells in the vestibular or Scarpa's ganglion lose their myelin before they penetrate the basement membrane of the neuroepithelium. Within the neuroepi- thelium these unmyelinated axons branch to form a complicated neural plexus which innervates the receptor hair cells (Fig. 4). A chalice-shaped nerve ending surrounds the entire subsurface of one or more type I hair cells. Type II cells are innervated by bouton-type nerve endings. In addition to afferent endings there are highly granulated boutons which abut both type I and type II hair cells. These endings are thought to belong to the vestibular efferent system (Smith and Rasmussen, 1968). Efferent fibers appear to synapse directly and *en passant* onto the nerve chalices of type I hair cells and onto the somas of the type II hair cells. Afferent fibers form axosomatic connections on single or multiple hair cells (Engström *et al.*, 1972). This complicated innervation pattern may be partly responsible for the different spontaneous discharge patterns (see Correia and Landolt, 1977; cf. Goldberg and Fernandez, 1977) which have been observed traveling on vestibular primary afferent fibers.

From the apical surface of both types of hair cells protrude a bundle (60–100) of stereocilia and a lone kinocilium. Stereocilia of different lengths are systematically configured in curved rows like the pipes of a pipe organ. The row of longest stereocilia is next to the single kinocilium. A histological section through the hair cell cilia at the level of the cell surface reveals that they form a geometric pattern. When viewed from above, the stereocilia form a hexagonal pattern on the cell surface. The lone kinocilium, located at one of the points of the hexagon, provides a morphological indication of the physiological directional polarization of sensory cells in the neuroepithelia of the cristae and maculae (Lowenstein and Wersall, 1959).

MORPHOLOGICAL AND PHYSIOLOGICAL POLARIZATION. In the neuroepithelia of the cristae ampullares, all hair cells are polarized in the same direction, i.e., the kinocilia are on the same side of the hair bundle on all cell surfaces. On the crista of the lateral ampulla, the kinocilia point to the utricle.[2] On the cristae of the anterior and posterior ampullae, the kinocilia point away from the utricle. A more complex pattern of polarization occurs in the utricular and saccular maculae. The kinocilia point in opposite directions on either side of the hook-shaped striola which runs along the long axis of the macula sacculi. In the macula utriculi, the kinocilia face each other on either side of the striola (see Fig. 4).

The morphological polarization of hair cells on the cristae and maculae and their physiological response as indicated by modulation of primary afferent discharge are related as follows: The primary afferent discharge from a hair cell is increased relative to its spontaneous discharge rate, when its stereocilia are deflected toward its kinocilium and is decreased when its stereocilia are deflected away from its kinocilium. Thus in the ampulla of the lateral duct where all hair cells are polarized in the same direction (toward the utricle) bending of the cilia toward the utricle (utriculopetal deflection) causes an increase in the neural discharge above the spontaneous level; conversely, deflection in the opposite direction (utriculofugal) decreases the neural discharge below the spontaneous level. In the vertical semicircular ducts, hair cells are polarized in such a way (kinocilia point away from utricle) that afferent discharge is increased by utriculofugal cilia bending and decreased by utriculopetal cilia bending (e.g., Lowenstein and Wersall, 1959). It appears that hair cells on the maculae are also physiologi-

[2]The lumens of all semicircular duct ampullae join the lumen of the utricle (see Fig. 3). Therefore, the utricle forms a pole on one side of each ampulla and the semicircular duct arm forms another pole on the opposite side of each ampulla. In the remainder of this chapter reference will be made to such things as endolymph flow, cupula deflection, and hair cell bending within each of the semicircular ducts as being toward the utricle (utriculopetal) or away from the utricle (utriculofugal).

cally polarized (Fernandez *et al.*, 1972; Loe *et al.*, 1973), but the more complex pattern of morphological polarization prohibits a general statement regarding a single direction of physiological polarization.

MECHANOELECTRICAL TRANSDUCTION WITHIN THE VESTIBULAR APPARATUS

The biophysics of the transduction process of the vestibular system involves two major considerations: (1) the dynamic mechanical response of the peripheral end organs to acceleration and (2) the principles which govern how the bending of cilia modulates spontaneous activity of the primary vestibular afferent neurons.

THE CUPULA-ENDOLYMPH SYSTEM. Each of the semicircular ducts with its ampulla and the utricle can be conceptualized as a circular, fluid-filled tube (toroid) of varying diameter with an internal valve or partition, the cupula, across it at one spot (see Fig. 5). Because these idealized circular tubes or membranous rings are fastened to the bony labyrinth and therefore to the cranium, they move

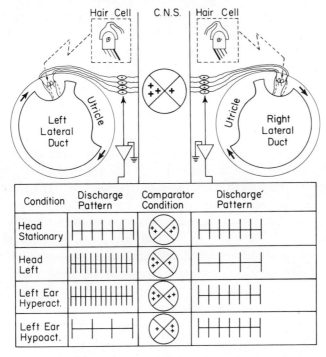

Fig. 5. Suspected response of the lateral semicircular ducts to an angular acceleration of the head to the left (as viewed from above). The arrows indicate direction of endolymph flow; the dashed lines indicate direction of cupula distortion; the inset hair cell illustrates deflection of the stereocilia relative to the kinocilium (dark hair) and to the utricle. Also illustrated are responses where the head is stationary but a pathological insult has occurred to the sensory end organ. The results of an "irritative" insult are illustrated in the left ear hyperactive panel; those of an "ablative" insult are illustrated in the left ear hypoactive panel. Note that if a CNS comparator utilizes *relative difference* in neural discharge from the left and right ampullary nerves (indicated by + signs inset into the CNS comparator) to execute cristoocular, cristocollic, and cristospinal reflexes, it is not able to distinguish physiological head motion neural information from an imbalance in neural discharge due to pathology. Modified from Correia and Landolt (1978).

MANNING J. CORREIA
AND
FRED E. GUEDRY, JR.

with the head as it moves. However, the endolymph inside the membranous ring tends to remain stationary by its inertial properties to the degree that the plane of the ring projects into the plane of rotation (see Groen, 1957; Landolt *et al.*, 1975). Thus, until the walls of the ring drag the endolymph along with them, there is endolymph movement relative to the ring. This movement produces distortion or sliding of the cupula relative to the underlying hair-bearing neuroepithelia. The range of cupula displacement has been speculated to be 0.01 μm at threshold to 3.0 μm at the upper limit of physiological head motions (Money *et al.*, 1971; Oman and Young, 1972). As the cupula distorts, the hair cell cilia which are embedded in it bend (respond to a shearing force) relative to their cell bodies. By some mechanism which is not yet clear (see Goldberg and Fernandez, 1975*a*) this bending presumably causes the hair cell to become depolarized or hyperpolarized relative to its resting potential. The extent of depolarization and hyperpolarization in turn regulates the release of excitatory transmitter substance into the hair cell–primary afferent synaptic cleft. Supposedly, depolarization of the hair cell produces a greater release of excitatory transmitter substance whereas hyperpolarization produces a decreased release of excitatory transmitter substance. The former condition appears to produce an increase in firing in vestibular primary afferents, whereas the latter condition appears to produce a decrease in vestibular primary afferent discharge (cf. Lowenstein, 1955).

The following example summarizes the transduction process just presented. Assume that a person decides to turn his head 90° to the left to look for the source of a loud sound. While the head is stationary, the majority of the vestibular primary afferents in the right and left lateral ampullary nerves are spontaneously active. As the head begins to turn, utriculopetal endolymph flow occurs in the lateral semicircular duct of the left labyrinth, bending rows of stereocilia toward their kinocilia (see Fig. 5). Consequently, the hair cells depolarize, increasing the rate of transmitter release, which in turn increases the neural discharge in the left vestibular nerve (see head left condition, Fig. 5). Utriculofugal endolymph movement in the right labyrinth hyperpolarizes the hair cells and neural activity in the right vestibular nerve decreases (see head left condition, Fig. 5). As the head stops, at the end of the head motion, the deceleration is equivalent to head acceleration in the opposite direction. This serves to reverse the steps just described and return the cupula-endolymph system to its resting position. Consequently, activity in the vestibular nerves returns to its spontaneous state as the head stops.

THE TORSION PENDULUM ANALOGY. A model based on an analogy has been developed which predicts the response of the cupula-endolymph system to various angular acceleration waveforms. This analogy likens the fluid-filled idealized ring of the semicircular duct to an angular accelerometer and the cupula-endolymph system to a highly damped torsion pendulum (Steinhausen, 1933; van Egmond *et al.*, 1949). This analogy leads to the following differential equation:

$$\theta \ddot{\xi}(t) + \pi \dot{\xi}(t) + \Delta \xi(t) = \theta \alpha(t) \tag{1}$$

where $\xi(t)$ is the angular displacement of the cupula-endolymph system relative to the semicircular duct, $\dot{\xi}(t)$ is the velocity of the cupula-endolymph system relative to the semicircular duct, $\ddot{\xi}(t)$ is the acceleration of the cupula-endolymph system relative to the semicircular duct, $\alpha(t)$ is the driving function which produces angular acceleration of the head and equivalently the semicircular duct, θ is the moment of inertia, π is the coefficient of the viscous drag moment of cupula-endolymph system, and Δ is the elastic restoring coefficient of the cupula-endolymph system. Equation (1) can be developed by returning to the example just discussed. As the semicircular duct is turned to the left by a voluntary head movement, for example, whose acceleration waveshape can be expressed as $\alpha(t)$, the mass of the cupula-endolymph system causes an inertial response to its acceleration equal to $\theta\beta(t)$. This inertial moment opposes cupula-endolymph movement relative to the Earth and causes it to lag or move in a direction opposite that of the membranous duct. This endolymph movement relative to the duct is denoted by arrows in Fig. 5. In opposition to the inertial moment, however, there are two moments which tend to pull the endolymph along with the semicircular duct. The first is a viscous drag moment, which, for special reasons (see Melvill Jones, 1972), is proportional to the velocity of cupula-endolymph movement relative to the semicircular duct, and equal to $\pi\dot{\xi}(t)$. The second opposing moment comes from the elasticity of the cupula, $\Delta\xi(t)$, which acts to restore the "distorted" cupula (dashed lines in Fig. 5). Thus the forces acting on the cupula-endolymph system may be expressed as

$$\pi\dot{\xi}(t) + \Delta\xi(t) = \theta\beta(t) \tag{2}$$

where $\beta(t)$ is the acceleration of the cupula-endolymph system in inertial space. Equation (2) may be expressed in terms of head acceleration. Acceleration of the cupula-endolymph system *relative* to the semicircular duct, $\ddot{\xi}(t)$, is equal to the acceleration of the semicircular duct, $\alpha(t)$, minus the acceleration of the cupula-endolymph system, $\beta(t)$. Thus

$$\ddot{\xi}(t) = \alpha(t) - \beta(t) \tag{3}$$

Solving equation (3) for $\beta(t)$ and substituting the result into equation (2), we obtain equation (1).

Numerous experiments (reviewed in Guedry, 1965, 1974; Clark, 1970; Goldberg and Fernandez, 1975a), using a variety of driving functions and a variety of response indicators of $\xi(t)$, have, in general, demonstrated that the torsion pendulum analogy, as a first approximation, describes the dynamics of the cupula-endolymph system. These experiments suggest that for man's lateral semicircular duct equation (1) can be written as

$$\ddot{\xi}(t) + 200\dot{\xi}(t) + 10\xi(t) = \alpha(t) \tag{4}$$

The behavioral implications of equation (4) become clear when we transfer it from the time domain into the frequency domain and, with certain assumptions (see Melvill Jones, 1972), rewrite it in the notation of the Laplace transform as (Outerbridge, 1969)

$$\frac{\xi}{\omega}(s) \cong \frac{\tau_1\tau_2 s}{(\tau_1 s + 1)(\tau_2 s + 1)} \tag{5}$$

where $s = j(2\pi f)$, $j = \sqrt{-1}$, ω is the angular velocity of the head, $\tau_1 \cong \pi/\Delta$, and $\tau_2 \cong \theta/\pi$. Equation (5) implies that over a range of frequencies, angular acceleration of the head is transduced into neural information concerning velocity of the head

MANNING J. CORREIA
AND
FRED E. GUEDRY, JR.

by a mechanical integration which takes place within the semicircular duct. Electrophysiological experiments (e.g., Fernandez and Goldberg, 1971; Melvill Jones and Milsum, 1971) tend to support this suggestion.

The region over which the cupula-endolymph system faithfully transduces information about angular head velocity is determined by the "long" (τ_1) and "short" (τ_2) time constants of equation (5). In man, estimates of τ_1 have been obtained from eye movement and sensation data. For example, Hixson (1974) estimated the long time constant τ_1 from horizontal eye movement to be 19 sec. Gilson et al. (1973), using a different stimulus, estimated τ_1 to be 16 sec from horizontal eye movement and 7.2 sec from vertical eye movement. If we assume that the long time constant for eye movement data is of the same order of magnitude as the long time constant for the cupula-endolymph system, we can arrive at an estimate $\tau_1 \simeq 20$ sec. Estimates of τ_2, which range from 0.005 to 0.002 sec, have been derived from physical measurements of endolymph (Money et al., 1971), and the semicircular ducts (Igarashi, 1966). Assuming $\tau_1 = 20.0$ and $\tau_2 = 0.005$, as in equation (4), equation (5) predicts that the cupula-endolymph system would faithfully transduce angular head velocity between a lower cutoff frequency, $f_1 = 0.008$ Hz, and an upper cutoff frequency, $f_u = 31.83$ Hz. This bandwidth would seem to include most physiological head motions in man. It has been suggested (Melvill Jones and Spells, 1963) that in other species the dimensions of the semicircular ducts (and therefore their frequency response) are "matched" to the behavior of that species, which in turn is dictated by environmental demands. This notion seems intuitively reasonable, since the range of head motions of a terrestrial animal like man is different from that of a monkey, which, as part of its natural behavior patterns, swings from tree to tree, or an animal like a bird (e.g., a hawk), which may encounter high-frequency turbulence in flight while trying to maintain visual fixation by the vestibuloocular reflex on a fleeing rodent.

It should be emphasized once again that the torsion pendulum model serves only as a first approximation of the behavior of the cupula–endolymph system. Significant departures from the responses predicted by this model have been noted at the level of the primary afferent system (see Goldberg and Fernandez, 1975a; O'Leary and Honrubia, 1976), and these departures are preserved throughout the central nervous system (see, e.g., Skavenski and Robinson, 1973).

THE STATOCONIORUM MEMBRANE SYSTEM. Since the statoconiorum membrane in both the utricle and saccule is denser than its surrounding medium, it slides relative to the macula when the head tips relative to gravity or when it is exposed to some other type of imposed linear acceleration (e.g., a sudden stop on the subway). The statoconiorum membrane is in part a gelatinous structure which should have elastic properties, and it is attached to the macula by the cilia of the hair cells, as well as other structures (Johnsson and Hawkins, 1967), which restrict its excursion further (6.0 μm displacement produced by a force of 10^{-5} Newton in the fish, de Vries, 1950).

THE MASS-SPRING-DASHPOT ANALOGY. The morphological conditions present in the utricle and saccule are analogous to a physical system of a mass which slides on lubricated guides but which is attached at one end to a support by a spring. Like the cupula-endolymph system, inertial, viscous, and elastic forces operate when the statoconiorum membrane is displaced. Unlike the cupula-endolymph system, however, the statoconiorum membrane and surrounding endolymph differ in specific gravity, a feature which provides sensitivity to linear acceleration.

A general equation which describes the conditions found in the utricle and saccule and which incorporates the density differences between the statoconiorum membrane and the surrounding endolymph may be written as (Goldberg and Fernandez, 1975a)

$$m_e\ddot{x}(t) + b\dot{x}(t) + kx(t) = A(t)m_e \frac{\rho_o - \rho_e}{\rho_o + \rho_e} \tag{6}$$

This equation relates statoconiorum membrane displacements, $x(t)$, to the forcing linear acceleration function, $A(t)$. The inertial, viscous, and elastic coefficients are m_e, b, and k, respectively. The difference in density between the statoconiorum membrane, ρ_o and the endolymph, ρ_e, is accounted for, and it also enters into the inertial coefficient, m_e. This coefficient, the effective mass of the otolith, includes not only the mass of the statoconiorum membrane but also the inertia of the endolymph which must be accelerated as the membrane moves. The system dynamics of equation (6) is determined by two parameters: a resonant frequency, $f_0 = [k(4\pi^2 m_e)^{-1}]^{1/2}$, and a damping factor, $c = b(4m_e k)^{-1/2}$. These parameters have been determined from physical measurements in the fish (de Vries, 1950) to be $f_0 = 50$ Hz and $c = 1.0$ (critical damping). Analysis of results from vestibular primary afferent recordings in the squirrel monkey (Fernandez and Goldberg, 1976b) suggests that the time constant which reflects the otolithic mechanical response is on the order of 10 msec. This result and the high resonant frequency parameter, which may be as high as 400 Hz in mammals (Fernandez and Goldberg, 1976b), have important behavioral implications. It suggests that the otoliths are a fast system and as such they are capable of transducing rapid dynamic head motion, as well as static head tilts. This further implies that the vestibular system uses all available input during conditions where both the otolith organs and the semicircular ducts are stimulated. The otolith organs and the semicircular ducts are almost always stimulated together since only on rare occasion does a head movement occur which is perfectly in the horizontal head plane so that the otoliths are not reoriented relative to gravity.

As well as sensing dynamic (time changing) linear acceleration, which occurs, for example, while running over rough terrain with the head pitching back and forth relative to the acceleration due to gravity, the otoliths must transduce static, maintained, head tilt relative to the acceleration due to gravity (g). This transduction process can be described by equation (6) for the special case where $\ddot{x}(t) = \dot{x}(t) = 0$.

Assuming $\rho_o \simeq 3.0\rho_e$, equation (6) becomes

$$kx(t) = \frac{1}{2}A(t)m_e \tag{7}$$

It has been shown in the classic behavioral fish studies of von Holst (1950) that the effective linear acceleration which acts on the statoconiorum membrane is not $A(t) = g \simeq 9.81$ m/sec² but that component of $A(t)$ which acts parallel to the plane of

MANNING J. CORREIA
AND
FRED E. GUEDRY, JR.

the hair cells in the macula. This component (the shear-directed component in the inclined plane problem in physics) can be expressed as $A(t) = g \sin \alpha$, where α is the angle that the head (and hence the statoconiorum membrane) has been tipped relative to gravity.

MECHANISMS OF COMMUNICATION OF INFORMATION FROM THE VESTIBULAR APPARATUS

THE LATERAL SEMICIRCULAR DUCTS. Figure 5 illustrates a simplistic mechanism by which the vestibular sensory end organs may communicate with the central nervous system (CNS). It suggests that a hypothetical comparator in the CNS constantly samples and weighs the relative amount of neural discharge in the right and left vestibular nerves. Although the same principles can be applied to the vertical semicircular ducts (see, e.g., Lowenstein and Sand, 1940), Fig. 5 illustrates the inputs from single nerve fibers of the right and left lateral ampullary nerves.

When the head is stationary, a balance of spontaneous neural activity is sensed by the comparator as indicated by an equal number of plus signs in the comparator condition column of the head stationary panel in Fig. 5. When the head is rotated to the left, neural activity increases in the left lateral ampullary nerve and decreases in the right lateral ampullary nerve. The comparator "senses" the imbalance (indicated by an unequal number of plus signs in comparator column for the head left panel in Fig. 5) and reflexive oculomotor and spinal responses are initiated. When the head stops, neural activity in each ampullary nerve returns to its spontaneous level and a balanced condition is "sensed" by the comparator. If the head were rotated to the right, the converse discharge patterns would occur and they would be "sensed" by the comparator as a head right rotation and appropriate reflexes would be initiated. The bottom two panels in Fig. 5 illustrate why dizziness, eye movement, and falling result from pathology of the peripheral labyrinth. Hyperactivity (caused, for example, by an irritative lesion) or hypoactivity (caused, for example, by an ablative lesion) in one nerve (left nerve in Fig. 5) is interpreted by the CNS comparator as an imbalance in neural activity or equivalently as a head motion. As in the case of head motion, reflexive motor responses are produced. Unlike head motions, however, the neural imbalance persists even with the head stationary. Therefore, the responses which are made are inappropriate, and postural and ocular disequilibrium occur. Specifically, spinal reflexes occur. However, since no head or body movement exists, these compensatory postural adjustments may cause one to fall. Compensatory vestibuloocular responses are made. However, since no head or body movement exists, these compensatory eye movements sweep objects which are in the visual field across the retina and the visual field blurs or appears to move. These inappropriate responses persist until the neural imbalance between ampullary nerves is compensated for by plasticity of the CNS. This central nervous system compensatory mechanism enables one to regain "the sense of equilibrium" with the loss of one of the labyrinths. While no one has isolated the structures which are directly responsible for "central" compensation, structures such as the cerebellum, reticular formation, and vestibular nuclei have been implicated (see McCabe et al., 1972).

Central compensation can occur following loss of one of the labyrinths because the right and left labyrinths are functionally redundant. A single semicircular duct, for example, can act as a bidirectional sensor of head motion within its plane. An increase in neural discharge above the spontaneous level signals one direction of rotation while a decrease below the spontaneous discharge level signals rotation in the opposite direction. A single semicircular duct signals various magnitudes of head acceleration bidirectionally as well. Its neural input-output or intensity function is sigmoid shaped (see Trincker, 1962) and is analogous to a transistor's base current–collector current transfer characteristic curve. The spontaneous discharge level is analogous to a transistor's base bias current and determines the operating point (point of operation with no input) on the transfer characteristic curve. Head accelerations which are excessive in one direction can lead to single unit neural discharge which is analogous to saturation of a transistor while excessive accelerations in the opposite direction can lead to the analogy of transistor cutoff (see, e.g., Figs. 4 and 7, Correia and Landolt, 1973).

The analogy between the output curves of each of the lateral cristae and a transistor amplifier can be carried one step further. For a given direction of angular acceleration of the head, the neural activity in the contralateral ampullary nerves is 180° out of phase (see Fig. 5) and provides a "push-pull" signal to the central nervous system. A push-pull amplifier circuit (with biased transistors) provides increased power, reduction of even harmonic distortion, continuity of signal during zero crossing, and decreased noise. All of these features are desirable for neural communication between the two-sided vestibular sensory system and the vestibular nuclei, the motor nuclei of the extraocular muscles and the motoneurons of the neck, torso, and limbs.

THE VERTICAL SEMICIRCULAR DUCTS. The vertical semicircular ducts, which are in the same plane (Fig. 3), appear to operate in a "push-pull" mode as do the lateral ducts. The anterior semicircular duct and its ampulla in one ear and the posterior semicircular duct and its ampulla in the contralateral ear are so arranged that head rotation which produces utriculofugal cupula distortion (increased ampullary nerve discharge) in the anterior ampulla produces utriculopetal cupula distortion (decreased ampullary nerve discharge) in the contralateral posterior ampulla. As with the lateral ducts, the vertical semicircular ducts in one ear can act as bidirectional sensors and their intensity functions are also analogous to a transistor transfer characteristic curve.

Unlike the lateral ducts, the vertical semicircular ducts must signal head movements in the vertical plane which can include either frontal or sagittal head motions. The mechanisms by which these types of head motions are communicated to the central nervous system were examined by Lowenstein and Sand (1940), who rotated isolated labyrinths of the thornback ray, *Raja clavata,* about the three major head axes and observed primary afferent neural discharge in the ampullary nerves. Their results are summarized in Table I. From Table I, it appears that head motions in the vertical plane produce opposite responses from the contralateral anterior and posterior ampullary nerves. Therefore, we need only consider the anterior and posterior ampullary nerves in the same labyrinth. It

MANNING J. CORREIA
AND
FRED E. GUEDRY, JR.

TABLE I.   RESPONSE OF EACH OF THE SIX AMPULLARY NERVES TO ANGULAR MOTION ABOUT THE THREE PRIMARY HEAD AXES[a]

	Rotation about the					
	Front-back head axis (x)		Left–right head axis (y)		Vertex–base head axis (z)	
Semicircular duct	Rightward (+x)	Leftward (−x)	Forward (+y)	Backward (−y)	Clockwise (−z)	Counterclockwise (+z)
Right anterior	+	−	+	−	−(0)	+(0)
Left anterior	−	+	+	−	+(0)	−(0)
Right posterior	+	−	−	+	+(0)	−(0)
Left posterior	−	+	−	+	−(0)	+(0)
Right lateral	0	0	0	0	+	−
Left lateral	0	0	0	0	−	+

[a]After Lowenstein and Sand (1940). +, increase in neural discharge; −, decrease in neural discharge; 0, no change in neural discharge. The zeroes in parentheses have been added because recent findings (see Estes *et al.,* 1975) suggest that when careful attention is given to placing the anterior and posterior ducts 98.7°, respectively, from the plane of z-axis rotation, their primary afferent neural response (in the cat) is nil.

may be noted that head motion in the sagittal plane is signaled by neural discharge of opposite polarity in the anterior and posterior ampullary nerves whereas head motion in the frontal plane is signaled by neural discharge of the same polarity. Thus bidirectional motion in either the sagittal or frontal head plane can be uniquely signaled by each of the labyrinths.

THE OTOLITH ORGANS. Stimulus-response or intensity functions have been obtained for the otolith organs (Loe *et al.,* 1973; Fernandez and Goldberg, 1976a). The hair cells on the otolith organs are morphologically and functionally polarized in different directions on the maculae. Therefore, intensity curves must be determined for each statoreceptor hair cell or cells innervated by a single primary afferent. For each receptor cell's preferred direction of sensitivity its primary afferent discharge generally appears to vary as a power function of the sine of angular head position or the magnitude of the shear force along the surface of the hair cell. Over an extended stimulus range, $\pm 4.92g$, the force–response relation, like that of the semicircular ducts, is analogous to a transistor's transfer characteristic curve. That is, it is sigmoid shaped and presumably displays both excitatory saturation and inhibitory cutoff.

VESTIBULOCOCHLEAR NERVE

GENERAL MORPHOLOGY

The vestibular portion of man's VIIIth cranial or vestibulocochlear nerve is composed of approximately 18,000 myelinated *afferent* fibers of bipolar ganglion cells which connect the sensory areas of the vestibular end organs primarily to the vestibular nuclei in the brain stem, but also to parts of the cerebellum. Statistics summarizing the distribution and size of fibers to the different vestibular sensory areas in man are listed in Table II, and illustrate two facts. First, ampullary nerve fibers are larger than macular nerve fibers, and, second, while both ampullary and macular nerve fibers generally innervate multiple hair cells, ampullary fibers innervate fewer hair cells. A small number of unmyelinated afferent fibers may be present in the vestibular nerve. Myelinated and unmyelinated *efferent* fibers, also present in the vestibular nerve, apparently originate bilaterally between the abducens and lateral vestibular nuclei (see Gacek and Lyon, 1974), and terminate on the sensory hair cells of the cristae and maculae. The ratio of myelinated afferent to myelinated efferent fibers is approximately 45:1.

The vestibulocochlear nerve exits the brain stem just below the pons and courses laterally through the acoustic porus, the internal auditory meatus, and into the labyrinth. The vestibular ganglion (Scarpa's ganglion) is located within the internal auditory meatus. It is divided into a superior and an inferior portion connected by a narrow isthmus (see Fig. 3). The superior portion contains ganglion cell bodies of fibers which innervate the lateral and anterior ampullae, the utricular macula, and a small portion of the saccular macula. The inferior portion contains ganglion cells for the posterior ampullary nerve and the saccular nerve. The majority of the myelinated vestibular ganglion cells in man are 30–40 μm in diameter (Bergström, 1973a). Lateral to the ganglion, the superior–inferior division of the vestibular nerve is maintained until each division branches to the specific neuroepithelia referred to above.

In the main, vestibular primary afferents act to provide fast neural information transfer between the hair cells of the vestibular neuroepithelia and their points of termination in the vestibular nuclei and cerebellum.

PRIMARY AFFERENT PROJECTIONS TO VESTIBULAR NUCLEI AND CEREBELLUM

Primary afferent vestibular projections to the cerebellum and to the vestibular nuclei have been mapped most extensively in two mammalian species, the cat and the monkey (e.g., Gacek, 1969; Brodal and Hoivik, 1964; Stein and Carpenter, 1967; Carpenter *et al.,* 1972). Since a larger body of work has been conducted on

TABLE II. DESCRIPTIVE STATISTICS OF MAN'S VESTIBULAR NERVE AND RELATED SENSORY NEUROEPITHELIA[a]

Sensory end organ	Sensory cells	Myelinated nerve fibers	Ratio cells/ fibers	Nerve diameter (%) (adult)	
				6–9 μm	>9 μm
Ant. and lat. amp.	15,200	5,899	2.6	61.5	15.9
Post. amp.	7,600	2,449	3.1	54.2	12.2
Utr. mac.	33,100	5,952	5.6	57.7	3.9
Sacc. mac.	18,800	4,046	4.6	52.2	6.8

[a]From the data of Bergström (1973a,b,c,d) and Rosenhall (1972a,b).

vestibular related *behavior* in the cat, the primary afferent projections in that species will be described in more detail, but exceptions for the monkey will be noted.

PROJECTIONS TO CEREBELLUM. Most vestibular primary afferents end ipsilaterally in the nodulus and adjoining areas in the uvula and flocculus. The ventral paraflocculus receives a moderate amount of fibers. A few fibers project to the lingula and dorsal paraflocculus. In the intracerebellar nuclei, fibers appear to terminate only in the small-celled ventral part of the lateral (dentate) nucleus.

Vestibular primary afferents which end in the cerebellum appear to originate primarily in the *ampullae* (Gacek, 1969). Carpenter *et al.* (1972) found that projections to the ipsilateral flocculus of the rhesus monkey arise from the ampullae (projections to folia 5–10), as well as the maculae (projections to folia 3–6). Vestibulocerebellar fibers traverse the superior vestibular nucleus and enter the cerebellum via the juxtarestiform body, where they end as mossy fibers (e.g., Shinoda and Yoshida, 1975).

PROJECTIONS TO VESTIBULAR NUCLEI. Brodal and Pompeiano (1957) clearly delimited the vestibular nuclei in the brain stem of the cat using cellular cytoarchitectural techniques. They delineated the four major vestibular nuclei, the superior vestibular nucleus (SVN), the lateral vestibular nucleus (LVN), the medial vestibular nucleus (MVN), and the inferior (or descending) vestibular nucleus (DVN), as well as other smaller cell groups, the interstitial nucleus of the vestibular nerve (NIV), and the small cell groups *x*, *y*, and *z* (see Brodal *et al.*, 1962, for specific anatomical locations). According to Gacek (1969), the projections to the vestibular nuclei from the maculae and cristae in the cat can be summarized as follows: The utricular and saccular nerve fibers course in the caudal one-third of the vestibular nerve and, after entering the brain stem, form ascending and descending branches. Some utricular fibers in the ascending branch terminate in the ventral part of the LVN, but mostly in the rostral part of the MVN. Utricular fibers in the descending branch give off collaterals to the caudal MVN and converge in the rostromedial part of the DVN. Saccular macula fibers project mainly to cell group *y* and to a lesser extent to the ventral LVN and the rostral DVN. Ampullary nerve fibers appear to occupy the rostral two-thirds of the vestibular nerve. Fibers from the lateral, anterior, and posterior cristae, in contrast to macular fibers, appear to give off collaterals to the vestibular interstitial nucleus (NIV) before bifurcating in the brain stem into ascending and descending branches. Most anterior-lateral ampullary fibers of the ascending branches terminate in the central-lateral and rostral regions of the SVN, while some appear to proceed on to the cerebellum. Posterior ampullary fibers terminate primarily in the central-medial and medial regions of the SVN. The descending ampullary branches send collateral fibers to the LVN, MVN, and DVN. Stein and Carpenter (1967) observed that in the monkey utricular and saccular fibers give off collaterals to the LVN and MVN while descending to terminate primarily in the DVN. A small number of descending utricular fibers actually pass beyond the DVN into the accessory cuneate nucleus. Central fibers which innervate the cristae, on the other hand, appear to project to portions of the SVN and oral parts of the MVN. Stein and Carpenter (1967) found that vestibular fibers from all receptors connect with NIV.

From the results of the above neuroanatomical studies, it appears that central projections from the maculae are primarily to areas concerned with mechanisms that modify muscle tone and are associated with spinal reflex activity; central projections from the cristae are primarily to areas which are concerned with control of the extraocular muscles. However, this apparent dichotomy does not preclude eye movements as a result of otolithic stimulation or spinal reflex activity as a result of semicircular duct stimulation (see below).

The previously discussed analogy of the physiological action of primary afferent neural activity from appropriate receptors in contralateral labyrinths to the behavior of a push-pull amplifier system is generally maintained in the neural responses of the vestibular nuclei. These and exceptional responses are detailed elsewhere (Precht, 1974).

Secondary Vestibular Fiber Projections

Secondary vestibular fibers which arise in the vestibular nuclei go to the cerebellum (nodulus, uvula, flocculus and the *fastigial nuclei*), the motor nuclei of the extraocular muscles, the mesencephalic nuclei, the reticular formation, as well as to all levels of the spinal cord. Commissural connections also exist between ipsilateral and contralateral vestibular nuclei. The vestibular nuclei, in turn, receive projections from these structures, either directly or indirectly. These connections are illustrated, in general, in Fig. 6.

Vestibuloocular Reflex

The pathways associated with the vestibuloocular reflex are illustrated for the vestibular nuclei, which are on the right side of Fig. 6. The basic vestibuloocular reflex is a simple three-neuron feedforward reflex arc; primary afferent ganglion cell → vestibular nucleus cell → motoneuron of the extraocular muscles. Recent evidence, however, which will be discussed in this section, suggests that the vestibuloocular reflex may be part of feedback systems. This aspect of the reflex system will be discussed following a description of the basic neural chain.

Neurobiological studies have shown that eye movements can be produced by electrical stimulation of either the ampullary nerves (Cohen and Suzuki, 1963) or the macular nerves (Fluur and Mellstrom, 1970a,b). However, the otolith organs and the semicircular ducts respond to different types of stimuli, have different mechanical response characteristics, produce different types of eye movement, and even have certain nonoverlapping neuroanatomical projections. Therefore, the vestibuloocular reflex arc associated with stimulation of the semicircular ducts

MANNING J. CORREIA
AND
FRED E. GUEDRY, JR.

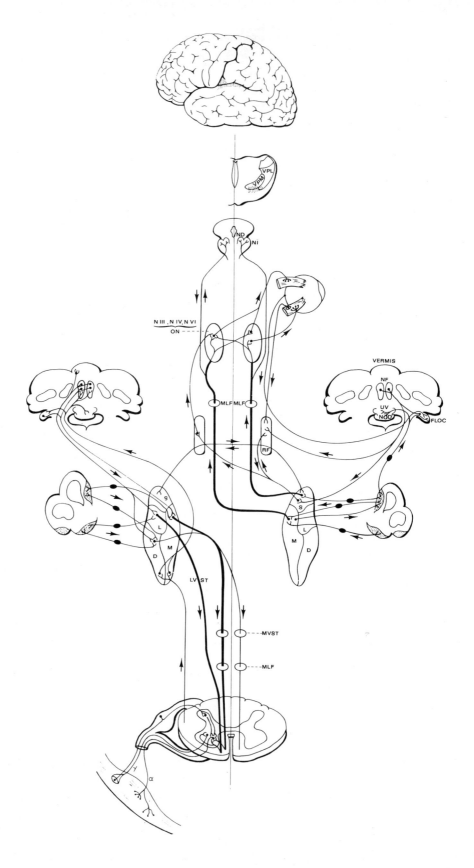

(cristoocular reflex) will be discussed separately from the reflex arc associated with
stimulation of the otolith organs (maculoocular reflex).

Both the cristoocular and maculoocular reflexes use the six extrinsic extraocular muscles of each eye as effectors of the reflex. These muscles and their
innervation are as follows: the superior rectus, inferior rectus, medial rectus, and
inferior oblique are supplied by the oculomotor nerve (cranial nerve III); the
superior oblique is supplied by the trochlear nerve (cranial nerve IV); the lateral
rectus is supplied by the abducens nerve (cranial nerve VI). The plane of eye
movement produced by contraction of these muscles is complex, and it is presented clearly elsewhere (e.g., see Willis and Grossman, 1973, Fig. 6–8, p. 293).
However, for the present it is sufficient to say that contraction of the following
muscles (and relaxation of their antagonists) produces the following deviations of
the eye: the medial and lateral recti move the eye toward (adduction) and away
from (abduction) the nose, respectively, in a plane parallel to the floor of the orbit;
the superior and inferior recti elevate and depress an abducted eye, respectively,
and intort and extort an adducted eye, respectively. Intorsion and extorsion
involve rotation of the top of the eye toward and away from the medial (nasal) wall
of the orbit, respectively. The superior oblique intorts an abducted eye and
depresses an adducted eye while the inferior oblique extorts an abducted and
elevates an adducted eye.

CRISTOOCULAR REFLEX

NEUROBIOLOGICAL ORGANIZATION. Projections to the motoneurons of the
extraocular muscles from the cristae of the semicircular ducts (in the cat and
monkey, Gacek, 1969; Tarlov, 1969, 1970) are by way of relays in the superior
vestibular nucleus (SVN) and the rostral portion of the medial vestibular nucleus
(MVN). From these nuclei, two pathways ascend to the Oculomotor Nuclei, ON
(the motor nuclei of cranial nerves III, IV, and VI, the oculomotor, trochlear, and
abducens nerves, respectively). The first pathway arises in the MVN. Between the
levels of the VIth and IVth nuclei, its fibers *cross* the midline into the medial
portions of the medial longitudinal fasiculus (MLF) where they ascend to the level

---

Fig. 6. Pathways and projection areas which are related to the vestibular system. Afferent and efferent
pathways, which are associated with the vestibuloocular reflex, are indicated for the vestibular nuclei
drawn on the right side of the figure. Afferent and efferent pathways, which are associated with the
vestibulospinal reflexes, are indicated for the vestibular nuclei drawn with the left side of the figure.
Vestibular projection areas in the thalamus and cerebral cortex are indicated by stippled areas. No
pathways, however, are drawn to these areas since they have not yet been clearly demonstrated.
Thalamus: VPL, ventral posterolateral nucleus; VPM, ventral posteromedial nucleus. Mesencephalic
nuclei: ND, nucleus of Darkschewitsch; NI, interstitial nucleus of Cajal. Motor nuclei of the extraocular
muscles: ON, oculomotor nuclei including the oculomotor nucleus (III), the trochlear nucleus (IV), and
the abducens nucleus (VI). Cerebellar structures: VERMIS; NF, fastigial nucleus; UV, uvula; NOD,
nodulus; FLOC, flocculus. Vestibular nuclei: S, superior; L, lateral; M, medial; D, descending.
Pathways: MLF, medial longitudinal fasciculus; LVST, lateral vestibulospinal tract; MVST, medial
vestibulospinal tract. Motoneurons: α, alpha; γ, gamma. Arrows in the figure indicate directions of
probable neural information flow.

MANNING J. CORREIA
AND
FRED E. GUEDRY, JR.

of the IIIrd nucleus. Projections of this pathway are bilateral to the abducens (VI) and oculomotor (III) nuclei and contralateral to the trochlear (IV) nucleus. These fibers have excitatory action[3] on all contralateral ON and the ipsilateral ON of the the medial rectus muscles. They have inhibitory action on the ipsilateral abducens (VI) nucleus. The second pathway originates in the SVN. Its fibers do not cross the midline until the level of the IIIrd nucleus and ascend in the lateral portions of the ipsilateral MLF. These fibers project to the oculomotor (III) nucleus bilaterally and to the trochlear (IV) nucleus ipsilaterally. Tarlov (1970), however, has reported bilateral projections to the trochlear (IV) nucleus. The SVN pathway appears to exert only inhibitory actions on the ON it innervates. A third pathway via the brachium conjunctivum (BC) to the oculomotor (III) nuclei has been observed in the rabbit (Highstein *et al.*, 1971). This pathway, which appears to exert excitatory effects on the extraocular motoneurons in the contralateral oculomotor (III) nucleus, has second-order cells in the lateral nucleus of the cerebellum and in the cell group *y* of the vestibular nucleus complex. These cell groups in the vestibular nuclei and cerebellum in the cat receive first-order projections from the macula of the saccule and possibly the utricle.

Electrical stimulation of the vestibular nerve in mammals (Sasaki, 1963; Baker *et al.*, 1969) produced excitatory postsynaptic potentials (e.p.s.p.'s) in the ON with latencies averaging 2.0 msec. Assuming that a synaptic delay is approximately 1.0 msec, this represents a disynaptic pathway [synapse on second-order cell (vestibular or cerebellar nuclear complex) and on oculomotor neuron] and confirms the above neuroanatomical observations.

In addition to the direct cristoocular pathways described above, a polysynaptic indirect route to the ON by way of the reticular formation is illustrated in Fig. 6 (Lorente de No, 1933; Ladpli and Brodal, 1968). This pathway may serve several important functions. For example, it provides a tract whereby descending control is exercised over the cristoocular reflex by higher centers (see next section). It may also play a role in the neural integration of head velocity information into head position information before this information reaches the level of the ON (see section "Behavioral Considerations"), and it may be involved in neural sharpening of the cristoocular reflex as, for example, when the "gain" of the cristoocular reflex is increased during "alerting" (Collins *et al.*, 1961)

CONTROL OF CRISTOOCULAR REFLEX. *Cerebellar Control.* Recent evidence suggests that the action of the cristoocular reflex can be moderated by other central structures. One such circuit involves the cerebellum (see Ito *et al.*, 1973). Ito (1970) suggests that Purkinje cells in the flocculus, which project to the vestibular nuclei (Angaut and Brodal, 1967), exert an inhibitory action on the vestibular nuclei cells, which in turn excite or inhibit motoneurons of the extraocular muscles. Thus

---

[3]Electrophysiological techniques have been used to determine the action of these pathways on the ON. Postsynaptic potentials (p.s.p.'s) recorded intracellularly in motoneurons of the ON have been used to determine whether vestibular nuclei axons exert an excitatory or inhibitory action on these motoneurons. Excitatory postsynaptic potentials (e.p.s.p.'s) have been assumed to indicate excitatory action, inhibitory postsynaptic potentials (i.p.s.p.'s) have been assumed to indicate inhibitory action. Studies which have used these techniques and on which the above summary statements are based include Baker *et al.* (1969, 1973), Highstein (1973), Highstein *et al.* (1971), and Sasaki (1963).

Purkinje cells in the flocculus provide an inhibitory or negative input at a summation point within the SVN, whereas vestibular primary afferent fibers provide an excitatory or positive input. It further appears that the inhibitory effect of floccular Purkinje cells may be modulated by a direct feedback route from the eye. That is, a circuit may exist which provides the vestibulocerebellum with sensory input regarding image position (or its mathematical derivatives) on the retina. Maekawa and Simpson (1973) have observed climbing fiber responses in the flocculus and nodulus of the rabbit following stimulation of the optic nerve and the retina. Ito *et al.* (1973) have suggested that eye movement which is driven by signals from the lateral semicircular duct is influenced by inhibitory control from floccular Purkinje cells which receive feedback from the ipsilateral retina via climbing fibers.

Thus, with certain assumptions, a feedback loop may exist whereby information from the visual system is routed back through the cerebellum to the vestibular nuclei (Fig. 6). This information could be useful for integration of visual and vestibular inputs in the regulation of the position of the eyes during natural head movements.

Control by Structures Rostral to the Vestibular Nuclei. A variety of studies (see Markham, 1972, for review) confirm the fact that cortical structures, diencephalic structures, and midbrain structures also influence vestibular-induced eye movements. However, just as it is not clear how vestibular information ascends to the cortex (see section "Vestibulocortical Projection Area"), it is not clear how the higher centers act on the vestibuloocular reflex arc. However, it does appear that, whatever the mechanism of action, it is primarily inhibitory. Two midbrain nuclei have been the subject of neurobiological studies. It has been shown that electrical stimulation of the nucleus of Darkschewitch has an inhibitory effect on eye movements of vestibular origin (Scheibel *et al.* 1961). Also, more specifically, it has been shown that electrical stimulation of the interstitial nucleus of Cajal inhibits certain types of ipsilateral neurons in the vestibular nuclei which are innervated by the lateral ampullary nerve (Markham *et al.*, 1966). These results suggest (Markham, 1972) that the midbrain nuclei may be relay stations for descending cortical control of the cristoocular reflex in cases where it is desired to have the eyes and the head move in the same direction and *not* in opposite directions as is dictated by the cristoocular reflex (see next section).

BEHAVIORAL CONSIDERATIONS: COMPENSATORY EYE MOVEMENT. The primary role of the cristoocular reflex is to ensure that during physiological head motions the eyes counterrotate an equal amount but in an opposite direction to angular head movement in any of the planes in which the head can move. Compensatory eye movements serve to stabilize images of the visual environment on the retina as the head turns.

This task of the cristoocular reflex involves a double mathematical integration of angular acceleration of the head which is sensed by the semicircular ducts. The first integration appears to occur in the semicircular ducts (see section "The Torsion Pendulum Analogy"). However, for the extraocular muscles to receive neural coded information so that they can move the eyes to an opposite position, a mathematical integration of head velocity information must take place. The

MANNING J. CORREIA
AND
FRED E. GUEDRY, JR.

anatomical site of this integrator is unknown. However, it appears to be located between the vestibular nuclei and the motoneurons of the extraocular muscles (e.g., abducens nucleus) since the former appears to carry head velocity information (Melvill Jones and Milsum, 1970) and the latter appears to carry head position information (Skavenski and Robinson, 1973). The cerebellum (Carpenter, 1972) and the pontine reticular formation (Cohen and Komatsuzaki, 1972) have been mentioned as possible sites of this integrator (see Robinson, 1974). The precision with which the cristoocular pathways produce this double integration and thus appropriate compensatory eye movement is remarkable and is discussed in detail in Chapter 10 of this volume.

Appropriate responses based on the cristoocular reflex are not restricted to any specific planes of head movement. For example, if you move your head in some plane other than the sagittal, frontal, or horizontal, equal and opposite eye movements occur. In fact, there is not a plane in which you can move your head and not obtain equal and opposite counterrotation of the eyes. This feat requires remarkable spatial resolution by the ampullary receptors and oculomotor effectors. This resolution for the cristoocular reflex appears to be based on the following considerations. The membranous labyrinth is a continuous closed system filled with endolymph. Therefore, endolymph can flow in more than one duct at the same time. It has been suggested, based on biophysical calculations (Groen, 1957; Landolt *et al.*, 1975) and verified by neurophysiological experiments (Estes *et al.*, 1975), that the pressure difference across the cupula (which causes cupula distortion and the consequent change in primary afferent neural activity) is directly proportional to the area of projection of the semicircular duct onto the plane of head rotation. Each ampullary nerve therefore must carry neural information proportionate to the extent to which its semicircular duct projects onto the plane of head rotation. This information is relayed to the extraocular muscles in a manner (see Wilson, 1972, for specific neural circuit of horizontal eye movements) which has the gross effect of producing eye movement in a plane determined by the proportionate neural discharge from each of the ampullary nerves. This effect is achieved because a spatial correspondence exists between eye movement plane and semicircular duct plane. That is, stimulation of semicircular ducts which lie in the same plane (e.g., right anterior and left posterior or right and left lateral) produces eye and head movement coplanar with the plane of these ducts. This spatial correspondence has been determined experimentally (Szenthagothi, 1950; Cohen and Suzuki, 1963; Suzuki *et al.*, 1969a; Cohen and Bender, 1966), and it is summarized in Table III. Figure 7 illustrates this important spatial correspondence on a more macroscopic level. Head movement produced by electrical stimulation of individual ampullary nerves clearly demonstrates that the head movement is coplanar with the semicircular duct whose ampullary nerve is stimulated (Fig. 7A,B). For eye movements, however, the planar correspondence is not so obvious. Stimulation of individual vertical ampullary nerves produces apparent disconjugate eye movement (Fig. 7B). However, as Suzuki *et al.* (1964) point out, this disconjugate eye movement actually compensates for the displacement of the optic axis of each eye from the midline and produces eye movement which is indeed coplanar with the vertical semicircular duct stimulated.

Thus two comparisons appear to permit the cristoocular reflex to achieve its objective, which is to produce counterrotation of the eyes in an equal and opposite direction but in the exact same plane as head motion. The first comparison is between the relative neural activity in each of the six ampullary nerves. This comparison apparently determines the plane of compensatory eye movements. The second comparison is between the neural activity in these nerves during head rotation and the spontaneous level of neural activity which is present during no head motion. This comparison may signal the magnitude of the head movement.

Since the cristoocular reflex causes the eyes to move in an equal but opposite direction to head movement, eye movement normally assumes the same waveshape as head movement, with one exception. That exception is a characteristic pattern of eye movements called *nystagmus*. During nystagmus the physiologically appropriate slow counterrotation of the eyes is interrupted by fast saccades in a direction opposite to the slow eye movements. These fast saccadic interruptions of the slow eye movements (slow phase) are called the fast phases. Nystagmus is the predominant cristoocular response to pathology or to excessive nonphysiological stimulation of the labyrinth. Nystagmus can occur, however, during normal head movements, particularly if they are of large amplitude and at submaximal rates. In the medical literature, the direction of nystagmus is defined by the direction of the fast phase. This is understandable since it is much easier for a physician who is looking at a patient's eyes to see the fast phase as compared to the slow phase, but it is unfortunate since it obscures the fact that the slow phase of nystagmus is the physiologically appropriate response of the vestibular apparatus, whereas the fast phase of nystagmus may be more closely associated with other neural structures (see Shimazu, 1972).

When head motion involves tipping the head relative to gravity (which occurs for all head motions except those which are in the Earth's horizontal plane), firing patterns from the otolith organs must also be considered since they also have neural projections to the extraocular motoneurons.

TABLE III. RELATIONSHIP BETWEEN AMPULLARY NEURAL DISCHARGE AND EXTRAOCULAR MUSCLE CONTRACTION

Mechanical stimulation (Szentagothai, 1950)			Electrical stimulation (Cohen *et al.*, 1964)	Major extraocular muscle which contracted[a]	
Semicircular duct	Direction of endolymph flow	Ampullary neural discharge	Effective ampullary discharge	Ipsilateral	Contralateral
Anterior	Utriculofugal	Increase	Increase	Sup. rectus	Inf. oblique
Posterior	Utriculofugal	Increase	Increase	Sup. oblique	Inf. rectus
Lateral	Utriculopetal	Increase	Increase	Med. rectus	Lat. rectus

[a] Generally it may be stated that electrical stimulation of an ampullary nerve results in excitation of one (see above) of the extraocular muscles in each eye and inhibition of the antagonistic muscle. This effect is mediated by excitation of the appropriate motoneurons in the contralateral ON and inhibition of the appropriate motoneurons in the ipsilateral ON (see Highstein, 1973, for an exception).

MANNING J. CORREIA
AND
FRED E. GUEDRY, JR.

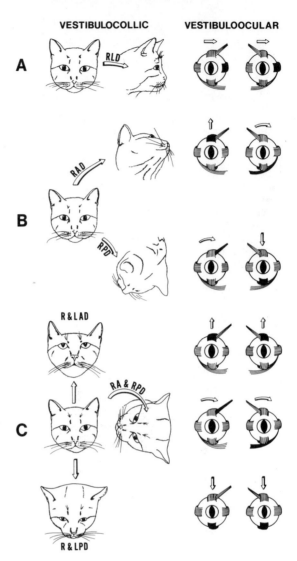

Fig. 7. Effects of electrical ampullary nerve stimulation on eye and head movement. Direction of movement of the head and eyes is illustrated for unilateral and bilateral stimulation of ampullary nerves from the anterior, posterior, and lateral semicircular ducts. R, Right; L, left; AD, anterior duct; PD, posterior duct; LD, lateral duct. Extraocular muscles which develop strong contractions are indicated by a black overlay. Note that plane of head movement and plane of eye movement are coplanar with the semicircular ducts whose ampullary nerves are stimulated or in planes which correspond to an appropriate response to angular head rotation. Based on the work of Suzuki and Cohen (1964), Cohen *et al.* (1964), and Cohen and Bender (1966).

Maculoocular Reflex

Neurobiological Organization. Stein and Carpenter (1967) observed that in the rhesus monkey utricular fibers project to the dorsolateral part of the MVN. A few saccular fibers were observed to enter the MVN. Gacek (1969) found that in the cat utricular fibers terminated in the rostral part of the MVN. In both species, therefore, few, if any, macular fibers were observed to project to the SVN, and those observed to project to the MVN appear to be rostral to the sites of origin of axons which project to the ON (Tarlov, 1972). Thus macular fibers do not project heavily to areas of origin of the two major vestibuloocular pathways. Macular fibers have been observed to project to the LVN and DVN (see section "Projections to Vestibular Nuclei"). However, Highstein and Ito (1971) were unable to observe any monosynaptic effects on the ON by fibers from the LVN and DVN. These anatomical and physiological results suggest that the maculoocular reflex is either a longer neural chain than the cristoocular reflex or that its route is not through the regions of the vestibular nuclei which provide the majority of projections to the ON. In the rabbit, an animal with laterally placed eyes, projections to the abducens motor nuclei have been observed from areas which receive primary afferent macular projections, namely, the group *y* of Brodal and Pompeiano (1957) and the lateral cerebellar nucleus (Highstein *et al.*, 1971). In this animal a disynaptic maculoocular pathway may exist.

The implications of current neuroanatomical studies discussed above are that (1) the otolith organs play a minor role in ocular reflexes and (2) the maculoocular reflex is a slower system than the cristoocular reflex. Neither of these implications is consistent with physiological or biophysical considerations. As indicated previously (see section "The Mass-Spring-Dashpot Analogy"), electrophysiological and biophysical studies indicate that the statoconiorum membrane system is a fast system. Additionally, Suzuki *et al.* (1969*b*) found that electrical stimulation of the whole utricular nerve induced countertorsion of both eyes. They also observed that stimulation of the *utricular nerve* induced changes in the eye muscles with a latency of 5.0 msec. Cohen and Suzuki (1963) reported extraocular muscle potential latencies of 5.0–6.0 msec following *ampullary nerve* stimulation. A comparison of latencies suggests that the maculoocular reflex is as fast as the cristoocular reflex.

BEHAVIORAL CONSIDERATIONS. Eye movements produced by physiological linear accelerations are of two types: static and dynamic eye movement. The static eye movement, ocular countertorsion, occurs when the head remains tipped relative to gravity. The eyes remain counterrotated as long as the head remains tilted. Dynamic eye movement, i.e., eye movement which changes with time, occurs in response to dynamic (time-changing) linear acceleration. For example, as a man runs across rough terrain, his head moves vertically up and down and pitches forward and backward relative to gravity. Thus the resultant linear acceleration vector (vector sum of forward linear acceleration and linear acceleration due to gravity) moves through the man's head. He must make compensatory eye movements to maintain the environment in focus.

Ocular Countertorsion. Static ocular countertorsion supposedly ensures that the environment remains "perceptually upright" during head tilt. However, some sort of amplification must occur at neural levels higher than the ON, since the magnitude of ocular countertorsion is much smaller than corresponding magnitudes of head tilt. Miller (1962) observed that counterrolling of the eyes in the frontal head plane increased with increasing angles of head tilt in the same plane up to head tilt angles of 45–90°. However, ocular counterrolling reached a maximum of 5–8° with head tilts of 45–90°. On the other hand, Correia *et al.* (1968) have observed that there is much less disparity between head tilt and

MANNING J. CORREIA
AND
FRED E. GUEDRY, JR.

adjustment of a luminour rod to one's *perception* of Earth vertical and Earth horizontal.

The disparity between static ocular compensation and head movement is much greater for the maculoocular reflex than the cristoocular reflex (see Chapter 10 of this volume). The mechanisms by which higher neural centers compensate for this disparity will become apparent with future neurobiological investigation.

Dynamic Ocular Responses. Studies which clearly demonstrate dynamic ocular responses to *pure* dynamic linear acceleration have been reviewed elsewhere (e.g., Benson and Barnes, 1973). Whether these eye movements result from pure otolithic stimulation is still a matter of controversy (see Correia and Money, 1970; Goldberg and Fernandez, 1975*b*). However, these studies have produced the following results which have behavioral implications: (1) Compensatory eye movement can be produced by change in linear acceleration of the head in the absence of any previous or coacting angular acceleration, i.e., without any confounding responses from the cristoocular reflex (Niven *et al.*, 1966; Benson and Barnes, 1973). (2) Compensatory eye movement produced by dynamic linear acceleration of the head does not appear to occur in all ocular planes as does compensatory eye movement which is produced by angular acceleration. Specifically, compensatory eye movement has been produced by dynamic linear acceleration acting in the horizontal or frontal head plane (xy or yz planes of Fig. 3), but no vertical compensatory eye movement has been noted for linear acceleration acting in the sagittal (xz) head plane (Niven *et al.*, 1966). (3) Horizontal eye movement produced by dynamic linear acceleration of the head terminates immediately following deceleration of the head (Benson and Barnes, 1973). Thus, whatever system which produces compensatory eye movement to dynamic linear acceleration, it may be presumed that it is a fast one (Niven *et al.*, 1966).

VESTIBULOSPINAL REFLEXES

The vestibulospinal reflexes are concerned with head motion, righting, balance, posture, and coordinated locomotion. As such, these reflexes, which have been categorized and thoroughly discussed elsewhere (Roberts, 1967) are of obvious behavioral importance. Neural information for vestibulospinal reflexive and purposive behavior is primarily mediated over two pathways.

NEUROBIOLOGICAL ORGANIZATION

The two major pathways illustrated for the vestibular nuclei on the left side of Fig. 6 mediate information from the labyrinth to the spinal musculature. These pathways are the medial vestibulospinal tract (MVST) and the lateral vestibulospinal tract (LVST). Other pathways, principally the reticulospinal and propriospinal tracts, which may receive collaterals from the LVST, may serve as important secondary pathways for conduction of vestibulospinal information to upper and particularly lower spinal levels (e.g., lumbosacral levels). The vestibulospinal reflexes consist of a three (sometimes more) neuron chain; primary afferent ganglion cell → vestibular nucleus cell → spinal motoneuron. In terms of behavior, it is convenient to further classify vestibulospinal reflexes into vestibulocollic reflexes (reflexes which involve the neck) and vestibulospinal reflexes of the limbs and torso.

THE MEDIAL VESTIBULOSPINAL TRACT. The MVST (Nyberg-Hansen, 1966) originates primarily in the MVN and to a lesser extent in the DVN (Wilson et al., 1967). Axons from these nuclei turn medially and course bilaterally (mostly uncrossed, however) in the MLF. In the spinal cord, MVST fibers course in the posterior part of the anterior funiculus and terminate in the medial part of the ventral horn, specifically in lamina VIII and adjacent parts of lamina VII (Nyberg-Hansen, 1964). Few, if any, MVST fibers have been traced below the cervical enlargement (McMaster et al., 1966). MVST fibers primarily exert an inhibitory effect (Wilson and Yoshida, 1969b) on neck muscle extensor motoneurons. However, Akaike et al. (1973) and Wilson and Maeda (1974) have shown that MVST fibers may also exert an excitatory effect contralaterally. It is probable that the inhibitory effects are modulated by descending control from the cerebellum, interstitial nucleus of Cajal (Markham, 1968), and other rostral structures. The MVN receives projections from the nodulus and flocculus (Angaut and Brodal, 1967), as well as from the fastigial nuclei (Brodal et al., 1962). The DVN receives projections from portions of the vestibulocerebellum as well as from the vermis of the anterior lobe (Walberg and Jansen, 1961).

THE LATERAL VESTIBULOSPINAL TRACT. The LVST arises in the LVN and courses purely ipsilaterally as far as the sacral segments of the cord. In the cervical cord the LVST is located in the periphery of the ventrolateral funiculus. The LVST courses dorsomedially in the thoracic cord to a medial position in the ventral funiculus (along the anterior median fissure) of the lumbar enlargement (Pompeiano and Brodal, 1957). LVST fibers, as shown in Fig. 6, make monosynaptic and polysynaptic connections with alpha and possibly gamma motoneurons (Wilson and Yoshida, 1969a; Pompeiano, 1972; Lund and Pompeiano, 1965). The neural circuitry exists for cerebellar control of vestibulospinal reflexes, just as was described earlier for the vestibuloocular reflexes. The LVN receives projections from the cerebellar cortex and the fastigial nuclei. Specifically, ipsilateral and contralateral axons project from the fastigial nucleus to the LVN (Brodal et al., 1962); cerebellar cortex fibers from the vermis of the anterior lobe, the flocculus, the nodulus, and the uvula also reach parts of the LVN (Angaut and Brodal, 1967). There is experimental evidence that activity from Purkinje cells in the anterior lobe vermis inhibits cells in the LVN (Ito and Yoshida, 1966; Ito et al., 1968), while stimulation of the fastigial nuclei is excitatory to LVN cells (Ito et al., 1970).

INTEGRATED ACTION OF THE LVST AND MVST. Wilson and Yoshida (1969a) observed disynaptic e.p.s.p.'s in upper cervical extensor alpha motoneurons with most latencies between 1.4 and 2.5 msec following ipsilateral electrical stimulation of the labyrinth. This stimulus also produced i.p.s.p.'s in cervical motoneurons which appeared to be disynaptic and mediated by the MVST (Wilson and Yoshida, 1969b). These results suggest that fast low-threshold pathways exist from the labyrinth to the neck and that excitatory fibers of the LVST and inhibitory fibers

MANNING J. CORREIA
AND
FRED E. GUEDRY, JR.

of the MVST provide the reciprocal excitatory and inhibitory innervation on the neck motoneurons necessary for a precise control system.

Wilson and Maeda (1974) (also summarized in Wilson, 1975) have further defined the neural circuits for the vestibulocollic reflex. They studied the cristocollic reflex. Generally, it appears that the MVST exerts primarily disynaptic inhibition of ipsilateral and disynaptic excitation and inhibition of contralateral neck motoneurons following ampullary nerve stimulation, while the LVST exerts disynaptic excitation to ipsilateral neck motoneurons. Thus the MVST exerts contralateral excitation and bilateral inhibition, and the LVST carries ipsilateral excitation.

BEHAVIORAL CONSIDERATIONS

VESTIBULOCOLLIC REFLEXES. The vestibulocollic reflex involves the labyrinth (semicircular ducts, Wilson, 1975; otolith organs, Wilson *et al.*, 1977) as the receptor and the neck muscles as the effectors. Suzuki and Cohen (1964) illustrated the cristocollic reflex by electrically stimulating ampullary nerves and observing head motion in an unanesthetized cat. Their results are summarized in Fig. 7 (from Cohen and Bender, 1966). It may be noted in Fig. 7 that the planes of the cristocollic head movement and cristoocular eye movement are nearly the same. This emphasizes the major roles of the vestibulocollic reflex, which may be summarized as follows: (1) The vestibulocollic reflex augments the vestibuloocular system in maintaining retinal image stabilization during whole body motion and during whole body tilt. Specifically, the cristoocular and cristocollic reflexes coact to stabilize vision relative to the axis of head turn; the maculoocular and maculocollic reflexes provide compensation for tilt of the axis of the head turn relative to gravity. Although it must be remembered that whenever the axis of rotation of the head is tilted, both maculo- and cristoreflexes are involved. (2) The vestibulocollic reflex seeks to maintain the head stationary in inertial space. To achieve this result, the vestibulocollic system involves a closed feedback loop. The vestibular apparatus, which is fixed in the head, is stimulated by head motion which is the result of the vestibulocollic reflex. Thus the control circuit exists for an error-activated system in which the head is driven to null labyrinthine input (i.e., maintain ampullary and macular discharge at its spontaneous level) and thereby maintain the head stationary in space (see Outerbridge, 1969). Dramatic behavioral consequences occur when this feedback loop is interrupted. For example, cats with their semicircular ducts mechanically deactivated (Money and Scott, 1962) have residual spontaneous discharge from the labyrinthine receptors. However, the inability of this discharge to be modulated (due to deactivation of end organs) produces uncontrolled pendular head motions in some animals for periods of up to several months (Money and Scott, 1962).

The vestibulocollic reflex appears to be highly developed in certain species where teleology dictates. In the cat, a strong vestibulocollic reflex can be inferred from studies on decerebrate rigidity. Destruction of the LVN considerably reduces the marked extensor rigidity produced by this procedure (Brodal *et al.*, 1962).

However, only opisthotonos is abolished in decerebrate-decerebellate cats when their labyrinths are destroyed (Batini *et al.*, 1957). Thus we may conclude that other systems which input to the LVN are responsible for facilitating postural tonus, whereas the labyrinthine input is closely related to the vestibulocollic reflex system. Birds of prey, particularly those with a poorly developed vestibuloocular reflex, such as the owl, have a highly developed vestibulocollic reflex. These animals are remarkable in their ability to maintain head (and hence eye) stability during different types of body motions (see Money and Correia, 1972). This clearly has survival value, for it allows the bird to maintain visual fixation on its prey during flight, particularly in turbulent air.

VESTIBULOSPINAL REFLEXES OF TORSO AND LIMBS. LVST fibers appear to be the primary excitatory and inhibitory pathway for forelimb and especially hindlimb motoneurons. Electrophysiological studies which involved stimulation of the LVN (see Pompeiano, 1972) produced monosynaptic e.p.s.p.'s in hindlimb extensor motoneurons of the ankle and knee; disynaptic and polysynaptic e.p.s.p.'s in most extensor motoneurons and a few flexor motoneurons, particularly pretibial motoneurons (Grillner *et al.*, 1970); and disynaptic and polysynaptic i.p.s.p.'s in many flexor motoneurons, particularly in the knee and ankle (Lund and Pompeiano, 1968; Wilson and Yoshida, 1969*a*), and a few extensor motoneurons, e.g., those of the hip (Grillner *et al.*, 1970). It appears that the flexor inhibition described above is produced by excitatory LVST fibers acting through segmental inhibitory neurons (Wilson, 1972).

In contrast to the vestibulocollic reflex, the vestibulospinal reflexes of the torso and limbs are generally at least trisynaptic, and axons of the final synapse appear to end on spinal interneurons (Maeda *et al.*, 1975). This neuroanatomical structure permits other systems to be integrated with the vestibular system to control postural reflexes. However, this arrangement may preclude the speed and precision of response which exists for the vestibulocollic reflex.

When an animal, such as a cat, stands on a platform which is tilted laterally to one side (e.g., see Wilson, 1975, Fig. 1), it extends its ipsilateral limbs and flexes its contralateral limbs. Man makes the same movements if the platform upon which he is crawling is tilted or if he starts to fall laterally. Roberts (1968) has confirmed this muscle flexion-extension pattern during head tilt in the forelimbs of decerebrate cats whose necks have been denervated. This study suggests that neural activity within the ipsilateral LVST increases during ipsilateral body tilts and decreases during contralateral body tilts. A similar but less definite pattern has been noted for the hindlimbs. It appears that ipsilateral tilt produces a diminished increase or a decrease in ipsilateral extensor activity (Erhardt and Wagner, 1970).

Human vestibulospinal reflex research has been conducted primarily along two lines. Both of these lines of research have exposed subjects to linear acceleration and observed either whole body compensatory responses or electrophysiological responses from certain selected muscles. Nashner (1972), for example, modeled the postural control system using body sway data obtained by tilting subjects on a platform. Watt and Melvill Jones (see, e.g., Melvill Jones, 1973) recorded e.m.g.'s from the gastrocnemius muscle before, during, and after unexpected release of subjects who were suspended at various heights above the floor.

SPINOVESTIBULAR PATHWAYS AND BEHAVIORAL CORRELATES. Somatic afferent impulses from muscle spindles, Golgi tendons, and other proprioceptors in ligaments, fascia, and joint capsules must be integrated with vestibular sensory information in the performance of reflexive and purposive behavior.

There is some evidence for a direct spinovestibular pathway (see Fig. 6), as well as more meager evidence for indirect pathways from the spinal cord to the vestibular nuclei via the reticular formation and the cerebellum (Brodal *et al.*, 1962). Spinovestibular fibers originate from the lumbrosacral levels of the spinal cord (Pompeiano and Brodal, 1957), and possibly from the cervical and thoracic levels as well. These fibers course ipsilaterally in the dorsal part of the lateral funiculus along with fibers of the dorsal spinocerebellar tract and terminate in the caudalmost regions of the DVN and the MVN, the dorsocaudal part of the LVN and in the vestibular complex cell groups x and z (Brodal and Pompeiano, 1957).

It has been suggested that proprioceptors which originate spinovestibular impulses are primarily located in the joints and signal joint displacement. Increased DVN, MVN, and LVN activity has been noted during joint movement but not during skin stimulation or deep muscle pressure (Fredrickson *et al.*, 1966*a;* Fredrickson and Schwarz, 1970). Recent behavioral experiments (Correia *et al.*, 1977) suggest that the spinovestibular contribution of muscle spindle afferents deserves reexamination.

It is evident that extralabyrinthine proprioception which is mediated by the spinovestibular pathways plays a role in the reflexive control of the head and body and probably in perception of motion and tilt of the head and body. However, the authoritative role of this sensory input in the perception of motion is illustrated by the following observation (Correia *et al.*, 1977). It has been repeatedly demonstrated in the vestibular literature that when a person sits on a rotating chair that decelerates from constant velocity rotation about an Earth vertical axis, perception of rotation is counter to the direction of previous rotation; i.e., the subject perceives the chair deceleration or equivalently acceleration in the opposite direction. Even after the rotator is stationary the perception of rotation continues. This illusionary perception has been called the "somatogyral illusion" and is discussed in Chapter 10. If, however, a person actively spins himself around in a pirouette maneuver for about 8 turns in 34 sec, the following unexpected sequence of events occurs when the person stops. His body may or may not twist about its long axis; i.e., he may assume a position which is a variation of the "discus-thrower's position" (see McNally and Stuart, 1967, Fig. 22, p. 73), and significantly he generally perceives body rotation in the same direction as previous rotation. This observation suggests that the cristospinal reflex produces a response that feeds back proprioceptive input from the spinal afferents which is mediated by ascending spinal pathways. The proprioceptive information appears to override the afferent input from the vestibular apparatus with regard to the perception of motion.

In general, however, during natural movements, the vestibular system and other proprioceptive systems work together to provide accurate information to higher centers about the location of the head and body in space. This synergistic action of the spinal afferents and vestibular afferents to provide information as to the orientation of head and body in space appears to be preserved in the rostral projections of these systems.

343

VESTIBULAR SYSTEM:
BASIC MECHANISMS

Rostral Projections of the Vestibular System

Neurobiological Organization

Vestibulocortical Projection Area. The VCPA (see Fig. 6) has been located in several species using electrophysiological techniques. In the cat, the VCPA is within the anterior suprasylvian sulcus immediately adjacent to the auditory area (Mickle and Ades, 1952). This area corresponds to the temporal lobe in primates. In man, in fact, electrical stimulation of portions of the superior temporal gyrus produces "dizziness," "swinging," and "spinning" (Penfield, 1957). However, in the rhesus monkey, vestibular fibers seem to project to a region of the postcentral gyrus between the primary and secondary somesthetic areas slightly posterior to Brodmann's area 2 (Fredrickson *et al.*, 1966*b*). This region is immediately posterior to the SI mouth field. Walzl and Mountcastle (1949) also found a similar projection area in the cat. In the guinea pig (Odkvist *et al.*, 1973*a*), rabbit (Odkvist *et al.*, 1973*b*), and squirrel monkey (*cf.* Odkvist *et al.*, 1973*a*), however, the VCPA appears to be located within the region of the sensory-motor forelimb field. This region corresponds to Brodmann's area 3a. The above results suggest that as evolutionary development proceeded the VCPA migrated from the somatosensory-motor area of the cortex toward the "associative" parietal cortex. In any event, it appears that in animals higher in evolutionary development, the cortical projections of the vestibular system become less associated with the auditory system and more closely associated with the proprioceptive systems. Throughout this chapter, the close relationship among the vestibular, the somesthetic and the kinesthetic systems have been indicated. It seems reasonable to conclude that in terrestrial animals, which are high in evolutionary development, the vestibular and auditory systems have in common only the eighth nerve whereas the vestibular system is completely intermeshed with proprioceptive systems from the sacral cord to the cortical projection areas.

In all the studies cited above, the latencies of evoked potentials in the cortex following vestibular nerve stimulation were at least trisynaptic (>3 msec). Gacek (1973) and Tarlov (1969) used neuroanatomical techniques (selective silver methods) to examine the rostral projections of the cat's and primate's (macaque, baboon, and chimpanzee) vestibular nuclei. Both authors concluded that a few fibers from this major waystation pass rostral to the complex of the oculomotor nuclei into the nuclei of the posterior commissure, the interstitial nuclei of Cajal, and the nuclei of Darkschewitsch (see Fig. 6). However, *no* vestibular nuclei fibers were observed to project to the thalamus (see Table I, Tarlov, 1969, for a literature review of conflicting results) *or* rostral to the level of the posterior commissure. Tarlov (1969) did confirm projections from the vestibular nuclei to the reticular formation. Therefore, he suggested that vestibular sensation might reach levels rostral to the posterior commissure by way of at least trisynaptic pathways. Specifically, he suggested that the reticulothalamic pathway might be a candidate to provide such a vestibuloreticulodiencephalic pathway.

VESTIBULOTHALAMIC PROJECTION AREA. While neuroanatomical studies have not identified the routes by which vestibular impulses reach the thalamus, electrophysiological evidence indicates that a thalamic representation of the vestibular system exists and that it corresponds to the VCPA (see Fig. 6). In the cat, long- and short-latency evoked potentials have been observed in the thalamus following electrical stimulation of the vestibular nerve (Mickle and Ades, 1954; Sans *et al.*, 1970). Mickle and Ades (1954) observed a short-latency evoked potential (4–5 msec) in an area between the medial geniculate body (MG) and the ventral posterolateral nucleus (VPL). Sans *et al.* (1970) observed a short-latency (1.5–2.0 msec) evoked potential in the VPL and a long-latency potential (3–10 msec) in the ventral lateral nucleus (VL). Sans *et al.* (1970) suggested that the cerebellum might provide a route for the long-latency potentials. In the rhesus monkey, Deecke *et al.* (1973) obtained long-latency and short-latency vestibular thalamic responses. A short-latency (2.5 msec) response was found in the ventral posteroinferior nucleus (VPI) which lies between and at the bottom of the ventral posterolateral nucleus (VPL) and the ventral posteromedial nucleus (VPM). A long-latency (4–5 msec) response was found in the medial geniculate body (magnocellular part), the ventrobasal (VB) complex, and the posterior and medial nuclei. The long-latency potentials observed by Deecke *et al.* (1973) persisted after cerebellectomy, thus providing contradictory evidence to the cerebellothalamic pathway suggested by Sans *et al.* (1970; see above). Deecke *et al.* (1973) observed that under barbituate anesthesia a few single neural units located in the VPI responded to both vestibular and kinesthetic inputs but not visual, acoustic, or skin stimulation. This observation has also been noted in the vestibular nuclei (Fredrickson, 1970) and the VCPA of the rhesus monkey (Schwarz and Fredrickson, 1971). Buttner and Henn (1976) appear to have confirmed the results of Deecke *et al.* (1973). They have observed rotation-sensitive single neural units in the VPI of the rhesus monkey.

BEHAVIORAL CONSIDERATIONS

The VCPA appears to serve two primary roles with respect to behavior. First, it acts as one of the loci for "sensory-sensory" and "sensory-motor" integration of messages concerned with spatial orientation, and, second, it provides for conscious perception of orientation in space. In Chapter 10, examples are given to illustrate veridical and illusionary perception of spatial orientation produced by vestibular stimulation alone as well as coacting with visual and somatosensory stimulation. Besides integrating these sensory inputs, the VCPA, as part of area 2 in the primate, is strongly interconnected to the motor cortex. It has been suggested by Kornhuber (1971) that the motor cortex adjusts motor signals generated by the cerebellum and basal ganglia by feedback from the somatosensory cortex (including VCPA) so that external objects can be accurately and appropriately handled.

It has been difficult to anatomically and physiologically locate the VCPA for several reasons. First, physiological studies on man have used electrical stimulation of cortical areas and required the patient to make the difficult distinction between vestibular sensations such as spinning and tilting from other body motion sensations which could result from stimulation of other proprioceptors. Second, with phylogenetic development the VCPA has assumed a more sophisticated role and therefore established more diffuse connections within the cortex. Its anatomical location may have even changed. These facts could explain the confusing results concerning the location and physiology of the VCPA in various species. Third, isolation of electrophysiological responses exclusively to vestibular stimulation is very difficult because, even before the level of the VCPA, the vestibular system has formed reciprocal relations with ascending and descending pathways which mediate proprioception and exteroception (vision, for example; see Grusser and Grusser-Cornehls, 1972).

It is probable that within several years, however, the VCPA will be anatomically delineated for different species by the use of neuronal marking techniques which utilize axonal transport. Elucidation of the physiology of the VCPA in its role of "sensory-sensory" and "sensory-motor" integration awaits years of neurobiological investigation.

CONCLUSIONS

As indicated in Figs. 1, 2, and 6, there are numerous diffuse interrelations of the vestibular apparatus and other structures within the nervous system. These interrelations are necessary to perform the complex tasks of retinal image stabilization, orientation, and smooth coordinated locomotion. During physiological head and body motions, the biophysics of the vestibular sense organs and their reflexive neural connections with various muscles of the head and body permit these tasks to be performed with speed and precision. This fidelity of response is further augmented by supplementary information from other sensory systems (e.g., vision, somesthesia). Unfortunately, unusual environmental or pathophysiological conditions can cause the vestibular system to produce inappropriate responses which can be disconcerting, incapacitating, or possibly fatal. One must appreciate both the physiological and nonphysiological aspects of the stimulus–response relations of the vestibular system since an acquaintance with one simplifies the understanding of the other. A more comprehensive summary which integrates these two aspects can be found at the end of Chapter 10 in this volume.

Acknowledgments

The artwork of R. W. Henricksen and Carolyn Martin and the secretarial assistance of Jan Arriola, Pat Groves, and Julie Breaux are gratefully acknowledged. Finally, sincere appreciation is expressed to those colleagues who kindly read and commented on various sections of this chapter.

MANNING J. CORREIA
AND
FRED E. GUEDRY, JR.

Akaike, T., Fanardjian, V. V., Ito, M., and Ohino, T. Electrophysiological analysis of the vestibulospinal reflex pathway of rabbit. II. Synaptic actions upon spinal neurones. *Exp. Brain Res.*, 1973, *17*, 497–515.

Angaut, P., and Brodal, A. The projection of the vestibulo-cerebellum onto the vestibular nuclei in the cat. *Arch. Ital. Biol.*, 1967, *105*, 441–479.

Anonymous. *Nomina Anatomica*, 3rd ed. Excerpta Medica Foundation, New York, 1968.

Anson, B. J., Harper, D. G., and Winch, T. R. The vestibular and cochlear aqueducts: Developmental and adult anatomy of their contents and parietes. In Third Symposium on the Role of the Vestibular Organs in Space Exploration. *NASA SP152*, 1967, pp. 125–146.

Baker, R. G., Mano, N., and Shimazu, H. Postsynaptic potentials in abducens motoneurons induced by vestibular stimulation. *Brain Res.*, 1969, *15*, 577–580.

Baker, R. G., Precht, W., and Berthoz, A. Synaptic connections to trochlear motoneurons determined by individual vestibular nerve branch stimulation in the cat. *Brain Res.*, 1973, *64*, 402–406.

Batini, C., Moruzzi, G., and Pompeiano, O. Cerebellar release phenomena. *Arch. Ital. Biol.*, 1957, *95*, 71–95.

Benson, A. J., and Barnes, G. R. Responses to rotating linear acceleration vectors considered in relation to a model of the otolith organs. In Fifth Symposium on the Role of the Vestibular Organs in Space Exploration. *NASA SP-314*, 1973, pp. 221–236.

Bergström, B. Morphology of the vestibular nerve. Part 1. *Acta Otolaryngol. (Stockholm)*, 1973*a*, *76*, 162–172.

Bergström, B. Morphology of the vestibular nerve. Part 2. *Acta Otolaryngol. (Stockholm)*, 1973*b*, *76*, 173–330.

Bergström, B. Morphology of the vestibular nerve. Part 3. *Acta Otolaryngol. (Stockholm)*, 1973*c*, *76*, 331–402.

Bergström, B. Morphological studies of the vestibular nerve. *Acta Univ. Upsaliensis*, 1973*d*, *159*, 1–41.

Brodal, A., and Hoivik, B. Site and mode of termination of primary vestibulo-cerebellar fibres in the cat: An experimental study with silver impregnation methods. *Arch. Ital. Biol.*, 1964, *102*, 1–21.

Brodal, A., and Pompeiano, O. The vestibular nuclei in the cat. *J. Anat. (London)*, 1957, *91*, 438–454.

Brodal, A., Pompeiano, O., and Walberg, F. *The Vestibular Nuclei and Their Connections: Anatomy and Functional Correlations.* Oliver and Boyd, Edinburgh, 1962.

Buttner, U., and Henn, V. Thalamic unit activity in the alert monkey during natural vestibular stimulation. *Brain Res.*, 1976, *103*, 127–132.

Carlstrom, D., Engstrom, H., and Hjorth, S. Electron microscopic and X-ray diffraction studies of statoconia. *Laryngoscope (St. Louis)*, 1953, *63*, 1052–1057.

Carpenter, M. B., Stein, B. M., and Peter, P. Primary vestibulo-cerebellar fibers in the monkey: Distribution of fibers arising from distinctive cell groups of the vestibular ganglia. *Am. J. Anat.*, 1972, *135*, 221–250.

Carpenter, R. H. S. Cerebellectomy and the transfer function of the vestibulo-ocular reflex in the decerebrate cat. *Proc. Roy. Soc. London Ser. B*, *181*, 1972, 353–374.

Clark, B. The vestibular system. *Ann. Rev. Psychol.*, 1970, *21*, 273–206.

Cohen, B., and Bender, M. B. The relationship of the semicircular canals to induced head and eye movements in mammals. In R. J. Wolfson (ed.), *The Vestibular System and Its Diseases.* University of Pennsylvania Press, Philadelphia, 1966, pp. 131–158.

Cohen, B., and Komatsuzaki, A. Eye movements induced by stimulation of the pontine reticular formation: Evidence for integration in oculomotor pathways. *Exp. Neurol.*, 1972, *36*, 101–107.

Cohen, B., and Suzuki, J. I. Eye movements induced by ampullary nerve stimulation. *Am. J. Physiol.*, 1963, *204(2)*, 347–351.

Cohen, B., Suzuki, J. I., Shanzer, S., and Bender, M. B. Semicircular canal control of eye movements. In M. B. Bender (ed.), *The Oculomotor System.* Harper & Row, New York, 1964, pp. 163–173.

Collins, W. E., Crampton, G. H., and Posner, J. B. Effects of mental activity on vestibular nystagmus and the electroencephalogram. *Nature*, 1961, *190*, 194–195.

Correia, M. J., and Landolt, J. P. Spontaneous and driven responses from primary neurons of the anterior semicircular canal of the pigeon. *Adv. Oto-Rhino-Laryngol.*, 1973, *19*, 134–148.

Correia, M. J., and Landolt, J. P. A point process analysis of the spontaneous activity of anterior semicircular canal units in the anesthetized pigeon. *Biol. Cybern.*, 1977, *27*, 199–213.

Correia, M. J., and Landolt, J. P. Neurophysiological response mechanisms in the vestibular afferent system. In J. Pulec (ed.), *Menieres Disease.* Palisades Pub. Co., Los Angeles, 1978.

Correia, M. J., and Money, K. E. The effect of blockage of all six semicircular canal ducts on nystagmus produced by dynamic linear acceleration in the cat. *Acta Otolaryngol. (Stockholm)*, 1970, *69*, 7–16.

Correia, M. J., Hixson, W. C., and Niven, J. I. On predictive equations for subjective judgments of vertical and horizon in a force field. *Acta Otolaryngol. (Stockholm), Suppl.*, 1968, *230*, 1–30.

Correia, M. J., Nelson, J. B., and Guedry, F. E. Antisomatogyral Illusion. *Aviat. Space Environ. Med.*, 1977, *48(9)*, 859–862.

Deecke, L., Schwarz, D. W. F., and Fredrickson, J. M. Vestibular thalamus in the rhesus monkey. *Adv. Oto-Rhino-Laryngol.*, 1973, *19*, 210–219.

de Vries, H. The mechanics of the labyrinth otoliths. *Acta Otolaryngol. (Stockholm)*, 1950, *38*, 262–273.

Dohlman, G. The attachment of the cupulae, otolith and tectorial membranes to the sensory cell areas. *Acta Otolaryngol. (Stockholm)*, 1971, *71*, 89–105.

Engström, H., Bergström, B., and Ades, H. W. Macula utriculi and macula sacculi in squirrel monkey. In H. W. Ades and H. Engstrom (eds.), Inner Ear Studies. *Acta Otolaryngol. (Stockholm) Suppl.*, 1972, *301*, 75–126.

Erhardt, K. J., and Wagner, A. Labyrinthine and neck reflexes recorded from single spinal motoneurons in the cat. *Brain Res.*, 1970, *19*, 87–104.

Estes, M. S., Blanks, R. H. I., and Markham, C. H. Physiologic characteristics of vestibular first-order canal neurons in the cat. I. Response plane determination and resting discharge characteristics. *J. Neurophysiol.*, 1975, *38*, 1232–1249.

Fernandez, C., and Goldberg, J. M. Physiology of peripheral neurons innervating semicircular canals of the squirrel monkey. II. Response to sinusoidal stimulation and dynamics of peripheral vestibular system. *J. Neurophysiol.*, 1971, *34*, 661–675.

Fernandez, C., Goldberg, J. M., and Abend, W. K. Response to static tilts of peripheral neurons innervating otolith organs of the squirrel monkey. *J. Neurophysiol.*, 1972, *35*, 978–997.

Fernandez, C., and Goldberg, J. M. Physiology of peripheral neurons innervating otolith organs of the squirrel monkey. II. Directional selectivity and force–response relations. *J. Neurophysiol.*, 1976a, *39*, 985–995.

Fernandez, C., and Goldberg, J. M. Physiology of peripheral neurons innervating otolith organs of the squirrel monkey. III. Response dynamics. *J. Neurophysiol.*, 1976b, *39*, 996–1008.

Fluur, E., and Mellstrom, A. Utricular stimulation and oculomotor reactions. *Laryngoscope*, 1970a, *80*, 1701–1712.

Fluur, E., and Mellstrom, A. Saccular stimulation and oculomotor reactions. *Laryngoscope*, 1970b, *80*, 1713–1721.

Fredrickson, J. M. Vestibular nerve projection to association fields of the cerebral cortex in the monkey. In J. Stahle (ed.), *Vestibular Function on Earth and in Space*. Pergamon Press, Oxford, 1970.

Fredrickson, J. M., and Schwarz, D. Multisensory influence upon single units in the vestibular nucleus. In Fourth Symposium on the Role of the Vestibular Organs in Space Exploration. *NASA SP-187*, 1970.

Fredrickson, J. M., Schwarz, D., and Kornhuber, H. H. Convergence and interaction of vestibular and deep somatic afferents upon neurons in vestibular nuclei of the cat. *Acta Otolaryngol. (Stockholm)*, 1966a, *61*, 168–188.

Frederickson, J., Figge, U., Scheid, P., and Kornhuber, H. H. Vestibular nerve projection to the cerebral cortex of the rhesus monkey. *Exp. Brain Res.*, 1966b, *2*, 318–327.

Gacek, R. The course and central termination of first order neurons supplying vestibular endorgans in the cat. *Acta Otolaryngol. (Stockholm) Suppl.*, 1969, *254*, 5–64.

Gacek, R. R. Anatomical studies of the vestibulo-ocular pathways in the cat. *Adv. Oto-Rhino-Laryngol.*, 1973, *19*, 66–75.

Gacek, R. R., and Lyon, M. Localization of vestibular efferent neurons in the kitten with horseradish peroxidase. *Acta Otolaryngol. (Stockholm)*, 1974, 77, 92–101.

Gilson, R. D., Stockwell, C. W., and Guedry, F. E. Nystagmus responses during triangular waveforms of angular velocity about the y- and z-axes. *Acta Otolaryngol. (Stockholm)*, 1973, *75*, 21–26.

Goldberg, J. M., and Fernandez, C. Vestibular mechanisms. *Ann. Rev. Physiol.* 1975a, *37*, 129–162.

Goldberg, J. M., and Fernandez, C. Responses of peripheral vestibular neurons to angular and linear accelerations in the squirrel monkey. *Acta Otolaryngol. (Stockholm)*, 1975b, *80*, 101–110.

Goldberg, J. M., and Fernandez, C. Conduction times and background discharge of vestibular afferents. *Brain Res.*, 1977, *122*, 545–550.

Grillner, S., Hongo, T., and Lung, S. The vestibulospinal tract: Effects on alpha-motoneurones in the lumbosacral spinal cord in the cat. *Exp. Brain Res.*, 1970, *10*, 94.

Groen, J. J. The semicircular canal system of the organs of equilibrium. II. *Phys. Med. Biol.*, 1957, *1(3)*, 225–242.

MANNING J. CORREIA
AND
FRED E. GUEDRY, JR.

Grusser, O. J., and Grusser-Cornehls, U. Interaction of vestibular and visual inputs in the visual system. *Prog. Brain Res.*, 1972, *37*, 573–583.

Guedry, F. E., Jr. Psychophysiological studies of vestibular function. In W. D. Neff (ed.), *Contributions to Sensory Physiology*. Academic Press, New York, 1965, pp. 63–135.

Guedry, F. E., Jr. Psychophysics of vestibular sensation. In H. H. Kornhuber (ed.), *Handbook of Sensory Physiology*, Vol. I/2, Springer-Verlag, Berlin, 1974, pp. 3–154.

Hardy, M. Observations on the innervation of the macula sacculi in man. *Anat. Rec.*, 1934, *59*, 403–418.

Highstein, S. M. The organization of the vestibulo-oculomotor and trochlear reflex pathways in rabbit. *Exp. Brain Res.*, 1973, *17*, 285–300.

Highstein, S. M., and Ito, M. Differential localization within the vestibular nuclear complex of the inhibitory and excitatory cells innervating 3rd nucleus oculomotor neurons in rabbit. *Brain Res.*, 1971, *29*, 358–362.

Highstein, S. M., Ito, M., and Tsuchiga, T. Synaptic linkage in the vestibulo-ocular reflex pathway of rabbit. *Exp. Brain Res.*, 1971, *13*, 306–326.

Hixson, W. C. Frequency response of the oculovestibular system during yaw oscillation. *NAMRL 1212.* Naval Aerospace Medical Research Laboratory, Pensacola, Fla., 1974.

Hixson, W. C., Niven, J. I., and Correia, M. J. Kinematics nomenclature for physiological accelerations with special reference to vestibular applications. Naval Aerospace Medical Institute, Pensacola, Fla., *NASA Monograph 14.* 1966.

Igarashi, M. Dimensional study of the vestibular end organ apparatus. In The Role of the Vestibular Organs in Space Exploration. *NASA SP-115*, 1966, pp. 47–54.

Ito, M. The cerebello-vestibular interaction in the cat's vestibular nuclei neurons. In Fourth Symposium on the Role of the Vestibular Organs in Space Exploration. *NASA SP-187*, 1970, 183–199.

Ito, M., and Yoshida, M. The origin of cerebellar-induced inhibition of Deiter's neurones. I. Monosynaptic initiation of the inhibitory postsynaptic potentials. *Exp. Brain Res.*, 1966, *2*, 330–349.

Ito, M., Kawai, N., and Udo, M. The origin of cerebellar-induced inhibition of Deiter's neurones. III. Localization of the inhibitory zone. *Exp. Brain Res.*, 1968, *4*, 310–320.

Ito, M., Udo, M., Mano, N., Kawai, N. Synaptic action of the fastigiobulbar impulses upon neurones in the medullary reticular formation and vestibular nuclei. *Exp. Brain Res.*, 1970, *11*, 29–47.

Ito, M., Nisimaru, N., and Yamamoto, M. Specific neural connections for the cerebellar control of vestibulo-ocular reflexes. *Brain Res.*, 1973, *60*, 238–243.

Johnsson, L. G., and Hawkins, J. E., Jr. Otolithic membranes of the saccule and utricle in man. *Science*, 1967, *157*, 1454–1456.

Kornhuber, H. H. Motor functions of cerebellum and basal ganglia: The cerebello-cortical saccadic (ballistic) clock, the cerebello-nuclear hold regulator, and the basal ganglia ramp (voluntary speed smooth movement) generator. *Kybernetik*, 1971, *8*, 157–162.

Ladpli, R., and Brodal, A. Experimental studies of commissural and reticular formation projections from the vestibular nuclei in the cat. *Brain Res.*, 1968, *8*, 65–96.

Landolt, J. P., Correia, M. J., Young, E. R., Cardin, R. P. S., and Sweet, R. C. A scanning electron microscopic study of the morphology and geometry of neural surfaces and structures associated with the vestibular apparatus of the pigeon. *J. Comp. Neurol.*, 1975, *159*, 257–287.

Lindeman, H. H. Studies on the morphology of the sensory regions of the vestibular apparatus. *Ergeb. Anat. Entwicklungsgesch.*, 1969, *40(1)*, 1–110.

Loe, P. R., Tomko, D. L., and Werner, G. The neural signal of angular head position in primary afferent vestibular nerve axons. *J. Physiol. (London)*, 1973, *230*, 29–50.

Lorente de No, R. Anatomy of the eighth nerve. I. The central projection of the nerve endings of the internal ear. *Laryngoscope*, 1933, *43*, 1–38.

Lowenstein, O. The effect of galvanic polarization on the impulse discharge from sense endings in the isolated labyrinth of the thornback ray (*Raja clavata*). *J. Physiol. (London)*, 1955, *127*, 104–117.

Lowenstein, O., and Sand, A. The individual and integrated activity of the semicircular canals of the elasmobranch labyrinth. *J. Physiol. (London)*, 1940, *99*, 89–101.

Lowenstein, O., and Wersäll, J. A functional interpretation of the electron microscopic structure of the sensory hairs in the cristae of the elasmobranch *Raja clavata* in terms of directional sensitivity. *Nature*, 1959, *184*, 1807–1810.

Lund, S., and Pompeiano, O. Descending pathways with monosynaptic action on motoneurones. *Experientia*, 1965, *21*, 602–603.

Lund, S., and Pompeiano, O. Monosynaptic excitation of alpha motoneurones from supraspinal structures in the cat. *Acta Physiol. Scand.*, 1968, *73*, 1–21.

Maeda, M., Maunz, R. A., and Wilson, V. J. Labyrinthine influence on cat forelimb motoneurons. *Exp. Brain Res.*, 1975, *22*, 69–86.

Maekawa, K., and Simpson, J. I. Climbing fiber responses evoked in vestibulo-cerebellum of rabbit from visual system. *J. Neurophysiol.*, 1973, *36*, 649–666.

Markham, C. H. Midbrain and contralateral labyrinth influences on brainstem vestibular neurons in the cat. *Brain Res.*, 1968, *9*, 312–333.

Markham, C. H. Descending control of the vestibular nuclei: Physiology. *Prog. Brain Res.*, 1972, *37*, 589–600.

Markham, C. H., Precht, W., and Shimazu, H. Effect of stimulation of interstitial nucleus of Cajal on vestibular unit activity in the cat. *J. Neurophysiol.*, 1966, *29*, 493–507.

McCabe, B. F., Ryu, J. H., and Sekitani, T. Further experiments on vestibular compensation. *Laryngoscope*, 1972, *82*, 381–396.

McMaster, R., Weiss, A., and Carpenter, M. Vestibular projections from the nuclei of the extraocular muscles: Degeneration resulting from discrete partial lesions of the vestibular nuclei in the monkey. *Am. J. Anat.*, 1966, *118*, 163–194.

McNally, W. J., and Stuart, E. A. *Physiology of the Labyrinth.* American Academy of Ophthalmology and Otolaryngology, Rochester, N.Y., 1967.

Melvill Jones, G. Transfer function of labyrinthine volleys through the vestibular nuclei. *Prog. Brain Res.*, 1972, *37*, 139–156.

Melvill Jones, G. Is there a vestibulo-spinal reflex contribution to running? *Adv. Oto-Rhino-Laryngol.*, 1973, *19*, 128–133.

Melvill Jones, G., and Milsum, J. H. Characteristics of neural transmission from the semicircular canal to the vestibular nuclei of cats. *J. Physiol. (London)*, 1970, *209*, 295–316.

Melvill Jones, G., and Milsum, J. H. Frequency response analysis of central vestibular unit activity resulting from rotational stimulation of the semicircular canals. *J. Physiol. (London)*, 1971, *219*, 191–215.

Melvill Jones, G., and Spells, K. E. A theoretical and comparative study of the functional dependence of the semicircular canal upon its physical dimensions. *Proc. Roy. Soc. London Ser. B,* 1963, *157*, 403–419.

Mickle, W. A., and Ades, H. W. A composite sensory projection area in the cerebral cortex of the cat. *Am. J. Physiol.*, 1952, *170*, 682–689.

Mickle, W. A., and Ades, H. Rostral projection pathway of the vestibular system. *Am. J. Physiol.*, 1954, *176*, 243–246.

Miller, E. F. Counter-rolling of the human eyes produced by head tilt with respect to gravity. *Acta Otolaryngol. (Stockholm)*, 1962, *54*, 479–501.

Money, K. E., and Correia, M. J. The vestibular system of the owl. *Comp. Biochem. Physiol.*, 1972, *42A*, 353–358.

Money, K. E., and Scott, J. W. Functions of the separate sensory receptors of nonauditory labyrinth in the cat. *Am. J. Physiol.*, 1962, *202*, 1211–1220.

Money, K. E., Bonen, L., Beatty, J., Kuehn, L., Sokoloff, M., and Weaver, R. Physical properties of fluids and structures of vestibular apparatus of the pigeon. *Am. J. Physiol.*, 1971, *220*, 140–147.

Nashner, L. M. Vestibular postural control model. *Kybernetik*, 1972, *10*, 106–110.

Niven, J. I., Hixson, W. C., and Correia, M. J. Elicitation of horizontal nystagmus by periodic linear acceleration. *Acta Otolaryngol. (Stockholm)*, 1966, *62*, 429–441.

Nyberg-Hansen, R. Origin and termination of fibers from the vestibular nuclei descending in the medial longitudinal fasciculus: An experimental study with silver impregnation methods in the cat. *J. Comp. Neurol.*, 1964, *122*, 355–367.

Nyberg-Hansen, R. Functional organization of descending supraspinal fibre systems to the spinal cord: Anatomical observations and physiological correlations. *Ergeb. Anat. Entwicklungsgesch.*, 1966, *39(2)*.

Odkvist, L. M., Rubin, A. M., Schwarz, D. W. F., and Fredrickson, J. M. Vestibular and auditory cortical projection in the guinea pig (*Cavia porcellus*). *Exp. Brain Res.*, 1973*a*, *18*, 279–286.

Odkvist, L. M., Rubin, A. M., Schwarz, D. W. F., and Fredrickson, J. M. Vestibular cortical projection in the rabbit. *J. Comp. Neurol.*, 1973*b*, *149*, 117–120.

O'Leary, D. P., and Honrubia, V. Analysis of afferent responses from isolated semicircular canal of the guitarfish using rotational acceleration white-noise inputs. II. Estimation of linear system parameters and gain and phase spectra. *J. Neurophysiol.*, 1976, *39*, 645–659.

Oman, C. M., and Young, L. R. Physiological range of pressure difference and cupula deflections in the human semicircular canal: Theoretical considerations. *Acta Otolaryngol. (Stockholm,)* 1972, *74*, 324–331.

Outerbridge. J. S. Experimental and theoretical investigation of vestibularly-driven head and eye movement. Thesis, Department of Physiology, McGill University, Montreal, Canada, July 1969.

Penfield, W. Vestibular sensation and the cerebral cortex. *Ann. Oto-Rhino-Laryngol. (Paris)*, 1957, *66*, 691–698.

Pompeiano, O. Vestibulo-spinal relations: Vestibular influences on gamma motoneurons and primary afferents. *Prog. Brain Res.*, 1972, *37*, 197–232.

Pompeiano, O., and Brodal, A. Spinovestibular fibers in the cat: An experimental study. *J. Comp. Neurol.*, 1957, *108*, 353–382.

Precht, W. The physiology of the vestibular nuclei. In H. H. Kornhuber (ed.), *Handbook of Sensory Physiology*, Vol. I/1. Springer-Verlag, New York, 1974.

Rauch, S., and Koestlin, A. Aspects chimiques de l'endolymphe et de la périlymphe. *Pract. Oto-Rhino-Laryngol. (Basel)*, 1958, *20*, 287.

Roberts, T. D. M. *Neurophysiology of Postural Mechanisms*. Butterworths, London, 1967.

Roberts, T. D. M. Labyrinthine control of the postural muscles. In Third Symposium on the Role of the Vestibular Organs in Space Exploration. *NASA SP-152*, 1968, pp. 149–168.

Robinson, D. A. The effect of cerebellectomy on the cat's vestibulo-ocular integrator. *Brain Res.*, 1974, *71*, 195–207.

Rosenhall, U. Vestibular macular mapping in man. *Ann. Otol.*, 1972a, *81*, 339.

Rosenhall, U. Mapping of the cristae ampullares in man. *Ann. Otol.*, 1972b, *81*, 882.

Sans, A., Raymond, J., and Marty, R. Résponses thalamiques et corticales à la stimulation électrique du nerf vestibulaire chez le chat. *Exp. Brain Res.*, 1970, *10*, 265–275.

Sasaki, K. Electrophysiological studies on oculomotor neurons of the cat. *Jap. J. Physiol.*, 1963, *13*, 287–302.

Scheibel, A., Markham, C., and Koegler, R. Neural correlates of the vestibulo-ocular reflex. *Neurology (Minneapolis)*, 1961, *11*, 1055–1065.

Schwarz, D. W. F., and Fredrickson, J. M. The vestibular cortex: A bimodal primary projection field. *Science*, 1971, *172*, 280–281.

Shimazu, H. Vestibulo-oculomotor relations: Dynamic responses. *Prog. Brain Res.*, 1972, *37*, 493–506.

Shinoda, Y., and Yoshida, K. Neural pathways from the vestibular labyrinths to the flocculus in the cat. *Exp. Brain Res.*, 1975, *22*, 97–111.

Skavenski, A. A., and Robinson, D. A. Role of abducens neurons in vestibulo-ocular reflex. *J. Neurophysiol.*, 1973, *36*, 724–738.

Smith, C. A., and Rasmussen, G. L. Nerve endings in the maculae and cristae of the chinchilla vestibule, with special reference to the efferents. In Third Symposium on the Role of the Vestibular Organs in Space Exploration. *NASA SP-152*, 1968, pp. 183–200.

Smith, C. A., Lowry, O. H., and Wu, M. L. The electrolytes of the labyrinthine fluids. *Laryngoscope*, 1954, *64*, 141.

Stein, B. M., and Carpenter, M. B. Central projections of portions of the vestibular ganglia innervating specific parts of the labyrinth in the rhesus monkey. *Am. J. Anat.*, 1967, *120*, 281–318.

Steinhausen, W. Über die Beobachtung der Cupula in den Bogengangsampullen des Labyrinths des lebenden Hechts. *Arch. Ges. Physiol.*, 1933, *232*, 500–512.

Suzuki, J. I., and Cohen, B. Head, eye, body and limb movements from semicircular canal nerves. *Exp. Neurol.*, 1964, *10*, 393.

Suzuki, J. I., Cohen, B., and Bender, M. B. Compensatory eye movements induced by vertical canal stimulation. *Exp. Neurol.*, 1964, *9*, 137–160.

Suzuki, J. I., Goto, K., Tikumasu, K., and Cohen, B. Implantation of electrodes near individual vestibular nerve branches in mammals. *Ann. Oto-Rhino-Laryngol. (St. Louis)*, 1969a, *78*, 815–826.

Suzuki, J. I., Tokumasu, K., and Goto, K. Eye movements from single utricular nerve stimulation in the cat. *Acta Otolaryngol. (Stockholm)*, 1969b, *68*, 350–362.

Szentagothai, J. The elementary vestibulo-ocular reflex arc. *J. Neurophysiol.*, 1950, *13*, 395–407.

Tarlov, E. The rostral projections of the primate vestibular nuclei: An experimental study in macaque, baboon and champanzee. *J. Comp. Neurol.*, 1969, *135*, 27–56.

Tarlov, E. Organization of vestibulo-oculomotor projections in the cat. *Brain Res.*, 1970, *20*, 159–179.

Tarlov, E. Anatomy of the two vestibulo-oculomotor projection systems. *Prog. Brain Res.*, 1972, *37*, 471–491.

Trincker, D. The transformation of mechanical stimulus into nervous excitation by the labyrinthine receptors. *Symp. Soc. Exp. Biol.*, 1962, *16*, 289–316.

van Egmond, A. A. J., Groen, J. J., and Jonkees, L. B. W. The mechanics of the semicircular canals. *J. Physiol. (London)*, 1949, *110*, 1–17.

von Holst, E. Die Arbeitsweise des Statolithenapparates bei Fischen. *Z. Vergl. Physiol.*, 1950, *32*, 60–120.

Walberg, F., and Jansen, J. Cerebellar corticovestibular fibers in the cat. *Exp. Neurol.*, 1961, *3*, 32–52.

Walzl, E. M., and Mountcastle, V. B. Projection of vestibular nerve to cerebral cortex of the cat. *Am. J. Physiol.,* 1949, *159,* 595–603.

Werner, C. F. Die Differenzierung der Maculae im Labyrinth insbesondre bei Saugetieren. *Z. Anat. Entwicklungsgesch.,* 1933, *99,* 696–709.

Wersall, J. Studies on the structure and innervation of the sensory epithelium of the cristae ampullares in the guinea pig: A light and electron microscopic investigation. *Acta Otolaryngol. (Stockholm) Suppl.,* 1956, *126,* 1–85.

Willis, W. D., Jr., and Grossman, R. G. *Medical Neurobiology.* Mosby, St. Louis, 1973.

Wilson, V. J. Physiological pathways through the vestibular nuclei. *Int. Rev. Neurobiol.,* 1972, *15,* 27–81.

Wilson, V. J. The labyrinth, the brain, and posture. *Am. Sci.,* 1975, *63,* 325–332.

Wilson, V. J., and Maeda, M. Connections between semicircular canals and neck motoneurons in the cat. *J. Neurophysiol.,* 1974, *37,* 346–357.

Wilson, V. J., and Yoshida, M. Comparison of effects of stimulation of Deiter's nucleus and medial longitudinal fasciculus on neck, forelimb and hindlimb motoneurons. *J. Neurophysiol.,* 1969a, *32,* 743.

Wilson, V. J., and Yoshida, M. Monosynaptic inhibition of neck motoneurons by the medial vestibular nucleus. *Exp. Brain Res.,* 1969b, *9,* 365–380.

Wilson, V. J., Wylie, R. M., and Marco, L. A. Projection to the spinal cord from the medial and descending nuclei of the cat. *Nature,* 1967, *215,* 429–430.

Wilson, V. J., Gacek, R. R., Maeda, M., and Uchino, Y. Saccular and utricular input to cat neck motoneurons. *J. Neurophysiol.,* 1977, *40,* 63–73.

Young, E. R., Correia, M. J., and Landolt, J. P. The marginal fiber mass in the utricle of the pigeon. *Brain Res.,* 1974, *81,* 533–542.

10

Vestibular Function in Normal and in Exceptional Conditions

Fred E. Guedry, Jr., and Manning J. Correia

Introduction

Whereas the preceding chapter dealt primarily with the structure and response mechanisms of the vestibular receptors and their neural pathways, this chapter deals with vestibular function as it relates to various aspects of our daily living. As indicated in Chapter 9, the two classes of receptors in the vestibular system, the semicircular canals and the otolith organs, respond, respectively, to angular and linear accelerations of the head. These detectors of motion and orientation relative to the Earth operate automatically whenever the head is moved, irrespective of whether the motion is actively or passively produced. Early in life they operate automatically in close harmony with the visual and proprioceptive systems to improve coordination and control of movement. Whereas the presence of vestibular sensations is seldom recognized in natural movement, they become the center of attention in some pathological conditions and in some exceptional states of motion.

Developmental Considerations

Phylogeny and Ontogeny of the Vestibular System

Sensory systems become functional in a regular order which holds for various species of mammals and birds: first the somesthetic system, followed by the

Fred E. Guedry, Jr.   Naval Aerospace Medical Research Laboratory, Naval Air Station, Pensacola, Florida 32508.   Manning J. Correia   Departments of Otolaryngology, Physiology, and Biophysics, University of Texas Medical Branch, Galveston, Texas 77550.

FRED E. GUEDRY, JR.,
AND MANNING J.
CORREIA

vestibular, auditory, and visual systems (Gottlieb, 1976). The vestibular system develops early both ontogenetically and phylogenetically (Lowenstein, 1973; Krause, 1903). Its early differentiation, its sensitivity to passive motion, and its eventual pervasive interrelations with sensory-motor systems suggest that it may play a significant role in prenatal development.

In man, the semicircular ducts develop between the fourth and fifth weeks of gestation, the anterior first, then the posterior, and finally the lateral. The utricle and saccule are formed by 6 weeks, and the cochlea appears to develop from the saccule. By 10 weeks, the vestibulocochlear nerve of the human embryo has differentiated to that of the adult (Streeter, 1906/1907). Primary vestibular neurons are among the earliest in the nervous system to myelinate (Langworthy, 1933). The "vestibulocerebellum," the flocculonodular lobe, develops as an outgrowth of the vestibular nuclei in the brain stem (Larsell and Jansen, 1972; Brodal, 1969). As with other CNS structures, neural connections within the cerebellum continue to form and re-form during life, a process that first may accommodate patterning of movements to growing and developing sensory and motor systems, and later may compensate for losses of function.

The vestibular system appears associated with older structures of the brain concerned with (1) automatic regulation of posture and movement relative to the Earth and (2) automatic integration of respiration and other vital functions with changes in states of motion (Smith and Smith, 1962). The survival value of this functional association becomes obvious when it is considered that movements become skilled, coordinated, and fast when they become automatic and not "thought through" and that changes in orientation and states of motion require respiratory and circulatory changes. The vestibular-autonomic system association becomes most obvious when vestibular stimuli are unnatural or when their interaction with other sensory inputs relevant to states of motion is unnatural. These messages set off startle reactions (e.g., fear of falling) and nonspecific emergency reactions because they constitute threats to the control of motion which throughout phylogenetic history have constituted threats to survival. The hyperarousal thus induced galvanizes somatic nervous system response involved in the control of motion, with the result that these two aspects of man's response to the sensory detection of motion, the somatic nervous system responses and the autonomic nervous system responses, are intimately interrelated. While novel stimuli to other sensory systems also set off arousal reactions, the vestibular system, because it automatically signals changes in states of motion and orientation which require respiratory and cardiovascular adjustments, may be more intimately involved with the autonomic system than some of the other sensory systems (Preber, 1958; Usami, 1962; Watanabe and Egami, 1973).

THE VESTIBULAR SYSTEM AND MATURATION

In early infancy, motion is predominantly passive, and its quantity and quality depend on the exigencies of life. The possibility that early differences in exposure to motion might have developmental implications has been a matter of substantial interest recently (Peto, 1970; Ornitz, 1970; Prescott, 1971; Guedry, 1972), although the idea that proprioceptive and vestibular stimulation in early life may be important in development of personality (Schilder, 1933) and of equilibration, motion skills, and judgments of spatial relations is not new (Petersen and Rainey, 1910). There are several basic ideas which can be considered in this connection: (1) Deprivation of passive motion early in life may prevent normal neurological development of motion control systems. The effects of sensory deprivation on neurological systems such as the visual system (Kolata, 1975; Greenough, 1972) could be expected to apply to this system as well, considering its close interrelation with both the visual system and motor systems. (2) The quality of early handling might condition idiosyncratic arousal reactions to motion which in turn could influence neurobiological and behavioral development. (3) Differences in development of the skilled control of motion could influence many aspects of human behavior.

Minkowski (1922) pointed out that the fetus, supported in amniotic fluid, is capable of more responses to vestibular stimulation than the newborn. Thus premature infants may realize two disadvantages: (1) after birth they are deprived of the amount of motion and vestibular stimulation that would have occurred as a result of the motion of the mother, and (2) they are partially deprived of the ability to respond reflexly to motions they experience. Recently it has been indicated that passive, gentle oscillation of premature infants improves general motor maturation, visual fixation and pursuit, and, in general, overall health (Neal, 1968). A series of studies (Korner and Thoman, 1972; Pederson and ter Vrught, 1973; Pomerleau-Malcuit and Clifton, 1973) offer general support for these findings and suggest that regimens of vestibular stimulation in early life may have more developmental significance than special regimens of auditory or cutaneous stimulation. The possibility that reading disabilities and some psychiatric disorders may involve anomalies in vestibulocerebellar development has also been indicated (Frank and Levinson, 1973; Holzman *et al.*, 1973; Hallpike *et al.*, 1951) but not without some controversy (Stockwell *et al.*, 1976). The stereotyped rocking behavior of psychiatric cases and of monkeys in sensory deprivation experiments and the instability and "swimming feelings" reported by mentally disturbed individuals have been cited as evidence supporting the general idea that deficiencies in equilibration systems, either genetically or environmentally determined, may somehow be involved in the etiology of behavioral disturbances. While a range of evidence can be adduced in support of these theoretical positions, more specific hypotheses and neurobiological experiments relevant to these are needed.

Both motion sickness susceptibility[1] (Reason and Brand, 1975) and the vestibuloocular response seem to change with maturation. Groen (1965) referred to an increased central control of vestibular nystagmus with maturation. He inferred this from finding that the "long time constant" (cf. Chapter 9) of the nystagmus response became shorter with age in a human infant, and assumed that the developing visual system might be responsible for altering the vestibular response.

---

[1]Vestibular nerve fibers may decrease in number fairly linearly with age from about 19,000 in young people to about 11,000 in octogenarians (Bergstrom, 1973). This may account in part for the decreased motion sickness susceptibility in advanced age groups. (However, compare Bruner and Norris, 1971, and Van der Laan and Oosterveld, 1974.)

FRED E. GUEDRY, JR.,
AND MANNING J.
CORREIA

The fact that such shaping can occur has been clearly demonstrated in adults (Gonshor, 1974; Melvill-Jones and Gonshor, 1974), and it probably occurs naturally in the developing child during early passive motion and later during voluntary whole-body movement. Tibbling (1969) did not confirm Groen's finding in regard to the long time constant, but she did find a very high response/stimulus gain ratio in newborn relative to that found in adults. A more extensive recent study of various age groups by Van der Laan and Oosterveld (1974) confirms the high gain ratios in young children indicated by Tibbling. There have been other indications of changes in vestibular responses during maturation (Galebsky, 1928; Lawrence and Feind, 1953; McGraw, 1941). Testing the vestibuloocular and vestibulocerebellar systems in young children is not a simple matter, and it is to be noted that tests of vestibular function, although sufficient to determine the presence or absence of vestibular function, are not sufficient to determine whether or not vestibuloocular responses are functionally efficient within the range of movements involved in everyday life. Within this range, unrecognized difficulties in vestibuloocular control may lead to inappropriate remedial actions and frustration for both child and parent. In sections that follow, experiments are described which serve to illustrate the kinds of difficulties that might arise in an individual with inadequate vestibuloocular responses during natural movements. Experiments are also described which demonstrate that it is possible to restructure vestibuloocular responses. It may be that procedures involved in these experiments will eventually prove useful in detecting and reshaping maladaptive vestibuloocular responses in both children and adults.

Vision and the Vestibuloocular Reflex

Relative Motion between Head and Target

In the normal adult during natural voluntary transport movements, vestibular responses to motion work synergistically and automatically with visual and proprioceptive responses to set off reflexes which serve to stabilize the eyes, head, and body. In the mature state, this category of response has a direct effect on the motion control of the body, and such somatic nervous system responses have vectorial attributes which must be reasonably matched in direction, magnitude, and timing to their stimulus analogues in order to be functionally effective. Hence precise measures of the dynamics of the stimulus-response relationship, e.g., gain ratios and phase relations at various stimulus frequencies, are of primary significance.

HEAD FIXED, TARGET MOVING. Natural head movements, as in nodding "yes" or "no" and as occur in walking and running, can introduce oscillatory velocities of the head relative to the Earth which exceed the limits of voluntary visual tracking. The reader can demonstrate this to himself by shaking his head rapidly about the z axis,[2] as in saying "no," while holding this page stationary. The

---

[2]See Chapter 9 for definition of x, y, and z axes.

print remains clear because both visual and vestibular inputs serve to stabilize the eyes relative to an Earth-fixed reference. Now hold the head stationary while oscillating the page at the same amplitude and frequency. The print is blurred. Above certain frequencies and amplitudes of angular oscillation, the visual tracking system operating alone fails to track the moving target, and vision blurs (Huddleston, 1969; Melvill-Jones and Drazin, 1962). Performance (digit identification) by Earth-fixed observers viewing displays oscillating at various frequencies is illustrated in the lower curve of Fig. 1 (Benson, 1972; Benson and Barnes, 1978).

TARGET FIXED, HEAD MOVING. The ability to see Earth-fixed targets during natural whole-body movements is substantially aided by the vestibuloocular reflex. During sinusoidal oscillation at 1–2 Hz, when the head velocity is maximal in one direction, the eye velocity from the vestibuloocular reflex is maximal in the other direction, so that the eye tends to remain stable relative to the environment, thereby improving dynamic vision for Earth-fixed targets. The upper curve in Fig. 1 shows that visibility of Earth-fixed targets remains very good during passive whole-body oscillation at frequencies which far exceed the tracking capacities of the visual system alone (lower curve, Fig. 1). This vestibuloocular stabilization provides a reference from which voluntary eye movements can be executed as the eye searches for and then holds visual details during natural movements of the head and body relative to the Earth.

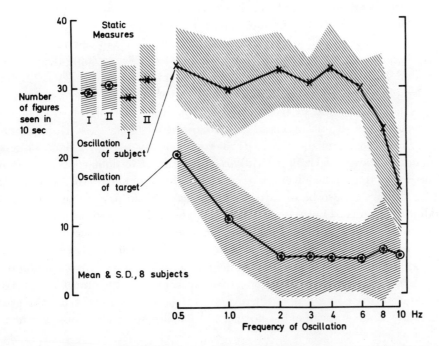

Fig. 1. Number of digits seen in 10 sec during relative movement between observer and target at various frequencies of angular oscillation at peak velocities of ±20°/sec. Lower curve: Observer is Earth-fixed and target oscillates relative to observer. Upper curve: Target is Earth-fixed and observer oscillates relative to target. Courtesy A. J. Benson. From Benson (1972) and Benson and Barnes (1978). Reprinted by permission of *Aviat. Space Environ. Med.*

FRED E. GUEDRY, JR.,
AND MANNING J.
CORREIA

Variations in the gain of the vestibuloocular reflex seem to complement limitations in the gain of the visual smooth tracking system response at certain frequencies. Figure 2 shows that at low frequencies of oscillation (0.5 Hz and below) the gain of the vestibuloocular reflex in the dark is about 0.6.[3] In other words, during oscillation at this frequency in the dark, as the head is turning at a rate of 30°/sec in one direction, the velocity of the eyes is about 0.6 (30°/sec) = 18°/sec in the opposite direction; thus in man vestibular compensation in the dark is insufficient to stabilize the eye relative to the Earth at this frequency of stimulation, and there would be a "retinal slippage" of 12°/sec. However, this is in the frequency range in which visual following is very good (Fig. 1, lower curve), so that when the head oscillates at these low frequencies in relation to a visible target, the synergy of the visual and vestibular systems provides a gain of 1.0. At higher frequencies where visual tracking deteriorates, the vestibular gain goes up, as shown in Fig. 2, and thus these two systems working together serve to maintain visual acuity over a substantial range of frequencies which far exceeds the response capabilities of either system operating independently.

Head movements generated during natural whole-body activities, recorded by Gresty and Benson (1976), are illustrated in Fig. 3. Noteworthy is the fact that higher frequencies (which require vestibular inputs for adequate visual tracking) are prominent among the head oscillations occurring in natural movement. This suggests that reduction or loss of vestibular function would reduce visual acuity during natural movement, especially since at the higher frequencies the gain of ocular stabilization by neck reflexes is very low in man (Meiry, 1971).[4] Individuals with bilateral labyrinthine loss complain of jumbled vision during passive motion (Whitteridge, 1960). Following recovery from bilateral loss of vestibular function, acuity loss during active head movements may be offset to some degree by an increased gain of neck-to-eye control, as reported by Dichgans *et al.* (1974) in the rhesus monkey. However, Atkin and Bender (1968) found deficits in vestibulo-ocular stabilization and in visual acuity during voluntary high-frequency (high peak velocity) head oscillations in man following vestibular loss. During passive whole-body oscillation there is marked loss of acuity for Earth-fixed targets at frequencies above 0.5 Hz in individuals with bilateral vestibular loss; i.e., performance is like that in the lower curve instead of the upper curve of Fig. 1 (Benson, 1972). Vision can also be disturbed during active head movements by adaptive modification of vestibular input/output relations. For example, the coupling between the vestibular input from head movements and the oculomotor response can be substantially modified by prolonged wearing of dove prisms, which produce a right-left reversal of the visual field. Once adjustment to this condition has been achieved, vestibular stimulation from head movements produces eye movements appropriate for the optically reversed direction of motion. When the glasses are removed, the individual has normal visual acuity for moving objects when his

[3]Barr *et al.* (1976) found a gain of 0.65, but noted that it was subject to voluntary control. For oscillation angles ±48° or less, efforts to imagine an Earth-fixed target (in darkness) increased gain almost to 1.0, and efforts to imagine a head-fixed target reduced gain.
[4]Meiry fixed the head relative to Earth and oscillated the trunk; gain may be higher during voluntary head turning.

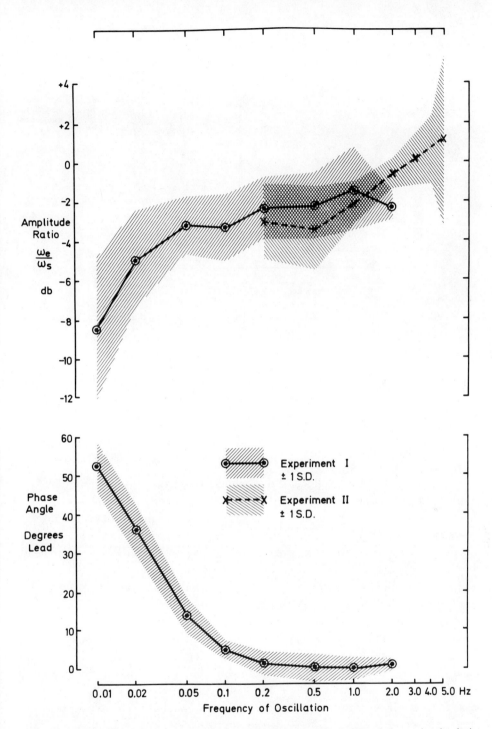

Fig. 2. Gain (upper curve) and phase (lower curve) of lateral eye velocity relative to head velocity during sinusoidal angular oscillation about the yaw axis (z axis). Peak stimulus angular velocity (ω_s) was $\pm 30°$/sec at all frequencies. Ratio of peak eye velocity (ω_e) to ω_s was used to calculate the gain, which is expressed in db units. Courtesy of A. J. Benson. From Benson (1970) and Benson and Barnes (1978). Reprinted by permission of *Aviat. Space Environ. Med.*

FRED E. GUEDRY, JR.,
AND MANNING J.
CORREIA

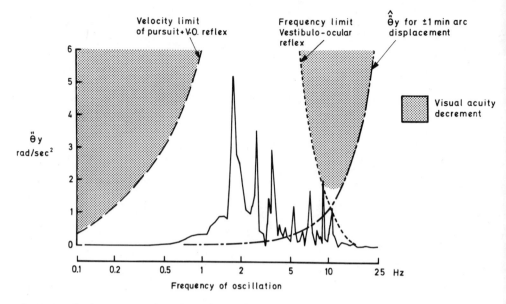

Fig. 3. Amplitude spectrum of head angular accelerations about the pitch axis (y axis) during whole-body activities. Courtesy of Gresty and Benson (1976).

head is stationary, but has greatly reduced vision during active head oscillations. This very impressive adaptive plasticity of the vestibuloocular reflex has been demonstrated by Gonshor (1974) (cf. Melvill-Jones and Gonshor, 1974).

HEAD AND TARGET MOVE IN UNISON

In the preceding section, the beneficial effects of the vestibuloocular responses for visibility of Earth-fixed targets during head and body motion were described. This section deals with situations in which an individual is required to read instruments within a turning or oscillating vehicle. In this case, the vestibuloocular reflex tends to drive the eyes relative to targets which move with the head, thereby interfering with the visibility of these head-fixed targets.

Even a small head-fixed visible target is sufficient to substantially suppress the vestibuloocular reflex (vestibular nystagmus) when the vestibular stimulus is a low-frequency sinusoidal oscillation or a constant angular acceleration of, say, $10°/sec^2$ maintained for about 10 or 12 sec. For example, during sinusoidal oscillation at a frequency of 0.04 Hz where the peak angular velocity of the head is 120°/sec, the mean peak velocity of vestibular nystagmus in the dark in man is about 80°/sec. When three-digit sets (visual angle $17' \times 48'$, luminance level 0.32 cd/m²) fixed relative to the head are viewed, the mean peak slow phase velocity is reduced to about 12°/sec; otherwise expressed, the suppression ratio is about 0.15. After about 10 min of practice, the suppression increases, the ratio becomes about 0.11, and the ability to read three-digit sets improves as shown in Fig. 4. Thus in a short time the beginnings of the adaptive plasticity demonstrated by Gonshor in longer exposures to unnatural conditions may be manifest (cf. Guedry and Ambler, 1973; Marshall and Brown, 1967).

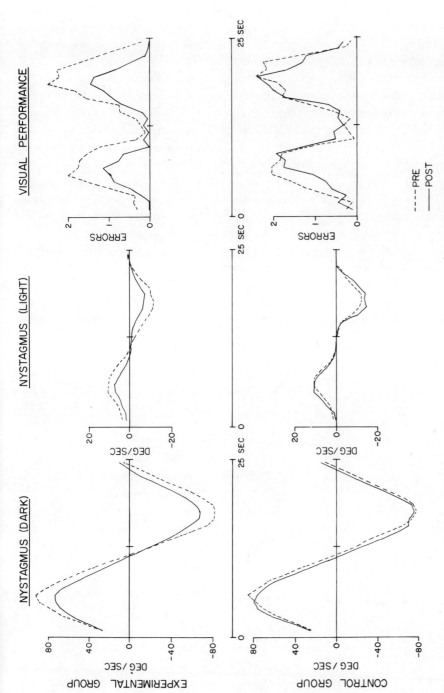

Fig. 4. Nystagmus slow phase velocity (°/sec) and visual performance in seeing three-digit sets during each second of angular oscillation at 0.04 Hz with peak angular velocity of ±120°/sec. Nystagmus was recorded with head-fixed visual display illuminated (light) and darkened (dark). Between the pre- and post-tests, the experimental and control groups oscillated for 9 min. During this interval, visual suppression of nystagmus was induced in the experimental group by a visual task requiring viewing of a head-fixed flight instrument; the control group oscillated in darkness. From Guedry and Ambler (1973).

FRED E. GUEDRY, JR.,
AND MANNING J.
CORREIA

Although some rolling maneuvers of aircraft may generate a sufficient vestibular stimulus to overcome visual fixation and degrade vision for aircraft instruments (Melvill-Jones, 1957), it would indeed be an unusual vehicle, other than a laboratory device, that would rotate sinusoidally at a frequency of 0.04 Hz with a peak angular velocity as high as ±120°/sec. However, the ability to see head-fixed targets during whole-body oscillation over a range of frequencies has been studied recently (Barnes *et al.*, 1978) and, as shown in Fig. 5, visual suppression of the vestibuloocular reflex is frequency dependent. At low frequencies, below 1.0 Hz, visual suppression of vestibular nystagmus is, as just indicated, very effective; but as frequency increases, visual suppression diminishes. During low-amplitude high-frequency ($f > 1.5$ Hz) angular oscillation, eye movements lose their nystagmoid character, and it is principally the slow phase component that remains. Thus at these higher frequencies, vestibular eye movements in the dark become sinusoidal in waveform (see Fig. 5), the gain (ratio of the output eye velocity to input stimulus velocity) increases to about 1.0, and the phase lead decreases to 0 (Figs. 2 and 5). It is at these frequencies that the capacity of the visual system to follow sinusoidal visual inputs fails (lower curve in Fig. 1). Therefore, it is not surprising that, in this stimulus range where visibility of Earth-fixed targets is quite good, visibility of head-fixed targets becomes very poor as shown in Fig. 6.

Thus far, interactions between visual and vestibular oculomotor control have been considered (1) when the individual was stationary (Earth-fixed) while the visual targets were in motion, (2) when the individual was moved while visible

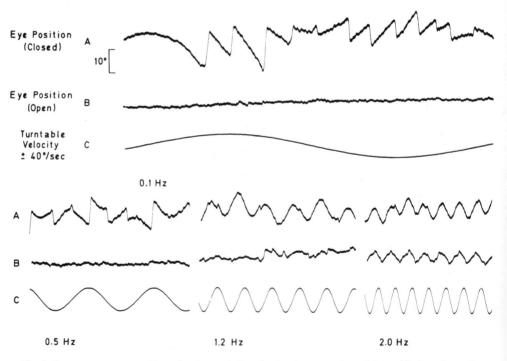

Fig. 5. Eye movement recordings showing variations in visual suppression of the vestibuloocular reflex and variations in the nystagmoid character of the reflex at different frequencies of angular oscillation. From Barnes *et al.* (1978). Reprinted by permission of *Aviat. Space Environ. Med.*

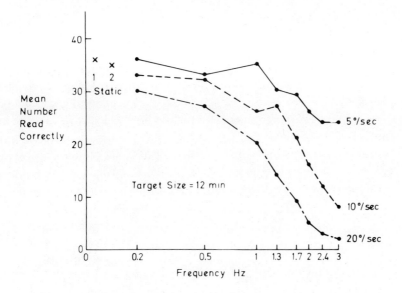

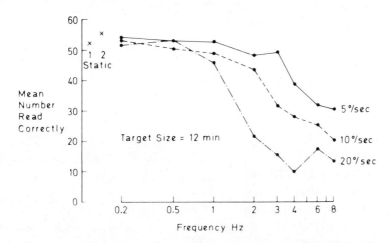

Fig. 6. Visibility of head-fixed targets during angular oscillation about the pitch or y axis (top) and about the yaw or z axis (bottom) at various frequencies with peak angular velocities of 5, 10, or 20°/sec. From Barnes *et al.* (1978). Reprinted by permission of *Aviat. Space Environ. Med.*

targets were stationary, and (3) when the individual was moved and the targets were fixed relative to his head. One way in which condition 1 is often studied is to rotate vertical black and white stripes past the eyes of a stationary observer; when the motion is unidirectional, this stimulus induces optokinetic nystagmus. The character of this nystagmus changes, depending on whether the individual attempts to voluntarily follow particular stripes or gazes at the moving visual field. The former response is thought to involve central vision and perhaps higher neural systems than the latter, which is regarded as more reflexlike, perhaps not involving the cerebral cortex. Condition 2, in which the person views the external scene during angular acceleration, can be used to observe both concordant

FRED E. GUEDRY, JR.,
AND MANNING J.
CORREIA

vestibular and visual oculomotor stimulation and also purely optokinetic stimulation. This can be accomplished by acceleration to some constant rotation speed which is then maintained. During angular acceleration to a velocity of, e.g., 90°/sec, the cupula is deflected, setting off vestibular nystagmus which is supplemented by optokinetic nystagmus from the passing stripes. Under these circumstances, the slow phase eye velocity (which in the dark would only be about 0.6 of head velocity) almost exactly compensates for the head velocity so that the eye is fixed relative to the Earth during each slow phase. When constant velocity is attained, however, the cupula begins to return toward null position, and the slow phase velocity of nystagmus commences a decline toward the level that is produced by the optokinetic stimulation alone (Mclvill-Jones, 1966).

HEAD AND CENTRAL VISUAL DISPLAY MOVE IN UNISON RELATIVE TO A VISIBLE BACKGROUND

A fourth situation involves a combination of situations 2 and 3 in which a head-fixed target in the center of the visual field (central target) is viewed during whole-body angular acceleration, but with the rotating structure not enclosed, so that the Earth-fixed background is visible in the peripheral visual field. This situation produces an interesting and somewhat surprising result. Optokinetic stimulation from the peripherally visible background might be expected to act in concordance with the vestibular input to drive the eyes relative to the head-fixed visual target and degrade vision for this target more than would the vestibular drive alone in the enclosed structure. However, just the opposite happens. The relative movement of the background improves the ability to fixate the central target and presumably to suppress the vestibular nystagmus. The effect has been observed only at low frequencies (0.033 Hz, ±90°/sec) of angular oscillation (Benson and Cline, 1975), and effects at higher frequencies remain to be observed. This apparent paradox in the interaction between the visual and vestibular systems probably reflects a necessary coordination between the central and peripheral visual tracking systems, as, for example, when we follow the flight of a ball or a bird against a complex background, or when we are riding or running and select an object to view against various parts of the visible background which move at different velocities relative to the eye. In these cases, central target tracking must predominate over peripheral field optokinetic stimuli (generated by the eye movement) in order for visual acuity of the central target to be sustained. Since vision for the central visual display during whole-body rotation was substantially improved by the peripheral optokinetic stimuli, it appears that the optokinetic peripheral stimuli either strengthened visual still-fixation of the head-fixed central visual display or diminished the vestibular influence on the oculomotor system.

There are many sites of interaction between the visual and vestibular systems which influence oculomotor control, but one of particular interest is the flocculonodular lobe of the cerebellum (Ito *et al.*, 1974; Lisberger and Fuchs, 1974; Takemori and Cohen, 1974). There is evidence suggesting that some Purkinje cells in the flocculus fire exclusively when there is discord between vestibular and visual control of the oculomotor system (Lisberger and Fuchs, 1974; Miles and Fuller, 1975). For example, these cells increase firing rates when targets are moved relative to a stationary head or when the head and targets are oscillated in unison relative to the Earth, but the firing rate is relatively unaffected when the head is oscillated relative to Earth-fixed targets, i.e., the only condition in which visual smooth tracking and the vestibuloocular reflex operate synergistically. It would be interesting to determine the response of Purkinje units during whole-body oscillation with a head-fixed central target moving relative to an Earth-fixed peripheral field.

Several methods of driving oculomotor responses have been described in this section to illustrate the functional importance of synergistic interactions between the visual and vestibular systems during whole-body motion. It is important to note, however, that there is a partial independence among systems of oculomotor control (Robinson, 1968) which is of diagnostic value. With the head stationary, voluntary inspection of two or more fixation points on a page is accomplished by high-speed saccadic eye movements, while observation of a slowly moving visual target is usually accomplished by a smooth oculomotor tracking response. Either of these types of response can be disrupted by CNS lesions which do not necessarily influence the other (Corvera *et al.*, 1973). Some conditions, such as mild alcohol intoxication (Guedry *et al.*, 1975), do not obviously influence vestibular nystagmus in the dark or saccadic excursions between fixation points but substantially impair both the visual suppression of vestibular nystagmus and the smooth visual tracking of a moving spot of light. Considering some of the experimental results referred to in the preceding paragraph, deviant responses under both of these conditions could be a sign of dysfunction in the flocculus of the cerebellum. While such a specific localization of dysfunction would be questionable in the absence of other confirming signs, it is to be noted that responses such as these, i.e., visual suppression of vestibular nystagmus (Ledoux and Demanez, 1970), smooth eye following (Corvera *et al.*, 1973), saccadic excursions between fixation points (Kornhuber, 1974; Haring and Simmons, 1973), and vestibular nystagmus in darkness, are used in the diagnostic evaluation of vertiginous patients (Baloh *et al.*, 1975).

PATHOLOGY OF THE VESTIBULAR SYSTEM AND PROBLEMS OF DIVERS

Description of vestibular pathology and its evaluation are beyond the scope of this chapter. A convenient summary of this subject is outlined by Henriksson *et al.* (1972), and only a few comments will be included here.

The complex neural organization of the vestibuloocular and vestibulospinal systems which operate so efficiently during natural head and body movements prohibits simplicity in localizing sites of pathology within the peripheral and central vestibular pathways. Three common symptoms of disease of the peripheral labyrinth are spontaneous nystagmus (nystagmus in the absence of head motion or tilt), ataxia, and vertigo. Each of these three symptoms can also be produced by lesions within the vestibuloocular or vestibulospinal pathways or within associated structures such as the cerebellum or mesencephalic nuclei. To

FRED E. GUEDRY, JR.,
AND MANNING J.
CORREIA

properly evaluate a patient with symptoms of vestibular pathology, a battery of tests, including some not specific to vestibular function, must be used. A knowledge of vestibular mechanisms facilitates interpretation of these tests. For example, suppose a patient is vertiginous, nauseous, has leftbeating nystagmus (slow phase to the right), and tends to fall to the right when his eyes are closed. Additionally, with his eyes closed, his finger and arm deviate to the right (past point) when he attempts to point "dead ahead." These signs and symptoms suggest reduced vestibular function on the right side for the following reasons: Reduced neural activity in the right vestibular nerve relative to that of the left produces the same net difference to the central nervous system (cf. Fig. 5 in Chapter 9) as would be produced by a leftward whole-body rotation, which also produces leftbeating nystagmus (compensatory slow phase right), a sensation of turning left, and a tendency to point rightward (past point) in attempting to point "dead ahead." Generally, compensatory eye and body movements are in a direction toward a hypoactive vestibular nerve. However, the sensation of motion and even compensatory body motion can be variable depending on concomitant input from other proprioceptors. Since the sensation of direction of motion following vestibular stimulation can be reduced or reversed by competing spinovestibular input (see later), a patient may perceive one direction of rotation while standing, a different one while sitting, and none while lying in bed.

A hyperactive left vestibular nerve (irritative condition) can cause the same responses as a hypoactive right vestibular nerve (ablative condition), since it can produce the same comparator condition (see Fig. 5, Chapter 9) in the CNS. Therefore, it is desirable to test each ear separately. Rotation stimulates both labyrinths, but the caloric test permits selective stimulation of each labyrinth. This involves irrigation of the external auditory meatus with cold or hot fluid while the head is tilted backward 60°, so that the plane of the lateral semicircular canals is aligned with gravity. The labyrinth and the external meatus of each ear are coupled by the surrounding temporal bone. By conduction, cooling or heating the external auditory meatus eventually also cools or heats the semicircular canals, most particularly a lateral portion of the lateral semicircular canal. Applying water 7°C below body temperature to the right external auditory meatus for 20–40 sec causes the endolymph in the lateral portion of the canal to become cool and more dense than elsewhere in the labyrinth. Because of gravity, this dense mass of endolymph tends to fall, so that the cupula is deflected in the right lateral canal just as when a leftward head turn is initiated. Cupula deflection in opposite direction can be produced by irrigating the right ear with warm water (7°C above body temperature). Warm endolymph in the lateral aspect of the semicircular canal, being less dense than endolymph in the other portions, tends to rise. The caloric test is useful because utriculopetal and utriculofugal cupula deflection can be produced in either of the two lateral semicircular canals separately. It is a simple diagnostic tool which may be used in conjunction with rotatory tests, positional tests, and oculomotor tests (e.g., pendular eye tracking or optokinetic tests). Usually if responses to both hot and cold calorization in one ear are considerably below normal while normal responses are elicited from the other ear, a lesion on the "weak" side would be suspected. However, the picture can in time be complicated by adaptive mechanisms which adjust the CNS for disordered imbalanced sensory inputs. These adaptive repair mechanisms, which serve to restore automatic control of motion and posture and coincidentally complicate interpretation of clinical tests, are quite likely the same mechanisms that provide habituation and suppress nausea during prolonged exposure to unnatural motion.

One popular activity that can produce nonphysiological stimulation of the vestibular system and, in some cases, irreversible labyrinthine disorders is scuba diving. Nystagmus, spatial disorientation, vertigo, and lesions within the peripheral and central nervous system have been reported in swimmers, divers, and caisson workers (Kennedy, 1972) following exposure to hyperbaric conditions. In addition to hyperbaria, other conditions in "subsurface" environments that can influence equilibration include unusual temperatures (e.g., cold air or cold water), reduced vision due to darkness or reduced somatosensory input due to the neutral buoyancy of the body in water, and unusual gas pressures or mixtures (see Edmonds, 1973).

During a scuba dive, caloric irrigation of one ear may occur if the external auditory canal of one ear is obstructed or if cold water gains access to one of the middle ear spaces because of perforation of the tympanic membrane. The vestibular endorgans can be stimulated mechanically by unequal ambient pressures within the middle ear cavity during change in pressure; a similar condition yields "pressure vertigo" in rapid ascents or descents in aircraft. Excessive pressures in the middle ear may produce barotrauma to the middle ear structures or, if severe enough, may rupture the round window with a consequent alteration of the perilymph/endolymph interface within the bony labyrinth. Inner ear barotrauma can cause sensorineural hearing loss and/or vestibular damage. Bubbles may be formed in the labyrinth or its vascular supply during decompression. The biochemical composition of the endolymph and perilymph may be altered by the breathing of gas mixtures required to sustain life at great pressure depths. Either of these last two conditions could alter the viscous, inertial, and frictional properties as well as the neural transduction process of the vestibular endorgans.

There are hazards in subsurface environments other than those which may stimulate or produce a lesion in the vestibular endorgans and their neural supply. All of the pathways and structures associated with the vestibular system are susceptible to vascular emboli, oxygen toxicity, carbon dioxide toxicity, anoxia, and carbon monoxide poisoning. Any of these conditions can occur during subsurface activities and cause problems with equilibrium and spatial orientation.

Vestibular System and Aviation

In aviation, "spatial disorientation" usually refers to inaccurate perception by the pilot of the attitude or motion of his aircraft relative to the fixed coordinate system constituted by the Earth's surface and gravitational vertical. Because of high potential for orientation error in flight, "all-weather" aircraft are equipped with instruments which provide sufficient information for the experienced pilot to

FRED E. GUEDRY, JR.,
AND MANNING J.
CORREIA

maintain control of the attitude and flight path of the aircraft even during periods of disorientation. However, undetected disorientation can endanger flight safety, and conflicts between perceived aircraft attitude and instrument information can be sufficiently disturbing to impair control. Spatial disorientation has been estimated to account for between 4–10% of major aircraft accidents and even higher percentages of fatal accidents (Gillingham and Krutz, 1974, p. 66; Hixson and Spezia, 1975). Some aspects of vestibular responses which contribute to pilot disorientation are considered in this section.

IMPORTANCE OF VISION TO ORIENTATION IN FLIGHT

The single most important cause of pilot disorientation is the absence of adequate visual reference to the Earth because of darkness or because of weather conditions such as rain, clouds, or snow. Certain flying conditions can also introduce misleading visual information such as sloping cloud banks, but the crucial factor in the human response is that, without good visual reference (or with misleading visual reference) to the Earth's surface, the remaining sensory data on spatial orientation are not sufficiently reliable to permit safe piloting of aircraft.

VISIBILITY OF COCKPIT INSTRUMENTS. In preceding sections, it has been shown that at certain frequencies the vestibuloocular reflex blurs vision for head-fixed targets. Loss of visibility of cockpit instruments has been indicated as a factor in disorientation in aviation (Melvill-Jones, 1965; Tormes and Guedry, 1975). Malcolm and Money (1972) include inability to read flight instruments during vibration and turbulence as one of the conditions common to the "jet upset phenomenon," a situation in which pilots of large jet aircraft have gone into severe and disastrous nose-down attitudes to compensate for erroneous sensations of extreme nose-up attitudes (cf. Martin and Melvill-Jones, 1965). The visibility of flight instruments may be degraded by several factors including the breakdown in visual tracking of vibrating instruments (Guignard, 1965), the brightness and wavelength of light from the instruments (Gilson, 1971), and the complexity of the instrument display. Any of these conditions would be further complicated by tendencies toward "grayout" from changing g loads exacerbated by vestibular stimuli (Sinha, 1968).

VISIBILITY OUTSIDE THE COCKPIT. Visibility of the Earth's surface could actually be improved by the vestibuloocular reflex in some circumstances (upper curve in Fig. 1), although there is no certainty that the complex vibratory motions in flight would set off optimal oculomotor stabilization for Earth-fixed or other external visual targets. Some maneuvers such as several consecutive complete turns can produce vestibular aftereffects which tend to degrade vision because of nystagmus while also disorienting the pilot. Despite good visual suppression of such effects, if maneuvers are sufficiently strong, e.g., five turns in 20 sec, the vestibular nystagmus after stopping such a turn can blur vision briefly for both cockpit instruments and Earth reference (Melvill-Jones, 1957; Benson and Guedry, 1971). In addition, an anticompensatory eye movement reflex, apparently dependent on vestibular stimulation, moves the eye to a goal before short high-velocity head movements are completed, with the compensatory reflex then aiding the eye in locking onto the target. Anticompensatory reflexes may on occasion blur vision from the cockpit for the external world (Melvill-Jones, 1964). Finally, vestibuloocular accommodation reflexes have been implicated in degrading vision in some aircraft maneuvers (Clark *et al.*, 1975).

ILLUSIONS PRODUCED BY CONDITIONS ENCOUNTERED IN AVIATION

So much emphasis has been placed on vestibular illusions in aviation that the impression is sometimes given that all vestibular information is misleading and useless. It should be apparent from earlier sections that this is an inappropriate conclusion. However, aircraft maneuvers may involve both unnatural turns and unusual changes in the direction and magnitude of resultant linear force vectors. Moreover, the seated pilot does not necessarily continually update his orientation assessment as one does automatically while walking or running. Thus both the pattern of vestibular stimulation and the response to it differ from those encountered in natural movement.

SOMATOGYRAL AND OCULOGYRAL ILLUSIONS. Aircraft maneuvers involving several complete revolutions (turns, rolls, or spins) tend to produce an illusion of turning in opposite direction just after the maneuver is completed. Contributing to this effect are semicircular canal responses illustrated in Fig. 7. The cupula-endolymph system responds to inertial torque imparted by angular acceleration (shown in Fig. 7 by the slope of the ω-change) which commences the rotation. The curves in Fig. 7 may be thought of as cupula deflection plotted with respect to time and sensation magnitude as the difference between these plotted curves and a theoretical cupula "threshold zone" (not shown) which gradually rises from the baseline whenever the cupula remains deflected in a given direction (cf. Guedry, 1974, p. 58*f*). If rotation at constant angular velocity continues, the cupula, without angular acceleration to sustain its deflection, commences a return toward null position by virtue of its elasticity. When the returning cupula intersects the increasing threshold zone, in about 20–40 sec. the sensation of rotation stops even though rotation continues. This has been referred to as the "per-rotary" primary effect of semicircular canal stimulation.[5] Then the cupula, because it is near null position as the stop commences, will be deflected in opposite direction by the deceleration, thereby eliciting a sensation of turning in opposite direction (a "postrotational" primary effect), which also persists for some 20–40 sec.

Stimulus and vestibular response characteristics which control the magnitude of the per- and postrotary vestibular effects are the velocity of rotation achieved, the duration of the rotation, and, with some stimuli, the particular set of canals stimulated (Gilson *et al.*, 1973*a;* Guedry *et al.*, 1971). Note that constant velocity need not be maintained during the turn for some illusory aftereffect to occur. Whenever angular acceleration of constant direction is applied for several seconds, the continued cupula displacement is opposed by the elastic restoring force

---

[5]A secondary effect involving sensation of rotation and nystagmus of opposite direction follows the primary effect. Secondary effects and some other discrepancies from predictions based on theoretical cupula mechanics are commonly attributed to adaptation effects which have been conceptualized as a shifting threshold zone (cf. Guedry, 1974).

of the cupula, whereas when the deceleration commences, the elastic restoring couple works with the inertial torque from the "stopping" stimulus to produce cupula overshoot. Information from the semicircular canals would therefore signal stop before the actual maneuver ends, and would signal reversed turn from the cupula "overshoot" for any long triangular or sinusoidal waveform of angular velocity, even though no period of constant velocity is interposed between the starting and stopping acceleration.

This sequence of perceptual events when observed in complete darkness has been called the "somatogyral illusion" (Benson and Burchard, 1973). Essentially the same sequence, when observed in darkness with only a small head-fixed visual display in view, has been called the "oculogyral illusion" (Graybiel and Hupp, 1946). In the latter case, the perceived motion of the body is referred to the visible display, which therefore seems to be turning with the observer. However, the display may appear to lead slightly, i.e., be displaced from "apparent dead ahead" in the direction of the apparent motion; the display may be slightly blurred while the vestibular signal is strong enough to generate nystagmus in spite of visual suppression; and the threshold for detection of angular acceleration seems to be lower for the oculogyral illusion than for the somatogyral illusion (Clark and Stewart, 1969; Guedry, 1974). From the point of view of aviation, it is important to

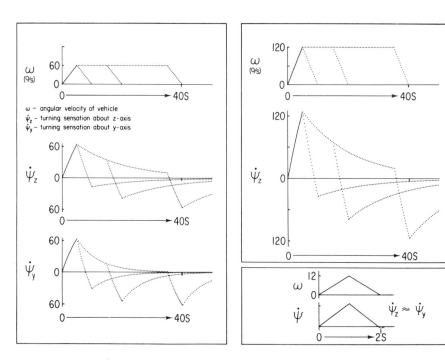

Fig. 7. Dependence of aftereffects (dotted lines below baselines) on (1) interval between acceleration and deceleration: compare afterresponse when interval of constant velocity is 0 sec, 10 sec, and 30 sec in left panel or in upper right panel; (2) set of canals stimulated: compare $\dot{\psi}_z$ (horizontal canal) responses and $\dot{\psi}_y$ (vertical canal) responses in left panel; (3) peak angular velocity (ω) attained: compare $\dot{\psi}_z$ responses in upper right and in left panel; (4) duration of a triangular angular velocity stimulus waveform: compare afterresponses to 10-sec period ω-waveform in left panel with negligible afterresponse to 2-sec ω-waveform in lower right panel.

note that these illusory effects occur even in the presence of a well-illuminated cockpit if external visual reference is absent or ill-defined.

The distinction between the somatogyral and oculogyral illusions assumes additional import in view of the curious difference in aftersensations produced by active vs. passive turning, described in Chapter 9. When a standing person, with eyes closed, turns himself actively, say, eight turns in 30 sec, he will, upon stopping, experience rotation in the same direction as the previous rotation. In many people, the head, torso, and legs twist in the same direction as the preceding turn, i.e., the vestibular effects on the motor system produce the expected compensatory response for the deceleratory reversal of response, but the sensation in the same direction as the previous turning apparently comes from feedback from the motor response, rather than from vestibular sensations. It is not the standing posture which produces this effect because standing individuals rotated passively experience aftersensations in a direction opposite the preceding rotation (Correia et al., 1977; Guedry et al., 1977). Opening the eyes after active turning tends to dispel or confuse the sensation aftereffect.

This difference in aftersensation between active and passive turning may be important in aviation. Pilots actively generate unusual vestibular stimuli, and, of course, continue to control the aircraft after maneuvers are completed.[6] The sensations of experienced pilots may be shaped to some extent by their active control functions and hence may be a little different than would be deduced from passive stimulation in laboratory devices. There have been several indications that pilots' reactions to flight simulators (Reason and Brand, 1975; Miller and Goodson, 1960) and to laboratory devices (Dowd et al., 1966) differ from those of nonpilot populations, and this could well be attributable in part to the pilots' tendency to react and exert control over unexpected motion inputs.

SOMATOGRAVIC AND OCULOGRAVIC ILLUSIONS. The somatogravic and oculogravic illusions are frequently regarded as being of otolith origin. They are apt to occur when the head and body are in a force field which is not in alignment with gravity, a condition that occurs frequently during flight and that is usually studied in the laboratory by means of a centrifuge. Although otolith stimulation plays a role in the effects of such stimuli, certainly other somatosensory receptors are also involved. Individuals without vestibular function experience these "illusions," although their perceptions differ somewhat from those of individuals with vestibular function (Graybiel and Clark, 1965; Guedry, 1974).

According to Einstein's equivalence principle, a vehicle, far away from the gravitational field of the Earth or other large mass, would, if it accelerated at 9.81 m/sec^2 in a straight line, generate a force field that would be indistinguishable from the gravitational field at the Earth's surface. When the otolith system and body are in a particular orientation relative to a force field which is the resultant of gravity and a constant linear acceleration, the response of these systems is as though they had the same orientation relative to gravity, except that there are magnitude differences between gravity at the Earth's surface and the resultant

---

[6] This effect may also contribute, in part, to some of the controversial findings concerning responses of ice skaters following spins (cf. Collins, 1966).

FRED E. GUEDRY, JR.,
AND MANNING J.
CORREIA

force field. The occupant of an aircraft in a sustained coordinated bank and turn experiences a force, the resultant of gravity and the centripetal linear acceleration vector, which is apt to be perceived as the upright direction because it is the "vertical" dimension of the existing force field. This perception of feeling upright during a coordinated bank and turn, or its converse of feeling tilted while seated upright on a rotating centrifuge, has been referred to as the "somatogravic illusion" (Benson and Burchard, 1973) when observers have indicated apparent body tilt without the use of visual reference cues; for situations in which an observer adjusts a line of light to indicate his perception of apparent vertical, the perceptual error has been called the "oculogravic illusion" (Graybiel, 1952). There has been some academic disagreement as to whether these effects should be referred to as illusion, since the individual is *upright* relative to the resultant-force "vertical" in the sustained bank and turn and is *tilted* relative to the resultant-force "vertical" on the centrifuge. However, the important point for the aviator is that accelerations in flight can yield a resultant force vector which may be perceived as upright, even though it is substantially "tilted" relative to gravity.

While the direction of the resultant force vector provides a fairly close approximation of the subjective vertical in "steady-state" conditions (i.e., conditions in which the observer experiences prolonged static tilt relative to the resultant force vector), there are a number of definite departures from this rule:

1. One departure results from conditions of dynamic (changing over time) linear and angular accelerations. During horizontal linear acceleration of an upright forward-facing observer, the resultant linear acceleration vector rotates in the pitch plane of the head and body. The otolith stimulation is as though the head and body had rotated backward relative to gravity, but because the head is fixed in upright position there is no angular acceleration to stimulate the vertical semicircular canals. Under these circumstances, the immediately perceived change in orientation is usually less than that which would be calculated from the immediate stimulus to the otolith (cf. Stockwell and Guedry, 1970; Guedry, 1974, p. 105*f*). This kind of situation occurs in linearly accelerating (or braking) aircraft, and although some change in attitude is experienced, if the head does not rotate on the neck during the linear acceleration or deceleration, then the experienced change in attitude is probably less than the dynamic rotation of the linear acceleration resultant vector, and hence closer to the actual attitude of the aircraft (Fig. 8). Even so, there can be enough change in perceived attitude to introduce dangerous reactions in flight (Collar, 1946). An extreme example of this kind of stimulus occurs during catapult takeoff from an aircraft carrier.

2. A second circumstance, in which judgments of vertical are apt to depart from alignment with the existing force field, occurs in the presence of a structured visual field. A prominent visual frame of reference with linear dimensions tilted relative to the direction of existing force field will frequently produce a compromise estimate of verticality between visual and force field cues.

Perceived tilt with discordant visual and force field cues has usually been studied in fairly static situations, whether by use of centrifuges or by simply tilting the body and/or visual field in different orientations relative to gravity (Guedry, 1974). Much attention has been devoted to the contention that there are idiosyn-

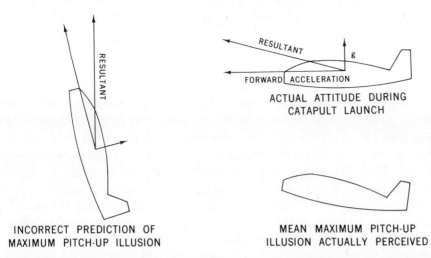

ACTUAL ATTITUDE DURING
CATAPULT LAUNCH

INCORRECT PREDICTION OF
MAXIMUM PITCH-UP ILLUSION

MEAN MAXIMUM PITCH-UP
ILLUSION ACTUALLY PERCEIVED

Fig. 8. Difference between the mean maximum illusory nose-high attitude actually perceived during a simulated catapult launch and the maximum illusory attitude predicted from the direction of the peak resultant vector. Maximum forward acceleration during catapult launch is about 4.5 g units, which, when resolved with gravity, yields a resultant vector that is displaced about 77° from the direction of gravity. In simulated catapult launches, subjects experienced lesser pitch-up than would be predicted from the 77° change in the resultant (*cf.* Cohen *et al.*, 1972).

cratic differences in regard to the use of visual versus body (force field) cues in the setting of a line of light to apparent vertical. Individuals who are more influenced in this task by the visual field than others are said to be field dependent (visual-field dependent), and scores on tests of field dependence/field independence have been reported to have some relationship to personality tests, to specialties in aviation (Brictson, 1975; Kennedy, 1975) and degree of disturbance exhibited in some motion situations (Barrett and Thornton, 1968; Long *et al.*, 1975). As in most areas where attempts are made to predict complex behavior from results of fairly simple tests, there are some inconsistencies in the findings.

Recently there has been renewed interest in the investigation of effects of large moving displays on perception of body rotation, body tilt, and the setting to vertical of lines of light. Effects of central field motion (visual angle less than 30°) are slight, but large moving peripheral fields can induce the sensation of body motion within 3 sec and substantial sensations of body tilt (Dichgans and Brandt, 1972, 1973; Dichgans *et al.*, 1972; Held *et al.*, 1975; Brandt *et al.*, 1971, 1973). Of considerable interest are apparently related findings that large moving visual fields modulate neural activity in the vestibular nuclei even when the head and body remain stationary (Dichgans *et al.*, 1973; Henn *et al.*, 1974). It has also been found that vestibular stimulation appears to modulate responses in central visual projection fields even when the retinal image is fixed (Grüsser and Grüsser-Kornehls, 1972; Horn and Hill, 1969; Horn *et al.*, 1972; Bisti *et al.*, 1974; Wiersma, 1970) and that single-stage bilateral labyrinthine destruction eliminates optokinetic afternystagmus in monkeys (Cohen *et al.*, 1973). These various results again point to the intimate relations between the visual and vestibular systems in both "feedforward" and "feedback" loops and indicate the importance of studying the somatogravic and oculogravic "illusions" as separate phenomena (see also Bauermeister, 1964). In aviation either a large tilted frame of reference from cloud formations, etc., or uniform motion in the pilot's visual field can induce illusory perceptions of the attitude of the aircraft. Dynamic visual stimuli can induce both illusory attitudes and illusory motion.

3. A third circumstance in which judgments of vertical may depart from alignment with the resultant force field occurs when the magnitude of the force field exceeds $1.0g$ (or is less than $1.0g$). Systematic departures, which appear to be attributable to otolith function, have been observed even in static or steady-state conditions. That component of the total force which acts in alignment with the mean plane of the utricle (the utricular shear component) is regarded as the effective stimulus to the utricle (cf. von Békésy, 1966; Fernandez et al., 1972). When the head is positioned so that the resultant force is maintained perpendicular to the utricular plane, then changes in the magnitude of the resultant force would not introduce a utricular shear component, and such changes do not alter the perception of verticality (Schone, 1964; Correia et al., 1968). However, when the head is in a position of 30° lateral tilt relative to a $2.0g$ field, then lateral displacement of the utricular otoliths relative to the underlying sensory hair cells is greater, because of the greater utricular shear component, than it would be with the same head tilt in a $1.0g$ field, and estimates of the visual vertical are systematically displaced as a result (Schöne, 1964; Miller and Graybiel, 1966; Correia et al., 1968). Thus the magnitude of the utricular shear component seems to have a definite effect on the perception of verticality. However, such perceptions are not perfectly predictable from calculations of this component, possibly because of nonlinear saturation effects[7] (Schöne and Parker, 1967) or to interacting responses of the sacculus. In a $1.0g$ field, a lateral head tilt of 30° would introduce an increase of utricular shear, but saccular shear would decrease. In a $2.0g$ field, both utricular and saccular shear would be increased. The input from the saccular displacement may partially cancel the effects of the increased utricular signal and account for some of the systematic departures of perceived tilts from those predicted from a simple utricular-shear model (cf. Guedry, 1974, pp. 96–103).

ILLUSIONS ASSOCIATED WITH HEAD MOVEMENTS. Nuttall (1958) attributed a series of fatal aircraft accidents to pilots' head movements required by necessity to shift radio frequencies during procedural turning maneuvers at low altitudes. Several illusory effects can be elicited by head movements during turning maneuvers in aircraft.

The Cross-Coupling Coriolis Illusion. When a vehicle rotates at some angular velocity, ω_1, about one axis while an individual within the vehicle tilts his head about an orthogonal axis at some angular velocity, ω_2, the head undergoes an angular acceleration of magnitude, $\omega_1\omega_2$, about a third axis, orthogonal to the other two axes. If the ω_1 and ω_2 axes are not orthogonal, the magnitude of the cross-coupled angular acceleration is $\omega_1\omega_2 \sin \phi$, where ϕ is the angle between the

---

[7]Saturation effects do not appear in accord with recent neurophysiological data of Fernandez and Goldberg (1976), who found peripheral otolith neurons increasing firing rates linearly as acceleration was progressively increased from 0 to $4g$ in the shear plane.

ω_1 and ω_2 axes and ω_1 and ω_2 are expressed in radians per second. As the head is turned about the ω_2 axis, different sets of semicircular canals are being stimulated: the plane of the $\omega_1\omega_2$ acceleration can be visualized as being perpendicular to the rotation plane of the vehicle, and the sets of semicircular canals are changing position relative to that plane. A specific example will serve to clarify the effects that such a stimulus produces. Assume that an observer, on a turntable which has been rotating in counterclockwise direction at constant velocity (ω_1) of 60°/sec for 20 or 30 sec, has his head fixed in tilted position toward his left shoulder. If he then moves his head to upright position, he experiences a forward tumble and a slight leftward rotation. Vestibular nystagmus produced by the canal stimulus is primarily down (fast phase) and slightly to the left. An important point to note here is that just after the head is upright the otolith system would signal the veridical head position relative to gravity, yet the fairly strong residual effects from the stimulus to the vertical canals would give a sensation of forward tumble (angular velocity) and a perceived attitude change (angular displacement) of the body and entire vehicle relative to Earth-vertical. Here, then, is a situation in which veridical information regarding orientation relative to the Earth provided by the otoliths is compromised by misleading canal signals resulting in an illusory change in attitude. The perception is confusing in that it seems to have too much velocity for the amount of tilt perceived (Guedry and Montague, 1961), but substantial tilts are reported (Clark and Stewart, 1967; Collins, 1968).

This effect is sometimes referred to as a Coriolis effect because the inertial torque which stimulates each canal can be derived by integrating the components of the linear Coriolis acceleration which act in alignment with the canal walls. From a practical point of view, the conditions that control the magnitude of this disturbing effect in aviation are the starting position of the head, the total angle through which the head is turned (the greater the angle, the greater the total integrated stimulus), the angular velocity (ω_1) of the aircraft, and time elapsed since onset of vehicle turn. Aircraft in a bank and turn commonly do not have a very high angular velocity (ω_1), and under these conditions the magnitude of cross-coupled (Coriolis) effects from head movements may be relatively slight, although in the unstable conditions of flight even slightly disorienting effects can be dangerous if external visual reference is either absent or misleading. In higher-rate sustained turns, the cross-coupled effects can be strong.

The "g-Excess" Illusion. There is another effect during head movements in aircraft which is apt to occur whenever the aircraft is generating an abnormal force field. This effect was observed during coordinated 2.0g turns about a large radius (r) of several miles. In this maneuver, the aircraft speed (tangential linear velocity) is very high, but the angular velocity (ω_1) is very low, about 4°/sec or 0.07 rad/sec.[8] This means that the cross-coupling (Coriolis) effects described in the preceding paragraphs would be almost negligible, yet during head movements in such turns observers have reported experiencing peculiar sensations sometimes

---

[8]The center of turn may be at a radial distance of 1 or 2 miles from the aircraft. The 2g resultant is obtained by resolving the gravity vector with the centripetal vector ($\omega_1^2 r$). To calculate centripetal acceleration, ω_1 must be expressed in radian units.

involving sudden shifts in the apparent attitude of the aircraft, together with nausea which would undoubtedly culminate in sickness in some individuals if frequent head movements were made in this situation. This has been called a "g-excess effect" because sensory signals from the otolith system when the head is moved in a high-g field would exceed those produced by the same head movement in a $1.0g$ field. The extra input may be perceptually attributed to a sudden maneuver of the aircraft, in which case a change in aircraft attitude in the plane of the head movement would be experienced. The perceived attitude change would be at right angles to the cross-coupled (Coriolis) effects. It is comparable to the effects of force field magnitude on estimates of verticality described previously, except that head movement introduces a dynamic stimulus to the otolith system and the perception is more confusing and less consistently reported (Gilson *et al.*, 1973*b*).

AUTOGYRAL AND AUTOKINETIC ILLUSIONS. It is well known that a small single light in an otherwise dark room will appear to move in a more or less random path and that the direction and extent of apparent movement can be influenced by suggestion or the expectations of the observer. Perhaps less well known is the fact that individuals in a rotatable but stationary structure frequently perceive rotation of the entire structure. This "autogyral" effect, which occurs in darkness or in illuminated but enclosed devices, indicates that absence of specific motion cues does not ensure perceived stability when motion expectations are high. Such effects are further evidence of the fact that disorientation can occur in aviation without any immediately preceding disorienting visual or vestibular stimuli. The extent to which autogyral effects might occur about axes other than an Earth-vertical axis has not been studied in laboratory situations except in the presence of misleading visual cues, in which case substantial errors of verticality can be induced. A number of instances in which pilots have mistaken stars and other fixed light sources as moving aircraft have probably involved autokinetic effects (Benson, 1965).

VESTIBULAR INSENSITIVITY AND PILOT DISORIENTATION

As in the preceding autogyral and autokinetic effects, many instances of pilot disorientation are less attributable to some overwhelming misleading vestibular response than to some subtle perceptual inconsistency or even to perceptual insensitivity to the acceleration environment.

PERCEPTION OF TILT. Typically, mean judgments of verticality indicated by psychophysical studies suggest fairly accurate perceptions, but the range of judgments usually includes a few large errors even though the observer can devote his entire attention to this one task. In long flights where vibration and a number of momentary accelerations from turbulence do not demand corrective responses from the pilot, the threshold of response to vestibular stimuli may increase because of the "acceleration noise level." Perceptual errors may then approach the occasional extreme errors encountered in laboratory experiments and also those found in water immersion studies where very large errors in the perceived vertical have been noted (Ross *et al.*, 1969; Nelson, 1968; cf. Guedry, 1974, pp. 88–92).

Even without a background of "acceleration noise" or water immersion, there are large mean errors in estimates of verticality when tilts occur very slowly; e.g., pitch and/or roll attitudes of 10° are typically regarded as upright, whereas sensitivity to detection of slow tilt increases substantially if the subject is rotated about the axis that is being tilted (Benson *et al.*, 1975), as shown in Fig. 9. Very slow or sustained tilts diminish rate information from the otoliths (Roberts, 1967) and corroborative information from the semicircular canals, and increase likelihood of adaptation effects (Passey and Guedry, 1949).

In flight, therefore, a gradual roll or pitch away from straight and level flight sometimes occurs at rates below the semicircular canal or otolith threshold perceptual levels. Adaptation to a tilt position so that this position seems upright yields a definite sensation of tilt in opposite direction when an individual returns to upright position. If a flight slowly entered a coordinated bank and turn, alignment of the resultant vector with the head-to-seat axis would allow for still further undetected deviation from straight and level flight. If the pilot should then become aware of the aircraft attitude from instrument information or external reference, his corrective actions could introduce vestibular stimuli considerably above threshold levels, indicating a definite change from an attitude which had just been perceived as straight and level. Circumstances such as these produce "the leans," one of the most common forms of disorientation reported by pilots (Clark,

VESTIBULAR
FUNCTION

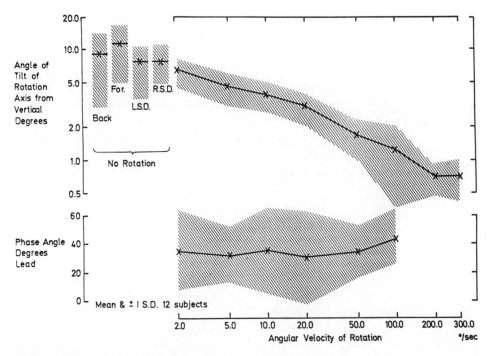

Fig. 9. Large mean errors in detection of very slow tilt (0.08°/sec) when there was no rotation about a slowly tilting axis, and increase in sensitivity to detection of tilt (wobble) as a function of rotation rate about the slowly tilting axis. Back, For., L.S.D., and R.S.D. in the "no rotation" condition refer to backward, forward, left-side-down, and right-side-down tilts, respectively. Phase lead of apparent nose-up position relative to true nose-up position is shown in lower curve. Data from Benson *et al.* (1975).

1971). The cockpit instruments show that the aircraft is straight and level, yet the pilot feels that he is in a "bank and turn." Though the pilot may be able to fly successfully by his instruments, prolonged perceptual conflicts can eventually degrade his performance. Curiously, the leans may persist for 30 min or more, much longer than any known normal afterresponse of the vestibular system. It is as though once the perceived vertical is displaced from the initially not very compelling sensory information about upright, then this displaced perception may sustain itself until the pilot attends for a while to some other aspect of the flight task or until there is a good visual reference to the Earth (Benson and Burchard, 1973). Emotional disturbance may further degrade "position sense" (cf. Stigler, 1912). Considering the range of positions which may be judged to be vertical in the absence of clearly misleading information, it should not be surprising that "the leans" could also be provoked by misleading visual stimuli such as sloping cloud banks, slanting rays of sunlight through clouds, rows of lights erroneously believed to be horizontal, and even the edge of the instrument glare shield sloping over the attitude gyro (Tormes and Guedry, 1975). Pilots occasionally find themselves in nearly inverted flight when just prior to the discovery they had believed themselves to be in normal, level flight. The probability of this kind of error is enhanced by the fact that man's estimates of vertical are relatively poor in some tilt positions and especially when he is inverted (Graybiel and Clark, 1962; Guedry, 1974, pp. 81–94). In these positions, visual cues assume a more predominant role (Young, 1973; Schöne and Udo de Haes, 1971; Udo de Haes and Schöne, 1970).

PERCEPTION OF VERTICAL LINEAR ACCELERATION. Vertical oscillations introduce linear accelerations that are aligned with gravity so that the magnitude of the resultant force field changes relative to the head, but its direction does not. If an erect observer is oscillated vertically, the changing linear acceleration is approximately perpendicular to the utricular otolith plane, and therefore it is ineffective as a utricular stimulus. Its approximate alignment with the saccular otolithic plane would introduce an effective saccular "shear" stimulus, but the saccular otoliths, already deflected by a $1g$ shear force, may be relatively insensitive to added acceleration in the same plane. From this theoretical point of view, otolithic insensitivity to vertical linear oscillation (VLO) as compared with its sensitivity to horizontal linear oscillation (HLO) might be expected. Von Békésy (1940) reported accurate amplitude estimates of high-frequency (up to 4 Hz) small-amplitude VLO, but his stimuli involved high peak accelerations at frequencies where otolith gain may be high. Recent neurophysiological findings (Fernandez and Goldberg, 1976) do not support the idea that otolithic neural input information would limit perception of VLO as compared to HLO, but some perceptual data suggest that there may be perceptual deficiencies with low-frequency stimuli. Walsh (1964) reported higher thresholds for 0.11 Hz VLO than he had previously reported (1961a,b, 1962) for HLO, although his data are not entirely consistent (*cf.* Benson *et al.*, 1975). Several recent experiments (Malcolm and Melvill-Jones, 1974; Melvill-Jones *et al.*, 1976) have indicated perceptual inaccuracies with VLO that seem excessive relative to fairly accurate perceptions of HLO in other studies (Guedry and Harris, 1963; Young and Meiry, 1968). Walsh (1964) reported large stimulus-response phase errors (individuals experienced maximum downward travel during upward travel) at 0.11 Hz and zero phase error at 1.0 Hz. Other phase data (Young and Meiry, 1968; Melvill-Jones *et al.*, 1976) for HLO and VLO are not consistent with those of Walsh (1962, 1964), probably because of differences in reporting methodology and in high-frequency stimulus artifacts, but averaged oculomotor responses of Melvill-Jones *et al.* (1976) exhibited stimulus-response phase angles at 0.11 Hz and 1 Hz consistent with Walsh's subjective data. Differences in body position (reclining in Walsh's studies, erect in other studies) may also contribute to some of the interexperiment differences. Spinovestibular interactions may modulate perceptual experience in the erect observer during VLO through mechanisms similar to those which produced the very different perceptual experiences noted above in the aftereffects of active vs. passive turning. If methodological differences and stimulus artifacts influence perceptual consistency in formal experiments, pilots of helicopters and VTOL aircraft would also be susceptible to occasional perceptual inconsistencies including large phase errors in the noisy acceleration environment of flight. Misjudgment of helicopter motion during low-altitude hover was found to be a prominent factor in a number of disorientation incidents during conditions of poor external visibility, and, moreover, extraneous motion stimuli such as visible "salt" spray through rotor blades, wave motion, ship motion during night landings, and even wind currents in the cockpit can exacerbate the situation in naval helicopter operations (Tormes and Guedry, 1975).

SENSORY INTERACTIONS IN FLIGHT AND FLIGHT SIMULATION

In foregoing descriptions of disorientation in aviation, some situations have sometimes been named and categorized as though the primary cause of the nominal event emanated from one wayward sensory input. For example, the oculogyral and oculogravic illusions have been discussed in relation to responses of the semicircular canals and to otolith organs, respectively. In practical flight situations, the independent occurrence of such effects almost never occurs and for that reason the effects of interactions among different sensory systems providing orientation information is important. Knowledge of the dynamic response of each sensory system to various frequencies of stimulation may eventually be sufficient for an engineering systems approach that will accurately predict patterns of input from motion sensors in complex flight. Unfortunately, the dynamics of otolith responses and the way in which the utricular and saccular otoliths coordinate to influence motor reflexes and perceptual responses are not very well agreed upon. Efforts have been made to relate certain perceptual measures to linear accelerations and to horizontal linear oscillations at several frequencies, but, at this juncture, it appears that perceptual "lags" may be as much dependent on central integration of inputs from several senses as on response characteristics of any one sensory system. Even the character of the perceptual experience, e.g., tilting sensations vs. linear velocity sensations, seems to depend on CNS interpretation of semicircular canal and otolith input patterns (cf. Guedry, 1974, pp. 68–79).

While this chapter has stressed disorienting effects of some motion stimuli, for perspective it should be noted that motion cue information is probably used subconsciously by experienced pilots in controlling aircraft. Addition of roll-motion cues to visual cues in experimental flight simulators has been shown to improve man-vehicle control in some conditions (Shirley and Young, 1968; E. Cohen, 1968), and to reduce simulator sickness (cf. Reason and Brand, 1975, p. 109*f*). The fact that experienced, as opposed to inexperienced, pilots become sick in fixed-base simulators suggests that pilots make use of body motion cues and are disturbed by their absence. Knowledge of the perceptual/motor effects of various sensory interactions is critical because simulation demands substitute patterns of sensory inputs for those that will occur in real flight.

Vestibular System and Space Exploration

The advent of the space age prompted increased study of vestibular function because of two potential problems of space operations. The first related to perceptual/motor and "motion" sickness effects that were anticipated for individuals living in the absence of our accustomed $1.0g$ force field. The second related to the possibility that a similar set of unwelcome effects could result from a counter-measure for weightlessness, namely, the rotation of space stations to produce "artificial gravity." Aside from vestibular effects of weightlessness, concerns about cardiovascular and neuromuscular deconditioning processes generated the distinct possibility that some artificial gravity (and hence a space centrifuge) might prove necessary. Since movement within a rotating structure was known to induce unusual vestibular stimulation and motion sickness, the vestibular system became a necessary consideration, irrespective of which mode of space flight was chosen (cf. Lansberg, 1960).

Weightlessness

The Inversion Illusion. Early in space flight, the Russian cosmonaut Titov reported an inversion illusion, i.e., he felt he was flying upside down, shortly after orbital flight was achieved (Billingham, 1966). Similar effects were also reported by other cosmonauts, sometimes with considerable persistence (Gazenko, 1964; Yuganov *et al.*, 1966). The inversion illusion has also been reported in parabolic flight both in normal observers and in individuals without labyrinthine function, but when these observers were restrained in their seats by straps then only individuals with normal vestibular function reported the phenomenon (Graybiel and Kellogg, 1967). While these results suggest that the weightless otolith receptors contributed to the inversion effect, it is noteworthy that astronauts have reported a "fullness in the head" like hanging upside down on Earth, apparently as a result of redistribution of the total circulating blood volume (Berry and Homick, 1973). Thus other physiological adjustments may contribute to the inversion illusion, and, moreover, reports of "hanging upside down" do not necessarily refer to a perception of being inverted (Berry and Homick, 1973). In stabilized orbital flight, there is of course no vertical up-down dimension because the resultant force field[9] is zero, and it appears that some cosmonauts were not especially disturbed by feeling inverted (Yuganov *et al.*, 1966). Some astronauts reported no sense of an external vertical, but rather that "up" is the headward direction (Jones, 1975). Degree of disturbance by these effects and even whether or not they are noticed may be dependent on the individual's direction of attention, e.g., toward an inverted visual display, and perhaps personality.

HEAD MOVEMENTS AND MOTION SICKNESS IN WEIGHTLESSNESS. In addition to his reports of the inversion illusion, Titov reported that head movements induced dizziness, vertigo, and nausea which culminated in emesis after about 6 hr in orbit (Gazenko, 1964; Graybiel *et al.*, 1974). Although there is some question about the possibility that rotation of the spacecraft may have contributed to Titov's "space sickness" by inducing cross-coupling effects during head movements (Billingham, 1966), subsequent cosmonauts reported unpleasant dizziness and nausea associated with head movements in stabilized spacecraft (Yuganov *et al.*, 1966). Early American astronauts in relatively small spacecraft did not report comparable effects, but space sickness induced by head and body movements became fairly common (Billingham, 1966) in the larger Apollo series spacecraft that permitted greater mobility of crew members. Nine of 25 astronauts (36% incidence) experienced space sickness associated with movement in Apollo command modules. Subsequently, a number of astronauts have had problems with space sickness associated with head and whole-body movements (Jones, 1975; Graybiel *et al.*, 1974) in Skylab missions, and this remains a problem to be overcome in future space operations by selection, training, conditioning, or medication. Unfortunately, it is difficult to account for individual differences in susceptibility to space sickness in Skylab crewmen, possibly because of individual precautions in making head and body movements and in anti-motion sickness medication used (Jones, 1975). It is noteworthy that some Russian scientists favor the use of vestibular selection tests and conditioning programs (Popov *et al.*, 1968; Yuganov *et al.*, 1969; Zasosov and Popov, 1958).

A PERSPECTIVE ON HEAD MOVEMENTS IN WEIGHTLESSNESS. To attain some understanding of the disturbance associated with head and whole-body motions within spacecraft during weightlessness, it is instructive to consider the vestibular signals which accompany natural head and body movements in a natural $1.0g$ environment and also some vestibular inputs and their effects when movements occur within an unaccustomed force field.

In our natural environment, the pattern of neural sensory inflow from the utricle and saccule provides information on orientation relative to gravity just *before* a head movement is made. During a head movement the initial and changing pattern of otolith information provides a coded message on instantaneous orientation relative to gravity, against which angular velocity information from the semicircular canals (and possibly rate information from the otolith

[9]The resultant of the centripetal acceleration (given by the square of the angular velocity of the spacecraft relative to the Earth times the distance of the craft from the center of the Earth) and the acceleration of gravity at the orbital radius is zero.

receptors) is "interpreted" by the central nervous system. As noted earlier, the semicircular canals, according to classical concepts, respond to angular acceleration and do not respond to linear acceleration or gravity; hence by themselves they cannot provide information on orientation relative to gravity. Therefore, the semicircular canals would respond in the same way when the head is rotated about its z axis, irrespective of whether the individual is upright with head erect, in which case the z axis would be aligned with gravity, or is lying on his side, in which case the z axis would be at right angles to gravity. In the former case (head upright), the initial head position relative to gravity does not change during the head movement, so that the signals from the horizontal (lateral) canals are unaccompanied by change-in-orientation information from the otolith organs. In the latter case (individual on one side), the signals from the horizontal semicircular canals are accompanied by change-in-position otolith information as the head is turned. From such analyses, it is quite clear that a given pattern of semicircular canal input can be accompanied by a variety of patterns of otolith inputs during natural movements on the Earth, but *ipso facto* it is also clear that the initial position information signaled by the otoliths and any change in it during a movement provide a ground (or a reference) against which the semicircular canal input (and any rate information from the otoliths) must be "interpreted" by the central nervous system to provide appropriate perceptual and motor responses during head motion relative to the Earth. While these natural head movements introduce a variety of patterns of inputs among the vestibular receptors, it is to be noted that they are typically highly synergistic. For example, after a person has leaned forward, if he rotates his head about his z axis, he is, in effect, turning his head about an axis which is tilted relative to gravity. In this case, the semicircular canals locate the axis (or plane) of rotation relative to the skull while the initial and final patterns of otolith signals locate this axis relative to gravity, and the changing otolith pattern probably locates it relative to the skull and to gravity during the movement. The axes of rotation located by the semicircular canals and otolith system are colinear. During the arcs of turn involved in natural head movements, typically 180° or less, semicircular canal information is from all indications essentially veridical; i.e., the amount of turn (angular displacement) can be accurately estimated from semicircular canal inputs alone (Guedry, 1974), and there would be little or no phase lead or lag or aftereffects (see lower right panel of Fig. 7). Thus the plane, magnitude, and temporal characteristics of angular velocity information from the semicircular canals would be consistent with the change-in-orientation information indicated by the otolith system.

When these temporally and geometrically precise patterns of input are disturbed by pathological conditions or by some form of unphysiological movements, then head movements frequently induce both illusory orientation information and nausea. This is a common report from individuals suffering from peripheral vestibular disorders, and some examples of unphysiological movements, mentioned in earlier sections, will be reviewed briefly here.

Head movements in a high-g field produce the illusory "g-excess effect" and nausea, probably because the otolith input during the head movement is excessive relative to the semicircular canal input. Head movements during continuous whole-body rotation (ω_1) induce cross-coupling (Coriolis) stimuli to the semicircular canals so that the angular velocity information they yield is mismatched in plane to the plane of orientation change indicated by the otolith system. Such stimuli induce both disorientation and nausea.[10] Repeated exposure to specific Coriolis cross-coupled stimuli results in a reduction of the disorientation, nausea, and nystagmus they initially produced. However, it is possible to induce essentially identical semicircular canal stimulation while introducing a different accompanying set of responses from the otolith system. When this is done with individuals habituated to the first stimulus pattern, disorientation, nystagmus, and nausea are elicited by the second stimulus pattern (Guedry *et al.*, 1964). Although a more general habituation may occur with prolonged habituation schedules (Guedry, 1965*a,b;* Patterson and Graybiel, 1974), the specificity of habituation to moderate schedules indicates the importance of coding or patterning of vestibular inputs to the immediate effects of novel stimulus conditions.

Another example of the importance of coding of vestibular inputs may be inferred from the effects of prolonged rotation about an Earth-horizontal axis. When rotation first starts, the messages from the semicircular canals and otoliths are matched, and there is no disorientation or nausea; but as such rotation continues, nausea is a common complaint. While the exact mechanism of the responses that occur during prolonged rotation in this situation is somewhat controversial (Benson, 1974), it is clear that nystagmus responses typically attributed to the semicircular canal input diminish as the cupula returns (theoretically) by its elasticity toward its resting position. They do not, however, diminish to zero, but rather continue at a low slow-phase velocity. One reasonable explanation for this continued response is that the continuous reorientation of the otolith system generates a sustained input to the central nervous system, which then drives the nystagmus response. The nausea and sickness induced here, then, may be attributable to continued otolith input with a diminished or missing input from the semicircular canals. When prolonged rotation about a horizontal axis stops, the opposite situation occurs. A strong semicircular canal stimulus indicates a turn in a direction opposite that indicated by the change-in-position information from the otoliths during the deceleration, and then just after the stop there is continuing sensory inflow from the semicircular canals because the cupula which was deflected by the stop returns only slowly to its position of static equilibrium. During this postrotation period, the otoliths (1) indicate no change in orientation and (2) signal a particular orientation relative to gravity which is incompatible with the continuing signal from the canals; viz., the direction of gravity is approximately in the plane of the responding canal instead of being perpendicular to it. Under these conditions, postrotation reactions (sensation of turning and nystagmus) are suppressed (Correia and Guedry, 1964, 1966; Koella, 1947), and many individuals report that the stopping either induces nausea or increases the nausea that had already developed during the rotation. That the postrotation ampullar

---

[10]If a head tilt is made during an angular acceleration (from zero velocity), there is no nausea at all despite a strong $\omega_1\omega_2$ cross-coupled (Coriolis) vector because the resultant of the total effect of this vector and that of the angular acceleration vector before the head movement is a vector that aligns perfectly with gravity (Guedry and Benson, 1976).

FRED E. GUEDRY, JR.,
AND MANNING J.
CORREIA

neural inflow from a deflected cupula is actually present but suppressed by the particular static position information from the otolith is strongly supported by the fact that postrotational nystagmus responses attain the normal unsuppressed rate of decay when the individual is repositioned so that the gravity vector is perpendicular to the plane of responding canals (Benson, 1974).

The augmented nystagmus response during rotation about an Earth-horizontal axis and the suppressed postrotation responses are very prominent effects when the horizontal semicircular canals are stimulated, but these effects are less evident, although present, when individuals are positioned so that the vertical semicircular canals are in the plane of rotation (Benson, 1974). This curious difference may reflect the way in which vertical, *vis-à-vis* horizontal, canal stimulation is coupled with otolith stimulation in daily activities. In man's normal active upright posture, the head and body are frequently turned about the z axis, stimulating the horizontal semicircular canals without changing head orientation relative to gravity. Conversely, almost all head movements from upright posture which stimulate the vertical semicircular canals also involve a change in orientation of the head relative to gravity and thus produce an otolith stimulus which is synergistic with the input from the vertical canals. It is possible that the driving of continuing dynamic "vertical" oculomotor responses by either the otolith system or the vertical semicircular canals alone may be rendered less effective because in natural head movements these responses are typically driven by synergistic inputs from both systems. In other words, the CNS coupling of sensory input to dynamic x- and y-axis outputs is adapted to synergistic inputs from the vertical canals and the otolith receptors. Thus a substantial amount of vertical canal stimulation in the absence of supplementary otolith stimulation may be considered as a relatively unnatural pattern of stimulation (Benson, 1974, p. 295) to which the central nervous system is relatively unadapted. This may serve to explain why sinusoidal oscillation about an Earth-vertical axis produced a high incidence of sickness when individuals were positioned on their sides to place the vertical canals in the plane of rotation but did not produce sickness when individuals were positioned in upright posture to place their horizontal canals in the plane of rotation (Benson and Guedry, 1971).

Experimental results such as these suggest a close interplay between the canals and otoliths in controlling dynamic positioning reflexes and perceptions of spatial orientation, and they also illustrate the fact that nausea and sickness are common in stimulus situations that induce antisynergistic and unusual inputs from the canals and otoliths. In this context it is not surprising that head movements have induced disorientation, nausea, and sickness during the weightlessness of orbital space missions, where "normal" semicircular canal responses are not accompanied by meaningful initial and final orientation and change-in-orientation information from the otolith system before, during, and after the movements. Precise patterns of information from the semicircular canal and otolith systems would be disrupted by the absence of the usual synergistic otolith inputs, and this might be especially troublesome for head movements that stimulate the vertical canals. Moreover, since the mechanics of the otolith system are not sufficiently established to predict its response in a weightless state to tangential acceleration generated by starting and stopping head and body movements, it is possible that both the absence of usual otolith responses during movements and some uncharacteristic otolith responses in starting and stopping such movements could contribute to antisynergistic intralabyrinthine responses, thereby yielding confusing orientation information and nausea.

HEAD MOVEMENTS DURING PASSIVE ROTATION IN WEIGHTLESSNESS. In recent space missions involving prolonged orbital flight (Skylab), specific experiments have been set up to study the effects of head movements during whole-body rotation in weightlessness (Graybiel *et al.*, 1974; Jones, 1975). The magnitude of disturbance produced by head movements on a rotating platform in the weightless condition was reported to be substantially less than that which had been observed on the Earth. This result may be attributable to the fact that in the weightless environment the semicircular canals would be stimulated by the cross-coupled stimulus as on the Earth, but conflictual otolith signals indicating simultaneous change in orientation in an orthogonal plane would be absent. The absence of this strong, orthogonal, intralabyrinthine mismatch could account for the diminished disturbance by this condition in Skylab.

If this conclusion could be reached without qualifications, it would indeed be significant because there have been suggestions that mismatches between "expected" sensory feedback from voluntary movements and actual feedback set off by the movement are important in the adaptive process (Guedry and Graybiel, 1962; Guedry, 1965*b,c*) and in "habituation sickness of space flight" (Melvill-Jones, 1974). Because the semicircular canal stimulation set off by head movements during rotation in weightlessness would be orthogonal to the expected feedback, one might anticipate some disturbance even in the absence of the conflictual orthogonal message from the otolith receptors. However, this conclusion and any deductions concerning the insignificance of expected feedback cannot be accepted without qualifications, for several reasons. First, head movements made on the rotation device in Skylab were accomplished by upper trunk movements. Thus there was a substantial linear head velocity component relative to the rotating platform which introduced an appreciable linear Coriolis acceleration vector, and, moreover, the radial distance achieved introduced a centripetal acceleration vector. Therefore, linear accelerations of transient magnitude and direction were introduced which, though less than the $1.0g$ orthogonal otolith stimulus on Earth, nevertheless introduced some specific otolith stimulation in Skylab. Second, these rotation experiments were carried out after the astronauts had been in orbit for 8 days. This means that many head movements had been made that involved semicircular canal inputs without normal synergistic otolith inputs. Such movements induced space sickness in some of the Skylab crewmen, but a considerable degree of adjustment occurred within this 8-day period, and it is even possible that some experience with head movements during whole-body tumbling had accrued. For this reason, the astronauts were, to a degree, already accustomed to conflicts similar in kind, although not necessarily identical to those produced when the tests were conducted on the rotating device in Skylab. Thus a reasonable explanation of the reduced disturbance during Coriolis cross-coupling stimulation in Skylab is twofold: (1) there was habituation in the preceding 8 days to head movements which produced semicircular canal inputs without synergistic inputs from the otolith receptors, and this habituation carried over to the head movements on the rotation device, which also produced semicircular canal inputs without synergistic otolith information; and (2) the magnitude of the geometric mismatch between the semicircular canal and otolith responses produced by head movements on the rotating device was probably less in Skylab because of the quasi-weightless condition than the magnitude of the mismatch that occurs on Earth.

EFFECTS OF ROTATING SPACE STATIONS

Because of anticipated problems of physiological "deconditioning" in weightlessness, the possibility of generating an artificial gravity by rotating the space station about its own central axis has been considered. The centripetal acceleration ($\omega^2 r$) would serve as an artificial gravity, in which case the astronauts would walk in the plane of rotation and the center of rotation would be "up" while the centrifugal direction would be "down." A number of configurations of such vehicles have been considered, but the aspect of the problem of interest here is the fact that head movements during rotation would produce the disturbing cross-coupling effects described in preceding sections. Since the magnitude of these effects is directly related to the rate of vehicle rotation, it was obvious initially that low rates of rotation would be desirable to reduce the discomfort and motion sickness that head movements would tend to induce, yet low rates of rotation would require a very large radius to produce an artificial gravity of $1.0g$ (see footnote 8). For this reason, the maximum feasible rate of rotation from the point of view of disturbance produced by unusual vestibular stimulation became important for designing the potential overall size of the space station. The problem is interlocked with other necessary determinations such as how much artificial gravity is necessary. If, for example, $0.5g$ as compared with $1g$ were sufficient to prevent cardiovascular and neuromuscular deconditioning, then the radius of the station could be halved for an otherwise acceptable rate of rotation. Note here that one cannot conclude from the reduced effects of head movements in the rotation chair in the Skylab experiments that there will be no problems from head movements in a rotating space station which produces a sustained artificial gravity. If the magnitude of the sustained artificial gravity were $1.0g$, the adjustment to disturbance produced by head movements could actually be greater in the rotating space station than on the Earth, due to the fact that when individuals stand in the plane of rotation a given head movement relative to the body will elicit a different semicircular canal reaction for every direction the man faces (Guedry, 1965a). In contrast, when an observer stands upright (approximately at right angles to the plane of rotation) on a rotating platform on Earth, a given head tilt relative to the body produces the same semicircular canal stimulus, irrespective of the direction the man faces in the room. Adaptation to this fairly consistent canal and otolith response for each movement executed from an upright position would probably be more readily accomplished than the variable combinations of canal and otolith input for a given head movement when individuals stand or sit "upright" (i.e., when they are in "active" orientations) within the plane of rotation. For this reason, some studies have been carried out with subjects "living" in the plane of rotation and moving about the floor of a slowly rotating room on Earth by means of air bearings. Adjustment to this condition seems to occur at about the same rate as for those studies carried out when individuals spent most of their active hours in upright position (Graybiel *et al.*, 1968; Graybiel, 1969). While such results serve to increase confidence that man can adjust to a rotating space station, they still do not settle the issue because in an Earthbound rotating laboratory the principal resultant linear acceleration vector (gravity and centripetal acceleration) is nearly perpendicular to the plane of rotation. This provides an otolith signal indicating position of the head relative to the plane of rotation immediately before each head movement is made and thus permits automatic "anticipation" of the incoming semicircular canal data that the head movement will produce. Such would not be the case in a rotating space station where the artificial gravity lies in the plane of rotation. There the orientation (heading) relative to the subjective horizontal plane of the platform would not come from otolith cues but would depend on visual cues that could be provided. Hence the issue remains to some degree unresolved. However, considering (1) man's impressive adaptive capacities, (2) the fact that visual cues play an important role in the shaping of vestibuloocular and perceptual responses (see below), and (3) the probable reduced canal/otolith conflict with low-magnitude artificial gravity, the vestibular adjustment problem may not be a limiting condition with selected crew members, especially if the rotation rate were fairly low ($\omega < 5$ rpm or 0.5 rad/sec).

FUNCTIONAL PLASTICITY OF THE VESTIBULAR SYSTEM. Spurred on by these conditions of potential space exploration, investigation of adjustment to rotating environments has uncovered many interesting facts about adaptation to unusual motion inputs. The response changes that occur during such adjustment may be very roughly divided into two categories: (1) responses under control of the somatic nervous system which have to do with the direct motor compensation for the experienced motion and (2) responses under autonomic nervous system control related to cardiovascular, respiratory, and emergency reactions elicited by unexpected changes in states of motion.

Adjustments in Somatic Nervous System Responses. Somatic nervous system responses, e.g., the vestibular nystagmus and illusory motion produced by the cross-coupling effects in rotating rooms, diminish with the repetitive stimulation induced by frequent head movements. The view of the room's interior tends to suppress the vestibular nystagmus set off by cross-coupled stimuli. With sufficient stimulation under conditions of visual suppression of nystagmus induced by head movements, both the vestibular nystagmus and the sensation of motion are reduced even when testing for the presence of these responses is carried out in darkness. Experiments have shown that the habituation of these responses is considerably facilitated by the presence of active visual suppression during the head movements, as compared with carrying out the same habituation schedule in darkness (Guedry, 1964). Because these individuals are living in an unusual force field, the initial somatic nervous system responses are maladaptive in that they degrade stabilization of vision during head movements, and the perceived motion is inappropriate for compensatory motor adjustments to the rotating room. With prolonged exposure to this condition, the plasticity of the nervous system results in a sensory-motor rearrangement which accommodates the individual's responses to the unnatural rotating environment. The rearrangement that takes place is perhaps best illustrated by compensatory responses which occur after 3–10 days of living in a continuously rotating room. Several hours after rotation has stopped, head movements made in darkness produce eye movements not in the plane of head rotation but rather in a plane at right angles to the plane of head rotation (thus in a direction at right angles to the normal response) and in a direction to oppose the nystagmus which had been produced when the individuals were first exposed to the rotating environment. Sensations and postural responses are similarly geometrically rearranged. This geometric rearrangement of response output to vestibular input indicates that the adaptive coupling of the central nervous system canceled out the functionally inappropriate responses which had occurred initially in the rotating environment. For further details concerning these experiments, the reader is referred to other sources (Guedry, 1965a,b,c; Patterson and Graybiel, 1974; Reason and Brand, 1975).

Another example of this kind of sensory-motor rearrangement involves not a rotating room but rather the effects of wearing dove prisms which produce right-left vision reversal. In an interesting series of experiments on this topic, Gonshor (1974) showed that prolonged sinusoidal oscillation in darkness did not produce nystagmus habituation to sinusoidal oscillation when mental arousal was maintained. However, when subjects wore right-left reversing prisms throughout the day and were tested from time to time by 2-min periods of passive sinusoidal oscillation in darkness during mental computation, nystagmus was reduced and became disorganized. After several days, nystagmus began to return, but there were marked changes in phase relations between nystagmus reversal and chair reversal; i.e., the ocular response to vestibular signals was phase shifted to accomplish a functional coordination of the vestibular responses to the optically shifted visual input. Phase shifts during passive oscillation at 0.17 Hz were about 130°, but during active head movements at frequencies of 0.58 Hz, phase shifts of 180° were observed. Thus the normal coordination among visual, vestibular, and proprioceptive inputs was rearranged (temporally shifted) by active voluntary movement while the subjects wore right-left reversing lenses, and evidence of this adaptive rearrangement was obtained from an involuntary response, vestibular nystagmus, recorded during passive angular oscillation in darkness with mentally aroused subjects.[11]

These examples of sensory-motor rearrangement, the one geometric and the other temporal, demonstrate the adaptive capacity of the nervous system and illustrate how central compensation may, in the case of vestibular lesions, especially permanent peripheral lesions, adjust eye movements and sensations during natural movement to those required for functional efficiency.

Changes in Autonomic Nervous System Responses. Many individuals who move about for a period of 30–60 min within an enclosed room rotating at a rate of 5–10 rpm exhibit responses associated with the autonomic nervous system. Pallor

---

[11]Mental arousal by computational tasks is necessary to assure that the nystagmus change has not occurred simply through reduced arousal. Nystagmus diminishes rapidly as subjects begin to relax after only a few repetitions of a semicircular canal stimulus even though the stimulation is carried out in darkness. Mental arousal will reinstate this kind of nystagmus habituation almost to its initial intensity in man (cf. Collins, 1974).

(and/or flushing), sweating, respiratory changes, salivation, and nausea are common. Since individuals without vestibular function do not exhibit these effects (Knoblock, 1965; Fregly and Kennedy, 1965), it appears that the unnatural vestibular stimulation in this environment is the critical factor. Although motion sickness (vomiting) is not exclusively an autonomic nervous system effect of vestibular stimulation (Borison, 1970; Money, 1970), the many autonomic signs that precede vomiting are symptomatic of the final objective somatic nervous sign of motion sickness, viz., emesis. With continued exposure, autonomic signs of motion sickness tend to follow a course similar to the changes in the somatic nervous system responses. For example, after 12 days aboard a room rotating at 10 rpm, subjects had no sensations of motion or nausea and very little measurable nystagmus (even in darkness) from cross-coupling effects when they tilted their heads while the room was still rotating (Guedry and Graybiel, 1962). However, head movements made hours after rotation stopped induced vestibuloocular responses and motion sensations which were inappropriate for the normal stationary environment. Nausea and vomiting occurred in some individuals 5 or 6 hr after rotation had ceased. Thus inefficient somatic and autonomic nervous system responses were suppressed during rotation, and both recurred upon return to a natural environment. When these subjects were again tested after 3 weeks in a normal environment, head movements during rotation produced sensations of motion and nystagmus (in darkness) which approached their initial intensity, but there was no nausea or motion sickness even after 2 hr of active movements within the rotating room (Guedry, 1965b,c). Here it appears that the somatic nervous system responses had returned toward their initial level while the autonomic responses to this unusual motion environment had remained suppressed. Possibly these maladaptive somatic nervous system responses were quickly suppressed after a brief return to active movement within the room, but unfortunately this was not adequately assessed. Thus it may be that the somatic and autonomic responses remained fairly closely associated, but it is also possible that the linkage between these two response systems was altered in the course of the adjustment (cf. Graybiel and Knepton, 1972).

The experiments within rotating rooms, which clearly involved an unnatural motion environment, are to be contrasted with those of Melvill-Jones and Gonshor (1974). The latter involved essentially natural voluntary movements relative to the Earth, while the visual feedback was distorted by right-left reversing lenses. Both conditions produced adaptive changes in the vestibuloocular reflexes, and both produced a substantial amount of motion sickness even though the latter did not involve unnatural vestibular stimuli.

VESTIBULAR SYSTEM AND MOTION SICKNESS

Given sufficient exposure to certain unaccustomed motions, any physiologically sound person can be made motion sick. In addition to nausea and emesis, signs and symptoms of motion sickness include drowsiness, poor motivation for work, mental depression, and a host of physiological effects with clear behavioral implications. Motion sickness has never been found in individuals lacking vestibular function, but among persons with normal function there are pronounced differences in susceptibility to the malady. A thorough review of this complex topic, although appropriate, would be prohibitively long for this chapter. Fortunately, excellent reviews are available by Reason and Brand (1975), Benson (1976), Dobie (1974), Lukomskaya and Nikol'skay (1974), Money (1970), Chinn and Smith (1955), and Tyler and Bard (1949) which include information on incidence in various transportation modes, various stimuli that produce sickness, psychological and physiological correlates of individual differences in susceptibility, and various preventive measures including personnel selection, drugs, and adaptation schedules.

There is no generally accepted model which provides quantitative prediction of the incidence of motion sickness in various conditions of motion. Two contrasting viewpoints are that (1) motion sickness results from discordant inputs among sensory detectors of whole-body motion and (2) motion sickness results from overstimulation of the vestibular system, an idea frequently coupled with attempts to identify that part of the vestibular system, the semicircular canals or the otoliths, responsible for the malady. Despite the general nature of these ideas, they have led to different conclusions about the significance of particular motion parameters in the production of motion sickness. For example, measurement of ship motions indicated that only low peak angular accelerations occur during rolling or pitching motions. This, coupled with the apparent absence of observed nystagmus, led to the conclusion that there was little or no stimulation of the semicircular canals in these provocative motion conditions. Unfortunately, this conclusion was misleading, at least to some proponents of the overstimulation (pick-a-receptor) viewpoint, who further inferred that the semicircular canals are not involved in the genesis of motion sickness in general, and that the malady results from overstimulation of the otolith system, particularly the utricle.[12] The factual basis of this generalization is now clearly questionable. To wit, voluntary head movements and involuntary head bobbing generated by vehicle motions produce semicircular canal stimuli, even though there is little or no angular acceleration in the motion of the vehicle itself; adequate, even strong, semicircular canal stimuli do not necessarily generate nystagmus, e.g., natural head movements through small arcs. Moreover, nystagmus may be suppressed by antisynergistic otolith or visual stimuli when motion stimuli are otherwise sufficient to produce it, and this kind of suppression is believed to be crucial to generating kinetosis in some situations. Thus proponents of conflict theories have been able to point out the likelihood of conflictual inputs from the semicircular canal and otolith systems in these motion conditions. These two viewpoints will be reconsidered briefly in this section.

PERIODIC MOTIONS THAT PRODUCE MOTION SICKNESS

Early laboratory studies of motion sickness were prompted by seasickness. Because ship motions are periodic, many investigators focused on frequencies of

[12]This replaced an earlier idea that the semicircular canals were primarily responsible for motion sickness.

oscillatory stimuli that produce sickness. Additionally, the idea that responding systems (such as the otolith system, stomach, and neuromuscular or cardiovascular system) might have maximal responses in specific frequency ranges increased the appeal of looking for provocative stimulus frequencies.

Studies of effects produced by two-pole swings and vertical linear oscillators indicate that the highest incidence of sickness occurs with oscillation in the frequency range of 0.15–0.33 Hz, and that incidence is directly related to the magnitude of the change in resultant linear acceleration (cf. O'Hanlon and McCauley, 1974; Johnson and Wendt, 1955; Fraser and Manning, 1950; Benson, 1973).[13]

Because the otoliths are stimulated by linear accelerations, it might be suspected that the high sickness index in the 0.15–0.33 Hz range signifies otolith resonance resulting in "overstimulation" of the otolith system. However, this conclusion would be questionable because (1) the otolith system is probably a fast-responding system (Goldberg and Fernandez, 1975) and if so there is no reason to expect resonance within the frequency range studied and (2) results in the swing studies are not really consistent with those of vertical linear oscillation because there are two rises and falls per cycle of swing oscillation. Swing oscillations of 0.25–0.33 Hz represent vertical linear oscillation frequencies of 0.50–0.66 Hz, i.e., above the "provocative range" found in the vertical linear oscillation studies, yet a high incidence of sickness was produced in the swing studies. When subjects' heads were carefully secured in a vertical oscillator, pure vertical oscillation at 0.58 Hz did not produce sickness (Manning, 1943). How, then, can we account for the high incidence of sickness on the two-pole swing at these frequencies?

The answer may well come from the fact that the two-pole swings in these studies introduced sinusoidally varying angular accelerations, peaking at 80–120°/sec^2, at the same frequency as the swing, i.e., in the provocative range, while the resultant linear acceleration remains aligned with the subject's z axis. Strong vertical semicircular canal responses thus elicited would not be matched by commensurate change-in-position signals from the otoliths (see Fig. 10), thereby yielding an intralabyrinthine conflict similar to that which occurs during cross-coupled (Coriolis) stimulation or during cessation of rotation about a tilted axis, or during head movements immediately after prolonged whole-body rotation. Each of these conditions is nauseogenic. The argument is strengthened by the fact that incidence of sickness on a parallel swing, which eliminates semicircular canal stimulation, was only about 50% of that obtained on a two-pole swing (Stewart and Manning, 1943). One is left to speculate on how much semicircular canal stimulation from head movements influenced the results of the vertical linear oscillation studies or studies of shipboard responses in which the head was either not fixed or only positioned against a headrest (cf. Johnson *et al.*, 1951), and then to add

---

[13]Similar dependence on magnitude of g-change and frequency has been reported in four men repeatedly tested by rotation about a tilted axis, a stimulus that also produces periodic otolith stimulation (Miller and Graybiel, 1973). However, results are insufficient to establish a clear trend; other data with this stimulus mode suggest that incidence may increase with frequency up to 0.5 Hz and higher (Benson, 1973; Benson *et al.*, 1975). Even data on vertical oscillation, although more extensive, require some tenuous interpolation to establish curves within 0.1–0.5 Hz range.

FRED E. GUEDRY, JR.,
AND MANNING J.
CORREIA

further speculation as to why different head positions produced very different sickness indices on two-pole swings (Howlett *et al.*, 1943; Manning and Stewart, 1949).

At one time, it was widely believed that the saccule was irrelevant to motion sickness, that the utricle was stimulated by linear accelerations perpendicular to its plane, i.e., by changes in pressure of the otoliths on the underlying sensory hair cells, and was the generator of motion sickness (cf. Howlett and Brett, 1943). Because of this belief, angular accelerations of two-pole swings and those produced by head movements on ships or linear oscillators tended to be neglected. Today "shear" rather than "compression" is considered the effective direction of otolith stimulation, and therefore the saccule can hardly be summarily dismissed. Saccular responses during vertical accelerations are more pronounced than utricular responses (Fernandez *et al.*, 1972). By emphasizing antisynergistic patterns of canal and otolith input as likely contributors to many instances of motion sickness, we may be neglecting other interactions of significance. Walsh (1964) indicated that sensations during vertical linear acceleration were phase advanced by about

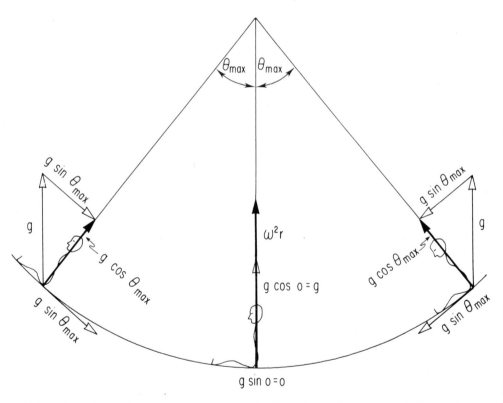

Fig. 10. Linear acceleration components on a two-pole swing. The resultant vector varies in magnitude but its direction remains approximately normal to plane of utricular maculae, presumably yielding little or no change in utricular stimulation (cf. Correia *et al.*, 1968; Fernandez *et al.*, 1972). Note that the constancy of the resultant alignment with the utricle would be altered only slightly due to head-to-seat distance (cf. Cipriani, 1942). At the center of the arc, angular velocity (ω) and centripetal acceleration ($\omega^2 r$) are at maximum magnitude.

90° relative to the stimulus with stimuli of low frequency (in the motion sickness range), whereas sensations were more nearly in phase with the stimulus at higher nonprovocative frequencies. If these sensations reflect saccular inputs, then at 0.25 Hz they would elicit vestibulospinal reflexes (cf. Melvill-Jones *et al.*, 1974) about 1 sec before the muscle and cutaneous receptors would be stimulated directly by the force change, e.g., by the peak *g* at the trough of a wave. However, the direct physical force on the muscles, joints, and cutaneous receptors would elicit ascending spinal messages to the vestibular nuclei, cerebellum, and reticular formation (cf. Pompeiano, 1975; Wilson, 1975) before the direct vestibular inputs to the same centers. Because each of these neuroanatomical sites has been identified as necessary for motion sickness, speculations (cf. Fukuda, 1976) about neuro-muscular/vestibular mismatches deserve serious consideration in the continuing effort to understand a variety of findings such as the influence of head position on swing sickness (Howlett *et al.*, 1943; Manning and Stewart, 1949), the influence of pilot training on simulator sickness, etc.

Nonperiodic Motions That Produce Motion Sickness

While some periodic motions, simple and complex, can cause a high incidence of motion sickness, many motions of no apparent periodicity can also cause sickness. A few random head movements during whole-body rotation or in hyper- or hypo-*g* fields produce nausea and sickness in some individuals. Particular maneuvers in acrobatic flight are identified by some individuals as a provocative condition, even though there is no obvious periodicity in the sequence of the maneuvers. Some of the conditions of visual stimulation which cause or exacerbate motion sickness have not involved visual or body motion stimuli with any particular periodicity. From observations such as these, it would appear that searches for "the provocative stimulus frequency" are based on an oversimplified concept of motion sickness. From the conflict point of view, periodic motions which generate motion sickness do so because the periodicity of the motion sets up phase mismatches between different sensory detectors of motion. Provocative motions without any particular periodicity usually involve immediately conflictual sensory inputs; i.e., the presence of conflict does not depend on the periodicity of the stimulus. It is, of course, not unlikely that such stimuli would produce a higher incidence of sickness if delivered at some particular frequency, but curiously this has not been studied systematically. In addition to frequency dependence of interactions among sensory transducers, it is possible that the less specific, more systemic reaction to motion is frequency dependent. In this connection, an empirical model predictive of incidence from stimulus frequency and magnitude (McCauley *et al.*, 1976) appears specific to vertical linear oscillation, the stimulus from which it was derived, but more generality may obtain if the imputed frequency dependence should be generated at least partially by dynamics of the emetic process.

Nonperiodic motions that produce sickness may be sufficiently spaced so that only relatively susceptible individuals become sick. Some such motions may also be inherently escapable, and therefore subject to voluntary control. For example,

FRED E. GUEDRY, JR.,
AND MANNING J.
CORREIA

sickness can be escaped in a rotating room or space laboratory if head movements are made very infrequently; individuals may program their exposure to the disturbing condition so that their adaptive mechanisms keep pace with their levels of exposure. Individuals exposed to disturbing visual-vestibular interactions can escape by closing their eyes and limiting provocative stimulation to within their tolerance levels. Other motions, however, afford minimal escape or ameliorative options. The complex multi-degree-of-freedom periodic motions experienced in life rafts in rough seas may exceed an individual's immediate adaptive potential, and they may not abate to a degree which would permit development of adaptive coupling capable of overcoming the malady. These various forms of provocative stimuli constitute different kinds of adjustment problems which remain a challenging practical problem.

SUMMARIZING COMMENTS ON MOTION SICKNESS

The review of motion sickness is complicated by various criteria of motion sickness, subject populations, provocative stimuli, and "psychological" sets and tasks of subjects involved in different studies. It is clear that the vestibular overstimulation theory alone is adequate to account for many instances of motion sickness. Motions which ordinarily do not induce sickness can be highly provocative when visual inputs are distorted. On the other hand, the effects of some motions which do provoke a fairly high incidence of motion sickness may be ameliorated by a wide-field view of a stable visual reference (Guedry, 1977; Reason and Diaz, 1973; Brandt *et al.*, 1971). Some forms of repetitive and prolonged vestibular "overstimulation" produce little or no motion sickness. Individuals who have become adapted to some unusual forms of motion, such as rotating rooms or ship motion, sometimes experience motion sickness upon returning to natural environment. Here, natural movement in a natural environment causes nausea and occasional emesis. These and other similar findings must be accounted for by any theory of motion sickness, and some version of the "conflict hypothesis" seems a more viable alternative than any single "vestibular overstimulation theory."

Several neuroanatomical sites associated with motion sickness are (1) the vestibular apparatus (motion sickness does not occur without it) and probably the vestibular nuclei (cf. Money, 1970); (2) the vestibular parts of the cerebellum; (3) a chemoreceptor emetic trigger zone in the superficial region of the floor of the fourth ventrical, which acts as a chemical transducer for agents in the bloodstream and cerebrospinal fluid and sets off vomiting (cf. Money, 1970); (4) a vomiting center deep in the bulbar reticular formation (Borison, 1970), which is necessary for vomiting and hence for the vomiting of motion sickness; (5) the cerebrum and cerebral cortex, which, although they have not been identified as necessary to the occurrence of motion sickness (Bard *et al.*, 1947), may have suppressive or facilitative influences on motion sickness (Reason and Brand, 1975; Money, 1970, p. 20); (6) the visual system, which is necessary for motion sickness induced by large-field moving scenes (Crampton and Young, 1953; Kottenhoff and Lindahl,

1958, 1960) with the body stationary and for the increases and decreases in incidence of motion sickness that occur when different visual stimuli are used during particular body motions. Since large moving visual fields modulate activity in the vestibular nuclei (Dichgans *et al.,* 1973; Henn *et al.,* 1974), visually induced motion sickness may involve mechanisms in common with those involved in motion sickness induced by body motion, although some authors have considered visually induced sickness as a separate entity.

While some previously held ideas are no longer accepted today, it is likely that their clear exposition served well in the orderly examination of ideas and in stimulating the amassing of data available for consideration today. With the admonition that our speculations may share a fate like some of those of the past, we offer the following generalizations concerning motion sickness and the stimuli that produce it.

1. Stimuli that produce motion sickness seem to fall in the following categories:

    a.   Motions that simultaneously produce sensory stimuli to the semicircular canals and otoliths which would, if they occurred separately, elicit somatic nervous system compensatory reactions of different planes or directions are productive of motion sickness.

    b.   Large moving visual fields that tend to set off compensatory reactions of planes or directions differing from reactions to coacting dynamic vestibular stimuli are productive of motion sickness.

    c.   Visual or vestibular signals indicating a state of motion differing from motion expected as a result of voluntary control actions tend to produce motion sickness.

    d.   Vestibular stimuli that superimpose reflexive saccades on saccadic eye movements involved in visual data acquisition from complex visual displays are productive of motion sickness (cf. Benson *et al.,* 1976). Activity in the cerebellar vermis precedes eye movements and apparently controls amplitude of voluntary saccadic movements (Wolfe, 1971). When the saccades of vestibular nystagmus conflict with voluntary saccades during inspection of a complex visual display, the incidence of motion sickness is substantially increased.

    e.   Oscillatory stimuli that induce any of the above conditions or that induce periodic mismatches between vestibulospinal reactions and *g*-load changes are productive of motion sickness, especially in the frequency range 0.1–0.4 Hz.

2. Neural centers responsible for the automatization of neuromuscular compensatory reactions to states of motion are important in motion sickness. Changes in states of whole-body motion, whether actively or passively induced, are detected by the vestibular system as part of a servosystem involved in the control of motion. The chain of reflexive actions set off by coacting vestibular, visual, and proprioceptive motion stimuli serves in an automatic manner to adjust the organism to the state of motion. When these servoactions are inadequate to compensate

FRED E. GUEDRY, JR.,
AND MANNING J.
CORREIA

for states of unnatural motion, arousal reactions involving both the autonomic and somatic nervous systems are set off which commit more, or in some cases substantially less, energy to the overall reaction. The signs and symptoms of motion sickness are by-products of inadequate servocompensatory actions, and they are signs of the process of adjustment to motion.

3. Adjustment to unnatural motions occurs as servocompensatory actions are modified. Neural centers responsible for automatization of skilled movement are important in this adjustment and in motion sickness. These include the extrapyramidal centers in the brain stem and the vestibular centers of the cerebellum. The flocculonodular lobe of the cerebellum is an important site of interactions of inputs from the semicircular canals, otoliths, and visual systems (Ito *et al.*, 1974: Miles and Fuller, 1975; Lisberger and Fuchs, 1974; Takemori and Cohen, 1974). The vestibular part of the cerebellum is also important to motion sickness (Money, 1970). Voluntary movements become skilled in the natural world as dependence on feedback from the external world is replaced by a miniaturized, programmed, fast feedback loop in the neocerebellum (cf. Ito, 1970). Skilled motion sequences can be executed when the cerebellum is intact in the absence of proprioceptor feedback from the body (Llinas, 1975). With prolonged exposure to unfamiliar motions, learning occurs in which original cerebellar bypass loops associated with voluntary movements are replaced by rearranged loops. As voluntary movement continues to occur in the unnatural environment, cerebellar loops are altered to correspond with the new feedback, and arousal levels thereby return toward normality and motion sickness is reduced. The "repair" mechanism may be the same as the central nervous system recoding that serves to normalize reactions when pathological conditions create disordered sensory inputs.

Return to a natural environment reinstates motion sickness because cerebellar fast feedback loops no longer correspond with the sensory feedback from motion in the natural environment. This would also account for the enhanced simulator sickness of the experienced pilot as compared with the novice (cf. Reason and Brand, 1975, p. 112).

In many respects the ideas just outlined are similar to the "sensory-rearrangement" motion sickness theory of Reason (1974). When an individual's perceptual and neuromuscular reactions are inappropriate for his state of motion, the central nervous system must either disregard part of the input or develop new sensory-motor patterns appropriate to the situation. Vomiting is one of several apparently nonfunctional reactions that occur in the course of adjustment. The nonfunctional autonomic aspects of the reaction tend to be reduced as the more specific somatic nervous system reactions are modified to fit the state of motion, but a close correlation has not always been demonstrated. The two sets of reactions may follow separate rates of adjustment and recovery. Immediate autonomic reactions, as well as adjustment rates, may differ markedly in individuals with very similar initial somatic nervous system reactions. The coupling between the direct sensory-motor adjustments and the less direct autonomic and general systemic reaction is subject to idiosyncratic factors that remain a challenging problem (cf. Graybiel, 1969; Reason and Brand, 1975).

Pervasive neurobiological relations with other sensory-motor systems characterize the vestibular system which responds to tilt and to changes in states of motion of the head relative to the Earth. When moved passively in early life, the ontogenetically primordial vestibular system activates developing motor and sensory processes which in later life function as an integrated automatized whole involved in the control of motion. As active voluntary movement develops, reflexes elicited by this system serve to stabilize the eyes, head, and body relative to the Earth. Thus the complexity of the neurobiological interrelations outlined in Chapter 9 is a salient characteristic of this system which operates reflexively through several motor systems that can be activated by other sensory systems and that are also under voluntary control. Typically, the vestibular system is stimulated by motion that has been initiated to orient another sensory system such as the eyes, ears, or nose toward something in the environment; i.e., it often functions as a silent partner in acts involving attention to other sensory inputs. An interesting possible developmental function relates to the fact that the information it provides is integral to the interpretation of changes in other sensory inputs resulting from head movement, and thus it may be instrumental in the development of concepts of spatial relations and of perceptual constancy.

Principal neural pathways from the endorgans course to four vestibular nuclei in the floor of the fourth ventricle, a part of the brain stem which lies just under the cerebellum, and an offshoot goes directly to the cerebellum. In the nuclei, pathways lead to and from the oculomotor nuclei, the cerebellum, and spinal tracts. These pathways influence motor responses and participate reflexively in the control of motion. The semicircular canals project to all four nuclei, but their oculomotor influence arises primarily from the superior vestibular nucleus and the rostral medial nucleus. Utricular and saccular pathways project prominently to parts of the lateral, descending, and medial nuclei which influence muscle tone and spinal reflex activity and provide lesser projections to the superior nucleus. It is clear that the reticular activating system is influenced by and influences the vestibular system and that autonomic responses are influenced through complex pathways by vestibular stimulation. Efferent tracts appear capable of adjusting peripheral vestibular inflow, and it is likely that reticular, cerebellar, and cortical mechanisms influence the adaptive coupling between spinal, vestibular, and visual inputs to influence gain, timing, and direction of perceptual motor responses relative to the magnitude, timing, and direction of stimuli generated by frequently encountered states of motion of the head and body.

The dynamic response of the semicircular canals to angular acceleration, predicted from the classical "torsion pendulum" analogy, has been related to functional responses (primarily oculomotor) over a frequency range encountered in natural movement and also to nonfunctional responses produced by unusual motion conditions. Responses of the otolith receptors, assumed to operate like density-difference linear accelerometers, can be predicted, but with less confidence because of doubts concerning the dynamic response of the receptor itself or

FRED E. GUEDRY, JR., AND MANNING J. CORREIA

of readily measured "output" responses which reflect its dynamics. Nevertheless, it is generally agreed that several systems (the semicircular canal, otolith, visual, and proprioceptor systems) operate in close coordination to influence control of motion and dynamic spatial orientation. This is relevant to recent interest in the developmental implications of early vestibular stimulation as well as to many activities in adult life. Dynamic vestibular and visual stimuli produced by whole-body movement can have profound effects on performance. The normal vestibu-loocular reflex can provide a substantial improvement in vision for Earth-fixed targets during natural whole-body movements involving high-frequency head oscillation, and individuals without it are handicapped in ways not commonly appreciated. However, during high-frequency head oscillation, this same reflex can degrade visual acuity for head-fixed targets. It can, for example, interfere with an aviator's visual scan of his flight instruments. Some unusual vestibular stimuli are also conducive to pilot disorientation. Here another form of visual-vestibular interaction is often involved; viz., visual information can either exacerbate or counteract pilot disorientation. Fortunately, clear visual reference to the Earth is usually sufficient to overcome disorientation.

Either unusual motion conditions or pathological processes can alter the highly coordinated information from the semicircular canals, otoliths, eyes, and proprioceptive systems that usually accompanies motion. These altered input patterns may be conflictual in that inputs from different sensory receptors call for responses that are mutually incompatible in timing, direction, or magnitude, and they constitute threats to the control of motion and hence to survival. Changes in states of motion also require respiratory and cardiovascular adjustments, and so it should not be surprising that sensory inputs that signal unusual states of motion may elicit strong autonomic responses. One of the more interesting results of vestibular experimentation is the elucidation of the adaptive changes in responses that occur when an unusual pattern of motion stimuli is frequently repeated. Repetitive stimulation that would elicit maladaptive responses eventually yields changes in sensory-motor and autonomic responses. Some of these changes indicate a simple reduction in response arousal, but others indicate a recoding in the nervous system such that a given motion input yields a different response output adjusted in plane, direction, and timing to the new motion condition. These changes in the input–output adaptive coupling probably reflect the presence of repair mechanisms that are available to compensate for pathological processes which also can alter the patterning of sensory-motor input/output relations. While such mechanisms clearly serve useful biological functions, their presence in slowly developing disease processes complicates the clinical evaluations of responses; i.e., the adaptation mechanisms suppress the symptoms that would otherwise reveal the disease state. However, by the same token, elucidation of mechanisms of habituation of vestibular responses in relation to systematically altered input patterns can serve to elucidate principles that may also apply to clinical diagnosis.

Before habituation or adjustment occurs, unusual motion conditions sustained for more than a few minutes can induce a high degree of disturbance. In addition to pathological states, some of the conditions that may elicit disorientation, inappropriate sensory-motion reactions, and motion sickness are ship motion, deep-sea diving, aviation, space flights, and devices such as flight simulators. This chapter has considered each of these problem areas, placing greatest emphasis on vestibular function in aviation and in space operations. Because motion sickness has been encountered in each of these situations, a separate section of this chapter is devoted to this subject. Tremendous individual differences in the ability to adjust to unusual motions are not well understood and remain a challenging neurobiological problem. Motion sickness, when it occurs, is regarded herein as one of several signs of an ongoing, but as yet inadequate, adjustment to a sustained unnatural motion.

Acknowledgments

The authors gratefully acknowledge the helpful suggestions of distinguished colleagues, Dr. Alan J. Benson, RAF Institute of Aviation Medicine, and Dr. Brant Clark, San Jose State College, in the preparation of this chapter.

REFERENCES

Atkin, A., and Bender, M. C. Ocular stabilization during oscillatory head movements. *Arch. Neurol.,* 1968, *19,* 559–566.

Baloh, R. W., Konrad, H. R., and Honrubia, V. Vestibulo-ocular function in patients with cerebellar atrophy. *Neurology,* 1975, *25,* 160–168.

Bard, P., Woolsey, C. N., Snider, R. S., Mountcastle, V. B., and Bromiley, R. B. The limitation of central nervous mechanisms involved in motion sickness. *Fed. Proc.,* 1947, *6,* 72.

Barnes, G. R., Benson, A. J., and Prior, A. R. J. Visual suppression of inappropriate eye movements induced by vestibular stimulation. *Aviat. Space Environ. Med.,* 1978, *49* (4), 557–564.

Barr, C. C., Schultheis, L. W., and Robinson, D. A. Voluntary, non-visual control of the human vestibulo-ocular reflex. *Acta Otolaryngol. (Stockholm),* 1976, *81,* 365–375.

Barrett, G. V., and Thornton, C. L. Relationship between perceptual style and simulator sickness. *J. Appl. Psychol.,* 1968, *52,* 304–308.

Bauermeister, M. Effect of body tilt on apparent verticality, apparent body position, and their relation. *J. Exp. Psychol.,* 1964, *67,* 142–147.

Benson, A. J. Spatial disorientation in flight. In J. A. Gillies (ed.), *A Textbook of Aviation Physiology.* Pergamon, New York, 1965.

Benson, A. J. Interactions between semicircular canals and gravireceptors. In *Recent Advances in Aerospace Medicine: Proceedings of the 18th International Congress of Aviation and Space Medicine, Amsterdam, 1969.* D. Reidel, Dordrecht-Holland, 1970, pp. 250–261.

Benson, A. J. Effect of angular oscillation in yaw on vision. *Proc. Aerospace Med. Assoc. Sci. Meet.,* 1972, pp. 43–44.

Benson, A. J. *Physical Characteristics of Stimuli Which Induce Motion Sickness: A Review.* IAM Rept. 532. RAF IAM, Farnborough, England, 1973.

Benson, A. J. Modification of the response to angular accelerations by linear accelerations. In H. H. Kornhuber (ed.), *Handbook of Sensory Physiology,* Vol. V1/2: *Vestibular System,* Part 2. Springer-Verlag, New York, 1974.

Benson, A. J. Motion sickness. In *RAF Textbook of Aviation Medicine.* RAF IAM, Farnborough, England, 1976.

Benson, A. J., and Barnes, G. R. Vision during angular oscillation: The dynamic interaction of visual and vestibular mechanisms. *Aviat. Space Environ. Med.,* 1978, *49*(2), 340–345.

Benson, A. J., and Burchard, E. Spatial disorientation in flight. In *A Handbook for Aircrew.* AGARDograph AG-170. Technical Editing and Reproduction, Ltd., London, 1973.

Benson, A. J., and Cline, G. Personal communication, 1975.

Benson, A. J., and Guedry, F. E. Comparison of tracking task performance and nystagmus during sinusoidal oscillation in yaw and pitch. *Aerospace Med.,* 1971, *42*, 593–601.

Benson, A. J., Diaz, E., and Farrugia, P. The perception of body orientation relative to a rotating linear acceleration vector. In H. Schöne (ed.), *Mechanisms of Spatial Perception and Orientation as Related to Gravity.* Gustav Fisher-Verlag, Stuttgart, 1975.

Benson, A. J., Guedry, F. E., and Moore, H. J. Influence of a visual display and frequency of angular oscillation on incidence of motion sickness. In preparation, 1978.

Bergstrom, B. Morphology of the vestibular nerve. III. Analysis of the calibers of the myelinated vestibular nerve fibers in man at various ages. *Acta Otolaryngol. (Stockholm),* 1973, *76*, 331–338.

Berry, C. A., and Homick, J. L. Findings on American astronauts bearing on the issue of artificial gravity for future manned space vehicles. *Aerospace Med.,* 1973, *44*, 163–168.

Billingham, J. Russian experience of problems in vestibular physiology related to the space environment. In *Second Symposium on "The Role of the Vestibular Organs in Space Exploration."* NASA SP-115. U.S. Government Printing Office, Washington, D.C., 1966.

Bisti, S., Maffei, L., and Piccotino, M. Visuovestibular interactions in the cat superior colliculus. *J. Neurophysiol.,* 1974, *37*, 146–155.

Borison, H. L. Résumé of sessions on motion sickness. In *Fourth Symposium on "The Role of the Vestibular Organs in Space Exploration."* NASA SP-187. U.S. Government Printing Office, Washington, D.C., 1970.

Brandt, Th., Wist, E., and Dichgans, J. Optisch induzierte Pseudocoriolis-Effekte und Circularvektion. *Arch. Psychiat. Nervenkr.,* 1971, *214*, 365–389.

Brandt, Th., Dichgans, J., and Koenig, E. Differential effects of central versus peripheral vision on egocentric and exocentric motion perception. *Exp. Brain Res.,* 1973, *16*, 476–491.

Brictson, C. A. *Evaluation of the Special Senses for Flying Duties: Perceptual Abilities of Landing Signal Officers (LSO'S).* AGARD CP-152. Technical Editing and Reproduction, Ltd., London, 1975.

Brodal, A. *Neurological Anatomy in Relation to Clinical Medicine.* Oxford University Press, New York, 1969.

Bruner, A., and Norris, T. W. Age related changes in caloric nystagmus. *Acta Otolaryngol. (Stockholm),* 1971, Suppl. 282.

Chinn, H. I., and Smith, P. K. Motion sickness. *Pharmacol. Rev.,* 1955, *7*, 33–82.

Cipriani, A. An analysis of the forces encountered on the simple swing used in the study of motion sickness. In *Proceedings of the Committee on Seasickness.* National Research Council of Canada Rept. No. C2246, Appendix C, 1942.

Clark, B. Pilot reports of disorientation across fourteen years of flight. *Aerospace Med.,* 1971, *42*, 708–712.

Clark, B., and Stewart, J. D. Attitude and Coriolis motion in a flight simulator. *Aerospace Med.,* 1967, *38*, 936–940.

Clark, B., and Stewart, J. D. Effects of angular acceleration on man, thresholds for the perception of rotation, and the oculogyral illusion. *Aerospace Med.,* 1969, *40*, 952–956.

Clark, B., Randall, R., and Stewart, J. D. Vestibulo-ocular reflex in man. *Aviat. Space Environ. Med.,* 1975, *46*, 1336–1339.

Cohen, B., Takemori, S., and Uemura, T. Visual-vestibular interaction: The role of the labyrinth in the production of optokinetic nystagmus and optokinetic afternystagmus. In *The Use of Nystagmography in Aviation Medicine.* AGARD CP-128. Technical Editing and Reproduction, Ltd., London, 1973.

Cohen, E. Simulation of aircraft motion. Presented at Annual Meeting of the Human Factors Society, Chicago, 1968.

Cohen, M. M., Crosbie, R. J., and Blackburn, L. H. Disorienting effects of aircraft catapult launches. In *The Disorientation Incident.* AGARD CP-95, Part 1. Technical Editing and Reproduction, Ltd., London., 1972.

Collar, A. R. *On an Aspect of the Accident History of Aircraft Taking off at Night.* Aeronautical Res. Council Repts. and Memoranda No. 2277. HMSO, London, August 1946.

Collins, W. E. Vestibular responses from figure skaters. *Aerospace Med.,* 1966, *37*, 1098–1104.

Collins, W. E. Coriolis vestibular stimulation and visual surrounds. *Aerospace Med.,* 1968, *39*, 125–138.

Collins, W. E. Arousal and vestibular habituation. In H. H. Kornhuber (ed.), *Handbook of Sensory Physiology,* Vol. VI. Springer-Verlag, New York, 1974.

Correia, M. J., and Guedry, F. E. *Influence of Labyrinth Orientation Relative to Gravity on Responses Elicited by Stimulation of the Horizontal Semicircular Canals.* NSAM-905, Rept. No. 100. Naval School of Aviation Medicine, Pensacola, Fla., 1964.

Correia, M. J., and Guedry, F. E. Modification of vestibular responses as a function of rate of rotation about an Earth-horizontal axis. *Acta Otolaryngol. (Stockholm),* 1966, *62*, 297–308.

Correia, M. J., Hixson, W. C., and Niven, J. I. On predictive equations for subjective judgments of vertical and horizon in a force field. *Acta Otolaryngol. (Stockholm),* 1968, Suppl. 230, pp. 1–20.

Correia, M. J., Nelson, J. B., and Guedry, F. E. Antisomatogyral illusion. *Aviat. Space Environ. Med.,* 1977, *48*, 859–862.

Corvera, J., Torres-Courtney, G., and Lopez-Rios, G. The neurotological significance of alterations of pursuit eye movements in the pendular eye tracking test. *Ann. Otol.,* 1973, *82*, 855–867.

Crampton, G. H., and Young, F. A. The differential effect of a rotary visual field on susceptibles and non-susceptibles to motion sickness. *J. Comp. Physiol. Psychol.,* 1953, *46*, 451–453.

Dichgans, J., and Brandt, Th. The visual–vestibular interaction and motion perception. *Bibl. Ophthalmol.,* 1972, *82*, 327–338.

Dichgans, J., and Brandt, Th. The psychophysics of visual induced perception of self-motion and tilt. In I. O. Schmidt and F. G. Worden (eds.), *The Neurosciences.* MIT Press, Cambridge, Mass., 1973.

Dichgans, J., Held, R., Young, L. R., and Brandt, Th. Moving visual scenes influence the apparent direction of gravity. *Science (New York),* 1972, *178*, 1217–1219.

Dichgans, J., Schmidt, C. L., and Graf, W. Visual input improves the speedometer function of the vestibular nuclei in goldfish. *Exp. Brain Res.,* 1973, *18*, 319–322.

Dichgans, J., Bizzi, E., Morasso, T., and Tagliasco, V. The role of vestibular and neck afferents during eye–head coordination in the monkey. *Brain Res.,* 1974, *72*, 225–232.

Dobie, T. G. *Airsickness in Aircrew.* AGARDograph AG-177. Technical Editing and Reproduction, Ltd., London, 1974.

Dowd, P. J., Moore, E. W., and Cramer, R. L. Effects of flying experience on the vestibular system: A comparison between pilots and non-pilots to Coriolis stimulation. *Aerospace Med.,* 1966, *37*, 45–47.

Edmonds, C. Vertigo in diving. In *The Use of Nystagmography in Aviation Medicine.* AGARD CP-128. Technical Editing and Reproduction, Ltd., London, 1973.

Fernandez, C., and Goldberg, J. Physiology of peripheral neurons innervating otolith organs of the squirrel monkey. *J. Neurophysiol.,* 1976, *39*, 970–1008.

Fernandez, C., Goldberg, J., and Abend, W. Response to static tilt of peripheral neurons innervating otolith organs of the squirrel monkey. *J. Neurophysiol.,* 1972, *35*, 978–997.

Frank, J., and Levinson, H. Dysmetric dyslexia and dyspraxia: Hypothesis and study. *J. Am. Acad. Child Psychiat.,* 1973, *12*, 690–701.

Fraser, A. M., and Manning, G. W. Effect of variation in swing radius and arc on incidence of swing sickness. *J. Appl. Physiol.,* 1950, *2*, 580–584.

Fregly, A. R., and Kennedy, R. S. Comparative effects of prolonged rotation at 10 rpm on postural equilibrium in vestibular normal and vestibular defective human subjects. *Aerospace Med.,* 1965, *36*, 1160–1167.

Fukuda, T. Postural behavior and motion sickness. *Acta Otolaryngol. (Stockholm),* 1976, *81*, 237–241.

Galebsky, A. Vestibular nystagmus in newborn infants. *Acta Otolaryngol. (Stockholm),* 1928, *11*, 409–423.

Gazenko, O. *Medical Studies on the Cosmic Spacecrafts "Vostok" and "Voskhod."* NASA TTF-9207. National Aeronautics and Space Administration, Washington, D.C., 1964.

Gillingham, K. K., and Krutz, R. W. *Effects of the Abnormal Acceleratory Environment of Flight.* SAM TR-74-57. USAF School of Aerospace Medicine, Brooks AFB, Tex., 1974.

Gilson, R. D. Lighting factors affecting the visibility of a moving display. *Percept. Psychophys.,* 1971, *10*, 400–402.

Gilson, R. D., Stockwell, C. W., and Guedry, F. E. Nystagmus responses during triangular waveforms of angular velocity about the *y*- and *z*-axes. *Acta Otolaryngol. (Stockholm),* 1973a, *75*, 21–26.

Gilson, R. D., Guedry, F. E., Hixson, W. C., and Niven, J. I. Observations on perceived changes in aircraft attitude attending head movements made in a 2-*g* bank and turn. *Aerospace Med.,* 1973b, *44*, 90–92.

Goldberg, J., and Fernandez, C. Vestibular mechanisms. *Ann. Rev. Physiol.,* 1975, *37*, 129–162.

Gonshor, A. An investigation of plasticity in the human vestibulo-ocular reflex arc. Doctoral dissertation, Department of Physiology, McGill University, Canada, September 1974.

Gottlieb, G. Conceptions of prenatal development: Behavioral embryology. *Psychol. Rev.,* 1976, *83*(3), 215–234.

Graybiel, A. Oculogravic illusion. *AMA Arch. Ophthalmol.*, 1952, *48*, 605–615.

Graybiel, A. Structural elements in the concept of motion sickness. *Aerospace Med.*, 1969, *40*, 351–367.

Graybiel, A., and Clark, B. Perception of the horizontal or vertical with the head upright, on the side, and inverted under static conditions, and during exposure to centripetal force. *Aerospace Med.*, 1962, *33*, 147–155.

Graybiel, A., and Clark, B. The validity of the oculogravic illusion as a specific indicator of otolith function. *Aerospace Med.*, 1965, *36*, 1173–1181.

Graybiel, A., and Hupp, D. I. The oculogyral illusion. *J. Aviat. Med.*, 1946, *3*, 1–12.

Graybiel, A., and Kellogg, R. S. The inversion illusion in parabolic flight: Its probable dependence on otolith function. *Aerospace Med.*, 1967, *38*, 1099–1102.

Graybiel, A., and Knepton, J. Direction-specific adaptation effects acquired in a slow rotation room. *Aerospace Med.*, 1972, *43*, 1179–1189.

Graybiel, A., Thompson, A. B., Deane, F. R., Fregly, A. R., Colehour, J. K., and Ricks, E. L. Transfer of habituation of motion sickness on change in body position between vertical and horizontal in a rotating environment. *Aerospace Med.*, 1968, *39*, 950–962.

Graybiel, A., Miller, E. F., and Homick, J. L. Experiment M-131 human vestibular function. In *Proceedings of Skylab Life Sciences Symposium.* NASA Technical Memorandum JSC-09275, "Susceptibility to Motion Sickness," November 1974.

Greenough, W. T. The nature and nurture of behavior—Development psychobiology. In *Readings from Scientific American.* Freeman, San Francisco, 1972.

Gresty, M., and Benson, A. J. Movement of the head in pitch during whole-body activity. Personal communication, 1976.

Groen, J. J. Central regulation of the vestibular system. *Acta Otolaryngol. (Stockholm)*, 1965, *59*, 211–218.

Grüsser, O.-J., and Grüsser-Kornehls, U. Interaction of vestibular and visual inputs in the visual system. *Progr. Brain Res.*, 1972, *37*, 573–583.

Guedry, F. E. Visual control of habituation to complex vestibular stimulation in man. *Acta Otolaryngol. (Stockholm)*, 1964, *58*, 377–389.

Guedry, F. E. Comparison of vestibular effects in several rotating environments. In *The Role of the Vestibular Organs in the Exploration in Space.* NASA SP-77. U.S. Government Printing Office, Washington, D.C., 1965*a*.

Guedry, F. E. Habituation to complex vestibular stimulation in man: Transfer and retention of effects from twelve days of rotation at 10 rpm. *Percept. Mot. Skills*, 1965*b*, *21*, 459–481, Monogr. Suppl. 1-V21.

Guedry, F. E. Psychophysiological studies of vestibular function. In W. D. Neff (ed.), *Contributions to Sensory Physiology.* Academic Press, New York, 1965*c*.

Guedry, F. E. *The Theory of Development of Reactions to Whole-Body Motion Considered in Relation to Selection, Assignment, and Training of Flight Personnel.* AGARD CP-95, Part I. Technical Editing and Reproduction, Ltd., London, 1972.

Guedry, F. E. Psychophysics of vestibular sensation. In H. H. Kornhuber (ed.), *Handbook of Sensory Physiology*, Vol. VI. Springer-Verlag, New York, 1974.

Guedry, F. E. *Visual Counteraction of Nauseogenic and Disorienting Effects of Some Whole-Body Motions—A Proposed Mechanism.* NAMRL-1232. Naval Aerospace Medical Research Laboratory, Pensacola, Fla., 1977. *Aviat. Space Environ. Med.*, 1978, *49* (1), 36–41.

Guedry, F. E., and Ambler, R. K. Assessment of reactions to vestibular disorientation stress for purposes of aircrew selection. In *Predictability of Motion Sickness in the Selection of Pilots.* AGARD CP-109. Technical Editing and Reproduction, Ltd., London, 1973.

Guédry, F. E., and Benson, A. J. Coriolis cross-coupling effects: Disorienting and nauseogenic or not? NAMRL-1231. Naval Aerospace Medical Research Laboratory, Pensacola, Fla., 1976. *Aviat. Space Environ. Med.*, 1978, *49*, 29–35.

Guedry, F. E., and Graybiel, A. Compensatory nystagmus conditioned during adaptation to living in a rotating room. *J. Appl. Physiol.*, 1962, *17*, 398–404.

Guedry, F. E., and Harris, C. W. *Labyrinthine Functions Related to Experiments on the Parallel Swing.* NSAM-874, Rept. No. 86. Naval School of Aviation Medicine, Pensacola, Fla., 1963.

Guedry, F. E., and Montague, E. K. Quantitative evaluation of the vestibular Coriolis reaction. *Aerospace Med.*, 1961, *32*, 487–500.

Guedry, F. E., Collins, W. E., and Graybiel, A. Vestibular habituation during repetitive complex stimulation: A study of transfer effects. *J. Appl. Physiol.*, 1964, *19*, 1005–1015.

Guedry, F. E., Stockwell, C. W., and Gilson, R. D. Comparison of subjective responses to semicircular canal stimulation produced by rotation about different axes. *Acta Otolaryngol. (Stockholm)*, 1971, *72*, 101–106.

Guedry, F. E., Gilson, R. D., Schroeder, D. J., and Collins, W. E. Some effects of alcohol on various aspects of oculomotor control. *Aviat. Space Environ. Med.*, 1975, *46*, 1008–1013.

Guedry, F. E., Mortensen, C. E., Nelson, J. B., and Correia, M. J. A comparison of nystagmus and turning sensations generated by active and passive turning. Presented at Extraordinary Meeting of the Bárány Society, London, September 1977.

Guignard, J. C. Vibration. In J. A. Gillies (ed.), *A Textbook of Aviation Physiology*, Chap. 29. Pergamon, Oxford, 1965.

Hallpike, C. W., Harrison, M. S., and Slater, E. Abnormalities of the caloric test results in certain varieties of mental disorders. *Acta Otolaryngol. (Stockholm)*, 1951, *39*, 151–160.

Haring, R. D., and Simmons, F. B. Cerebellar defects detectable by electronystagmography calibration. *Arch. Otolaryngol.*, 1973, *98*, 14–17.

Held, R., Dichgans, J., and Bauer, J. Characteristics of moving visual scenes influencing spatial orientation. *Vision Res.*, 1975, *15*, 357–365.

Henn, V., Young, L. R., and Finley, C. Vestibular nucleus units in alert monkeys are also influenced by moving visual fields. *Brain Res.*, 1974, *71*, 144–149.

Henriksson, N. G., Pfaltz, C., Torok, N., and Rubin, W. *A Synopsis of the Vestibular System: An Effort to Standardize Vestibular Conceptions, Tests, and Their Evaluation.* Gasser & Cie, Basel, 1972.

Hixson, W. C., and Spezia, E. *Major Orientation Error Accidents in Regular Army UH-1 Aircraft during Fiscal Year 1971: Accident Factors.* NAMRL-1219 USAARL 76-1. Naval Aerospace Medical Research Laboratory, Pensacola, Fla., 1975.

Holzman, P. S., Proctor, L. R., and Hughes, D. W. Eye tracking patterns in schizophrenia. *Science,* 1973, *181*, 179–181.

Horn, G., and Hill, R. M. Modifications of receptive fields of cells in the visual cortex occurring spontaneously and associated with bodily tilt. *Nature,* 1969, *221*, 186–188.

Horn, G., Steckler, G., and Hill, R. M. Receptive fields of units in the visual cortex of the cat in the presence and absence of bodily tilt. *Exp. Brain Res.*, 1972, *15*, 113–132.

Howlett, J. G., and Brett, J. R. A speculation on the mechanism of utricular response to stimulation and motion sickness. National Research Council of Canada Rept. No. C2509, Appendix F. In *Proceedings of the Conference on Motion Sickness.* National Research Council of Canada, Ottawa, 1943.

Howlett, J. G., Wardill, T. E. M., Brett, J. R. The effect of position on the incidence of swing sickness. National Research Council of Canada Rept. No. C2507, C2508, Appendix E. In *Proceedings of the Conference on Motion Sickness.* National Research Council of Canada, Ottawa, 1943.

Huddleston, H. F. Oculomotor pursuit of vertical sinusoidal targets. *Nature,* 1969, *222*, 572–574.

Ito, M. The cerebellovestibular interaction in the cat's vestibular nuclei neurons. In *Fourth Symposium on "The Role of the Vestibular Organs in Space Exploration."* NASA SP-187. U.S. Government Printing Office, Washington, D.C., 1970.

Ito, M., Shiida, T., Yagi, N., and Yamamoto, M. Visual influence on rabbit horizontal vestibulo-ocular reflex presumably effected via the cerebellar flocculus. *Brain Res.*, 1974, *65*, 170–174.

Johnson, C., and Wendt, G. R. Studies of motion sickness. XVII. The effects of temperature, posture, and wave frequency upon sickness rates. *J. Psychol.*, 1955, *39*, 423–433.

Johnson, W. H., Stubbs, R. A., Kelk, G. F., and Frenks, W. R. Stimulus required to produce motion sickness. *J. Aviat. Med.*, 1951, *22*, 365–374.

Jones, W. A summary of Skylab findings of interest to life science scientists. In *Current Status in Aerospace Medicine.* AGARD CP-154. Technical Editing and Reproduction, Ltd., London, 1975.

Kennedy, R. S. *A Bibliography of the Role of the Vestibular Apparatus Under Water and Pressure: Content-Oriented and Annotated.* U.S. Naval Medical Research Institute, Bethesda, Md., 1972.

Kennedy, R. S. Motion sickness questionnaire and field independence scores as predictors of success in naval aviation training. *Aviat. Space Environ. Med.*, 1975, *46*, 1349–1352.

Knoblock, E. C. Biochemical responses to vestibular stimulation. In *The Role of the Vestibular Organs in the Exploration of Space.* NASA SP-77. U.S. Government Printing Office, Washington, D.C., 1965.

Koella, W. Experimentell-physiologischer Beitragzun Nystagmusproblem. *Helv. Physiol. Pharmacol. Acta,* 1947, *5*, 154–168.

Kolata, G. B. P. Behavioral development: Effects of environments. *Science,* 1975, *189*, 207–209.

Korner, A. F., and Thoman, E. B. Relative efficacy of contact and vestibular proprioceptor stimulation in soothing neonates. *Child Dev.,* 1972, *43*, 443–453.

Kornhuber, H. H. The vestibular system and the general motor system. In *H. H. Kornhuber (ed.), Handbook of Sensory Physiology.* Springer-Verlag, New York, 1974.

Kottenhoff, H., and Lindahl, L. E. H. Visual and emotional factors in motion sickness: Preliminary communication. *Percept. Mot. Skills,* 1958, *8*, 173–174.

Kottenhoff, H., and Lindahl, L. E. H. Laboratory studies on the psychology of motion sickness. *Acta Psychol.,* 1960, *17*, 89–112.

Krause, R. Entwickelungsgeschichte des Gehörorgans. In *Handbuch der Entwickelungslehre,* Lief. 4 and 5. O. Hertwig, June 1903.

Langworthy, O. R. Developing of behavioral patterns and myelinization of the nervous system in the human fetus and infant. *Contrib. Embryol.,* 1933, *24*, 3–57.

Lansberg, M. P. *A Primer of Space Medicine.* Elsevier, Amsterdam, 1960.

Larsell, O., and Jansen, J. *The Comparative Anatomy and Histology of the Cerebellum; The Human Cerebellum, Cerebellar Connections, and Cerebellar Cortex.* University of Minnesota Press, Minneapolis, 1972.

Lawrence, M. M., and Feind, C. R. Vestibular responses to rotation in the newborn infant. *Pediatrics,* 1953, *12(381)*, 300–306.

Ledoux, A., and Demanez, J.-T. "Ocular fixation" index in the caloric test. In J. Stahle (ed.), *Vestibular Function on Earth and Space.* Pergamon, Oxford, 1970.

Lisberger, S. G., and Fuchs, A. F. Response of flocculus Purkinje cells to adequate vestibular stimulation in the alert monkey: Fixation versus compensatory eye movements. *Brain Res.,* 1974, *69*, 347–353.

Llinas, R. R. The cortex of the cerebellum. *Sci. Am.,* January 1975.

Long, G. M., Ambler, R. K., and Guedry, F. E. Relationship between perceptual style and reactivity to motion. *J. Appl. Psychol.,* 1975, *60*, 599–605.

Lowenstein, O. The labyrinth in the making—A study of morphological and physiological features of the labyrinth in cyclostomes. *Adv. Oto-rhino-laryngol.,* 1973, *19*, 31–34.

Lukomskaya, N., Ya., and Nikol'skay, M. I. *Search for Drugs Against Motion Sickness.* Translation Bureau, Secretary of State Department of Canada, Defence and Civil Institute of Environmental Medicine, Downsview, Ontario, Canada, 1974.

Malcolm, R., and Melvill-Jones, G. Erroneous perception of vertical motion by humans seated in the upright position. *Acta Otolaryngol. (Stockholm),* 1974, *77*, 274–283.

Malcolm, R., and Money, K. E. Two specific kinds of disorientation incidents: Jet upset and giant hand. In *The Disorientation Incident.* AGARD CP-95, Part I. Technical Editing and Reproduction, Ltd., London, 1972.

Malcolm, R., Money, K. E., and Anderson, P. *Peripheral Vision, Artificial Horizon Display.* AGARD CP-145. Technical Editing and Reproduction, Ltd., London, 1975.

Manning, G. W. *Failure of a Vertical Accelerator to Produce Motion Sickness.* National Research Council of Canada Rept. No. C2649, App. H., Dec. 10, 1943.

Manning, G. W., and Stewart, W. G. Effect of body position on incidence of motion sickness. *J. Appl. Physiol.,* 1949, *1*, 619–628.

Marshall, J. E., and Brown, J. H. Visual-arousal interaction and specificity of nystagmus habituation. *Aerospace Med.,* 1967, *38*, 597–599.

Martin, J. F., and Melvill-Jones, G. Theoretical man–machine interactions which might lead to loss of aircraft control. *Aerospace Med.,* 1965, *36*, 713–717.

McCauley, M. E., Royal, J. W., Wylie, C. D., O'Hanlon, J. F., and Mackie, R. R. *Motion sickness incidence: Exploratory Studies of Habituation, Pitch, and Roll, and the Refinement of a Mathematical Model.* Tech. Rept. 1733-2. Human Factors Research, Inc., Santa Barbara Research Park, Goleta, Calif., April 1976.

McGraw, M. B. Development of rotary, vestibular reactions in the human infant. *Child Dev.,* 1941, *12*, 17.

Meiry, J. L. The vestibular and proprioceptive stabilization of eye movement. In P. Bach-y-rita, C. Collins, and J. Hyde (eds.), *The Control of Eye Movements.* Academic Press, New York, 1971.

Melvill-Jones, G. *Current Problems Associated with Disorientation in Man-Controlled Flight.* FPRC Rept. 1021, 1957.

Melvill-Jones, G. Predominance of anticompensatory oculomotor response during rapid head rotation. *Aerospace Med.,* 1964, *35*, 965–968.

Melvill-Jones, G. Disturbance of oculomotor control in flight. *Aerospace Med.,* 1965, *36*, 461–465.

Melvill-Jones, G. Interactions between optokinetic and vestibulo-ocular response during head rotation in various planes. *Aerospace Med.,* 1966, *37*, 172–177.

Melvill-Jones, G. Adaptive neurobiology in space flight. *Proc. Skylab Life Sci. Symp. L. B. Johnson Space Center, Houston, Tex., Aug. 27–29, 1974.* NASA TMX-58154, Vol. II, November 1974, pp. 847–859.

Melvill-Jones, G., and Gonshor, A. Goal-directed flexibility in the vestibuloocular reflex arc., In *1974 International Symposium on "Basic Mechanisms of Ocular Motility and Their Clinical Implications."* Wenner Gren Symposium Series, Vol. XXIV, Stockholm, 1974.

Melvill-Jones, G., and Drazin, D. H. Oscillatory motion in flight. In A. B. Barbour and H. E. Whittingham (eds.), *Human Problems of Supersonic Flight*. Pergamon, London, 1962.

Melvill-Jones, G., Watt, D. G. D., and Rossignol, S. Eighth nerve contributions to the synthesis of locomotor control. In R. B. Stein, K. B. Pearson, R. S. Smith, and J. B. Redford (eds.), *Control of Posture and Locomotion*. Plenum, New York, 1974.

Melvill-Jones, G., Rolph, R., and Downing, G. H. Human subjective and reflex responses to sinusoidal vertical acceleration. In *DRB Aviat. Med. Res. Unit Repts.*, Vol. V, 1974–1976. Report No. DR 225. Defence Research Board, Ottawa, 1976.

Miles, F. A., and Fuller, J. H. Visual tracking in the primate flocculus. *Science*, 1975, *189*, 1000–1002.

Miller, E. F., and Graybiel, A. Magnitude of gravito-inertial force, an independent variable in egocentric visual localization of the horizontal. *J. Exp. Psychol.*, 1966, *71*, 452–460.

Miller, E. F., and Graybiel, A. Perception of the upright and susceptibility to motion sickness as functions of angle of tilt and angular velocity in off-vertical rotation. In *Fifth Symposium on "The Role of the Vestibular Organs in Space Exploration."* NASA SP-314. U.S. Government Printing Office, Washington, D.C., 1973.

Miller, J. W., and Goodson, J. E. Motion sickness in a helicopter simulator. *Aerospace Med.*, 1960, *31*, 204–211.

Minkowski, M. Über frühzeitige Bewegungen: Reflexe und muskulare Reaktionen beim menschlichen Fötus und ihre Beziehungen zum totalen Nerven- und Muskelsystem. *Schweiz. Med. Wochenschr.*, 1922, *52*, 721–724, 751–755.

Money, K. E. Motion sickness. *Physiol. Rev.*, 1970, *50*, 1–39.

Money, K. E., and J. Friedberg. The role of the semicircular canals in causation of motion sickness and nystagmus in the dog. *Can. J. Physiol. Pharmacol.*, 1964, *42*, 793–801.

Neal, M. Vestibular stimulation and developmental behavior of the small immature infant. In *Nursing Research Report 3*, pp. 1–4. American Nurses Foundation, New York, 1968.

Nelson, J. E. Effects of water immersion and body position upon the perception of gravitational vertical. *Aerospace Med.*, 1968, *39*, 806–811.

Nuttall, J. B. The problem of spatial orientation. *J. Am. Med. Assoc.*, 1958, *166*, 431–438.

O'Hanlon, J. F., and McCauley, M. E. Motion sickness incidence as a function of the frequency and acceleration of vertical sinusoidal motion. *Aerospace Med.*, 1974, *45*, 366–369.

Ornitz, E. M. Vestibular dysfunction in schizophrenia and childhood autism. *Comp. Psychiat.*, 1970, *11*, 159–173.

Passey, G. E., and Guedry, F. E. Perception of the vertical. II. Adaptation effects in four planes. *J. Exp. Psychol.*, 1949, *39*, 700–707.

Patterson, J. L., and Graybiel, A. Acceleration, gravity, and weightlessness. In N. Balfour Slonim (ed.), *Environmental Physiology*, Chap. VI. Mosby, St. Louis, 1974.

Pederson, D. R., and ter Vrugt, D. The influence of amplitude and frequency of vestibular stimulation on the activity of 2-month-old infants. *Child Dev.*, 1973, *44*, 122–128.

Petersen, S., and Rainey, L. H. The beginnings of mind in the newborn. *Bull. Lying-In Hosp. New York*, 1910, *7*, 99–122.

Peto, A. To cast away—A vestibular forerunner of the superego. *Psychoanal. Stud. Child*, 1970, *25*, 401–416.

Pomerleau-Malcuit, A., and Clifton, R. K. Neonatal heart rate response to tactile, auditory and vestibular stimulation in different states. *Child Dev.*, 1973, *44*, 485–496.

Pompeiano, O. Vestibulo-spinal relationships. In R. E. Naunton (ed.), *The Vestibular System*. Academic Press, New York, 1975.

Popov, N. I., Solodovnic, F. E., and Khlebnikov, G. F. Vestibular training of test pilots by passive methods. In V. V. Parin and M. D. Yemel'yanov (eds.), *Physiology of the Vestibular Analyzers*. NASA Technical Translation NASA TT F-616, June 1970. (Book published by Nauka Press, Moscow, 1968.)

Preber, L. Vegetative reactions in caloric and rotation tests. *Acta Otolaryngol. (Stockholm)*, 1958, Suppl. 144.

Prescott, J. W. Early somatosensory deprivation as an ontogenetic process in the abnormal development of the brain and behavior. In I. E. Goldsmith and J. Moor-Jankowski (eds.), *Medical Primatology*. Karger, Basel, 1971.

Reason, J. T. Motion sickness, space sickness. In *Man in Motion*. Weidenfeld and Nicholson, London, 1974.

Reason, J. T., and Brand, J. J. *Motion Sickness*. Academic Press, New York, 1975.

Reason, J. T., and Diaz, E. Effects of visual reference on adaptation to motion sickness and subjective responses evoked by graded cross-coupled angular accelerations. In *Fifth Symposium on "The Role of the Vestibular Organs in Space Exploration.*" NASA SP-314. U.S. Government Printing Office, Washington, D.C., 1973.

Roberts, T. D. M. *Neurophysiology of Postural Mechanisms.* Plenum, New York, 1967.

Robinson, D. A. Eye movement control in primates. *Science,* 1968, *161*, 1219–1224.

Ross, H. E., Crickmore, S. D., Sills, N. V., and Owen, E. T. Orientation to the vertical in free divers. *Aerospace Med.,* 1969, *40*, 728–732.

Schilder, P. The vestibular apparatus in neurosis and psychosis. *J. Nerv. Ment. Dis.,* 1933, *78*, 1–23, 137–164.

Schöne, H. On the role of gravity in human spatial orientation. *Aerospace Med.,* 1964, *35*, 764–772.

Schöne, H., and Parker, D. E. Inversion of the effect of increased gravity on the subjective vertical. *Naturwissenschaften,* 1967, *54*, 288–289.

Schöne, H., and Udo de Haes, H. Space orientation in humans with special reference to the interaction of vestibular, somesthetic and visual inputs. In *Biokybernetik 3: Materialen des II. Internationalen Symposiums "Biokybernetik," Leipzig, 1969.* Gustav Fisher-Verlag, Jena, 1971.

Shirley, R., and Young, L. R. Motion cues and man-vehicle control. Effects of roll motion cues on operators' behavior in compensatory systems with disturbance inputs. *IEEE Trans. Man-Machines Syst.,* 1968, *MMS-9,* 121–128.

Sinha, R. Effect of vestibular Coriolis reaction on respiration and blood-flow changes in man. *Aerospace Med.,* 1968, *39*, 837–844.

Smith, K. U., and Smith, W. M. *Perception and Motion.* Saunders, Philadelphia, 1962.

Stewart, W. G., and Manning, G. W. The effect of tilting the head back on the incidence of sickness on the four-pole swing. National Research Council of Canada Rept. C2510, App. G, June 1943.

Stigler, R. Experiments dealing with the participation of the sensation of gravity in the orientation of man in space. *Arch. Ges. Fisiol.,* 1912, *148*, 573–594. (Transl. by A. Woke, NMRI, 1972.)

Stockwell, C. W., and Guedry, F. E. The effects of semicircular canal stimulation during tilting on the subsequent perception of the visual vertical. *Acta Otolaryngol. (Stockholm),* 1970, *70*, 170–175.

Stockwell, C. W., Sherard, E. S., and Schuler, J. V. Electronystagmographic findings in dyslexic children. *Tr. Am. Acad. Ophthalmol. Otolaryngol.,* 1976, *82* (2), ORL, 239–243.

Streeter, G. L. On the development of the membranous labyrinth and the acoustic and facial nerves in the human embryo. *Am. J. Anat.,* 1906/1907, *6*, 139–166.

Takemori, S., and Cohen, B. Loss of visual suppression of vestibular nystagmus after flocculus lesions. *Brain Res.,* 1974, *72*, 213–244.

Tibbling, L. The rotary nystagmus response in children. *Acta Otolaryngol. (Stockholm),* 1969, *68*, 459–467.

Tormes, F. R., and Guedry, F. E. Disorientation phenomena in naval helicopter pilots. *Aviat. Space Environ. Med.,* 1975, *46*, 387–393.

Tyler, D. B., and Bard, P. Motion sickness. *Physiol. Rev.,* 1949, *29*, 311–369.

Udo de Haes, H., and Schöne, H. Interaction between statolith organs and semicircular canals on apparent vertical and nystagmus. *Acta Otolaryngol. (Stockholm),* 1970, *69*, 25–31.

Usami, M. Study of the influence of rotary stimulation on respiration. *J. Oto-rhino-laryngol. Soc. Japan,* 1962, *65*, 662–671. (Transl. by E. R. Hope, DRB Canada, September 1964.)

Van der Laan, F. L., and Oosterveld, W. J. Age and vestibular function. *Aerospace Med.,* 1974, *45*, 540–547.

Von Békésy, G. Über die Stärke der Vibrationsempfindung und ihre objektive Messung. *Akust. Z.* 1940, *5*, 113–124.

Von Békésy, G. Pressure and shearing forces as stimuli of labyrinthine epithelium. *Arch. Otolaryngol.,* 1966, *84*, 26–130.

Walsh, E. G. Role of the vestibular apparatus in the perception of motion on the parallel swing. *J. Physiol. (London),* 1961*a*, *155*, 506–513.

Walsh, E. G. Sensations aroused by rhythmically repeated linear motion-phase relationships. *J. Physiol. (London),* 1961*b*, *155*, 53P–54P.

Walsh, E. G. The perception of rhythmically repeated linear motion in the horizontal plane. *Br. J. Physiol.,* 1962, *53*, 439–445.

Walsh, E. G. The perception of rhythmically repeated linear motion in the vertical plane. *Q. J. Exp. Physiol.,* 1964, *49*, 58–65.

Watanabe, I., and Egami, T. Effects of loading to the autonomic nervous system on equilibrium function of normal and pathological subjects. *Second Symp. Smolence,* September 1973.

Whitteridge, D. Central control of eye movements. In *Handbook of Physiology,* Section 1: *Neurophysiology,* Vol. II. American Physiological Society, Washington, D.C., 1960.

Wiersma, C. A. G. Neuronal components of the optic nerve of the crab, *Carcinus maenas. Proc. Kon. Ned. Akad. Wet.,* 1970, *C73*, 24–34.

Wilson, V. J. Physiology of the vestibular nuclei. In R. F. Naunton (ed.), *The Vestibular System.* Academic Press, New York, 1975.

Wolfe, J. W. Relationship of cerebellar potentials to saccadic eye movements. *Brain Res.,* 1971, *30,* 204–206.

Young, L. R. On visual-vestibular interaction. In *Fifth Synposium on "The Role of the Vestibular Organs in Space Exploration."* NASA SP-314. U.S. Government Printing Office, Washington, D.C., 1973.

Young, L. R., and Meiry, J. L. A revised dynamic otolith model. *Aerospace Med.,* 1968, *39,* 606–608.

Yuganov, E. M., Gorshkov, A., Kasyan, I., Bryanov, I., Kolosov, I., Kopanev, V., Lebedev, V., Popov, N., and Solodovnik, F. Vestibular reaction of cosmonauts during the flight in the Voskhod space ship. *Aerospace Med.,* 1966, *37*, 691–694.

Yuganov, Ye M., Markaryan, S. S., Lapayev, E. V., and Sidel'Nikov, I. A. Outlook for the development of vestibular selection methods in aviation. *Voyemo Med. Zh.,* 1969, *12*, 57–61. (Tr. J-7902, pp. 65–69.)

Zasosov, R., and Popov, A. Vestibultarnaya Tranirovka M. *Bol'Shaya Meditsinskaya Entsiklopediyz,* 1958, *5*, 275–279. (ATCIN IAI Rept. No. 1255904, June 29, 1959.)

11

Functional Properties of the Auditory System of the Brain Stem

J. M. HARRISON

INTRODUCTION

For purposes of exposition, the ascending auditory system is herein divided into three levels: the acoustic nerve and the cochlear nucleus, the superior olivary complex, and the inferior colliculus. A fourth section deals with the descending auditory system.

Information on various auditory structures varies. Most is known about what is sometimes called the principal ascending auditory system of the brain stem. This consists, essentially, of the acoustic nerve, the anterior and middle parts of the ventral cochlear nucleus, the three major nuclei of the superior olivary complex, and the central nucleus of the inferior colliculus. The principal ascending system is not, in fact, a single system, but is composed (beyond the acoustic nerve) of multiple ascending pathways having different connections within the principal system and involving nerve cells of various morphological types. In addition to the principal system, the ascending auditory system has at least two other pathways about which relatively little is known.

Each section contains an outline of the principal anatomical nuclei and tracts whose functions are being considered. The system has been extensively analyzed using pure-tone stimuli (sine waves of slow rise and decay time), and the majority of studies considered in this chapter are concerned with this kind of analysis.

J. M. HARRISON   Department of Psychology, Boston University, Boston, Massachusetts 02215; New England Regional Primate Research Center, Harvard Medical School, Southborough, Massachusetts.

The cochlea is not considered in this chapter. Since the pioneering work of von Békésy (1960), the cochlea has probably been the most intensely studied part of the auditory system, and an adequate presentation of this material requires a separate chapter. Information on the middle ear and the cochlea can be found in Keidel and Neff (1974), Miller (1970), Spoendlin (1966), Wever and Wever (1964), and Whitfield (1967).

ACOUSTIC NERVE AND COCHLEAR NUCLEI

It is convenient to think of the auditory system as consisting of three major components: (1) a principal ascending system, (2) a secondary ascending system (stria of Held) which is partially interconnected with the descending system, and (3) a secondary ascending system consisting of the dorsal cochlear nucleus and the dorsal acoustic stria (stria of Monoltow). The majority of the physiological and behavioral work has been done on the principal system, the secondary ascending systems being little understood. The principal system itself is complex insofar as it consists of multiple ascending systems.

The three systems are innervated by the acoustic nerve. Ninety-five percent of the axons of the nerve are in contact with the inner hair cells of the cochlea, the remaining 5% being in contact with the outer hair cells. The ascending systems are thus essentially inner hair cell systems.

In addition to the ascending components, the auditory system has a descending system from the inferior colliculus to the cochlea, the descending axons innervating principally the outer hair cells. Like the secondary ascending systems, the descending system is also poorly understood because of the relatively small amount of physiological and behavioral work. For a general review of the auditory system of the brain stem, see Morest (1973), Harrison and Feldman (1970), Harrison and Howe (1974 *a,b*), and Galambos (1954).

ANATOMY

The acoustic nerve is composed of the centrally directed axons of the spiral ganglion cells (located in the cochlea). About 95% of the peripheral processes of these cells innervate the inner hair cells, the remaining 5% making contact with the outer hair cells (Spoendlin, 1966, 1973). The acoustic nerve also contains efferent axons of the crossed and uncrossed olivocochlear bundles (Rasmussen, 1946, 1953). These efferent axons innervate principally the outer hair cells. They also make contact with the afferent fibers of the acoustic nerve which innervate the inner hair cells. The general arrangement is shown in Fig. 1 (Spoendlin, 1973).

The acoustic nerve enters the central nervous system at the cochlear nucleus. Upon entry, the axons of the nerve bifurcate into an ascending and a descending branch, the general arrangement being shown in Fig. 2. The axons of both branches keep their positions relative to each other, suggesting that the nucleus is tonotopically innervated (Ramon y Cajal, 1952; Feldman and Harrison, 1969; van Noort, 1969; Harrison and Feldman, 1970; Lorente de No, 1933). Results of

anatomical experiments in which lesions were made in the cochlea in order to
study the resulting degeneration of the axons of the cochlear nerve also suggest
that the projection of the cochlea upon the cochlear nucleus is tonotopic (Sando,
1965; van Noort, 1969; Webster, 1971; Moskowitz and Liu, 1972). The degree of
tonotopicity between the afferent axons and the groups of nerve cells in the
cochlear nucleus varies from group to group, and will be considered further
below. The distribution of the afferent axons is such that the base of the cochlea
(high frequencies) is represented dorsally and the apex (low frequencies) ventrally, with intermediate parts of the cochlea being represented at intermediate
positions between the dorsal and ventral extremes (Fig. 2).

411

FUNCTIONAL
PROPERTIES OF THE
AUDITORY SYSTEM OF
THE BRAIN
STEM

The cochlear nucleus is divided into the dorsal and ventral cochlear nuclei
(Ramon y Cajal, 1952). The ventral cochlear nucleus is further divided by the
region of bifurcation of the acoustic nerve axons into anterior and posteroventral
cochlear nuclei (Fig. 2). The anteroventral, middle (interstitial nucleus of Lorente
de No), and anterior parts of the posterior ventral cochlear nuclei form the
principal ascending system at this level. The ventral cochlear nucleus is a complex
structure composed of nerve cells of different types (Harrison and Warr, 1962;
Osen, 1969; Lorente de No, 1933; Brewer *et al.*, 1974; Ramon y Cajal, 1952;
Strominger and Strominger, 1971; Strominger and Bacsik, 1972; Webster, 1971;
Moskowitz and Liu, 1972). While the parcellation of the ventral cochlear nucleus is
not fully understood (Morest *et al.*, 1973), certain anatomical arrangements have
been established (Fig. 2).

The anteroventral cochlear nucleus contains nerve cells (principal cells) which
are innervated by two or three large synaptic endings called the bulbs of Held.
These endings arise from the axons of the ascending branch of the acoustic nerve,
and they presumably form a secure synapse between the nerve and the principal
cells of the nucleus (Lenn and Reese, 1966; Brewer and Morest, 1975; Ramon y
Cajal, 1952; Harrison and Warr, 1962; Harrison and Irving, 1965; Reese, 1966;
Stotler, 1953; Osen, 1970; MacDonald and Rasmussen, 1971; Feldman and
Harrison, 1969; van Noort, 1969). In the region of bifurcation of the acoustic

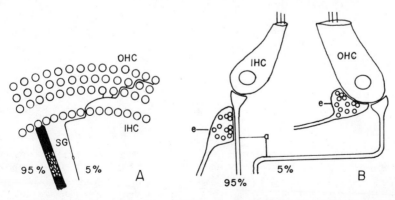

Fig. 1. A: Afferent innervation of the inner (IHC) and outer (OHC) hair cells by the acoustic nerve.
Only about 5% of the afferent axons reach the outer hair cells. SG, Spiral ganglion cells. B: Efferent
innervation of the inner and outer hair cells. a, Afferent axons; e, efferent axons and endings. After
Spoendlin (1973).

nerve and extending into the anterior and posterior ventral cochlear nuclei are a second class of cells (the globular cells of Harrison and Warr, 1962) which, in the rat, also receive large synaptic endings from the acoustic nerve. The globular cells give rise to large-diameter axons which enter the trapezoid body. These two groups of cells form part of the principal ascending system.

Located in the posterior ventral cochlear nucleus are a group of cells (the type k cells of Harrison and Irving, 1966a; the octopus cells of Osen, 1969) the dendrites of which lie across the axons of the descending branch of the acoustic nerve. The cell bodies and proximal dendrites are densely covered with two types of small synaptic endings which arise from collaterals of the descending branch (Cohen Kane, 1973). Since, for many of the type k cells, the dendrites lie across the axons of the descending branch, the cells may be innervated from the length of the cochlea and show a lesser degree of tonotopicity (broader tuning curves) than cells of the anteroventral and middle regions of the ventral cochlear nucleus (see inset of Fig. 2).

The dorsal cochlear nucleus is a complex laminated structure and is innervated by the descending branch of the acoustic nerve (Cohen et al., 1972; Osen, 1970; Powell and Erulkar, 1962; Powell and Cowan, 1962; Webster, 1971).

Axons leave the cochlear nuclei via three major tracts or pathways: the trapezoid body (ventral acoustic stria), the stria of Held (intermediate acoustic stria), and the dorsal acoustic stria. The principal system ascends via the trapezoid body.

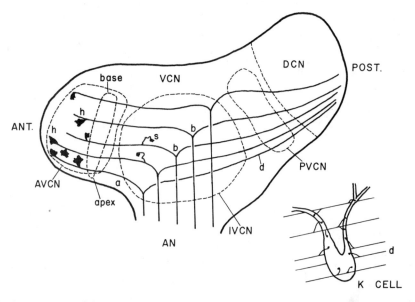

Fig. 2. Arrangement of the acoustic nerve (AN) in the cochlear nuclei in sagittal section. Axons of acoustic nerve bifurcate (b) into ascending (a) and descending (d) branches. The ascending branch gives rise to bulbs of Held (h), large synaptic endings (s), and other endings (not shown). The anteroventral cochlear nucleus (AVCN) and intermediate ventral cochlear nucleus (IVCN) form the principal part of the ascending auditory system at this level. The posterior ventral cochlear nucleus (PVCN) contains the type k cells (see inset) (octopus cells of Osen). The dorsal cochlear nucleus (DCN) is innervated by the descending branch of the acoustic nerve. The projection of the cochlea is shown in dotted outline in the AVCN. VCN, Ventral cochlear nucleus. After Harrison and Feldman (1970).

The trapezoid body is composed principally of axons which arise from the nerve cells of the anteroventral and intermediate parts of the ventral cochlear nucleus (Warr, 1966, 1972; Harrison and Warr, 1962; Harrison and Irving, 1965, 1966a; van Noort, 1969). The intermediate stria arises from the type k cells of the posterior ventral cochlear nucleus (Harrison, 1966; Warr, 1972) and forms the secondary ascending system which makes contact with the descending system at the periolivary nuclei and which also ascends to the contralateral inferior colliculus. The axons of the dorsal acoustic stria arise from the dorsal cochlear nucleus (Ramon y Cajal, 1952) and pass principally to the contralateral inferior colliculus.

413

FUNCTIONAL
PROPERTIES OF THE
AUDITORY SYSTEM OF
THE BRAIN
STEM

PHYSIOLOGY OF ACOUSTIC NERVE

A number of the functional properties of axons of the acoustic nerve have been well established using microelectrodes to measure the activity of single axons. The majority of the work has been carried out on the cat, and this review relies heavily on those data. When data from other species are referred to, this will be indicated.

The axons of the acoustic nerve show spontaneous activity in the absence of any experimental stimulus. They discharge at spontaneous rates which vary from about 6 spikes per minute to about 100 spikes per second for different axons. While the possibility that background noise is producing this activity cannot be excluded, it is believed that this is not the case (Kiang, 1965b). Spontaneous activity depends on the integrity of the hair cells of the cochlea. If these are destroyed then spontaneous activity ceases, although the sensitivity of the nerve fibers remains unaltered as shown by their responses to electric shocks applied to the cochlea (Kiang et al., 1970).

All axons of the acoustic nerve show the same general response pattern to tone or noise bursts of long risedecay time. This discharge pattern can be shown conveniently in post stimulus time (PST) displays. This display consists of a diagram of the number of spikes during each of a series of time intervals after the onset of the stimulus (Kiang, 1961). A typical discharge pattern is shown in Fig. 3. The response of the axons starts at a high rate, then rapidly declines to a steady rate which is maintained for the duration of the stimulus. At the termination of the stimulus, the spontaneous activity is reduced, to return to its stable level after 5–10 msec (Kiang, 1965a; Suga, 1973). While earlier experiments indicated that inhibitory responses might be found in acoustic nerve axons (Rupert et al., 1963), other work has failed to confirm this finding (Kiang et al., 1962; Kiang, 1965a).

Kiang (1965b) reports that after examining some 350 acoustic nerve units in the cat he could find no evidence of subpopulations of units, in terms either of spontaneous activity or of responses to various types of stimuli, which might correspond with the inner and outer hair cells of the cochlea. In view of the anatomical pattern of afferent innervation of the inner and outer hair cells discussed above (Spoendlin, 1973, Fig. 1), Kiang's observation suggests that virtually all the physiological data are probably best interpreted as reflecting activity of the inner hair cells. More recently, Pfeiffer and Kim (1972) have presented data on the responses of auditory nerve axons to clicks which reveal two populations of responses. Population I comprised about 93% of the axons and was presumed to represent activity of the inner hair cells. The remaining 7% were presumed to correlate with activity of the outer hair cells. This correlation, however, has not yet been demonstrated experimentally.

One way of representing the response of individual acoustic nerve axons is the tuning curve. To measure the tuning curve, an animal is exposed to tone bursts over a wide range of frequencies and intensities. At each frequency the threshold of the axon is determined and the results are plotted as a function of frequency (Kiang, 1965*b*). Two typical tuning curves are shown in Fig. 4. The frequency at which the threshold of a given axon is the lowest is termed the characteristic frequency (cf). As a rule, axons particularly sensitive to low-frequency tones have relatively broad tuning curves and are more symmetrical about their characteristic frequency than are higher-frequency axons. High-frequency axons have a narrow asymmetrical v-shaped portion and a long tail which extends into the low-frequency region. In addition to a cf (at the base of the V), high-frequency axons have a region of somewhat higher sensitivity in the tail portion of their tuning curve.

If thresholds at the characteristic frequency are plotted as a function of frequency for a large number of axons (Fig. 5), the line joining the most sensitive axons at each frequency corresponds approximately to the audibility function (threshold as a function of frequency) obtained by behavioral methods (Kiang, 1965*b*; Neff and Hind, 1955; Miller *et al.*, 1963; Elliott *et al.*, 1960). Inspection of the figure also reveals that for any given frequency the thresholds of individual axons vary over a 20–40 dB range.

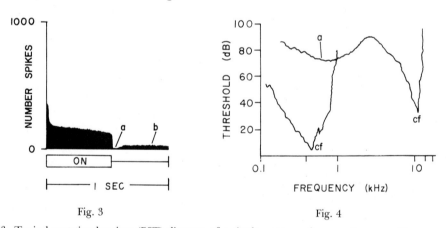

Fig. 3   Fig. 4

Fig. 3. Typical poststimulus time (PST) diagram of a single axon on the acoustic nerve. The axon discharged at a high rate at the onset of the tone (initial peak in the diagram). The rate then declined to a steady level. At the termination of the tone burst, the level of the spontaneous activity was reduced (a), to gradually return to a stable level (b). Acoustic nerve axons show a continuous discharge to even a long tone burst (13 min). cf = 1.82 kHz, tone burst = 1.82 kHz, 2.5 msec rise–decay time. After Kiang (1965*b*), his Fig. 6.1.

Fig. 4. Typical tuning curves of single axons of the acoustic nerve of the cat. The frequency at which the axon has its lowest threshold is called the characteristic frequency (cf). Note the difference in shape between the low-frequency and high-frequency axons. The latter (usually above 6 kHz) have long tails which extend into the low-frequency region and have a point of greater sensitivity (a) in this region. After Kiang and Moxon (1974), their Fig. 2.

415

FUNCTIONAL
PROPERTIES OF THE
AUDITORY SYSTEM OF
THE BRAIN
STEM

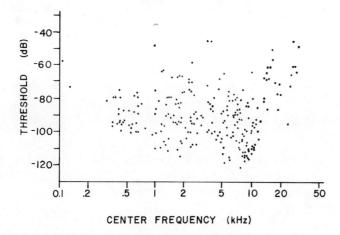

Fig. 5. Threshold at characteristic frequency for a large number of axons from 12 cats (the plot of individual cats is essentially the same). The most sensitive axons at each frequency correspond to the behavioral threshold for the cat. The threshold of axons at any given frequency varies over a range of 30–40 dB. After Kiang (1965*b*), his Fig. 7.8.

The relationship between the rate of discharge of individual axons of the acoustic nerve and the intensity of the tone burst (at cf) is highly variable, as shown in Fig. 6 (Kiang, 1965*b*; Rose *et al.*, 1971). For many axons this relationship is nonmonotonic.

For axons with characteristic frequencies below about 5 kHz, the discharge is time locked (phase locked) to the stimulus in cat and squirrel monkey (Kiang, 1965*b*; Rose *et al.*, 1971). That is, the spikes are grouped into clusters separated by time intervals equal to the period of the stimulus tone. Axons with high characteristic frequencies also show time-locked discharges when stimulated by low-frequency tones (below about 5 kHz) of sufficient intensity to reach the threshold of the tail portion of the tuning curve (Kiang and Moxon, 1974). Thus under the appropriate circumstances (essentially with tones below about 5 kHz of intensity at or above about 80 dB) virtually all axons of the acoustic nerve contain information concerning the period of the stimulus.

The functional properties of the acoustic nerve imply the following with respect to changes in the intensity and frequency of a stimulus. For all frequencies, as the intensity of a tone increases the number of axons responding also increases. The effect of increasing the intensity of a low-frequency tone (1 kHz) on the number of axons responding to the tone is shown schematically in Fig. 7B. Increasing intensity adds axons of increasingly divergent characteristic frequency until virtually all axons of the acoustic nerve are firing at about 90 dB, SPL. The discontinuity (indicated by "a") in Fig. 7B represents the point at which the intensity of the tone reaches the tails of the tuning curves of high-frequency units. In addition to the above, increasing intensity changes the rate of discharge of axons already discharging. A similar plot is shown in Fig. 7A for a 20 kHz tone. Once more, as the intensity increases, the number of axons responding increases. In the case of high-frequency tones, however, recruitment is principally of axons having high characteristics frequencies than the tone because of the asymmetrical shape of the high-frequency tuning curves. As for low-frequency tones, increasing intensity also changes the rate of discharge of axons which are already responding.

By comparing parts A and B of Fig. 7 the effect of changing the frequency of a tone of given intensity can also be derived. For all but near-threshold intensities an increase in frequency shifts the hatched portion of the diagram upward, decreases the total number of axons responding (especially at higher intensities) and narrows the range of cf's of responding axons. Changing both the intensity and frequency changes the populations of the axons responding, but for many values of intensity and frequency the populations will be overlapping (i.e., they will contain many of the same axons). Therefore, for the acoustic nerve, there is no independent coding of frequency and intensity of a given tone. Both frequency and intensity are encoded as a particular pattern of responding across many individual axons.

Because this fact once posed a problem for explanations of pitch and loudness discrimination, it is worth emphasis. Physically, the intensity and frequency of a tone may be independently varied. Furthermore, an animal may be trained to respond as a function of either the intensity or frequency of a tone. But it should be understood that these facts do *not* imply that the physical frequency and intensity of a sound are encoded independently by the acoustic nerve or that

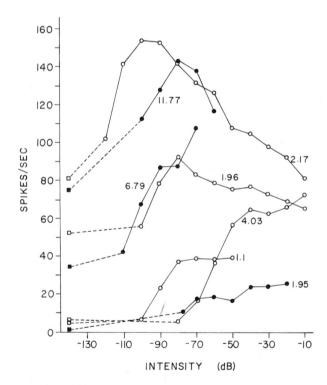

Fig. 6. Different axons have differently shaped rate–intensity functions. There is no relation between the form of the function (monotonic or nonmonotonic) and the characteristic frequency (cf) of the axon. The number at each function indicates the cf of the axon, and all measurements were made using a continuous tone at that frequency. After Kiang (1965*b*), his Fig. 6.10.

417

FUNCTIONAL
PROPERTIES OF THE
AUDITORY SYSTEM OF
THE BRAIN
STEM

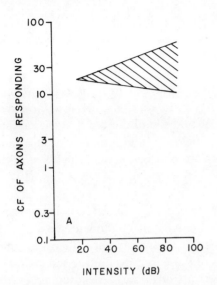
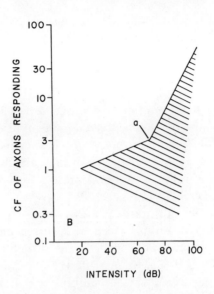

Fig. 7. Hypothetical plot of axons of a given characteristic frequency responding to a tone of a given intensity. A: 20 kHz tone. B: The same plot for a 1 kHz tone. The inflection of the curve at about 75 dB (a) is due to the tails of the high cf axons. All responses will be phase locked.

behavior appropriate to either stimulus parameter results automatically. The truth of the matter is that further neural mechanisms inside the animal's brain must operate on the response of the acoustic nerve before differential responding to either frequency or intensity changes can result, and this behavior is in no way elicited automatically by the physical parameters of the stimulus or the discharge characteristics of the nerve. In general, sounds of different frequency, intensity, and spectral content each produce different patterns of responding in overlapping subpopulations of axons in the acoustic nerve. Behavioral responses based on any of these parameters are the result of further analysis at later stages of the auditory system.

At frequencies below about 5 kHz, the responses of the axons are time locked to the frequency of the tone, a factor which may also be relevant in the production of the behavioral response. Whether the locking of discharges is relevant to frequency discrimination or to other behavioral auditory functions, such as localization by binaural phase (or time) differences, has not been determined at this time (Wever and Lawrence, 1954).

Physiology of Cochlear Nucleus

The physiological properties of nerve cells in the cochlear nucleus have been investigated using microelectrodes in conjunction with tone bursts. The following are the major findings under conditions in which the tone bursts (or long risedecay time) were at the characteristic frequency of the neuron being investigated.

Neurons of all frequencies are found in all divisions of the cochlear nuclei, although the nuclei have not been explored in sufficient detail to determine whether all anatomical cell types have center frequencies that cover the entire range of the cat. As would be expected from the anatomical connections between the acoustic nerve and the cochlear nuclei, the majority of parts of the ventral and the dorsal cochlear nucleus are tonotopically organized (Rose, 1960; Rose *et al.*, 1959; Kiang, 1965*a*; Mast, 1970*a*).

The distribution of thresholds of cochlear nucleus neurons is approximately like that found in the acoustic nerve (Pfeiffer, 1966, cat; Mast, 1970*a*, chinchilla), but the relation between the rate of discharge and stimulus intensity varies greatly in different neurons, some having monotonic and others nonmonotonic functions. In general, these functions are also similar to those found in the axons of the acoustic nerve (Fig. 6) (Moushegian and Rupert, 1970, kangaroo rat; Mast, 1970*a*, chinchilla).

The discharge patterns of nerve cells in the cochlear nuclei have been placed into four groups which are relatively independent of such parameters as intensity, duration, and repetition rate of tone bursts at center frequency (Pfeiffer, 1966; Kiang, 1965*a*; Kiang *et al.*, 1965). Examples of these four groups are shown in Fig. 8. All, except the on-neurons, discharge spontaneously and give sustained excitatory discharges to stimuli of long duration (Starr and Livingston, 1963; Gertain *et al.*, 1968; Suga, 1964, 1973; Mast, 1970*a*). If tone bursts at other than center frequency or noise bursts are used as the stimulus, the discharge patterns become much more complex and these characteristics will not be further discussed here (Greenwood and Goldberg, 1970; Suga, 1964).

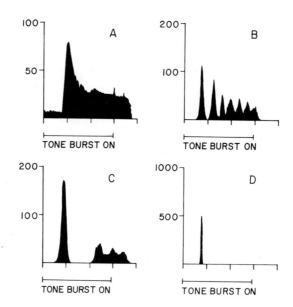

Fig. 8. Four types of discharge patterns found in the cochlear nuclei in cat. Each unit was stimulated at its cf's. A: Primarylike pattern, resembling pattern found in the acoustic nerve (cf = 3.5 kHz.) B: Chopper pattern, characterized by multiple peaks which are not related to the frequency of the stimulus (cf = 7 kHz). C: Pauser pattern, characterized by the slow onset of the sustained part of the pattern. The initial peak is not always present (cf = 6.6 kHz). D: "On" pattern. This type has no spontaneous activity (cf = 2.1 kHz). After Pfeiffer (1966), his Fig. 1.

419

FUNCTIONAL
PROPERTIES OF THE
AUDITORY SYSTEM OF
THE BRAIN
STEM

While it is not possible in every case to relate the type of discharge pattern to particular cell types in the cochlear nuclei, the following correlations have been found (for a summary, see Kiang *et al.*, 1973). Primarylike patterns (i.e., similar to patterns found in the acoustic nerve) are found in the anterior and globular cell (central) parts of the ventral cochlear nucleus, while chopper patterns are found predominantly in the middle and posterior regions of the ventral cochlear nucleus. The anterior and middle parts of the ventral cochlear nucleus form the principal ascending system at this level, and axons originating in these regions connect with the principal nuclei of the superior olivary complex and the inferior colliculus via the trapezoid body. Thus the principal ascending system is associated predominantly with primarylike patterns and with a lesser number of chopper patterns. Primarylike patterns are found in the principal nuclei of the superior olivary complex, while modified chopper patterns are found in one of these nuclei (the lateral superior olive) (Goldberg *et al.*, 1964; Kiang *et al.*, 1973).

On-type discharge patterns are found only in the posterior ventral cochlear nucleus, and they have been identified with the type k cells of Harrison and Irving (1966*a*) which are found in this region (octopus cells of Osen, 1969) (Pfeiffer, 1966; Kiang, 1973). These cells, part of one of the secondary ascending systems at this level, give rise to axons which form the intermediate acoustic stria (stria of Held) (Harrison, 1966; Warr, 1972), and on-type discharge patterns have been found in this tract (Kiang *et al.*, 1973).

Pauser-type patterns are found only in the dorsal cochlear nucleus (Pfeiffer, 1966; Kiang *et al.*, 1965; Mast, 1970*a*).

Primarylike, chopper, and pauser-type patterns have tuning curves which are essentially the same as those found in the axons of the acoustic nerve (Kiang, 1965*a*; Kiang *et al.*, 1965; Suga, 1964; Mast, 1970*a*). The on-type discharge patterns are associated with broad tuning curves (Fig. 9). This would be expected from the mode of innervation of the type k cells as has already been pointed out above (Fig. 2).

Chopper, pauser, and on-type discharge patterns are generated within the cochlear nuclei as a function of both the complex pattern of innervation from the acoustic nerve and the discharge characteristics of nerve cells with local connections. The measurement of intracellular potentials of cells in the cochlear nuclei shows that hyperpolarization and depolarization of the membrane occur during stimulation, indicating the complex nature of the innervation (Starr and Britt, 1970; Gerstein *et al.*, 1968). While the intracellular measurements have not been tied in with specific types of discharge patterns, they do indicate that some cells in the cochlear nuclei receive both excitatory and inhibitory synaptic endings. These cells, at least, are not simply relaying the input patterns of the acoustic nerve to the next level in the system.

Mast (1970*b*) has shown that about 20% of the nerve cells of the dorsal cochlear nucleus are inhibited by stimulation of the contralateral ear in addition to being excited by ipsilateral stimulation. This effect was not due to direct stimulation (via bone conduction or stimulus leakage) of one ear when the other was being stimulated. All the binaural neurons showed excitation by ipsilateral and

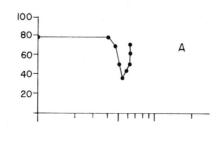

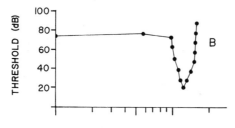

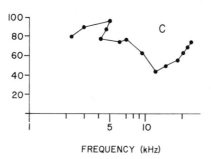

FREQUENCY (kHz)

Fig. 9. Typical tuning curves found in the cochlear nucleus and acoustic nerve. A: Tuning curve of acoustic nerve axon. B: Tuning curve associated with either primarylike, chopper, or pauser discharge patterns. Curves such as this are essentially the same as those found in the acoustic nerve. C: Broad tuning curve associated with "on"-type neurons. Curves such as this are associated with the type k cells (octopus cells) found in the posterior ventral cochlear nucleus. After Kiang *et al.* (1973), their Fig. 3.

inhibition by contralateral stimulation, and the level of inhibition was found to be 2–5 dB less sensitive than the level of excitation. The characteristic frequencies of the excitatory and inhibitory tuning curves were the same. The anatomical basis of this binaural interaction is not known, but Mast suggests that it may depend on the descending auditory system which has a prominent connection with the dorsal cochlear nucleus (see the section in this chapter entitled "Descending Auditory System").

COMPARATIVE VARIATION IN HEARING

Different species of mammals differ conspicuously in the frequency range of hearing as measured behaviorally. Shown in Table I is the approximate range of hearing (measured at approximately 40 dB above the most sensitive frequency) of representative species. At one extreme, for many species the upper frequency of hearing is at least 10 times (50 kHz or above) the frequency at which time locking ceases in the acoustic nerve and cochlear nuclei. Hence, for most of the range of hearing of these animals, time locking is of little significance. At the other extreme, tree shrew, man, chinchilla, and the four species of monkeys have hearing extending down to between 50 and 150 Hz, man being a conspicuously low-

421

FUNCTIONAL
PROPERTIES OF THE
AUDITORY SYSTEM OF
THE BRAIN
STEM

TABLE I.   APPROXIMATE RANGE OF HEARING[a] OF A RANGE OF DIFFERENT MAMMALIAN
SPECIES

Species	Range		Source
	High (kHz)	Low	
Dolphin (*Tursiops*)	130	2 kHz	Johnson (1966)
Bat (*Myotis*)	120	10 kHz	Dalland (1970)
Freshwater dolphin	80	1 kHz	Jacobs and Hall (1971)
Seal (*Phoca*)	64	1 kHz	Møhl (1968)
Rat	60	1 kHz	Harrison and Turnock (1975)
Hedgehog	50	1.5 kHz	Ravizza *et al.* (1969*a*)
Opossum	50	1.5 kHz	Ravizza *et al.* (1969*b*)
Cat	45	200 Hz	Neff and Hind (1955)
Bushbaby	45	250 Hz	Heffner *et al.* (1969*b*)
Tree shrew	40	50 Hz	Heffner *et al.* (1969*a*)
Killer whale	35	3 kHz	Hall and Johnson (1971)
Sea lion	35	250 Hz	Schusterman *et al.* (1972)
Guinea pig	30	150 Hz	Heffner *et al.* (1970)
Rhesus monkey	25	75 Hz	Stebbins (1970)
Squirrel monkey	25	75 Hz	Beecher (1974*a*)
Owl monkey	25	75 Hz	Beecher (1974*b*)
Chinchilla	20	75 Hz	Miller (1970)
Man	15	75 Hz	—

[a]To about +40 dB from the most sensitive frequency.

frequency species. In fact, as pointed out by Masterton *et al.* (1969), man is almost unique in this regard.

Time locking between the stimulus and axon discharges only takes place at frequencies below about 4 kHz. Mammalian species with an extremely high-frequency range of hearing (and a high-/low-frequency cutoff) will have a smaller (or possibly zero) part of the range in which time locking takes place. The reverse will be true for species with predominantly low-frequency hearing. The anatomical study of the cochlear nuclei of species at these two extremes may indicate that certain neuron types or certain regions of the nucleus are associated with time locking. At this time, there are insufficient data to draw any conclusions on this point.

It is clear from the data of Table I that many species live in quite different acoustic worlds. Sounds of significance to a bat are virtually undetected by man, and *vice versa*. It is possible that this is one of the factors that make the design of behavioral experiments on hearing in different species difficult, since the designer of the experiments is at the low frequency end of the spectrum.

SUPERIOR OLIVARY COMPLEX

ANATOMY AND PHYSIOLOGY

The superior olivary complex consists of three principal nuclei (the medial and lateral superior olivary nuclei and the medial nucleus of the trapezoid body) and a number of surrounding cell groups (see Fig. 10). The three principal nuclei are part of the principal ascending auditory system while the surrounding nuclei, the periolivary nuclei of Morest (1968), are part of both the secondary ascending and descending systems (Harrison and Howe, 1974a,b).

The lateral superior olivary nucleus consists of fusiform cells which possess voluminous polar dendrites (Ramon y Cajal, 1952, his Fig. 343), arranged in the form of a normal or inverted N in many species. The cells are located in such a way that their long axis is approximately normal to the edge of the nucleus (Taber, 1961; Stotler, 1953; Harrison and Feldman, 1970; Morest, 1968; Boudreau and Tsuchitani, 1970).

The lateral superior olive is innervated from the anteroventral cochlear nucleus of the same side, and anatomical and physiological studies show that this innervation is tonotopic (Boudreau and Tsuchitani, 1970; West and Harrison, 1973; Tsuchitani and Boudreau, 1966; Guinan et al., 1972b; Warr, 1966; Goldberg and Brown, 1968; Stotler, 1953; van Noort, 1969; Harrison and Irving, 1965; Galambos et al., 1959). Units of the lateral superior olive are excited by ipsilateral stimulation and give a modified primarylike response (which contains some chopper characteristics) to tone bursts presented to the ipsilateral ear. The tuning curves of these units are narrow and essentially like those found in the acoustic nerve (Kiang et al., 1973). The lateral superior olive is also innervated from the contralateral ventral cochlear nucleus via the medial nucleus of the trapezoid body (see below). This innervation is inhibitory and tonotopic (Galambos et al., 1959; Goldberg and Brown, 1968; Boudreau and Tsuchitani, 1968) for frequencies above about 1 kHz in the cat (Fig. 11).

The excitatory (ipsilateral) and inhibitory (contralateral) tuning curves correspond closely for each unit, and the excitatory and inhibitory effects are approxi-

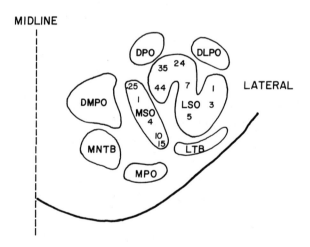

Fig. 10. Schematic illustration of the right superior olivary complex in transverse section. The numbers indicate the distribution of characteristic frequencies (in kHz) in the medial and lateral superior olivary nuclei. DLPO, Dorsolateral periolivary nucleus; DMPO, dorsomedial periolivary nucleus; DPO, dorsal periolivary nucleus; LSO, lateral superior olive; LTB, lateral nucleus of trapezoid body; MNTB, medial nucleus of the trapezoid body; MPO, medial periolivary nucleus; MSO, medial superior olive.

423

FUNCTIONAL
PROPERTIES OF THE
AUDITORY SYSTEM OF
THE BRAIN
STEM

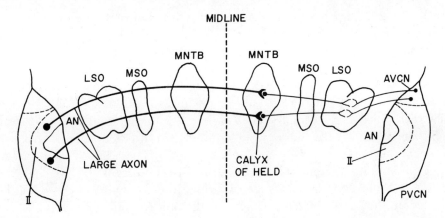

Fig. 11. Bilateral innervation of the lateral superior olivary nucleus in horizontal section. At LSO, ipsilateral projection is excitatory and contralateral is inhibitory. AN, Acoustic nerve; AVCN, anterior ventral cochlear nucleus; LSO, lateral superior olive; MNTB, medial nucleus of the trapezoid body; MSO, medial superior olive; PVCN, posterior ventral cochlear nucleus; II, region two of the ventral cochlear nucleus. After Harrison and Feldman (1970), his Fig. 9.

mately equal and opposite for binaural stimuli of equal intensity and frequency (above about 1 kHz) (Tsuchitani and Boudreau, 1969). If an external sound source is placed at various angles in the horizontal plane of an animal, the measured intensity of stimulation at the two ears is a function of the angle of the speaker (Harrison and Downey, 1970). If the speaker is to the left of the midline, the left ear is stimulated at a greater intensity than the right (for frequencies above about 2 kHz for the cat). Under these conditions, the left lateral superior olive will receive a larger excitatory input than inhibitory and its appropriate units will respond. The right lateral superior olive, on the other hand, will receive a larger inhibitory than excitatory input and its units will be inhibited (no response). When the stimulus is on the midline, both lateral superior olives will receive approximately equal excitatory and inhibitory inputs, and both will give a small or no response. Thus units in the lateral superior olive indicate (among other things) on which side of the midline a sound source is located on the basis of the intensity difference at the two ears. A singe unit in these nuclei, however, does not indicate the particular angle of the speaker, that is, its actual angular location. However, the responding population of units possibly do.

The medial superior olivary nucleus consists of a column of cells, the major (polar) dendrites of which are directed medially and laterally (Stotler, 1953; Ramon y Cajal, 1952, his Figs. 346 and 345; Clark 1969a,b; Harrison and Warr, 1962). The medial superior olive is innervated directly and tonotopically, from the anteroventral cochlear nucleus of both sides, the laterally directed dendrites receiving ipsilateral axons and the medial dendrites receiving contralateral axons (Stotler, 1953; Goldberg and Brown, 1968; van Noort, 1969; Warr, 1966; Guinan et al., 1972b).

While the innervation is tonotopic, the majority of the units have center frequencies below about 10 kHz; hence the medial olive may be considered a low- to intermediate-frequency nucleus (Goldberg and Brown, 1968; Guinan et al.,

1972*b*). Like the lateral superior olive, the units of the medial superior olive give primarylike responses and have narrow tuning curves similar to those of the acoustic nerve (Kiang, 1973). The ipsilateral and contralateral tuning curves for the same unit may not correspond closely.

About 50% of the units are excited by stimulation of either ear (excite-excite, E-E, units) and the remainder are either monoaural or complex forms of excite-inhibit, E-I, units. These complex units may be E-E for one frequency, E-I for a second, and E-I for white noise. Goldberg and Brown (1968) suggest that E-E units, since they respond to stimulation of either ear, will be relatively insensitive to changes in interaural intensity (in contrast to E-I cells) because, as excitation on one side is diminished (by movement in azimuth of a sound source), it will be increased on the other, the net excitation to the unit remaining constant.

The medial nucleus of the trapezoid body contains three types of nerve cell, of which the principal cell is the type usually recognized as constituting the nucleus. The principal nerve cells are each innervated by a single very large synaptic ending called a calyx of Held. The calyx arises from a single large-diameter axon which, in turn, arises from globular cells of the intermediate part of the contralateral ventral cochlear nucleus (see Fig. 2) (Harrison and Irving, 1964, 1966*a*; Harrison and Warr, 1962; type g cells located in region II of the ventral cochlear nucleus). The large-diameter axon is a rapid conductor, and the calyx of Held, being so massive, is probably a synapse of certain action. The transmission through the principal cells of the medial nucleus of the trapezoid body is thus of short latency (Kiang *et al.*, 1973), certain, and on a one-to-one basis from axon to cell body.

The nucleus is tonotopically organized, and the vast majority of the units respond only to contralateral stimulation, as would be expected from their anatomical connections (Guinan *et al.*, 1972*b*). The units give parimarylike responses and have tuning curves similar to those found in the acoustic nerve (Kiang *et al.*, 1973). The axons of the principal cells of the medial nucleus of the trapezoid body pass to the lateral superior olive of the same side (see Fig. 11), supplying the contralateral innervation for that nucleus (Harrison and Warr, 1962; Rasmussen, 1965). The medial nucleus contains at least two other types of neuron (Morest, 1968), one of which probably responds only at the termination of the stimulus (Kiang *et al.*, 1973).

COMPARATIVE VARIATION IN THE SUPERIOR OLIVARY COMPLEX

It was first pointed out by Harrison and Irving (1966b) that there is a systematic variation in the relative and absolute size (measured by the number of cells in the nucleus) of the medial and lateral superior olives in different mammalian species. The medial olive is completely absent in some forms (hedgehog, *Erinaceous europus,* and the bats *Myotis* and *Carollia,* for example) and large in others (cat and rhesus monkey, for example). The variation in size of the medial olive in a range of different species is given in Table II. In attempting to understand this size variation, a number of other neural structures have been examined and a correlation has been found between the size of the medial olive

425

FUNCTIONAL
PROPERTIES OF THE
AUDITORY SYSTEM OF
THE BRAIN
STEM

TABLE II. NUMBER OF NERVE CELLS IN THE MEDIAL AND LATERAL SUPERIOR OLIVES
(WHEN AVAILABLE) AND THE HIGH- AND LOW-FREQUENCY CUTOFF OF HEARING

Animal	Medial olive	Lateral olive	High frequency	Low frequency
Bat *(Myotis)*	0	3850	120 kHz	10 kHz
Hedgehog	0	1090	50 kHz	1.5 kHz
Bat *(Phyllostomus)*	100	4340	120 kHz	10 kHz
Mouse	210	1190		
Hamster	300	980		
Rat	690	1480	60 kHz	1 kHz
Gerbil	1100	1220		
Squirrel	1240	1160		
Guinea pig	2300	3780	30 kHz	150 Hz
Chinchilla	3090	3220	20 kHz	75 Hz
Tamarin	3100			
Bushbaby	4000		45 kHz	250 Hz
Owl monkey	4558		25 kHz	75 Hz
Squirrel monkey	4600	1300	25 kHz	75 Hz
Macaque	5100	1830	25 kHz	75 Hz
Cat	5900	3360	45 kHz	200 Hz
Capybara	6600			
Gibbon	7000			
Lion	12,100			
Zebra	21,000			

and the size of the eye and eye-movement or visuomotor system as represented by either the diameter of the eye or the number of nerve cells in the VIth (abducens) nucleus. This initial work was expanded to cover additional species, and essentially the same relationships were found (Irving and Harrison, 1967; Harrison and Feldman, 1970; Feldman and Harrison, 1971; Feldman, quoted in Harrison and Howe, 1974a; Harrison, 1974). Typical observations are shown in Fig. 12. It will be noted that the slope of the function differs for nocturnal and diurnal animals and that the general correlation holds for both classes. The high correlation between the size of the medial superior olive and the sixth nuclei implies that the medial olive and the pathways associated with it are related to interactions between the auditory and visual systems, in particular with the orientation of the head and eyes toward a source of sound (Harrison and Irving, 1966b).

It is particularly interesting that the medial superior olivary nucleus is absent in some echolocating forms (Microchiroptera and Cetacea). Since on the basis of natural and experimental observations (Turner and Norris, 1966; Simmons and Vernon, 1971; Simmons, 1973) it is known that these animals are excellent sound locators, it is clear that the medial superior olive and its associated pathways are not essential for localization in either the horizontal or the vertical axis.

The lateral superior olivary nucleus also varies in size in different species, although, unlike the medial olive, is probably present in all species. In man and gorilla it is difficult to detect in some specimens and may be vestigial (Noback, 1959; Olszewski and Baxter, 1954). In bats (*Myotis* and *Phyllostomus*), excellent localizers, the lateral superior olive is large in an absolute sense (in spite of the small size of the animal and its nervous system). Since mammalian species have, at least, the medial or the lateral superior olive (and most species probably have both), either, in the absence of the other, may be an essential part of the localizing mechanism (Table II).

On the basis of the relative sizes of the medial and lateral superior olivary nuclei, mammalian species can be categorized into three groups as indicated in Table III. Group 1, species lacking the medial superior olive, includes small animals with poor vision but good localizing abilities (the echolocators). The inclusion of the dolphin in this group would seen to negate the possibility that animals of this group are necessarily small in body size. However, the dolphin operates in a marine environment in which sounds travel about 5 times as fast as in the air. This means that the size of the dolphin's head is effectively one-fifth its real size with respect to the production of interaural intensity and time differences, making the animal fit better in group 1 in terms of functional head size. Since the lateral superior olive is found in all the forms studied (although it may be vestigial and difficult to recognize), group 2 is not so sharply divided from group 3 as is group 1. Probably, the majority of species fall into group 3, the mixed group, where both the medial and lateral olivary systems are well developed.

Masterton and Diamond (1967) have suggested, on the basis of the comparative data, that the medial and lateral superior olives may be associated with the two cues on which the ability to respond to the position of a stimulus in azimuth is based: binaural time (Δt) and binaural intensity (ΔI) differences. Some of the considerations on which this idea is based are the following.

The magnitude of the time cue is a function of the distance between the two ears. The interaural time difference (Δt) is maximum when a sound is on one side of the animal (90° azimuth). This value is about 90 μsec for the rat and 900 μsec for man. For other azimuthal positions of a sound the corresponding times

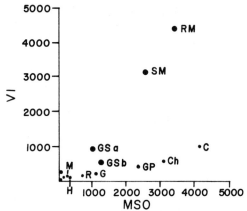

Fig. 12. Relationship between the size of the medial superior olive (MSO) and the number of neurons in the VIth nucleus. Large dots represent species with cone retinas and small dots animals with predominantly rod retinas. The species not indicated with letters are two species of bats and hedgehog. C, Cat; Ch, chinchilla; GP, guinea pig; GS a, ground squirrel *(tridecemlineatus)*; GS b, ground squirrel *(beecheyi)*; H, Hamster; G, gerbil; M, mouse; R, rat, RM, rhesus monkey; SM, squirrel monkey. After Harrison and Feldman (1970), their Fig. 25.

427

FUNCTIONAL
PROPERTIES OF THE
AUDITORY SYSTEM OF
THE BRAIN
STEM

TABLE III. CLASSIFICATION OF MAMMALS IN TERMS OF THE RELATIVE SIZE OF THE MEDIAL AND LATERAL SUPERIOR OLIVES

Group[a]	Typical species	Comments
1. No MSO	Bats, hedgehog, mole, blindmouse, dolphin	Small animals with reduced vision, well-developed high-frequency hearing, and poor low-frequency sensitivity; includes echolocators (exception of the dolphin, see text)
2. Small or vestigial LSO	Gorilla, man	Relatively large animals with good vision; man and chimpanzee have poor high-frequency hearing but sensitive low-frequency hearing
3. Both LSO and MSO well developed	Cat, dog, chinchilla	Hearing well developed over wide frequency range

[a]LSO, Lateral superior olive; MSO, medial superior olive.

differences will be less (Masterton *et al.*, 1969). If the magnitude of Δt at the threshold of angular detection is about the same for rat and man, the angular threshold (based on Δt) must be larger for rat than for man. In other words, Δt is less useful as the basis for responding to the position of the stimulus in rat compared with man. Stated generally, the smaller the distance between the animal's ears, the less useful are interaural time differences for localization. Thus, for very small animals, it is possible that the neural mechanisms on which the use of interaural time differences depends may have either atrophied or never developed.

The interaural intensity difference produced by a sound is a function of the size of the head, shape and placement of the ears, and ear movement. As a first approximation it is usually stated that interaural intensity differences become large (and consistent) enough for localization as the wavelength of the sound equals or is smaller than the size of the head (Casseday and Neff, 1973). Actual measurements of interaural intensity differences in different species show that, for a given species, there is a frequency below which the interaural intensity differences are not large (or consistent) enough to act as a cue for responses to stimulus position. This frequency, however, may be lower than that expected simply on the basis of the size of the head (Harrison and Downey, 1970). The reason for this may be that the magnitude of the interaural intensity difference depends on the acoustic properties of the pinna as well as simply head size (Fattu, 1969). The range of species over which interaural intensity differences have been measured as a function of frequency is small (bat, cat, rat, rabbit, squirrel monkey, man), but the data tend to support the assumption that for a large range of head sizes there is a negative correlation between head size and the minimum frequency for an effective head shadow (Harrison and Downey, 1970; Sivian and White, 1933; Wiener, 1947; Masterton *et al.*, 1969). In the general case, the smaller the head and the less effective the pinna as a directional organ, the higher will be the minimum frequency of a sound to produce a sufficiently large and reliable interaural intensity difference for localization.

Summarizing the preceding two paragraphs, it appears that as the interaural distance and hence the maximum Δt decrease, interaural time difference becomes an increasingly unreliable cue for a response to stimulus position. An animal with a small Δt will have to depend increasingly (the smaller the animal is) on interaural intensity differences. But as the head gets smaller, the minimum frequency for the production of an effective interaural intensity difference increases, requiring that the animal have well-developed hearing over a high-frequency range. In the limit, an animal with a very small Δt may not even develop the internal mechanism for response to stimulus position by interaural time differences, and may depend entirely on the interaural intensity differences. Such an animal would necessarily have well-developed high-frequency hearing. These speculations are supported by the large negative correlation (-0.86) between maximum Δt and the high-frequency cutoff of hearing over a range of 19 mammalian species reported by Masterton *et al.* (1969).

Masterton (1974) has related these comparative data to the development of the nuclei of the superior olivary complex. It can be seen from Table III that it is small animals which lack the medial superior olive (for a discussion of the exception of the dolphin, see above). These animals also have well-developed high-frequency hearing (Dalland, 1965; Masterton *et al.*, 1969). This suggests that the lateral superior olive (well developed in this group of animals) is associated with both high-frequency hearing and responding to stimulus position by interaural intensity differences.

As we have seen, single unit physiological studies of lateral superior olivary nucleus show that units are excited by ipsilateral and inhibited by contralateral auditory stimulation. In the absence of stimulation of either ear the units are silent. The balance of excitation and inhibition is such that when stimuli of equal intensity and frequency are applied to the two ears, the balance is about equal. If the intensity of the stimulus of one side, say the left, is increased relative to the other (right) side, units in the left lateral olive will fire while units in the right lateral olive will be inhibited. If this type of interaction is translated into lateral olivary responses to a stimulus which is of high enough frequency to produce a sound shadow of the head and which is moved in the azimuth plane from one side of the animal to the other, then when the stimulus is on the left side (left ear receiving a stronger stimulus than the right) units of the left lateral olive will be firing while those of the right olive will be silent. When the stimulus is on the midline, units of both olives will be weakly firing or silent. When the stimulus moves to the right side of the animal, units of the right lateral olive will be silent. Thus activity of units of the lateral superior olive is correlated with whether a stimulus is on the right or left side of the midline of an animal, while relative inactivity of the units is correlated with midline stimuli. This correlation is based on interaural intensity differences. It should be noted that the angular position of a stimulus when it is on one side of the animal is not represented by differential firing patterns in the lateral superior olive. The lateral superior olive responds, essentially, to high-frequency stimuli off the midline of the animal and is inactive to stimuli on the midline, that is, to stimuli to which the animal is oriented.

429

FUNCTIONAL
PROPERTIES OF THE
AUDITORY SYSTEM OF
THE BRAIN
STEM

The possible role of the medial superior olivary nucleus in responding to the position of a stimulus is less clear. Animals having a small interaural distance and therefore a small Δt include species in which the medial olive is either absent or small (Table II). From inspection of Table II it can be seen that there is a relation between the size of the animal (that is, the size of maximum Δt) and the number of nerve cells in the medial superior olivary nucleus. This is not simply a reflection of the fact that the size of the nervous system as a whole is also roughly correlated with the size of the mammal, since in a range of primates from marmoset to man, for example, the number of cells in the medial olive increases with animal size while the number of cells in the lateral olive does not increase (Moore and Moore, 1971).

There is no clear evidence from physiological studies of the relation between response of the medial olive and responding to stimulus position. Three types of cells have been found in the medial olive: cells (the majority) which are excited by the stimulation of either ear (E-E cells), E-I cells similar to those found in the lateral superior olive, and cells whose discharge pattern is a function of the time intervals between pairs of stimuli presented to the two ears (Guinan *et al.*, 1972*a*; Goldberg and Brown, 1968; Galambos *et al.*, 1959). The discharge characteristics of a cell, however, depend on the parameters of the stimuli. For example, a cell which is excited by stimulation of either ear over one intensity range may have excite-inhibit characteristics over a second intensity range. Physiological studies indicate that this nucleus is composed of units the majority of which have their best frequency below 10–12 kHz (Guinan *et al.*, 1972*a*; Goldberg and Brown, 1968). That is, the medial olive is principally concerned with the lower frequencies and it may be that this is the reason for the absence of this nucleus in the smaller animals, forms in which low-frequency hearing is often poorly developed (Masterton *et al.*, 1969).

While the comparative and physiological data do not strongly indicate that the medial superior olive is principally concerned with behavioral responding to stimulus position based on interaural time differences, Masterton (1974) has made use of the variation in size of the medial superior olive in a "natural ablation" experiment to see if differences in this kind of behavior in animals with and without medial olives could be detected (Masterton *et al.*, 1975). The medial superior olivary nucleus is absent in hedgehog and progressively larger in rat, tree shrew, and cat. These four species were trained on a behavioral task using a slow rise–decay time tone pip as the stimulus. The apparatus contained two speakers, each associated with a water spout for the delivery of water reinforcement. The sound could be presented through one or other of the two speakers on any given trial. A trial was initiated by the animal's licking a tube set facing and in front of the two speakers. This ensured that the animal's head was in a relatively constant position with respect to the speakers (which subtended an angle of 60° at the animal's head). The ability of the animals to respond to the position of the tone pip was measured at octave frequencies between 0.25 and 32 kHz.

The results are shown in Fig. 13. The interpretation of the results is based on the following considerations. Responding to the position of a tone pip can be

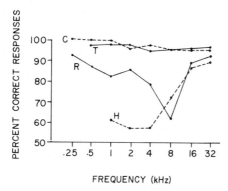

Fig. 13. Average performance of four species (C, cat; H, hedgehog; R, rat; T, tree shrew) responding to the position of a pure tone at various frequencies. After Masterton *et al.* (1975), their Fig. 4.

based on interaural intensity differences or interaural time differences. Which cue will be dominant (or even present) is a function of the frequency of the stimulus. Above a critical frequency (under the conditions of the experiments this was estimated as 4 kHz for the cat and 8 kHz for the other species) phase differences (that is, time differences) at the two ears provide ambiguous information concerning the position of the stimulus. Hence above these frequencies phase differences could not be the basis of correct responding. As can be seen from Fig. 13, all species were able to respond correctly to the position of tone bursts above the critical frequencies, so this behavior must have been based on interaural intensity differences. Since the medial olive is absent in hedgehog, this nucleus is not essential for correct responses based on interaural intensity differences. For stimuli below the critical frequencies, asymptotic performance is correlated with the size of the medial superior olivary nucleus. The hedgehog, in which the medial superior olive is absent, was unable to respond to the position of stimuli below the critical frequency, while the rat (small medial olive) performed at lower levels than the tree shrew or cat (both with larger medial olives). On the basis of these data Masterton argues that the medial superior olivary nucleus is necessary for responding to position based on interaural time (or phase) differences.

In assessing this conclusion it must be remembered that comparative studies reveal correlations between two variables but these correlations do not imply causal connections. The finding of one correlation does not preclude the existence of others. For example, in the four species used in this experiment the diameter of the eye is probably also correlated with performance on the low-frequency task. Which of the two correlations is viewed as the most significant depends on *a priori* considerations such as have been discussed in this section.

BEHAVIORAL STUDIES OF THE SUPERIOR OLIVARY COMPLEX

The effects of lesions of the auditory system of the medulla have been investigated with a view to determining the significance of the crossed auditory pathways at the level of the superior olivary complex in responding to stimulus position. In order to evaluate these experiments it is necessary to have a clear picture of the position of the various auditory pathways in the medulla. These are illustrated in their approximate positions in Fig. 14A. In the experiments to be discussed, three kinds of lesions have been made: section of the auditory system at the midline, as shown in Fig. 14B; destruction of the superior olivary complex of one side, as shown in Fig. 14C; and sectioning of the lateral lemniscus of one side, as shown in Fig. 14A.

In most of these experiments, cats were trained on a task which required them to go to one of two food boxes behind which a stimulus (buzzer or broad-band noise) had been sounded. Opening the door of the correct box was rein-forced with food. The angle between the food boxes was then gradually reduced

431

FUNCTIONAL
PROPERTIES OF THE
AUDITORY SYSTEM OF
THE BRAIN
STEM

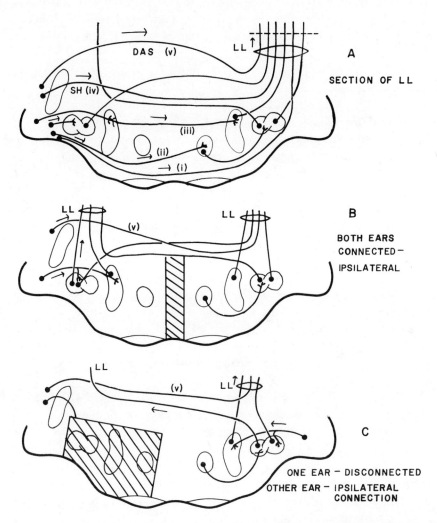

Fig. 14. Major ascending acoustic pathways in transverse section in the medulla at the level of the superior olivary complex and lateral lemniscus. Except for C, the connections of only one side are shown. A: Section of the lateral lemniscus on one side. Virtually all ascending connections on this side are cut. The corresponding connections on the other side remain intact. Note that the intact lateral lemniscus will contain binaural information. B: A deep midline lesion. All ascending binaural axons are severed, leaving only monoaural information in each lateral lemniscus. C: Effect of destroying one superior olivary complex. Only monoaural connections remain. CN, Cochlear nucleus; DAS, dorsal acoustic stria; LL, lateral lemniscus; SH, stria of Held.

until the minimum angle between the boxes which could support correct responding was determined. The major data reported in the experiments are the effects of the various lesions on the angular threshold between the food boxes.

In normal cats correct responding in the experimental apparatus depends on binaural cues, but it is possible that following one or more of the lesions animals may still perform correctly—presumably, however, on the basis of monaural cues. To rest the possibility of monaurally based correct responses, normal cats were trained to criterion and the minimum angular threshold was measured (typically, 4.5°). One cochlea was then destroyed and, after recovery, the animals were reintroduced into the apparatus. The preoperatively acquired behavior was lost. With extensive retraining (many more trials than are required by normal cats) the monaural cats were able to respond appropriately; however, the minimum angular threshold, was raised (typically 20° in a monaural cat).

Casseday and Neff (1975) achieved a complete midline section of virtually all the auditory pathways (except possibly the dorsal acoustic stria (v) (Fig. 14B) in one cat (No. 514). When tested postoperatively, it was found that the preoperatively acquired discrimination had vanished and that the cat could not be retrained to respond to the position of the broad-band noise. This cat was not deaf since it acquired an avoidance response based on a sounding speaker and had normal absolute intensity thresholds at 250 Hz, 1 kHz, and 8 kHz. Less extensive midline lesions were made in three other cats, one of which (No. 474) also failed to respond appropriately postoperatively. The other two cats showed virtually no postoperative loss of the behavior and had essentially normal minimum angular thresholds.

From inspection of the drawings of the lesions of the three cats with partial midline sections it is difficult to find any correlation between the size or placement of the lesion and the presence or absence of the ability to respond correctly. In these three animals the dorsal and intermediate acoustic striae were probably intact (whereas they were probably sectioned in cat 514). Since the behavior was lost in cat 474, these two pathways probably can be eliminated as being able to support the behavior following partial lesions of the more ventrally placed pathways.

Moore *et al.* (1974) made midline lesions in three cats (559, 517, 588). In two of the animals there was a slight increase in the minimum angular threshold but in none was the behavior abolished. However, destruction of the various crossing pathways in these cases proved to be incomplete. In a fourth cat (459) the superior olivary complex of one side was completely destroyed and the behavior was lost in this animal. This lesion has the effect of disconnecting one ear from the auditory system (Fig. 14C). With massive retraining the behavior was recovered, presumably on the basis of monaural cues.

On the basis of these experiments it is not possible to attribute the loss of the ability to respond to stimulus position to the damage of any particular pathway, or any structure in this part of the auditory system. A deep midline cut interrupts all crossed connections to the inferior colliculus and the superior olivary complex (with the exception of the crossed connections of the dorsal acoustic stria), and in the absence of these, sound localization behavior is lost. Following such a midline

433

FUNCTIONAL
PROPERTIES OF THE
AUDITORY SYSTEM OF
THE BRAIN
STEM

cut, the remaining axons in the lateral lemniscus arise from the ipsilateral medial and lateral superior olives, and these axons contain information from only one ear.

The unilateral destruction of the lateral lemniscus, in contrast to the midline lesion, leaves intact all the connections to the superior olivary complex (Fig. 14A). The remaining lemniscus contains the (binaural) output of both lateral superior olives and the ipsilateral medial superior olive. The crossed connections from the cochlear nucleus to the inferior colliculus are also intact. Thus the remaining lemniscus contains information from both ears. The complete destruction of the lateral lemniscus of one side abolished preoperatively learned responding to the position of the sounding speaker, but the task was rapidly relearned (with fewer trials than was required for initial training). The animals showed a slight increase in the minimum angular threshold (typically 2–5°) (Casseday and Neff, 1975). The destruction of the remaining lateral lemniscus in a second operation permanently abolished the behavior, showing that this behavior was dependent on the previously intact lemniscus. The effects of lesions of the lateral lemniscus on hearing are discussed in greater detail in the following section of this chapter.

The effect of lesions of the auditory system of the medulla on the ability to respond to stimuli on the basis of their interaural time difference (lateralization experiment) has been investigated by Masterton *et al.* (1967). In these experiments, cats, fitted with headphones, were required to discriminate a click pair in which the click to the left ear preceded the click to the right ear by 0.5 msec (LR) from a click pair in which the click to the right ear preceded the click to the left ear by 0.5 msec (RL). Control experiments showed that the discrimination of LR from RL could not be carried out by cats deprived of one cochlea and also that, in normal cats, the minimum time between the click pairs for correct responding was about 0.05 msec.

The complete destruction of the superior olivary complex and all the crossing pathways on the left side in one animal (329) permanently abolished the LR vs. RL discrimination (at a Δt of 0.5 msec). In this animal the left cochlear nucleus was effectively disconnected from the ascending auditory system except for some surviving axons of the dorsal and intermediate acoustic stria (Fig. 14A). Remeasurement of the threshold showed that RL could be discriminated from LR provided that the value of Δt was increased to about 0.9 msec, a value far greater than exists under natural conditions. Extensive, but subtotal, unilateral lesions of the superior olivary complex and ventral pathways did not affect the discrimination of Δt of 0.5 msec. That is, the behavior was not affected by such lesions, a finding similar to that of Casseday and Neff. Measurement of the Δt threshold, however, showed that this was increased from a normal of about 0.05 msec to about 0.2 msec.

The fact that the animals with subtotal lesions in the work of Casseday and Neff did not show large changes in the minimum angular threshold implies that the postoperative behavior in the threshold region was based on interaural intensity rather than time differences. The virtually complete destruction of the lateral lemniscus of one side did not prevent the acquisition of the Δt discrimination, nor was there an effective change in the Δt threshold value. These animals resemble those of Casseday and Neff, in that Δt discrimination was normal following unilateral lemniscal destruction.

The unilateral lesion of the lateral lemniscus did alter one aspect of the behavior; it abolished transfer from L vs. R (on which the cats were first trained) to LR vs. RL. Transfer between the two conditions occurs in normal cats. The reason for this loss is obscure.

Taken together, the ablation experiments on the medullary auditory structures and the lateral lemniscus show that if the axons ascending in the lemniscus contain only unilateral information (as occurs following the midline lesion) then the ability to respond to the position of the sound is abolished. In contrast, a single lemniscus having virtually normal connections is able to support this behavior. The behavior studied in these experiments does not require the bilateral interaction of the two lemnisci at the collicular or higher levels. The single lemniscus contains binaural information by virtue of the axons which arise from nerve cells in the medial and lateral superior olivary nuclei, and this would seem to be essential to support the behavior. Thus from these studies it appears that the superior olivary complex is part of the mechanisms for responding to the azimuth of an acoustic event.

As has already been mentioned, there is no evidence that the patterns of interaural interaction in the superior olivary complex represent the azimuth of an external sound. That is, there are no units in the superior olivary complex which fire when a sound is presented at, say, 10° to the left of the animal's midline but which remain entirely silent if the stimulus is presented a few degrees either side of 10°. However, experiments designed to test this possibility have not yet been done. Therefore, the question must remain open.

INFERIOR COLLICULUS

ANATOMY AND PHYSIOLOGY

The inferior colliculus forms part of the roof of the midbrain in mammals and consists of several major subdivisions or neuronal areas: a central, a pericentral, and an external nucleus (Fig. 15A). The inferior colliculus in the cat has been studied by a number of researchers and has been divided or parcelled in several different ways. The most extensive study on the cat is by Rockel and Jones (1973a), and their terminology and parcellation will be followed in this chapter.

The central nucleus is subdivided into two regions, a ventral (or principal) part and a dorsomedial part (corresponding to the dorsomedial nucleus of Geniec and Morest, 1971). The ventral part of the central nucleus consists of two types of principal cells (in addition to other cell types), and the dendrites of these cells are arranged in curved laminae of complex shape (Rockel, 1971; Rockel and Jones, 1973a,b; Morest, 1964, 1966a,b). Axons of the lateral lemniscus which arise from the contralateral ventral and dorsal cochlear nucleus, the ipsilateral medial superior olive, and the lateral superior olive of both sides enter the central nucleus ventrally and run in the laminae formed by the cells of the central nucleus. The axons terminate on the proximal dendrites of the principal cells.

435

FUNCTIONAL
PROPERTIES OF THE
AUDITORY SYSTEM OF
THE BRAIN
STEM

The laminar arrangement of the ascending axons and the dendrites of the principal cells suggests that the central nucleus is tonotopically organized (Osen, 1972; Morest, 1964, 1966*b;* Warr, 1966, 1969; Strominger and Strominger, 1971; Stotler, 1953; Fernandez and Karapas, 1967; Barnes *et al.,* 1943; Goldberg and Moore, 1967).

The lateral lemniscus, as already indicated, arises from several sources at lower levels. It has not been determined whether the axons from these several sources terminate on the same or different neurons of the central nucleus, or on different parts of the same neurons. If the principal cells do receive innervation from several sources, then it might be expected that the response patterns of the cells would be more complex than those of lower-level neurons.

The axons of the principal cells of the central nucleus form the major ascending auditory tract in the brachium of the inferior colliculus to the medial geniculate body, and we have already seen that axons of the lateral lemniscus terminate within the central nucleus. From this arrangement it can be seen that destruction of the inferior colliculus which includes the ventral central nucleus interferes with the major ascending auditory system by severing the connections between the lateral lemniscus and the medial geniculate bodies. This arrangement is shown schematically in Fig. 15B (Harrison and Howe, 1974*a,b*).

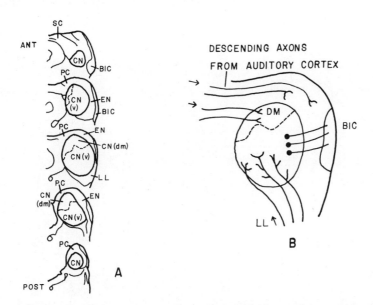

Fig. 15. Cytoarchitectonic subdivisions and major connections of the inferior colliculus. A: Schematic cross section through the inferior colliculus at different levels to show the major nuclei. After Rockel and Jones (1973*a*). B: Principal auditory connections through the inferior colliculus. BIC, Brachium of inferior colliculus; CN, central nucleus; CN(dm), central nucleus, dorsomedial part; CN(v), ventral part of central nucleus (principal ascending nucleus); EN, external nucleus; LL, lateral lemniscus; Pc, pericentral nucleus.

The pericentral nucleus and the dorsomedial part of the central nucleus (dorsomedial nucleus) are innervated by axons which descend from the various parts of the auditory cortex; thus these nuclei are part of a descending auditory system. Axons which descend to lower levels in the auditory system (dorsal cochlear nucleus and the periolivary nuclei) arise in the inferior colliculus, but their site of origin is not known.

The external nucleus is innervated by collaterals of the brachium of the inferior colliculus (Harrison and Howe, 1974b) (Fig. 15B), but little further is known about the auditory input to this area.

Electrophysiological studies of the inferior colliculus have shown that the central nucleus, and also possibly the pericentral nucleus, are tonotopically organized in cat and rat. As the microelectrode passes through the central nucleus, the center frequency of the neurons changes in a systematic way, going from low frequencies (lateral-dorsal) to high frequencies (ventral-medial). The arrangement is shown in Fig. 16. The tonotopic organization is presumably correlated with the anatomical arrangement of the laminae in the nucleus, but as yet there is no experimental confirmation of this speculation (Rose *et al.*, 1963; Geisler *et al.*, 1969; Aitkin *et al.*, 1970; Clopton and Winfield, 1974; Grinnell, 1963a).

Units in the central nucleus show more complexity and variation of discharge patterns than units at lower levels of the auditory system (with the exception of the nuclei of the lateral lemniscus). Both excitatory and inhibitory synaptic potentials are found, intracellularly, and these potentials may have sufficiently different patterns to reflect multiple inputs (Nelson and Erulkar, 1963). It is these multiple inputs which, presumably, produce the complex discharge patterns seen in the ventral nucleus.

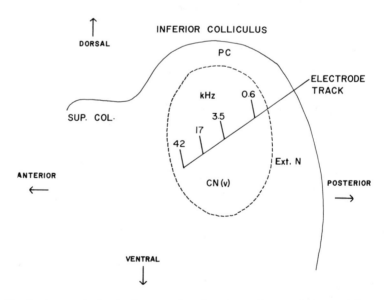

Fig. 16. Tonotopic organization in the central nucleus (ventral part) of the cat. Schematic sagittal section. CN(v), Central nucleus; Ext. N, external nucleus; PC, pericentral nucleus. After Rose *et al.* (1963), their Fig. 1.

437

FUNCTIONAL
PROPERTIES OF THE
AUDITORY SYSTEM OF
THE BRAIN
STEM

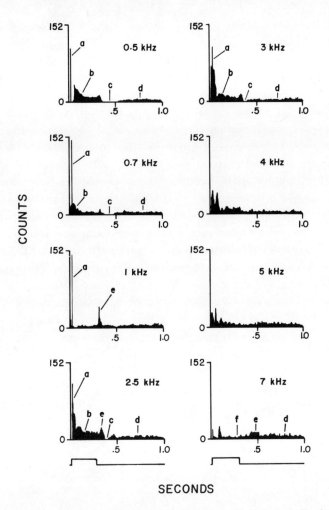

Fig. 17. Discharge pattern of a single unit in the central nucleus of the inferior colliculus in an alert cat when stimulated by tone bursts of different frequencies. Tones were presented through a single speaker on the cat's midline. a, "On" response; b, sustained response; c, inhibitory "off" response; d, spontaneous activity; e, "off" response; f, inhibitory sustained response. After Bock *et al.* (1972), their Fig. 3.

Because of the variability of discharge patterns it is not usual to classify units in the central nucleus into types. The patterns of response can be most easily understood in terms of three phases or components of the discharge which vary with such stimulus parameters as frequency, intensity, and rise–decay time of the stimulus (Suga, 1969a, 1971, 1973; Rose *et al.*, 1963; Bock *et al.*, 1972; Starr and Don, 1972). The three phases, each of which may be excitatory or inhibitory (reduction of spontaneous activity), consist of an "on" component, a "sustained" component (usually with a time interval between the "on" and the "sustained"), and an "off" component. The way these phases vary in one particular unit in an alert cat as a function of frequency is shown in Fig. 17. In other units the occurrence of the various phases is different.

The complexity of units in the inferior colliculus indicates that some may respond only to special features of the stimulus which are of significance to the animal species in question. Suga (1973) pointed out that many naturally occurring sounds can be broken down to noise, frequency-modulated tones, and pure tones. He has examined the inferior colliculus in bats for units showing signs of specialization for these characteristics. The majority of units (67%) had symmetrical tuning curves and responded equally to tone and noise bursts and to frequency-modulated tones. The response of the units could be predicted from a knowledge of their behavior with respect to pure tones. Units with very narrow tuning curves (8%) and with inhibitory areas on either side responded to pure tones but not to noise or frequency-modulated tones. A small percentage of units (1.6% and 1.2%) were found to be responsive to either frequency-modulated tones or noise only. Nelson *et al.* (1966) also found units in the cat which, under certain conditions, responded to frequency-modulated tones when sweeping in one direction but not the other. Thus, while there is some evidence for feature detection in the inferior

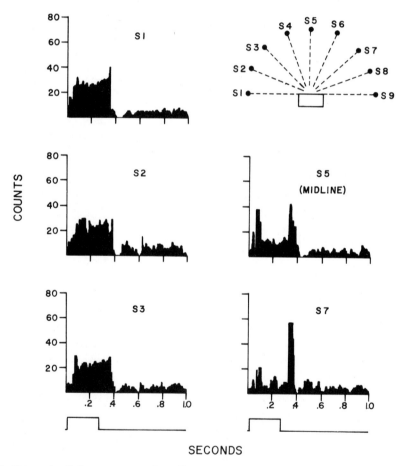

Fig. 18. Change in discharge pattern of a collicular unit with change in the position of the sounding speaker (tone burst, 1 kHz, 60 dB). S1, S2, etc., refer to speaker positions. After Bock and Webster (1974), their Fig. 3.

colliculus, either the majority of the units appear to be universal responders or the features they detect have not yet been discovered.

439

FUNCTIONAL
PROPERTIES OF THE
AUDITORY SYSTEM OF
THE BRAIN
STEM

The response of single units in the inferior colliculus to changes in the position of a sounding speaker or to changes in binaural time and intensity differences (lateralization) has been investigated in cat, bat (*Myotis*), rat, and kangaroo rat (Geisler *et al.,* 1969; Erulkar, 1959; Flammino and Clopton, 1975; Hind *et al.,* 1963; Friend *et al.,* 1966; Bock and Webster, 1974; Stillman, 1974; Grinnell, 1963*b*). In free field experiments in the alert (unanesthetized) cat (Bock and Webster, 1974) the animal was exposed to tones from speakers situated in nine positions (22.5° apart) arranged in a semicircle in front of and around the sides of the animal (Fig. 18). It was found that about 50% of units in the central nucleus were sensitive to the position of the sound.

Typical changes in the discharge pattern of a single unit to changes in the position of the sounding speaker are also shown in Fig. 18. It can be seen that the "on," "sustained," and "off" phases of the discharge vary with the position of the sound. From inspection of other units, it appears that position is not uniquely represented by any particular change in discharge characteristics since a pattern produced by one position of the sound can be produced in a second position by changing the intensity or the frequency of the stimulus (Bock and Webster, 1974).

In lateralization experiments, units sensitive to interaural time differences and interaural intensity differences have been found in the central nucleus (Geisler *et al.,* 1969; Flammino and Clopton, 1975; Benevento *et al.,* 1970; Hind *et al.,* 1963). Units sensitive to interaural time differences may be either excited by monoaural stimulation of either ear (E-E units) or excited by the stimulation of one ear (usually the contralateral) and inhibited by the stimulation of the other (E-I units). Units are about equally divided between these two types (Geisler *et al.,* 1969). Units which are sensitive to interaural intensity differences are of the E-I class (Benevento *et al.,* 1970). That is, the units fire maximally or minimally over a range of interaural time differences independently of the frequency and intensity of the stimulus.

Some units (with center frequency below about 4 kHz) show a characteristic delay with respect to interaural intensity differences. The relationship of the characteristic delay to the total discharge pattern may be complex, one phase of the pattern showing a relationship of interaural delay while a second phase may not. For the unit shown in Fig. 19, the "sustained" portion of the discharge is correlated with position while the "on" phase is not. Under natural conditions the maximum binaural time difference that can occur is fixed by the width of the animal's head, and this value is about 90 μsec for the rat and 250 μsec for the cat. While it is thought that the characteristic delay may be related to the ability to respond to the position of a sound, the value of the delay is frequently outside the maximum time difference that can occur under natural conditions (Clopton and Winfield, 1974). However, this does not preclude the possibility that when the characteristic delay is within natural limits it is related to the ability to respond to sound position. Units which show a characteristic delay usually discharge at a much lower rate when monoaurally stimulated, and they may have either E-E or E-I characteristics.

Collicular units which are sensitive to interaural intensity differences can be divided into two classes. In the first class the behavior of the unit is determined primarily by the interaural intensity difference, the absolute intensity of the stimuli having little effect on the firing rate (Fig. 20A). For units of the second class the discharge of the unit depends on both interaural intensity difference as well as the absolute intensity of the stimulus (Fig. 20B). The maximum interaural intensity difference in the cat under natural conditions is about 20 dB, so that the functions shown in Fig. 20 may be relevant to responding to stimulus position based on interaural intensity differences (Geisler *et al.*, 1969).

In summary, it can be seen that units in the central nucleus of the inferior colliculus show a higher order of complexity than units at lower levels (with the exception of the dorsal nucleus of the lateral lemniscus; see below). That is, active processing takes place within the nucleus. The various phases of the discharge patterns of the units vary with frequency, intensity, spectral content, and frequency and intensity modulation of tones. There is no clear evidence that any of these stimulus characteristics are uniquely represented in any particular units, and none of the units showed a one-to-one coding of particular positions of a sound in the azimuth plain. However, it is well known that the ability to respond to the position of pure tones is less precise than in the case of more complex sounds (Harrison and Beecher, 1969; Terhune, 1974). Therefore, for the physiological exploration of the response of single units to localize stimuli, pure tones may not be the optimum type of stimuli to use.

Practically nothing is known about the dorsomedial part of the central

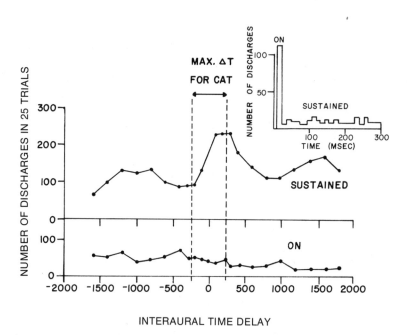

Fig. 19. Characteristic delay shown by the sustained phase of the discharge and not the on phase in a collicular unit. This was an E-E unit stimulated with a noise burst having a 400–4000 Hz pass band. The maximum interaural time delay that occurs under natural conditions in the cat is about 250 μsec. After Geisler *et al.* (1969), their Fig. 3.

441

FUNCTIONAL
PROPERTIES OF THE
AUDITORY SYSTEM OF
THE BRAIN
STEM

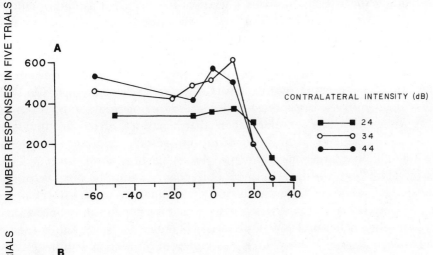

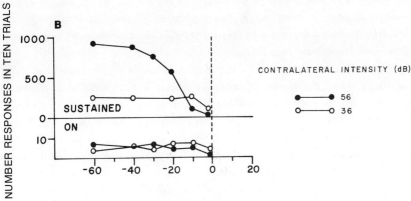

Fig. 20. A: Collicular unit sensitive to interaural intensity differences independently of the absolute intensity of the stimulus. This unit gave a sustained discharge under the stimulus conditions. Binaural stimulation at a characteristic frequency of 6.9 kHz. B: Unit sensitive to both absolute and interaural intensity differences (sustained part of discharge pattern). The "on" portion of the pattern was not sensitive to interaural intensity differences. 6.5 kHz tone burst. After Geisler *et al.* (1969), their Figs. 8 and 10.

nucleus, the pericentral nucleus, or the external nucleus except that they also seem to have a tonotopic representation.

The dorsal nucleus of the lateral lemniscus is similar, physiologically, to the central nucleus of the inferior colliculus. The nucleus shows tonotopic organization, and the discharge patterns of the units show the phases which are similar to those found in the central nucleus (Brugge *et al.*, 1970).

BEHAVIORAL STUDIES OF THE INFERIOR COLLICULUS

In considering the effects of lesions of the midbrain auditory system on behavior, two major points have to be kept in mind. First, the lesions have to be considered within the context of the known connections of the auditory system.

Thus cutting the lateral lemniscus interrupts the principal ascending auditory system and deprives higher levels (inferior colliculus, medial geniculate body, and auditory cortex) of input via this system. Behavioral changes which follow such a lesion reflect the effect of the interruption of this system and should be interpreted in this context. Any ability to respond to sounds which remains after the lesion must depend either on the activity of lower levels or on inputs to higher levels arriving over the remaining ascending auditory pathways. It is also usual to find in the experiments considered here that behavioral effects are found only after complete destruction of the structure in question. Because partial lesions, even though very large, may have no observable behavioral effect, adequate histological methods for the assessment of the damage must be used. Second, if a lesion destroys some particular behavior (for example, a frequency discrimination using a given procedure) this does not mean that it will necessarily have a similar effect on other behavioral procedures classed under the same rubric (i.e., frequency discrimination). This point is well known in connection with the effects of lesions of the auditory cortex on frequency discrimination and the reader is referred to the chapter on this topic.

ANATOMICAL CONSIDERATIONS. It has been shown that the principal auditory system at the level of the midbrain consists of the lateral lemniscus, the central nucleus of the inferior colliculus, and the brachium of the interior colliculus. The last structure consists of the axons of the principal neurons of the central nucleus which terminate in the ventral division of the medial geniculate body of the same and opposite sides (Harrison and Howe, 1974a) (Fig. 15B). In terms of these connections, whether the lateral lemniscus, central nucleus, or brachium is destroyed in an experimental lesion, the principal ascending system is being severed and the behavioral effects of all three lesions might be expected to be the same. Destroying the central nucleus, for example, means that the brachium has been destroyed and the lemniscus cut.

Interpretation, however, is complicated by the fact that the auditory system consists of ascending connections other than those of the principal system. The central nucleus sends axons to the pericentral nucleus of the inferior colliculus (Morest, 1966a,b) and possibly to the superior colliculus in addition to those to the brachium. These axons would not be cut by lesions of the brachium but would be by lesions of the central nucleus. The dorsal division and the magnocellular nucleus of the medial geniculate body and the suprageniculate nucleus receive auditory connections from the lateral tegmental system (Morest, 1965). This system ascends just medial to the brachium and is liable to be cut by brachial lesions, but not by lesions of the inferior colliculus. These systems may continue to function in the absence of the principal system and may be able to support certain aspects of hearing.

From what is known of the connections of the principal ascending system it is probably safe to say that if in three cats with different lesions (one of the lemnisci, one of the central nuclei, and one of the brachia) hearing is affected in the same way, then the effect is due to interruption of the principal system. If, however, other aspects of hearing are affected in different ways by the three lesions, then the differences will be due to interference with or the sparing of other connections of the structures involved.

443

FUNCTIONAL
PROPERTIES OF THE
AUDITORY SYSTEM OF
THE BRAIN
STEM

The behavioral effects of placing lesions in a given structure often depend on the structure in question being completely destroyed. Even small remnants may be sufficient to support the behavior. Again, it is necessary to emphasize that adequate means be used to assess the degree of damage produced by the lesion, and that these data be available for each animal on which the behavioral work has been done. Incomplete lesions of the lateral lemniscus, central nucleus, or brachium of the inferior colliculus have little or no behavioral effect on the kinds of behavioral tasks which have been used, and for this reason only those experiments in which the lesions were apparently complete are considered below (Casseday and Neff, 1975; Casseday, 1970; Suga, 1969b; Strominger and Oesterreich, 1970; Oesterreich et al., 1971).

While the results of most ablation studies are interpreted in terms of the destruction to the ascending auditory system, the same structures may be involved in the descending system. At the level of the inferior colliculus the two systems are apparently independent, the pericentral and dorsomedial nuclei being part of the descending system and the central nucleus part of the ascending system. Hence lesions of the inferior colliculus which are confined to the dorsal one-third are primarily interrupting the descending system, while lesions which are ventral enough to include the central nucleus are interrupting both systems. While there is no reason to think that the behavioral effects produced by lesions are due primarily to the interruption of the descending rather than the ascending system, the former interpretation can not always be excluded.

BEHAVIORAL EFFECTS OF LESIONS. In ablation studies it is not always useful to ask the question: what is the role of or the effects of lesion of a given auditory structure on a number of auditory discriminations classed under the same rubric (e.g., frequency discrimination or intensity discrimination)? This question implies that all members of the discrimination class will be affected in the same way by the lesion and that the class is unitary with respect to the nervous system. For example, it is common to class a number of different procedures as measuring frequency discrimination. However, it may be the case that a particular lesion which affects a frequency discrimination as measured by one behavioral procedure may have no effect on the same frequency discrimination as measured by a different procedure, even when the two procedures are used with the same animal (Thompson, 1960). What this probably means is that the lesion has produced a behavioral deficit or deficits which play some role in the procedure affected and no role in the procedure not affected. Without extensive experimental analysis it is not possible to say what this is, and as yet the necessary experimental analyses have not been carried out in connection with lesions of the brain stem auditory system.

Most of the work on the effects of ablation of midbrain structures on hearing has been done on the ability to respond to the position or temporal sequence of two stimuli (lateralization), and this will be considered first (see Erulkar, 1972, for a review of the literature).

EFFECT OF MIDBRAIN LESIONS ON LOCALIZATION. The majority of the experiments to be considered here have been carried out using behavioral methods developed by Neff et al. (1956). In these experiments the animal (cat) is placed in a starting box and is faced with two (sometimes more) food boxes. A sound (buzzer, noise burst, or pure tone) is sounded over or behind one of the boxes. At the termination of the stimulus the cat is released and allowed to approach one of the two boxes. If it opens the box at which the stimulus was sounded, it is reinforced. If it opens the other box, it is not reinforced and the trial is terminated. The animals rapidly reach a high level of correct responding using this procedure. When the training criterion has been reached, the angle between the boxes is gradually reduced to obtain a measure of the threshold (minimum angle between the boxes at which 75% correct response level is maintained). Following the measurement of threshold, lesions are made in the desired auditory structures and the animal is allowed to recover. Behavioral testing is then resumed, and the cat is retrained if necessary. Thresholds (if possible) are then remeasured.

There is complete agreement that unilateral lesions of the lateral lemniscus, central nucleus of the inferior colliculus, or the brachium have little permanent behavioral effects. In cats, the behavior was abolished postoperatively, but all animals were able to relearn the task to criterion. An increase in angular threshold of between 5° and 20° was usually found (Casseday, 1970; Casseday and Neff, 1971, 1975; Strominger and Oesterreich, 1970). With a different procedure, Suga (1969b) has studied the bat (*Myotis*) using echolocation. The animals were required to fly in a room containing vertically suspended wires. Wires of four different diameters were used (from 0.2 mm, about threshold for the normal bat, to 3.7 mm), and the number of contacts with the wires that the bat made in a test session was automatically recorded. Suga found that unilateral destruction of the inferior colliculus had no permanent behavioral effect on echolocation in bats.

In a lateralization experiment, Masterton *et al.* (1968) required cats (wearing earphones) to discriminate a click to the left ear from a click to the right ear (L vs. R). When the animals reached criterion on this task they were required to discriminate the sequence of a click to the left followed 0.5 mse later by a click to the right ear (LR vs. RL) from the reverse sequence. In normal cats the L vs. R discrimination transferred without additional training to the LR vs. RL task. Unilateral lesions of the lateral lemniscus did not interfere with training the animals on L vs. R but did prevent the transfer of this training to the LR vs. RL discrimination. However, the cats could be retrained to criterion on this latter discrimination and the Δt threshold was normal.

These experiments clearly show that responding to the position of a stimulus is possible after the unilateral destruction of the principal ascending auditory system, even under such natural conditions as echolocation. As pointed out by Masterton (1974) and Strominger and Oesterreich (1970), this does not mean that hearing has not been altered by such lesions, but simply that it has been altered in such a way that the animals are able to compensate for the deficiencies. It is possible, for example, that the left and right halves of auditory space are represented in the right and left sides of the auditory system at higher levels. Depriving the animal of the system on one side would abolish the ability to respond to the position of stimuli on the opposite side and force the animal to adopt postures that would ensure that the stimulus always falls on the unaffected side.

Neff and his collaborators have shown that such behavior following unilateral lesions of the principal system need not be based on monoaural stimulation. Cats can be trained to respond to stimulus position monoaurally, but the behavior is

445

FUNCTIONAL
PROPERTIES OF THE
AUDITORY SYSTEM OF
THE BRAIN
STEM

quite different from the behavior observed in the foregoing experiments. Mon-oaural animals, unlike normals, never perform at a level of 100% correct responses even for wide angles of the stimulus sources. The angular threshold is raised about 20°, and the monoaural animals require extensive training compared with normals (Casseday and Neff, 1975).

Bilateral lesions of the lateral lemniscus, central nucleus, or brachium of the inferior colliculus abolish (or severely affect) the ability to respond to stimulus position in cats, echolocation in bats, and head orientation to sounds in cats (Casseday and Neff, 1971, 1975; Casseday, 1970; Suga, 1969*b*; Strominger and Oesterreich, 1970; Belenkov and Goreva, 1969). Lateralization (LR vs. RL) is also abolished (Masterton *et al.*, 1968). Cats in which the behavior is abolished are able to discriminate a buzzer (or 1 kHz tone) from silence and are able to perform at an above chance level on the L vs. R discrimination. In the lateralization experiments it was shown that the cats could discriminate intensity differences by reducing the intensity of one of the stimuli in the L vs. R discrimination or the second stimulus in the sequence in the LR vs. RL discrimination.

Electrical stimulation of the central nucleus of the inferior colliculus produces orientation movements of the head (to the contralateral side) and also orienting movements of the eyes and pinnae. Weak stimulation produces movements of the contralateral pinna, and stronger stimulation produces movements of both pinnae (Gerken, 1970; Syka and Straschill, 1970). These data do not supply information on the functions of the inferior colliculus, but they do indicate that activity (although in this case involving unnatural discharge patterns) of the principal ascending system is accompanied by responses relevant to stimulus position.

Lesions confined to the upper part of the inferior colliculus (which destroy the pericentral, dorsomedial, and part of the external nuclei) and those which section the commissure of the inferior colliculus do not affect behavior in any of the behavioral tasks considered above (Suga, 1969*b*; Masterton *et al.*, 1968; Moore *et al.*, 1974). These lesions interfere predominantly with the descending auditory system, and the results indicate that disruption of this system does not interfere with localization behavior.

OTHER BEHAVIORAL EFFECTS OF MIDBRAIN LESIONS. A frequency discrimination (800 Hz vs. 1 kHz) was permanently abolished in cats following the bilateral destruction of the brachium of the inferior colliculus (Goldberg and Neff, 1961). These animals were still able to learn to avoid a shock at the onset of a buzzer. The auditory intensity difference limen was measured in cats at 65 dB prior to bilateral destruction of the brachium of the inferior colliculus. Destruction of the brachium raised the limen about 10 dB, while destruction of the inferior colliculus (in conjunction with destruction of the auditory cortex) raised the limen between 5 and 7 dB (Goldberg and Neff, 1961; Oesterreich *et al.*, 1971).

SUMMARY. The ability to respond to the position of a stimulus in the horizontal plane is the most affected of any of the aspects of hearing that have been investigated. While all preoperatively acquired auditory discriminations are abolished by bilateral midbrain lesions, intensity discriminations can be reacquired with only relatively small changes in the intensity limen. Response to stimulus position in the horizontal plane depends on binaural interaction in the principal auditory system that takes place in the superior olivary complex and the midbrain (as shown by physiological studies), and it appears that the whole principal ascending system is necessary for this behavior. At this stage it is not clear how responding to stimulus position in the horizontal plane is carried out in the nervous system. There are no units, up to the midbrain level, which give unique responses to particular positions of a stimulus. Under natural conditions binaural stimuli differ simultaneously in intensity, time, and also spectral content (for complex stimuli). These physical properties of the stimuli are correlated, and the discovery of units which show unique discharge patterns (should they exist) for particular positions of stimuli may require extensive examination of the physiology of the system under conditions in which the animal is presented with real stimuli originating in various positions.

The consideration of the ability of animals to respond to stimulus position is further complicated by the precedence effect (Wallach *et al.*, 1949). If two sounds with a short time interval between them (such as occur when a primary sound is followed by an echo) reach an animal, only the first of the pair exerts behavioral control in terms of position. This occurs even though (as is usually the case) the second sound comes from a different direction. Kelly (1974) has measured the time interval between two sounds over which the precedence effect holds and found the limits to be between about 30 μsec and 5 msec in the rat. The precedence effect allows an animal to distinguish between a primary sound and its echo provided that the echo-producing surface is so placed as to produce a delay of not greater than about 5 msec and not less than about 30 μsec. The physiological processes associated with the precedence effect are presumably set into activity by the first of the pair of sounds. It appears that these processes have not been distinguished from those associated with the control of responding by stimulus position, the observed action patterns of units in the midbrain usually being interpreted without the precedence effect in mind.

Electrophysiological data show that the central nucleus of the inferior colliculus responds in a complex way to the location, frequency, intensity, and other parameters of the stimulus. These complex responses have some role in hearing, but what this might be is not revealed by the ablation of the central nucleus and the effect that this lesion has on hearing. Such a lesion both destroys the complex responses of the nucleus and interrupts the pathway which includes the nucleus. What the behavioral experiments do show is whether or not the ascending pathway which was interrupted is essential for the auditory discrimination tested.

THE DESCENDING AUDITORY SYSTEM

ANATOMY AND PHYSIOLOGY.

It was first pointed out by Rasmussen (1946, 1953) that a bundle of efferent axons passes down the vestibular nerve, crosses to the acoustic nerve, and terminates among the hair cells of the cochlea. This bundle, the olivary peduncle of classical anatomy, was thought to arise in the vicinity of the superior olivary complex, and was shown to contain axons arising from both the ipsilateral (uncrossed olivocochlear bundle) and contralateral sides (crossed olivocochlear bundle). This discovery of the olivocochlear bundles led to work on both these axons and other components of what is now known as the descending auditory system. The central components of this system and its organization have been reviewed by Harrison and Howe (1974b), and Iurato (1974) has reviewed the work on the peripheral connections of the descending system in the cochlea.

The major nuclei and descending tracts of the descending system are shown in Fig. 21. Two descending systems start in area P (AI, AII, and Ep) of the auditory cortex in the cat. One system descends to the ventral division of the

447

FUNCTIONAL
PROPERTIES OF THE
AUDITORY SYSTEM OF
THE BRAIN
STEM

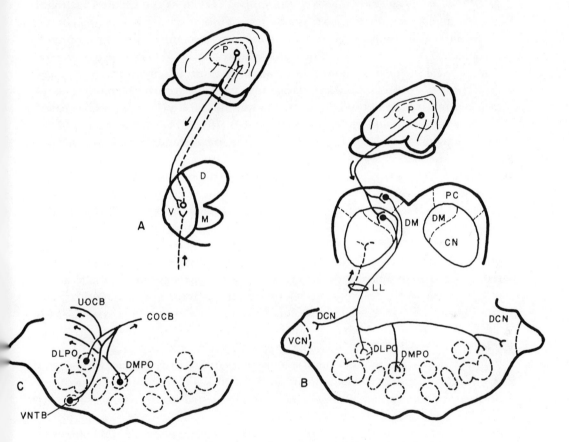

Fig. 21. Major components of the descending auditory system. A: The corticothalamic system. Axons descend to the ventral nucleus of the medial geniculate body. B: The cortico-inferior collicular system. Axons descend to the pericentral nucleus and the dorsomedial portion of the central nucleus. Axons descend from the inferior colliculus (site of origin uncertain) to the dorsal cochlear nucleus and the periolivary nuclei. Descending tracts in solid lines, ascending tracts in dashed lines. C: Origin of the crossed and uncrossed olivocochlear bundles. COCB, Crossed olivocochlear bundle; CN, central nucleus; D, dorsal division of the medial geniculate body; DCN, dorsal cochlear nucleus; DM, dorsomedial part of the central nucleus; DLPO, dorsolateral periolivary nucleus; DMPO, dorsomedial periolivary nucleus; P, principal auditory area of the cerebral cortex; PC, pericentral nucleus; LL, lateral lemniscus; M, medial nucleus of the medial geniculate body; UOCB, uncrossed olivocochlear bundle; V, ventral division of the medial geniculate body; VCN, ventral cochlear nucleus; VNTB, ventral nucleus of the trapezoid body. After Harrison and Howe (1974b), their Fig. 10A,B and Warr (1975).

medial geniculate body, where it terminates (Fig. 21A). The second descends from area P of the auditory cortex to the pericentral and dorsomedial nuclei of the inferior colliculus (Fig. 21B) (Diamond *et al.,* 1969). From these two nuclei axons descend to nerve cells located in and near the hilus of the lateral superior olivary nucleus (the dorsolateral periolivary nucleus) of both sides, to the dorsomedial periolivary nucleus of the same side, and to the dorsal cochlear nuclei of both sides. Warr (1975) has identified nerve cells in the hilus and vicinity of the lateral superior olive (part of the dorsolateral periolivary nucleus) and cells in the vicinity of the medial nucleus of the trapezoid body (the dorsomedial periolivary nucleus) as contributing to both the crossed and uncrossed olivocochlear bundles (Fig. 21C). He has also identified cells in the ventral nucleus of the trapezoid body as contributing principally to the crossed bundle. From this work it appears that the uncrossed bundle contains more axons than the crossed and that the total number is about 1800 axons in the kitten. The olivocochlear bundles also project to the anteroventral cochlear nucleus of both sides (Rasmussen, 1960).

The effect of electrically stimulating the crossed olivocochlear bundle (where it crosses in the floor of the IVth ventricle) was first shown to reduce whole action potentials of the cat auditory nerve by Galambos (1956). The N_1 component of the action potential to click stimuli was reduced. Galambos showed that this effect was not due to action of the middle ear muscles. The amount of inhibition under optimal conditions corresponds to a reduction of about 20 dB in the intensity of the stimulus. In the presence of a masking noise, the whole nerve action potential produced by tone burst stimulation may be unchanged, increased, or decreased depending on the intensity of the stimulus and the signal-to-noise ratio (Dewson, 1967; Nieder and Nieder, 1970; Klinke and Galley, 1974).

The response of single auditory nerve axons to clicks and tone bursts is also reduced by the stimulation of the crossed olivocochlear bundle. The maximum reduction occurs when the acoustic stimuli are of intermediate intensities, the effect being less at higher and lower intensities. The tails of tuning curves are also less affected than the V-shaped portion (Wiederhold, 1970; Teas *et al.,* 1972; Wiederhold and Kiang, 1970; Kiang *et al.,* 1970; Fex, 1962).

It is clear from the foregoing experiments that activity in the crossed (and possibly the uncrossed) olivocochlear bundle reduces the response of the acoustic nerve to auditory stimuli. This conclusion has suggested that the bundles are part of a feedback system (Rasmussen, 1955), which at the simplest level can be interpreted as adjusting the sensitivity of the cochlea as a function of the intensity and other parameters of the sound stimulus. Along the same lines, the effect of the system has also been seen as adjusting the sensitivity of the cochlea (and other levels in the auditory system) as a function of the state of the animal (sleepy, excited, habituated to a continuous sound, exposed to the sequence light–loud sound) (Galambos, 1960; Desmedt, 1960). A number of experiments, summarized by Whitfield (1967), have been carried out to test these ideas, but there is insufficient agreement among the findings to reach a conclusion. The evidence indicates, as Klinke and Galley point out, that sound may not even be the major source of stimulation of the bundles, since responses can be obtained in the

449

FUNCTIONAL
PROPERTIES OF THE
AUDITORY SYSTEM OF
THE BRAIN
STEM

crossed bundle only to sounds of greater than about 60 dB above threshold (Fex, 1962).

So far, little is known concerning the natural conditions under which the bundles are activated.

BEHAVIORAL STUDIES OF THE DESCENDING SYSTEM.

There have been few experiments on the behavioral functions of the crossed olivocochlear bundle. Galambos (1960) was unable to find changes in the absolute intensity or the differential intensity threshold in cats at 300 Hz, 1.5 kHz, and 5 kHz following cutting of the crossed bundle at the floor of the IVth ventricle. The differential frequency threshold was also unaffected. These measurements were made in the presence of a masking sound and the middle ear muscles were cut. Trahiotis and Elliott (1970) found no changes in the absolute intensity threshold (measured in silence in cats) or in the temporary threshold shift produced by exposure to a loud sound. They found a slight shift (3–7 dB) in masked intensity thresholds.

Dewson (1968) found behavioral changes following the cutting of the crossed bundle in rhesus monkeys. Masking of the discrimination of vowel sounds (i vs. u) was increased following the lesion by about 15 dB, while the discrimination in silence was unaffected. Capps and Ades (1968) found an increase in the differential frequency threshold in squirrel monkeys following transection of the crossed bundle. At 1 kHz the differential threshold was changed, typically, from 1.1 kHz to 1.5 kHz and at 4 kHz from 4.3 to 4.9 kHz.

We have already seen in the preceding section that the interruption of the descending system at the level of the pericentral and dorsomedial nuclei of the inferior colliculus has no effect on localization, lateralization, or echolocation.

There is simply insufficient information at this time to come to any firm conclusions regarding the behavioral functions of the descending systems.

CONCLUSIONS

The following speculations can be drawn from the material presented in this chapter.

TONOTOPIC ORGANIZATION

There is both anatomical and physiological evidence of tonotopic organization throughout the principal auditory system from the acoustic nerve to the inferior colliculus. That is, the receptor surface is represented in an orderly and approximately isomorphic manner at different levels in the system. In this regard the auditory system resembles the visual and somasthetic systems. Since isomorphism is the general rule in the sensory systems, it is presumably necessary for the same reasons in all three systems. The sensory surfaces of the three systems are bilateral, and since bilateral connections occur at various levels in all three systems, the isomorphic organization may ensure that corresponding regions of the respective sensory surfaces come together at the bilaterally innervated nerve cells. Since the ability of mammals to respond to the position of sounds depends principally upon binaural stimulation, the isomorphic organization in the auditory system may be essential for the appropriate bilateral innervation of nerve cells in the superior olivary complex and the inferior colliculus.

As in other systems, isomorphic organization in the auditory system is not physiologically sharp in the sense that a tone of given frequency fires only a narrow range of units at any level. There is no "point-to-point" functional projection of the cochlea on the auditory system. With the system as it is, stimuli of different parameters fire different (but necessarily overlapping) groups of neurons at each level. The bulk of the system is used with many stimuli, making its usage "efficient" compared with a system possessing "point-to-point" isomorphism in which only a small fraction of the system would be used in connection with the majority of stimuli.

The evidence presented in this chapter does not support the idea that tonotopic organization is uniquely related to frequency discrimination. The destruction of part of the system—for example, the base of the cochlea—prevents an animal from being controlled by any aspects of sounds which fall within the frequency range of the destroyed region, and which are of insufficient intensity to fire the remaining healthy portion of the cochlea (Stebbins, 1970). The animal is deaf at high frequencies. However, some aspects of hearing (loudness functions, for example) for frequencies which fall within the range of the undestroyed part of the cochlea may also be altered.

FIRING PATTERNS

At the level of the acoustic nerve and cochlear nucleus, nerve cells tend to fire in a sustained manner for the duration of the stimulus (except for the *on* units in the cochlear nucleus). The duration of the discharge to tones is about equal to the duration of the tone. However, at the level of the inferior colliculus the firing patterns are radically different. At the higher levels, many units may show only a transitory response or one or two spikes with a constant latency (depending upon stimulus parameters) while others may show both transitory and sustained responses. Others, again depending on particular stimulus parameters, may show only *off* responses. Many of these firing patterns show little resemblance to the initiating stimuli. The significance of the firing patterns at the various levels is not known, nor is there any clear evidence that such stimulus parameters as frequency, intensity and relative position to the animal's midline are independently coded.

RESPONSES TO THE POSITIONS OF EVENTS IN THE ACOUSTIC ENVIRONMENT

The ability of an animal to respond to the relative positions of events in its acoustic environment depends on binaural stimulation coupled with the rejection of responding to the apparent position of echos. The large amount of bilateral innervation found at all levels above the cochlea nucleus in the auditory system compared to other sensory systems may be a reflection of the translation of binaural stimulation into appropriate orientation and movement. The evidence indicates that bilateral innervation of nerve cells at the levels of the superior olivary complex and probably the inferior colliculus is necessary for an animal to respond to the position of an auditory event.

Comparative Variation

The auditory system differs radically in different mammalian species, as does the frequency range of hearing. These differences are in part probably adaptations of hearing to the size of the animal, especially with respect to the basis of its ability to respond to the positions of events in its acoustic environment.

Acknowledgments

The research of Harrison, Irving, Feldman, Downey, Segal, Howe, Beecher, and West referred to was sponsored by various National Science Foundation grants to Boston University. I thank Mary T. Turnock for her constructive criticism and advice on this chapter and its earlier drafts. I also thank her for the drafting of the figures.

References

Aitkin, L. M., Anderson, D. J., and Brugge, J. F. Tonotopic organization and discharge characteristics of single units in the inferior colliculus of the alert cat. *J. Neurophysiol.*, 1970, *33*, 421–440.

Barnes, W. T., Magoun, H. S., and Ranson, S. W. Ascending auditory pathways in the brainstem of the monkey. *J. Comp. Neurol.*, 1943, *79*, 129–152.

Beecher, M. D. Pure tone thresholds of the squirrel monkey. *J. Acoust. Soc. Am.*, 1974a, *56*, 139–144.

Beecher, M. D. Hearing in the owl monkey. I. Auditory sensitivity. *J. Comp. Physiol. Psychol.*, 1974b, *86*, 422–426.

Belenkov, N. J., and Goreva, O. A. Role of posterior colliculus in orienting reflexes. *J. Higher Nervous Activity*, 1969, *19*, 453–461 (Russian).

Benevento, L. A., Coleman, P., and Loe, R. R. Responses of single units at inferior colliculus to binaural click stimuli; contribution of intensity levels, time difference and intensity difference. *Brain Res.*, 1970, *17*, 387–404.

Bock, G. R., and Webster, W. R. Coding of spatial localization by single units in the inferior colliculus of the cat. *Exp. Brain Res.*, 1974, *18*, 387–398.

Bock, G. R., Webster, W. R., and Aitkin, L. M. Discharge patterns of single units in the inferior colliculus of the alert cat. *J. Neurophysiol.*, 1972, *35*, 265–277.

Boudreau, J. C., and Tsuchitani, C. Binaural interaction in the cat superior olive S-segment. *J. Neurophysiol.*, 1968, *31*, 442–454.

Boudreau, J. C., and Tsuchitani, C. Cat superior olive S-segment cell discharge to tonal stimuli. In W. D. Neff (ed.), *Contributions to Sensory Physiology*, Vol. 4. Academic Press, New York, 1970.

Brewer, J. R., and Morest, D. K. Relations between auditory nerve endings and cell types in the cat's anteroventral cochlear nucleus seen with the Golgi method and Nemarski optics. *J. Comp. Neurol.*, 1975, *160*, 491–506.

Brewer, J. R., Morest, D. K., and Kane, E. The neuronal architecture of the cochlear nucleus of the cat. *J. Comp. Neurol.*, 1974, *155*, 251–300.

Brugge, J. F., Anderson, D. J., and Aitkin, L. M. Response of neurons in the dorsal nucleus of the lateral lemniscus of cat to binaural tonal stimulation. *J. Neurophysiol.,* 1970, *33,* 441–459.

Capps, M. J., and Ades, H. W. Auditory frequency discrimination after transection of the olivocochlear bundle in squirrel monkeys. *Exp. Neurol.,* 1968, *21,* 147–158.

Casseday, J. H. Auditory localization; the role of the brainstem auditory pathways in the cat. Ph.D. dissertation, Department of Psychology, Indiana University, 1970.

Casseday, J. H., and Neff, W. D. Auditory localization; role of the lateral lemniscus. *J. Acoust. Soc. Am.,* 1971, *50,* 118.

Casseday, J. H., and Neff, W. D. Localization of pure tones. *J. Acoust. Soc. Am.,* 1973, *54,* 365–372.

Casseday, J. H., and Neff, W. D. Auditory localization; the role of the auditory pathways in the brainstem of the cat. *J. Neurophysiol.,* 1975, *38,* 451–462.

Clark, G. M. The ultrastructure of nerve endings in the medial superior olive in the cat. *Brain Res.,* 1969a, *14,* 293–305.

Clark, G. M. Vescicle shape versus type of synapse in the endings of the cat medial superior olive. *Brain Res.,* 1969b, *15,* 548–551.

Clopton, B. M., and Winfield, J. A. Unit responses in the inferior colliculus of the rat to temporal patterns of tone sweeps and noise bursts. *Exp. Neurol.,* 1974, *42,* 532–540.

Cohen, E. S., Brewer, J. R., and Morest, D. K. Projections of the cochlear nerve to the dorsal cochlear nucleus in the cat. *Anat. Rec.,* 1972, *172,* 294.

Cohen Kane, E. Octopus cells in the cochlear nucleus of the cat; heterotypic synapses upon hemeotypic neurons. *Int. J. Neurosci.,* 1973, *5,* 251–279.

Dalland, J. I. Hearing sensitivity in bats. *Science,* 1965, *150,* 1185–1186.

Dalland, J. I. The measurement of ultrasonic hearing. In W. C. Stebbins (ed.), *Animal Psychophysics.* Appleton-Century-Crofts, New York, 1970, pp. 21–40.

Dewson, J. H. Efferent olivocochlear bundle; some relationships to noise masking and to stimulus attenuation. *J. Neurophysiol.,* 1967, *30,* 817–832.

Dewson, J. H. Efferent olivocochlear bundle; some relationships to discrimination in noise. *J. Neurophysiol.,* 1968, *31,* 122–130.

Desmedt, J. E. Neurological mechanisms controlling acoustic input. In G. L. Rasmussen and W. W. Windle (eds.), *Neural Mechanisms of the Auditory and Vestibular Systems.* Thomas, Springfield, Ill., 1960, pp. 152–164.

Diamond, I. T., Jones, E. G., and Powell, T. P. S. The projection of the auditory cortex upon the dienrephalon and brainstem in the cat. *Brain Res.,* 1969, *15,* 305–340.

Downey, P., and Harrison, J. M. Control of responding by the location of auditory stimuli; role of differential and nondifferential reinforcement. *J. Exp. Anal. Behav.,* 1972, *18,* 453–464.

Elliott, D. N. Effect of peripheral lesions on acuity and discrimination in animals. In A. B. Graham (ed.), *Sensorineural Processes and Disorders.* Little, Brown, Boston, 1967, pp. 179–189.

Elliott, D. N., Stein, L., and Harrison, J. J. Determination of absolute intensity thresholds and frequency difference thresholds in cats. *J. Acoust. Soc. Am.,* 1960, *32,* 380–384.

Erulkar, S. D. Responses of single units of the inferior colliculus of the cat to acoustic stimulation. *Proc. Roy. Soc. London Ser. B,* 1959, *150,* 336–355.

Erulkar, S. D. Comparative aspects of spatial localization of sound. *Physiol. Rev.,* 1972, *52,* 237–360.

Fattu, J. Acoustic orientation of the rabbit pinna and external auditory meatus. *J. Acoust. Soc. Am.,* 1969, *46,* 124.

Feldman, M. L., and Harrison, J. M. The projection of the acoustic nerve to the ventral cochlear nucleus of the rat: A Golgi study. *J. Comp. Neurol.,* 1969, *137,* 267–294.

Feldman, M. L., and Harrison, J. M. The superior olivary complex in primates. In *Medical Primatology.* Karger, Basel, 1971.

Fernandez, C., and Karapas, F. The course of the striae of Monokow and Held in the cat. *J. Comp. Neurol.,* 1967, *131,* 371–381.

Fex, J. Auditory activity in centrifugal and centripetal cochlear fibers in the cat. *Acta Physiol. Scand.,* 1962, *55,* Supple. 189, 5–68.

Flammino, F., and Clapton, B. Neural responses in the inferior colliculus of albino rat to binaural stimuli. *J. Acous. Soc. Am.,* 1975, *57,* 692–695.

Friend, J. H., Suga, N., and Suthers, R. A. Neural responses in the inferior colliculus of echolocating bats to artificial orientation sounds and echos. *J. Cell Physiol.,* 1966, *67,* 319–332.

Galambos, R. Neural mechanisms of audition. *Physiol. Rev.,* 1954, *34,* 497–528.

Galambos, R. Suppression of auditory nerve activity by stimulation of efferent fibers to the cochlea. *J. Neurophysiol.,* 1956, *19,* 424–437.

453

FUNCTIONAL
PROPERTIES OF THE
AUDITORY SYSTEM OF
THE BRAIN
STEM

Galambos, R. Studies of the auditory system with implanted electrodes. In G. J. Rasmussen and W. W. Windle (eds.), *Neural Mechanisms of the Auditory and Vestibular Systems.* Thomas, Springfield, Ill., 1960, pp. 137–151.

Galambos, R., Schwartzkopff, J., and Rupert, A. Microelectrode study of the superior olivary complex. *Am. J. Physiol.,* 1959, *197*, 517–536.

Geisler, C. G., Rhode, W. S., and Hazleton, D. W. Responses of inferior colliculus neurons in the cat to binaural acoustic stimuli having wideband spectra. *J. Neurophysiol.,* 1969, *32*, 960–974.

Geniec, P., and Morest, D. K. The neuronal architecture of the human posterior colliculus. *Acta Otolaryngol (Stockholm).* 1971, Suppl. 295, 1–33.

Gerken, G. M. Electrical stimulation of the subcortical auditory system in behaving cat. *Brain Res.,* 1970, *17*, 483–497.

Gerstein, G. L., Butler, R. A., and Erulkar, S. D. Excitation and inhibition in cochlear nucleus. I. Tone burst stimulation. *J. Neurophysiol.,* 1968, *31*, 526–536.

Goldberg, J. M., and Brown, P. B. Functional organization of dog superior olivary complex; an anatomical and physiological study. *J. Neurophysiol.,* 1968, *31*, 639–656.

Goldberg, J. M., and Moore, R. Y. Ascending projections of the lateral lemniscus in the cat and monkey. *J. Comp. Neurol.,* 1967, *129*, 143–155.

Goldberg, J. M., and Neff, W. D. Frequency discrimination after bilateral section of the brachium of the inferior colliculus. *J. Comp. Neurol.,* 1961, *116*, 265–290.

Goldberg, J. M., Adrian, H. O., and Smith, F. D. Responses of neurons of superior olivary complex to acoustic stimuli of long duration. *J. Neurophysiol.,* 1964, *27*, 706–749.

Greenwood, D. D., and Goldberg, J. M. Responses of neurons in the cochlear nuclei to variations in noise bandwidth and tone–noise combinations. *J. Acoust. Soc. Am.,* 1970, *47*, 1022–1040.

Grinnell, A. D. The neurophysiology of audition in bats; intensity and frequency parameters. *J. Physiol. (London),* 1963a, *167*, 38–66.

Grinnell, A. D. The neurophysiology of audition in bats; directional localization and binaural interaction. *J. Physiol. (London),* 1963b, *167*, 97–113.

Guinan, J. J., Guinan, S. S., and Norris, B. E. Single auditory units in the superior olivary complex. I. Responses to sounds and classifications based on physiological properties. *Int. J. Neurosci.,* 1972a, *4*, 101–120.

Guinan, J. J., Norris, B. E. and Guinan, S. S. Single auditory units in the superior olivary complex. II. Location of unit categories and tonotopic organization. *Int. J. Neurosci.,* 1972b, *4*, 147–166.

Hall, J. D., and Johnson, C. S. Auditory thresholds of a killer whale. *J. Acoust. Soc. Am.,* 1971, *51*, 515–517.

Harrison, J. M. Cells of origin of the stria of Held. *Anat. Rec.,* 1966, *154*, 463–464.

Harrison, J. M. The auditory system of the medulla and localization. *Fed. Proc.,* 1974, *33*, 1901–1903.

Harrison, J. M., and Beecher, M. D. Control of responding by the location of an auditory stimulus. *J. Exp. Anal. Behav.,* 1969, *12*, 217–228.

Harrison, J. M., and Downey, P. Intensity changes at the ear as a function of the azimuth of a tone source; a comparative study. *J. Acoust. Soc. Am.,* 1970, *47*, 1509–1518.

Harrison, J. M., and Feldman, M. L. Anatomical aspects of the cochlear nucleus and superior olivary complex. In W. D. Neff (ed.), *Contributions to Sensory Physiology,* Vol. 4. Academic Press, New York, 1970, pp. 95–143.

Harrison, J. M., and Howe, M. Anatomy of the afferent auditory system of mammals. In W. D. Keidel and W. D. Neff (eds.), *Handbook of Sensory Physiology,* Vol. V/1. Springer, Berlin, 1974a, pp. 283–336.

Harrison, J. M., and Howe, M. Anatomy of the descending auditory system (mammalian). In W. D. Keidel and W. D. Neff (eds.), *Handbook of Sensory Physiology,* Vol. V/1. Springer, Berlin, 1974b, pp. 363–388.

Harrison, J. M., and Irving, R. Nucleus of the trapezoid body; dual afferent innervation. *Science,* 1964, *143*, 473–474.

Harrison, J. M., and Irving, R. The anterior ventral cochlear nucleus. *J. Comp. Neurol.,* 1965, *124*, 15–42.

Harrison, J. M., and Irving, R. The organization of the posterior ventral cochlear nucleus. *J. Comp. Neurol.,* 1966a, *126*, 391–402.

Harrison, J. M., and Irving, R. Visual and nonvisual auditory systems in mammals. *Science,* 1966b, *154*, 738–743.

Harrison, J. M., and Turnock, T. Animal psychophysics; improvements in the tracking method. *J. Exp. Anal. Behav.,* 1975, *23*, 141–148.

Harrison, J. M., and Warr, B. A study of the cochlear nucleus and ascending pathways of the medulla. *J. Comp. Neurol.*, 1962, *119*, 341–380.

Heffner, H. E., Ravizza, R. J., and Masterton, B. Hearing in primitive mammals. III. Tree shrew. *J. Aud. Res.*, 1969*a*, *9*, 12–18.

Heffner, H. E., Ravizza, R. J., and Masterton, B. Hearing in primitive mammals. IV. Bushbaby. *J. Aud. Res.*, 1969*b*, *9*, 19–23.

Heffner, R., Heffner, H., and Masterton, B. Behavioral measurements of absolute and frequency difference thresholds in guinea pig. *J. Acoust. Soc. Am.*, 1970, *49*, 1888–1895.

Hind, J. E., Goldberg, J. M., Greenwood, D. D., and Rose, J. E. Some discharge characteristics of single neurons in the inferior colliculus of the cat. II. Timing of discharges and observations on binaural stimulation. *J. Neurophysiol.*, 1963, *26*, 321–341.

Irving, R., and Harrison, J. M. Superior olivary complex and audition; a comparative study. *J. Comp. Neurol.*, 1967, *130*, 77–86.

Iurato, S. Efferent innervation. In W. D. Keidel and W. D. Neff (eds.), *Handbook of Sensory Physiology*, Vol. V/1. Springer, Berlin, 1974.

Jacobs, D. W., and Hall, J. D. Auditory thresholds of fresh water dolphins, *Inia geoffrensis. J. Acoust. Soc. Am.*, 1971, *51*, 530–533.

Johnson, C. S. Auditory thresholds in the bottle nosed dolphin. United States Naval Ordinance Test Station, TP 4178, 1966, 1–22.

Keidel, W. D., and Neff, W. D. (eds.). *Handbook of Sensory Physiology*, Vol. V/1. Springer, Berlin, 1974.

Kelly, J. B. Localization of paired sound sources in the rat; small time differences. *J. Acoust. Soc. Am.*, 1974, *55*, 1277–1284.

Kiang, N. The use of computers in the study of auditory neurophysiology. *Trans. Am. Acad. Ophthalmol. Otolaryngol.*, 1961, *65*, 735–747.

Kiang, N. Stimulus coding in the auditory nerve and cochlear nucleus. *Acta Otolaryngol.*, 1965*a*, *59*, 186–200.

Kiang, N. *Discharge Patterns of Single Fibers in the Cat's Auditory Nerve.* Research Monograph No. 35, MIT Press, Cambridge, Mass., 1965*b*.

Kiang, N., and Moxon, E. C. Tails of tuning curves of auditory nerve fibers. *J. Acoust. Soc. Am.*, 1974, *55*, 620–630.

Kiang, N., Pfeiffer, R. R., Warr, B., and Backus, A. S. N. Stimulus coding in the cochlear nucleus. *Ann. Otolaryngol.*, 1965, *74*, 463–485.

Kiang, N., Moxon, E. C., and Levine, R. A. Auditory nerve activity in cats with normal and abnormal cochleas. In G. E. W. Wolsterholme and J. Knight (eds.), *Sensorineural Hearing Loss.* J. A. Churchill, London, 1970, pp. 241–273.

Kiang, N., Watanabe, T., Thomas, E. C., and Clark, L. F. Stimulus coding in the cat's auditory nerve. *Ann. Otol. Rhinol. Laryngol.*, 1972, *71*, 2–18.

Kiang, N., Morest, D. K., Godfrey, D. A., Guinan, J. J., and Kane, E. C. Stimulus coding at caudal levels of the cat's auditory system. I. Response characteristics of single units. In A. R. Møller (ed.), *Basic Mechanisms in Hearing.* Academic Press, New York, 1973, pp. 455–478.

Klinke, R., and Galley, N. Efferent innervation of vestibular and auditory receptors. *Physiol. Rev.*, 1974, *54*, 316–357.

Lenn, N. J., and Reese, T. S. The fine structure of the nerve endings in the nucleus of the trapezoid body and the ventral cochlear nucleus. *Am. J. Anat.*, 1966, *118*, 375–389.

Lorente de No, R. Anatomy of the eighth nerve. III. General plan of structure of the primary cochlear nuclei. *Laryngoscope*, 1933, *43*, 327–350.

MacDonald, D. M., and Rasmussen, G. L. Ultrastructural characteristics of synaptic endings in the cochlear nucleus having acetylcholinesterase activity. *Brain Res.*, 1971, *28*, 1–18.

Mast, T. E. Study of single units of the cochlear nucleus of the chinchilla. *J. Acoust. Soc. Am.*, 1970*a*, *48*, 505–512.

Mast, T. E. Binaural interaction and contralateral inhibition in dorsal cochlear nucleus in chinchilla. *J. Neurophysiol.*, 1970*b*, *33*, 108–115.

Masterton, B. Adaptation for sound localization in the brainstem of mammals. *Fed. Proc.*, 1974, *33*, 1904–1910.

Masterton, B., and Diamond, I. T. Medial superior olive and sound localization. *Science*, 1967, *155*, 1696–1697.

Masterton, B., Jane, J. A., and Diamond, I. T. The role of brainstem auditory structures in sound localization. I. Trapezoid body, superior olive and lateral lemniscus. *J. Neurophysiol.*, 1967, *30*, 341–359.

455

FUNCTIONAL
PROPERTIES OF THE
AUDITORY SYSTEM OF
THE BRAIN
STEM

Masterton, R. B., Jane, J. A., and Diamond, I. T. Role of brainstem auditory structures in sound localization. II. Inferior colliculus and its brachium. *J. Neurophysiol.*, 1968, *31*, 960–1008.

Masterton, R. B., Heffner, H. E., and Ravizza, R. J. The evolution of human hearing. *J. Acoust. Soc. Am.*, 1969, *45*, 966–985.

Masterton, R. B., Thompson, G. C., Bechtold, J. K., and Robards, M. J. Neuroanatomical basis of binaural phase-difference analysis for sound localization; a comparative study. *J. Comp. Physiol. Psychol.*, 1975, *89*, 379–386.

Miller, J. D. Audibility curve in chinchilla. *J. Acoust. Soc. Am.*, 1970, *48*, 513–523.

Miller, J. D., Watson, C. S., and Covell, W. P. Deafening effects of noise on the cat. *Acta Orolaryngol.*, 1963, Suppl. 176, 1–28.

Møhl, B. Auditory of the common seal in the air and water. *J. Aud. Res.*, 1968, *8*, 27–38.

Møller, A. R. *Basic Mechanisms in Hearing.* Academic Press, New York, 1973.

Moore, C. N., Casseday, J. H., and Neff, W. D. Sound localization; the role of the commissural pathways of the auditory system of the cat. *Brain Res.*, 1974, *82*, 13–27.

Moore, J. K., and Moore, R. Y. A comparative study of the superior olivary complex in primate brains. *Folia Primatol.*, 1971, *16*, 35–51.

Morest, D. K. The laminar structure of the inferior colliculus of the cat. *Anat. Rec.*, 1964, *148*, 314.

Morest, D. K. The lateral tegmental system of the midbrain and medial geniculate body; a study with Nauta and Golgi methods in the cat. *J. Anat.*, 1965, *99*, 611–634.

Morest, D. K. The cortical structure of the inferior quadrigeminal lamina of the cat. *Anat. Rec.*, 1966a, *154*, 314.

Morest, D. K. The non-cortical neuronal architecture of the inferior colliculus of the cat. *Anat. Rec.*, 1966b, *154*, 477.

Morest, D. K. The collateral system of the medial nucleus of the trapezoid body of the cat; its neurological architecture and relation to the olivocochlear bundle. *Brain Res.*, 1968, *9*, 288–311.

Morest, D. K. Auditory neurons of the brainstem. *Adv. Oto-Rhino-Laryngol.*, 1973, *20*, 337–356.

Morest, D. K., Kiang, N., Kane, E. C., Guinan, J. J., and Godfrey, D. A. Stimulus coding at caudal levels in the cat's auditory system. II. Patterns of synaptic organization. In A. R. Møller (ed.), *Basic Mechanisms in Hearing.* Academic Press, New York, 1973, pp. 479–504.

Moskowitz, N., and Liu, J. C. Central projections of the spiral ganglion of the squirrel monkey. *J. Comp. Neurol.*, 1972, *144*, 335–344.

Moushegian, G., and Rupert, A. L. Response diversity of neurons in the ventral cochlear nucleus of kangaroo rat. *J. Neurophysiol.*, 1970, *33*, 351–364.

Neff, W. D., and Hind, J. E. Auditory thresholds in the cat. *J. Acoust. Soc. Am.*, 1955, *27*, 480–483.

Neff, W. D., Fisher, J. F., Diamond, I. T., and Yela, M. Role of auditory cortex in discriminations requiring localization of sound in space. *J. Neurophysiol.*, 1956, *19*, 500–512.

Nelson, P. G., and Erulkar, S. D. Synaptic mechanisms of excitation and inhibition in the central auditory pathway. *J. Neurophysiol.*, 1963, *26*, 908–923.

Nelson, P. G., Erulkar, S. D., and Byron, J. S. Responses of units of the inferior colliculus to time varying acoustic stimuli. *J. Neurophysiol.*, 1966, *29*, 834–860.

Nieder, P., and Nieder, I. Antimasking of crossed olivocochlear bundle stimulation with loud clicks in guinea pigs. *Exp. Neurol.*, 1970, *28*, 179–188.

Noback, C. R. Brain of gorilla. II. Brainstem nuclei. *J. Comp. Neurol.*, 1959, *111*, 345–386.

Oesterreich, R. E., Strominger, N., and Neff, W. D. Neural structures mediating differential sound intensity discrimination in the cat. *Brain Res.*, 1971, *27*, 251–270.

Olszewski, J., and Baxter, D. *Cytoarchitecture of the Human Brainstem.* Karger, Basel, 1954.

Osen, K. K. Cytoarchitecture of the cochlear nuclei in the cat. *J. Comp. Neurol.*, 1969, *136*, 453–448.

Osen, K. K. Course and termination of primary afferents in the cochlear nucleus of cat; an experimental anatomical study. *Arch. Ital. Biol.*, 1970, *108*, 21–51.

Osen, K. K. The projection of the cochlear nucleus on the inferior colliculus of the cat. *J. Comp. Neurol.*, 1972, *144*, 355–369.

Pfeiffer, R. R. Classifications of response patterns of spike discharges for units in the cochlear nucleus; tone burst stimulation. *Exp. Brain Res.*, 1966, *1*, 220–235.

Pfeiffer, R. R., and Kim, D. O. Response patterns of single cochlear nerve fibers to click stimuli; descriptions for cat. *J. Acoust. Soc. Am.*, 1972, *52*, 1669–1677.

Powell, T. P. S., and Cowan, W. M. An experimental study of the projections of the cochlea. *J. Anat.*, 1962, *69*, 269–284.

Powell, T. P. S., and Erulkar, S. D. Transneuronal cell degeneration in the auditory relay nuclei of the cat. *J. Anat.*, 1962, *69*, 249–268.

Ramon y Cajal, S. *Histologie du Systeme Nerveux de l'Homme et des Vertébrés,* Vol. 1. Instituto Ramon y Cajal, Madrid, 1952.

Rasmussen, G. L. The olivary peduncle and other fiber projections of the superior olivary complex. *J. Comp. Neurol.,* 1946, *84,* 141–219.

Rasmussen, G. L. Further observations on the efferent cochlear bundle. *J. Comp. Neurol.,* 1953, *99,* 61–74.

Rasmussen, G. L. Descending or "feedback" connections of auditory system of cat. *Am. J. Physiol.,* 1955, *183,* 653.

Rasmussen, G. L. Efferent fibers of the cochlea nerve and cochlear nucleus. In G. L. Rasmussen and W. W. Windle (eds.), *Neural Mechanisms of the Auditory and Vestibular System.* Thomas, Springfield, Ill., 1960, pp. 105–115.

Rasmussen, G. L. Efferent connections of the cochlear nucleus. In A. B. Graham (ed.), *Sensorineural Hearing Processes and Disorders.* Little, Brown, Boston, 1965.

Ravizza, R. J., Heffner, H. E., and Masterton, B. Hearing in primitive mammals. II. Hedgehog. *J. Aud. Res.,* 1969a, *9,* 8–11.

Ravizza, R. J., Heffner, H. E., and Masterton, B. Hearing in primitive mammals. I. Opossum. *J. Aud. Res.,* 1969b, *9,* 1–7.

Reese, T. S. Fine structure of the nerve endings in ventral cochlear nucleus of normal and experimental animals. *Anat. Rec.,* 1966, *154,* 408–409.

Rockel, A. J. Observations of the inferior colliculus of the adult cat stained by the Golgi technique. *Brain Res.,* 1971, *30,* 407–410.

Rockel, A. J., and Jones, E. G. The neuronal organization of the inferior colliculus of the adult cat. I. Central nucleus. *J. Comp. Neurol.,* 1973a, *147,* 11–60.

Rockel, A. J., and Jones, E. G. Observations of the fine structure of the inferior colliculus of the cat. *J. Comp. Neurol.,* 1973b, *147,* 61–92.

Rose, J. E. Organization of frequency units in the cochlear nucleus complex of the cat. In G. L. Rasmussen and W. W. Windle (eds.), *Neural Mechanisms of the Auditory and Vestibular Systems.* Springfield, Ill., 1960, pp. 116–136.

Rose, J. E., Galambos, R., and Hughes, J. Microelectrode studies of the cochlear nuclei of the cat. *J. Johns Hopkins Hosp.,* 1959, *104,* 211–251.

Rose, J. E., Greenwood, D. D., Goldberg, J. M., and Hind, J. E. Some discharge characteristics of single neurons in the inferior colliculus of the cat. I. Tonotopic organization relation of spike counts to the tone intensity and firing patterns of single elements. *J. Neurophysiol.,* 1963, *26,* 294–320.

Rose, J. E., Brugge, J. F., Anderson, D. J., and Hind, J. E. Phase locked response to low frequency tones in single auditory nerve fibers of the squirrel monkey. *J. Neurophysiol.,* 1967, *30,* 769–793.

Rose, J. E., Anderson, D. J., Hind, J. E., and Brugge, J. F. Some effects of stimulus intensity on response of auditory nerve fibers in the squirrel monkey. *J. Neurophysiol.,* 1971, *34,* 685–700.

Rupert, A., Moushegian, G., and Galambos, R. Unit responses to sound from auditory nerve of cat. *J. Neurophysiol.,* 1963, *26,* 449–465.

Sando, I. The anotomical interrelationships of the cochlear nerve fiber. *Acta Oto-Laryngol Suppl,* 1965, *59,* 417–436.

Schuknecht, H. F. Neuroanatomical correlates of auditory sensitivity and pitch discrimination in the cat. In G. L. Rasmussen and W. W. Windle (eds.), *Neural Mechanisms of the Auditory and Vestibular Systems.* Thomas, Springfield, Ill., 1960, pp. 76–90.

Schusterman, R. J., Balliet, R. F., and Nixon, J. Underwater audiogram of the California sea lion by the conditioned vocalization technique. *J. Exp. Anal. Behav.,* 1972, *17,* 339–350.

Simmons, J. A. The resolution of target range by echolocating bats. *J. Acoust. Soc. Am.,* 1973, *54,* 157–173.

Simmons, J. A., and Vernon, J. Echolocation; discrimination of targets by the bat. *J. Exp. Zool.,* 1971, *176,* 315–328.

Sivian, L. J., and White, S. D. On minimum audible auditory fields. *J. Acoust. Soc. Am.,* 1933, *4,* 288–321.

Spoendlin, H. The organization of the cochlear receptor. *Adv. Oto-Rhino-Laryngol.,* 1966, *13,* 1–115.

Spoendlin, H. The innervation of the cochlear receptors. In A. R. Møller, (ed.), *Basic Mechanisms in Hearing.* Academic Press, New York, 1973, pp. 185–234.

Starr, A., and Britt, R. Intracellular recording from cat cochlear nucleus during tone stimulation. *J. Neurophysiol.,* 1970, *33,* 137–147.

Starr, A., and Don, M. Responses of squirrel monkey medial geniculate body to binaural clicks. *J. Neurophysiol.,* 1972, *35,* 501–517.

457

FUNCTIONAL
PROPERTIES OF THE
AUDITORY SYSTEM OF
THE BRAIN
STEM

Starr, A., and Livingston, R. B. Long lasting nervous system responses to prolonged sound stimulation in waking cats. *J. Neurophysiol*, 1963, *26*, 416–431.

Stebbins, W. C. Studies of hearing and hearing loss in the monkey. In W. C. Stebbins (ed.), *Animal Psychophysics*. Appleton-Century-Crofts, New York, 1970, pp. 41–66.

Stillman, R. D. Responses of one type of neuron in the inferior colliculus of the kangaroo rat. *J. Acoust. Soc. Am.*, 1974, *47*, 76.

Stotler, W. S. An experimental study of the cells and connections of the superior olivary complex of the cat. *J. Comp. Neurol.*, 1953, *98*, 401–432.

Strominger, N. L., and Bacsik, R. D. The anteroventral cochlear nucleus in man and the rhesus monkey. *Anat. Rec.*, 1972, *172*, 413.

Strominger, N. L., and Oesterreich, R. E. Localization of sound after section of the brachium of the inferior colliculus. *J. Comp. Neurol.*, 1970, *138*, 1–18.

Strominger, N. L., and Strominger, A. I. Ascending brainstem projection of the anteroventral cochlear nucleus in the monkey. *J. Comp. Neurol.*, 1971, *143*, 217–232.

Suga, N. Single unit activity in cochlear nucleus and inferior colliculus of echolocating bats. *J. Physiol. (London)*, 1964, *172*, 449–474.

Suga, N. Classification of inferior colliculus neurons of bats in terms of responses to pure tones, frequency modulated sounds and noise bursts. *J. Physiol. (London)*, 1969a, *200*, 555–574.

Suga, N. Echolocation and evoked potentials of bats after ablation of the inferior colliculus. *J. Physiol. (London)*, 1969b, *203*, 707–728.

Suga, N. Responses of inferior colliculus neurons of bats to tone bursts with different rise times. *J. Physiol. (London)*, 1971, *217*, 159–177.

Suga, N. Feature extraction in the auditory system of bats. In A. R. Møller (ed.), *Basic Mechanisms in Hearing*. Academic Press, New York, 1973, pp. 675–742.

Syka, J., and Straschill, M. Activation of motor responses after electrical stimulation of the inferior colliculus. *Exp. Neurol.*, 1970, *28*, 384–392.

Taber, E. The cytoarchitecture of the brainstem of the cat. I. Brainstem nuclei of the cat. *J. Comp. Neurol.*, 1961, *116*, 27–69.

Teas, D. C., Konishi, T., and Neilsen, D. W. Electrophysiological studies on the spatial distribution of the crossed olivocochlear bundle along the guinea pig cochlea. *J. Acoust. Soc. Am.*, 1972, *51*, 1256–1264.

Terhune, J. M. Sound localization abilities of untrained humans using complex and sinusoidal sounds. *Scand. Audio.*, 1974, *3*, 115–120.

Thompson, R. F. Function of auditory cortex in cat in frequency discrimination. *J. Neurophysiol.*, 1960, *23*, 321–334.

Trahiotis, C., and Elliott, D. N. Behavioral investigation of some possible effects of sectioning the crossed olivocochlear bundle. *J. Acoust. Soc. Am.*, 1970, *47*, 592–596.

Tsuchitani, C., and Boudreau, J. C. Single units analysis of cat superior olive S-segment with tonal stimuli. *J. Neurophysiol.*, 1966, *29*, 684–697.

Tsuchitani, C., and Boudreau, J. C. Stimulus level of dichotically presented tones and superior olive S-segment cell discharge. *J. Acoust. Soc. Am.*, 1969, *46*, 979–988.

Turner, R. N., and Norris, K. S. Discriminative echolocation in the porpoise. *J. Exp. Anal. Behav.*, 1966, *9*, 535–546.

van Noort, J. *The Structure and Connections of the Inferior Colliculus*. Van Gorcum, The Netherlands, 1969.

von Békésy, G. *Experiments in Hearing*. McGraw-Hill, New York, 1960.

Wallach, H., Newman, E. B., and Rosenzweig, M. R. The precedence effect in sound localization. *Am. J. Psychol.*, 1949, *62*, 315–336.

Warr, B. Fiber degeneration following lesions in the anterior ventral cochlear nucleus of the cat. *Exp. Neurol.*, 1966, *14*, 453–474.

Warr, B. Fiber degeneration following lesions of the posterior ventral cochlear nucleus of the cat. *Exp. Neurol.*, 1969, *23*, 140–155.

Warr, B. Fiber degeneration following lesions in the multipolar and globular cell areas in the ventral cochlear nucleus of the cat. *Brain Res.*, 1972, *40*, 247–270.

Warr, B. Olivocochlear and vestibular efferent neurons of the feline brainstem; their location, morphology and number determined by retrograde axonal transport and acetylcholinesterase histochemistry. *J. Comp. Neurol.*, 1975, *161*, 159–181.

Webster, D. B. Projection of the cochlea to the cochlear nucleus in Merriam's kangaroo rat. *J. Comp. Neurol.*, 1971, *133*, 477–494.

West, C., and Harrison, J. M. Transneuronal cell atrophy in the congenitally deaf white cat. *J. Comp. Neurol.,* 1973, *151*, 377–399.

Wever, E. G., and Lawrence, M. *Physiological Acoustics.* Princeton University Press, Princeton, N.J., 1954, pp. 404–410.

Whitfield, I. *The Auditory Pathway.* Williams and Williams, Baltimore, 1967, pp. 125–126.

Wiederhold, M. L. Variations in the effects of electrical stimulation of the crossed olivocochlear bundle on cat single auditory nerve responses to tone bursts. *J. Acoust. Soc. Am.,* 1970, *48*, 966–977.

Wiederhold, M. L., and Kiang, N. Effects of electric stimulation of the crossed olivocochlear bundle on single auditory nerve fibers in the cat. *J. Acoust. Soc. Am.,* 1970, *48*, 950–965.

Wiener, F. M. On the diffraction of a progressive sound wave by the head. *J. Acoust. Soc. Am.,* 1947, *19*, 143–146.

12

Auditory Forebrain: Evidence from Anatomical and Behavioral Experiments Involving Human and Animal Subjects

RICHARD J. RAVIZZA AND SUSAN M. BELMORE

INTRODUCTION

In recent years, careful utilization of experimental and clinical data has permitted new insights into the basic organization of mammalian forebrain. The intent of the present chapter is to examine one aspect of this inquiry: the structure of auditory forebrain and its role in mammalian hearing. To achieve this goal, the discussion is built around three issues presented in three separate sections.

The first section presents anatomical evidence for the conclusion that the auditory forebrain is longitudinally subdivided into three thalamocortical systems corresponding to the ventral, medial, and dorsal nuclei of the medial geniculate and their respective cortical projection areas.

The second section turns to the function of auditory forebrain, the discussion focusing on ablation-behavior experimentation in nonhuman mammals. In this section it is argued that the available evidence indicates that auditory forebrain is *not* involved in the analysis of the physical parameters of sounds, such as frequency and intensity. Instead, the evidence already available indicates that audi-

RICHARD J. RAVIZZA Psychology Department, Pennsylvania State University, University Park, Pennsylvania 16802. SUSAN M. BELMORE Department of Psychology, University of Kentucky, Lexington, Kentucky 40506. This paper was supported in part by NINCDS research grant 11554.

tory cortex is involved in the natural process of localizing sounds in space and in the temporal aspects of hearing. The three longitudinal components of auditory forebrain may be involved in different aspects of these functions.

Finally, the third section centers on human auditory forebrain. The human auditory forebrain embraces two kinds of capacities: those shared with nonhuman mammals and those uniquely developed in man. Further, several of the auditory capacities shared with other mammals form the substrate for more uniquely human auditory functions such as speech perception. In particular, evidence is presented that a number of the functions for which nonhuman auditory cortex appears most essential may also play a crucial role in human speech perception: the analysis of brief, transient sounds and the capacity for storage of certain types of auditory information.

ANATOMICAL ORGANIZATION

The auditory system is usually described as a pathway consisting of six major levels: spiral ganglion, cochlear nucleus, superior olivary complex, inferior colliculus, medial geniculate, and auditory cortex. The initial accomplishment of neuroanatomists interested in auditory forebrain was to trace the auditory pathway from cochlea to cortex by describing the major connections between each level. In recent years, the development of new staining techniques such as the Nauta and Fink-Heimer procedures has added the important advantage of allowing unmyelinated as well as myelinated fiber systems to be described (Fink and Heimer, 1967). Further, the recent development of techniques for tracing the normal flow of proteins in both the anterograde and retrograde directions has markedly increased the resolving power of this anatomical analysis (Cowan *et al.,* 1972; LaVail and LaVail, 1974). Using these new techniques along with the Golgi technique, neuroanatomists have been extending the structural analysis of the auditory system to include a detailed description of the unique connections of the various subdivisions of each level of the auditory system. With this recent emphasis in mind, the overall goal of this part of the chapter is twofold: (1) to describe the normal architectonic structure of thalamic and cortical auditory centers, and their connections with each other and other parts of the brain, and (2) to summarize these new facts in terms of a three-part longitudinal subdivision of auditory forebrain.

THALAMIC AUDITORY CENTERS

The mammalian medial geniculate nucleus, the chief thalamic center for audition, consists of three major subdivisions: ventral, medial, and dorsal (*cf.* Morest, 1964; see also Fig. 1). Although each subdivision can be further subdivided, the present discussion focuses on these major subdivisions.

In the ventral division the neurons contain tufted dendrites and are organized into relatively discrete laminae or sheets. Electrophysiological evidence indicates that this division is tonotopically organized such that low frequencies are represented laterally and high frequencies medially (Aitkin and Webster, 1971).

In the dorsal division the neurons have a radiating pattern of dendrites and are loosely packed. Unlike the ventral division, this region is relatively insensitive to simple sounds such as pure tones (Lippe and Weinberger, 1973*a,b*). Instead, the dorsal division appears most responsive to complex sounds (Whitfield and Purser, 1972; Altman *et al.*, 1970).

Finally, the medial division is architectonically more complex than the other two. It is composed of both tufted and radial cell types and is electrophysiologically responsive to somatic and vestibular as well as to auditory stimuli (cf. Poggio and Mountcastle, 1960; Liedgren *et al.*, 1976).

RELATION OF ANATOMICAL CONNECTIONS TO ARCHITECTONIC SUBDIVISIONS. The architectonic parcellation of the medial geniculate into ventral, dorsal, and medial subdivisions is supported by the distribution of afferent projections to

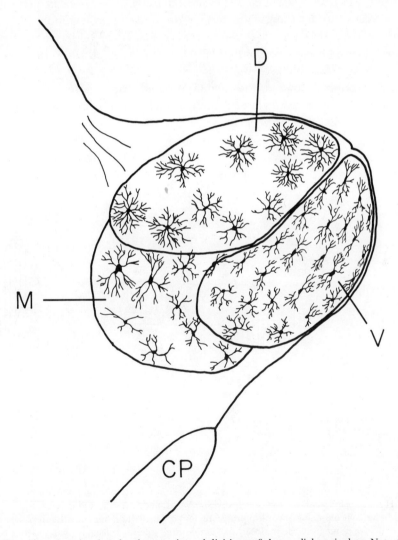

Fig. 1. Frontal section showing the three major subdivisions of the medial geniculate. Note that the ventral division (V) contains tufted neurons, the dorsal division (D) radial neurons, and the medial division(M) a combination of both types. After Morest's (1964) Golgi study of cat medial geniculate.

the medial geniculate from other parts of the brain (Fig. 2). The ventral division receives ascending fibers only from the inferior colliculus (cf. Moore and Goldberg, 1963; Morest, 1964, 1965; Oliver and Hall, 1975). Further, this projection to the ventral division appears to originate solely within the central nucleus of the inferior colliculus, which is the only portion of the inferior colliculus that receives direct projections from hindbrain auditory centers (see Chapter 11) (Casseday *et al.*, 1976; Rockel and Jones, 1973). The ventral division's only other known source of input is a reciprocal projection from its own cortical projection area AI and to a much lesser extent possibly AII and EP (Diamond *et al.*, 1969; Jones and Powell, 1968; Pontes *et al.*, 1975).

In contrast, the dorsal division receives input from the parabrachial region, the deep layers of the superior colliculus, the pericentral nucleus of the inferior colliculus, and the extensive reciprocal projection from its own cortical projection area—AII, EP, I, and T. Unlike the ventral division, the regions projecting to the dorsal division do *not* themselves receive direct input from hindbrain auditory structures. Instead, input to these centers is limited to midbrain or forebrain auditory nuclei (Moore and Goldberg, 1963; Morest, 1964, 1965; Diamond *et al.*, 1969; Harting *et al.*, 1973; Oliver and Hall, 1975).

Like the dorsal division, the medial division receives afferent fibers from a wide variety of sources, including many which are not directly connected to

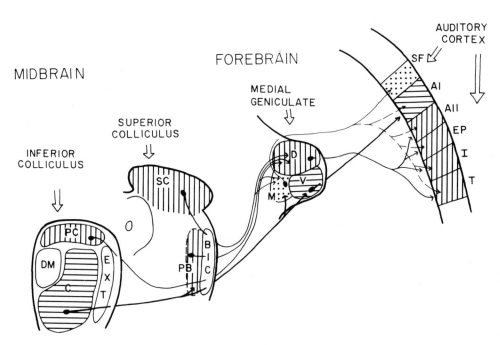

Fig. 2. Longitudinal subdivision of the ascending portion of the midbrain and forebrain auditory system. Horizontal lines indicate the ventral division(V), its midbrain input from the central division (C) of the inferior colliculus, and its cortical projection to AI. The vertical lines indicate the dorsal division (D), its midbrain input from the pericentral division of the inferior colliculus (PC), superior colliculus (SC), and the parabrachial region (PB), and its cortical projection areas AII, EP, I, and T. The stippled region indicates the medial division (M) and its cortical projection area SF and its lesser projection to the remainder of auditory cortex.

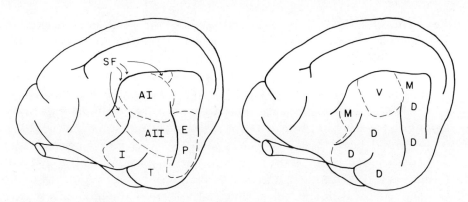

Fig. 3. Lateral view of cat cortex. On the left are shown the cortical subdivisions based on Woolsey's (1960) electrophysiological mapping of auditory cortex (AI, first auditory area; AII, second auditory area; EP, posterior ectosylvian area; I, insular area; T, temporal area; SF, suprasylvian fringe area). On the right are shown the *major* cortical targets of the three major subdivisions of the medial geniculate (V, ventral; D, dorsal; M, medial). Lesser projections from the medial division to virtually every part of auditory cortex are not shown.

auditory hindbrain. Some of these afferent projections, such as those from the central nucleus of the inferior colliculus, the deep layers of the superior colliculi, the parabrachial region, and auditory cortex, are shared with either the ventral or the dorsal division. However, other afferent projections (such as those arising in the dorsal column nuclei, fastigial nuclei, ventral spinal cord, and cortical area SF) are unique to the medial division and are probably not all auditory in function (Rinvik, 1968; Jones and Powell, 1968; Boivie, 1971; Carpenter, 1960; Nauta and Kuypers, 1958; Hand and Lui, 1966; Morest, 1965; Mehler, 1966; Moore and Goldberg, 1963; Casseday *et al.,* 1976; Oliver and Hall, 1975).

In the cat, this architectonic parcellation of the medial geniculate into three major parts is also paralleled by the organization of its major efferent projections. For the most part, fibers from each division of the geniculate terminate in relatively discrete cortical regions (Morest, 1964). The projection of the ventral division appears limited to only the central portions of auditory cortex—AI and to a lesser extent possibly AII and EP (Rose and Woolsey, 1949; Wilson and Cragg, 1969; Graybiel, 1973; Heath and Jones, 1971; Niimi and Naito, 1974) (Fig. 3). In fact, Diamond and his colleagues recently used the method of retrograde transport of HRP to study this projection and concluded that the vast majority of the ventral division's projection is probably limited to AI (Winer *et al.,* 1977). In contrast, the medial and dorsal divisions project primarily to an area surrounding this central part of auditory cortex. The medial division projects primarily to SF and to a much lesser extent to the remainder of auditory cortex (AI, AII, T, I, and EP), while the dorsal division projects mainly to AII, EP, I, and T (Locke, 1961; Mehler, 1966; Jones and Leavitt, 1973; Heath and Jones, 1971; Graybiel, 1973; Raczkowski *et al.,* 1976).

It should be emphasized that although the major features of the thalamocortical projection have been worked out, our present understanding is by no means complete. For example, in Morest's description of medial geniculate architectonics, he subdivides each major subdivision into several discrete regions. To date,

RICHARD J. RAVIZZA
AND SUSAN M.
BELMORE

further attempts to describe the locus and extent of these smaller subregions of medial geniculate have focused on the individual cortical projections of the various subregions of the dorsal division. For example, the caudal tip of the medial geniculate—a portion of the dorsal division—projects to temporal cortex (cf. Diamond *et al.*, 1958; Winer *et al.*, 1977). The medial part of the dorsal division— also referred to as the suprageniculate nucleus or part of the medial portion of the posterior group—sends its projections primarily to insular cortex (Graybiel, 1970, 1973; Jones and Leavitt, 1973; Winer *et al.*, 1977). Preliminary evidence also indicates that the remainder of the dorsal division may project mainly to AII and EP (Winer *et al.*, 1977). Although this detailed analysis has not yet turned to the ventral and medial divisions, Oliver and Hall (personal communication) have found that the rostral portions of the medial division of tree shrew medial geniculate project to a cortical region which may be homologous to SF in the cat, whereas the more caudal portions of the medial division may project over a much wider area of cortex. Finally, Winer *et al.*, (1977) suggest that the ventral extremity of the ventral division may be a separate nucleus which projects beyond AI to E.P.

The pattern of termination of the medial geniculate's projections in the individual layers of auditory cortex has been examined in several species. Microscopic analysis of auditory cortex in hedgehog, tree shrew, rat, and, more recently, monkey reveals that projections from the ventral and dorsal divisions of the medial geniculate terminate primarily in cortical layers III and IV (see Fig. 4). In contrast, those from the medial division terminate mainly in layer 1 in monkey (Jones and Burton, 1976), and in layers I and VI in hedgehog and tree shrew (Ravizza and Diamond, 1972; Casseday *et al.*, 1976), and are perhaps even more widespread in the rat (Ryugo and Killackey, 1974). This general pattern of

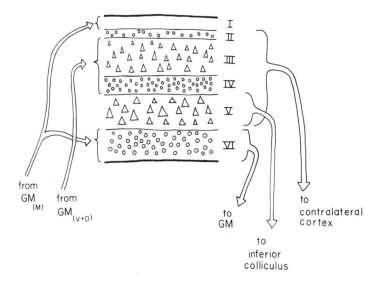

Fig. 4. A highly schematic cross-section of auditory cortex showing interlaminar pattern of termination of medial geniculate fibers in auditory cortex and the laminar origin of projections from auditory cortex to other parts of the brain. Based on data from hedgehog (Ravizza and Diamond, 1972), tree shrew (Casseday *et al.*, 1976), and hamster (Ravizza *et al.*, 1976).

different divisions projecting to different cortical layers is by no means unique to the auditory system; similar relationships have been described in other thalamo-cortical systems in rat, opossum, and hedgehog (cf. Killackey and Ebner, 1973).

SUMMARY OF THALAMIC ANATOMY. The architectonic organization of the mammalian medial geniculate and its connections with other brain structures indicate that it consists of three parts: (1) the ventral division, which receives ascending input solely from the central nucleus of the inferior colliculus and projects primarily to cortical area AI; (2) the dorsal division, which receives ascending input from the superior colliculus, the parabrachial region, and the pericentral nucleus of the inferior colliculus and projects to cortical areas AII, EP, I, and T; and (3) the medial division, which receives input from auditory, somatic, and vestibular pathways and projects mainly to auditory cortical area SF and to a lesser extent the remainder of auditory cortex.

CORTICAL AUDITORY CENTERS

Auditory cortex in cat can be subdivided into several discrete areas on the basis of its electrophysiological responses to sounds. For example, Woolsey (1960) employed electrophysiological criteria to subdivide auditory cortex into six major areas (AI, AII, EP, I, T, and SF; see Fig. 3). A fundamental question which this sort of physiological analysis raises is the correspondence between the various electrophysiological subdivisions and the structure of auditory cortex as reflected in cortical architectonics.

Anatomical studies reveal that cat auditory cortex can also be subdivided into several parts solely on the basis of its degree of architectonic specialization. AI is the most specialized region and has been characterized as "koniocortex"—that is, cortex with a high concentration of granular cells in layer 4 (Rose, 1949; Bremer and Dow, 1939). AII, EP, and parts of SF form a separate group of architectonically distinct regions. Each of these areas contains some koniocortical features, but is not true koniocortex and consequently has been characterized as a transitional belt between AI proper and surrounding cortical regions (Rose, 1949). Finally, the insular-temporal region and the remainder of SF exhibit even more primitive architectonic organization and consequently bear even less resemblance to AI (Rose, 1949). Available evidence indicates that AI, AII, and EP defined by architectonic criteria correspond reasonably well to electrophysiological subdivisions shown in the left-hand portion of Fig. 3 (Rose and Woolsey, 1949). Unfortunately, detailed comparisons of cortical architectonics and evoked potentials have not been made for the remainder of auditory cortex. Indeed, this entire sort of analysis would be enhanced if the evoked response technique employed by Woolsey were supplemented by a detailed microelectrode analysis of cat auditory cortex such as that already begun by Merzenich and his colleagues (*e.g.*, Merzenich *et al.*, 1975).

AFFERENT AND EFFERENT CONNECTIONS OF AUDITORY CORTEX. Auditory cortex has been shown to receive direct projections from two primary sources: the medial geniculate and contralateral auditory cortex. In contrast, auditory cortex sends efferent projections to many parts of the nervous system. First, it projects

RICHARD J. RAVIZZA
AND SUSAN M.
BELMORE

reciprocally to contralateral auditory cortex and to all three divisions of the medial geniculate. In addition, its projections terminate in caudate nucleus, putamen, amygdala, reticular nucleus of the thalamus, interstitial nucleus, parabrachial region, pretectal nuclei, inferior and superior colliculi, substantia nigra, and pontine nuclei.

RELATIONSHIP TO ARCHITECTONIC SUBDIVISIONS. The architectonic parcellation of auditory cortex into several discrete areas corresponds remarkably well with the organization of its afferent anatomical connections from the divisions of the medial geniculate and contralateral and auditory cortex (Figs. 2 and 3). The more specialized core region—AI—receives direct projections primarily from the medial geniculate's ventral division and from contralateral cortical area AI (Rose and Woolsey, 1949; Wilson and Cragg, 1969; Diamond et al., 1968; Winer et al., 1977). As we have already mentioned, SF receives direct projections mainly from the medial geniculate's medial division (Morrison et al., 1970; Locke, 1961; Jones and Leavitt, 1973; Heath and Jones, 1971; Graybiel, 1973). SF also receives direct cortical projections from only the SF portion of contralateral auditory cortex (Diamond et al., 1968). Finally, as mentioned above, the remainder of auditory cortex AII, EP, I, and T receives direct input from various parts of the dorsal division (Diamond et al., 1958; Jones and Leavitt, 1973; Graybiel, 1973; Winer et al., 1977). AII, EP, I, and T are also known to receive direct projections from contralateral AII, EP, I, and T, respectively (Diamond, et al., 1968, Cranford et al., 1976b).

Available anatomical evidence also indicates that those cortical regions differ in their projections to the remainder of the brain. To begin with, each cortical area sends an efferent projection to that division of the medial geniculate from which its thalamocortical afferent projection arises (Diamond et al., 1968; Jones and Powell, 1968; Pontes et al., 1975). Evidence from electron microscopic studies of the ventral division indicates that these descending projections terminate on the very same neurons which receive direct input from the inferior colliculus and which give rise to the thalamocortical projections (Majorossy and Réthelyi, 1968; Morest, 1975).

Corticotectal projections from all areas of auditory cortex terminate in the pericentral and dorsal medial divisions of the inferior colliculus (Diamond et al., 1968). Additional corticotectal projections from auditory cortex also terminate in the superior colliculus. However, the projections to superior colliculus do not arise from AI. Instead, they originate from auditory cortex surrounding AI, with AII and SF projecting to its superficial layers and IT and EP projecting to its deeper layers (Paula-Barbosa and Sousa-Pinto, 1973).

The efferent projections of auditory cortex to the basal ganglia have also been shown to be highly organized. Available evidence suggests that each cortical subdivision projects to a relatively restricted portion of caudate, putamen, and claustrum in such a way that the spatial organization between the cortical areas is topographically maintained (Webster, 1965; Otellin, 1972; Kemp and Powell, 1970).

Finally, auditory cortex sends a direct projection to the dorsal lateral pontine nuclei. The exact cortical areas from which this projection originates remain unknown at this time (Kusama et al., 1966).

Recent anatomical investigations employing retrograde transport of labeled protein indicate that the laminar distribution of neurons giving rise to these efferent projections is highly organized at least in hamster. Although not all efferent projection systems have been studied, available information indicates that neurons in layer VI of auditory cortex project to medial geniculate, those in layer V project to inferior colliculus, and, finally, neurons in layers II, III, IV, and V project to contralateral auditory cortex (Ravizza *et al.*, 1976) (Fig. 4).

SUMMARY OF CORTICAL ANATOMY. Like the medial geniculate, auditory cortex is neither anatomically nor electrophysiologically homogeneous. In the cat it consists of six discrete subdivisions (AI, AII, EP, SF, I, and T). Furthermore, the afferent and efferent connections of each cortical area are different. Each cortical area receives input from a given portion of the medial geniculate and the contralateral auditory cortex. In a similar way, each subdivision of auditory cortex projects either to different subcortical regions or to different portions of the same subcortical centers. As in the medial geniculate, the basic organization of these cortical areas seems to be into three major divisions: AI, which is closely related to the ventral division of the medial geniculate; AII, EP, I, and T, which are related to its dorsal division; and SF, which is related to its medial division.

COMPARATIVE CONSIDERATIONS

Although much work has been done on the anatomy of the cat auditory system, our understanding of the organization of the auditory system in other mammals is sparse. The comparative data already available indicate that the *overall* anatomical organization of thalamic and cortical auditory centers is remarkably similar in all mammals including man (cf. Jones and Burton, 1976; Harrison and Howe, 1974*a,b*).

There are, however, a growing number of facts which point toward some striking differences among extant mammals in the detailed organization of particular portions of auditory cortex. To begin with, architectonic and electrophysiological evidence indicates that there may be more subdivisions of auditory cortex in more specialized mammals than in more generalized mammals. For example, in the cat Woolsey (1960) found at least six tonotopic representations of the cochlea in auditory cortex of the cat, whereas in the rabbit Galli *et al.* (1971) report only two electrophysiological representations. Before placing great weight on these data from different laboratories, it should be stressed that comparative conclusions of this sort are strongest when the observations on different species are made in the same laboratory using identical recording procedures. Nevertheless, this same general conclusion is supported by architectonic studies. For example, in man auditory koniocortex is well developed, with a high concentration of granular cells in layer 4. In cat and monkey koniocortex is not so well developed, i.e., the proportion of granular cells is considerably lower, (Rose, 1949). The most generalized mammals, such as hedgehog and opossum, lack dense concentration of small granular cells so characteristic of auditory cortex in primates. These differences are so striking that when describing the cortical architectonics of generalized mammals, Sanides labeled the most specialized portion of auditory cortex in hedgehog and rat as "prokoniocortex" rather than koniocortex (Sanides, 1969,

RICHARD J. RAVIZZA
AND SUSAN M.
BELMORE

1970, personal communication). Thus one striking difference in the organization of auditory cortex among specialized mammals such as cat, monkey, and man is the appearance of well-developed koniocortex within the projection area of the medial geniculate's ventral division.

A second difference among mammals concerns the anatomical organization of the regions surrounding primary auditory cortex. Unlike other mammals, human auditory cortex is *not* anatomically asymmetrical. Differences have been observed in the size of the planum temporale—a flat area directly behind Heschel's transverse gyrus on the upper surface of the temporal lobe (cf. Geschwind and Levitsky, 1968; Wada, 1969; Yeni-Komshian and Benson, 1976) (see Fig. 5). In a study of 100 normal brains, Geschwind and Levitsky (1968) found the planum temporale larger on the left in 65 cases, equal in 24 cases, and larger on the right in only 11 cases.

Further, architectonic analysis indicates that this asymmetry mostly arises from a particular subdivision of human auditory cortex called "parakoniocortex" (Sanides, 1975). Although the exact thalamic projections to this portion of human cortex are not yet known, available evidence indicates that it receives direct input from the medial geniculate. That anatomical asymmetries of this sort might not be limited to man is revealed by recent evidence which indicates that the left sylvian fissure may be longer than the right in great apes as well as man (Yeni-Komshian and Benson, 1976; LeMay and Geschwind, 1975).

In summary, although the overall organization of auditory thalamus and cortex appears remarkably similar in all mammals including man, two major

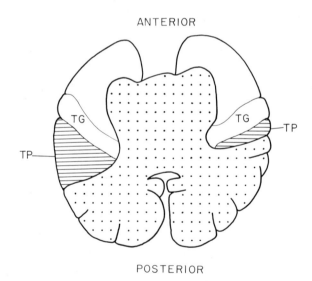

Fig. 5. Top view of the human brain following horizontal section in the plane of the sylvian fissure. Stippled region indicates cut upper surface of specimen. In man the transverse gyrus of Heschel (TG) contains the projection area of the ventral division system. The cross-hatched area indicates the extent of the planum temporale (TP), which is an extension of Wernicke's area and may be a portion of the dorsal division system. Note the greater extent of the planum temporale on the left side of a typical brain. After Geschwind and Levitsky (1968).

structural differences between generalized and specialized mammals have been identified in the organization of auditory cortex: (1) an increased number of architectonic subdivisions, including the appearance of true auditory koniocortex within the projection area of the ventral division in specialized mammals such as cat, monkey, and particularly man, and (2) a striking asymmetry in auditory cortex of man and to a lesser degree great apes. This expansion may reflect a unilateral expansion of secondary auditory cortex, which may in turn receive direct projections from the medial geniculate.

Although it remains too early to tell whether these differences between specialized mammals such as man and generalized mammals such as the hedgehog, rat, or rabbit reflect unique specialization, they may provide important clues about the evolution of the human auditory system. Indeed, if the cytoarchitectonic and thalamocortical systems of these experimental animals do represent accurate models of primitive and advanced mammalian brains, then one major change which took place in the evolution of human auditory cortex would be an increased number of parts of auditory cortex, reflected both in the number of architectonic subdivisions and in the asymmetrical expansion of certain portions of human auditory cortex.

Summary of Anatomical Preliminaries

The preceding anatomical analysis of thalamic and cortical hearing centers in the cat indicates that each level is composed of distinct subdivisions which differ both in normal cytoarchitecture and in their connections with the remainder of the brain. The ventral division of the medial geniculate forms a core or central portion of auditory forebrain. At each level, this system is topographically organized and receives direct input from the ascending auditory system. The medial division and its cortical projection area, SF, form a dorsal crescent, belt, or fringe surrounding the core of auditory cortex. Finally, the dorsal division and its projection areas AII, EP, I, and T form a ventral belt or fringe. At each level, these two belt or fringe regions are less topographically organized than the core system and receive input from nonauditory as well as from the ascending auditory system.

Although comparative data are quite limited, particularly for primates, available evidence indicates that this basic organization of auditory forebrain is common to all mammals. Thus it is on this basic mammalian organization of auditory forebrain that the known specializations which characterize human auditory cortex are superimposed: a highly granular koniocortex which makes up the core of human auditory cortex and the appearance of an asymmetrical expansion of the belt or fringe regions in the left auditory cortex of man.

Hearing and the Ablation Method

For over a century the close connection between forebrain and sensory receptors has been interpreted to mean that the forebrain makes important contributions to exteroceptive perception. Indeed, for generations the neocortical contribution to sensory processes has been thought to be the capacity for sensation itself. From this point of view, even the most simple psychological experience cannot be accomplished until sound-evoked impulses reach the auditory area in the cortex. This point of view also suggests that brain stem synapses in a sensory pathway—such as cochlear nucleus, superior olive, inferior colliculus, and medial geniculate—play a dual role mediating unlearned reflexive responses to stimuli and relaying sensory-evoked information toward the neocortex. Within the auditory system this concept implies (1) that the cortex is necessary for hearing and (2) that the synapses in the hindbrain and midbrain auditory systems provide connections between the ears and specific muscle groups required for simple reflexes to sound. Herrick summarized this conception of the neocortical contribution to audition:

> The central connections of the . . . cochlear nerve . . . effect both reflex connections in the brain stem and cortical connections through the lateral lemniscus, medial geniculate and auditory radiations, for conscious sensations of hearing. (Herrick, 1924, p. 228)

Herrick's cleavage of conscious sensations of hearing from reflexive responses to sound also denies the notion that, if an animal makes an overt response to a sound, it "hears"; because the overt response may be merely "reflexive" and in that case yields no information about true "hearing."

To avoid the possibility of confusing simple reflexive responses to sounds with "hearing," a conscious perception, investigations of hearing came to employ two sorts of behavioral tests. The first kind is a test of *reflex capacity* (ear wiggles, head turning, etc.). The second kind is a test of the potential of a sound to be used as a *conditioned stimulus*. The reasoning behind the second kind of test is that, if an animal "senses" the stimulus, the animal should be able to associate almost any response to it. Thus an animal's auditory sensitivity can once more be inferred from its behavior by redefining "hearing" as the ability to make learned responses to sound.

The fact that an animal's auditory sensitivity might be inferred from its ability to perform learned responses to sounds generates a variety of problems when it is put into practice, particularly following lesions within the central nervous system. These problems arise because the outcome of a postoperative test must be made by observing the animal's ability to learn: that is, an inability to learn might be confounded with an inability to hear. Obviously, any postoperative deficiencies in learning (such as intellectual incapacities), or responses in conflict with the responses to be learned (such as emotional disturbances), or an inability to perform the required response itself (such as a motor impairment) might each be mistakenly interpreted as a sensory deficit.

A second, almost opposite, set of problems often encountered while interpreting the effects of an ablation is that of failing to infer a sensory deficit from an animal's performance when a sensory deficit actually exists. This problem arises if an animal is able to employ a different set of sensory cues during postoperative testing from those it employed during preoperative testing. For instance, an animal trained to make a certain response to an auditory stimulus during preoperative training might learn to perform the required response postoperatively in an entirely different way, such as on the basis of sensory cues arising from kinesthetic stimuli from unaffected auditory reflexes.

In the following discussion the results of ablation-behavior experiments are reviewed. The problem of confusing sensory deficits with nonsensory deficits and the problem of compensating cues will be seen to play an important role in our understanding of neocortical contributions to mammalian hearing.

CONTRIBUTION OF THE AUDITORY CORTEX TO HEARING

The effect of modern animal training procedures on our understanding of neocortical contributions to hearing has been dramatic. The early idea that conscious sensations of sounds are dependent on cortex, as expressed in the quotation by Herrick, had virtually dominated the study of auditory cortex for years. By 1930, numerous reports of deafness resulting from bilateral destruction of the auditory cortex had appeared in both the human and animal literature (cf. Ferrier, 1886; Bramwell, 1927).However, in the 1930s the conclusion that auditory cortex is essential for the formation ·of a conditioned response to sound was beginning to be questioned (Mettler *et al.,* 1934; Bard and Rioch, 1937). By 1942 evidence to the contrary had accumulated to the point that Girden could state that, if long recovery times intervene between ablation and testing, no appreciable effects of lesions of the auditory cortex are evident in tasks involving simple sound detection tasks (Girden, 1942). Since Girden, an even larger number of experiments have demonstrated that auditory cortex is not necessary for an animal to make learned responses to sounds, nor is it necessary for absolute pure-tone sensitivity (Kryter and Ades, 1943; Stoughton, 1954; Wegener, 1954; Ravizza and Masterton, 1972; Heffner, 1973). Obviously, these facts mean that the removal of auditory cortex does not abolish the capacity to perform a learned response to the occurrence of a sound—certainly, auditory cortex ablation does not result in deafness or in an incapacity for "hearing."

PHYSICAL PARAMETERS OF SOUND: INTENSITY AND FREQUENCY. Once it became evident that, despite the massive projection of the auditory system to cortex, an animal without auditory cortex could still make conditioned responses to sound, it was suggested that perhaps an animal's ability to discriminate specifc physical parameters of sound such as intensity and frequency might be dependent on neocortex. Loudness sensitivity (that is, intensity DL) was soon tested by Raab and Ades (1946), Rosenzweig (1946), Meyer and Woolsey (1952), and later Oesterreich *et al.* (1971). They found that cats without auditory cortex showed normal sensitivity to variations in the loudness of sounds. Attention was then turned to pitch sensitivity.

By this time Woolsey and Walzl (1942) had already demonstrated the topographical arrangement of projections from the cochlea to auditory cortex. This fact was thought to indicate that the cortex might enable mammals to make pitch discriminations. At first, the idea seemed to be correct. Meyer and Woolsey (1952) removed auditory cortex (AI, AII, EP, I, T, and SII) from cats and found that the ability to discriminate pitch was apparently lost. What appeared to be a clear

RICHARD J. RAVIZZA
AND SUSAN M.
BELMORE

confirmation of a role of auditory cortex in hearing was soon shattered, however, when Butler *et al.* (1957) showed that the deficit discovered by Meyer and Woolsey was actually due to their method of stimulus presentation rather than a deficit in pitch discrimination itself. This alternative explanation of Meyer and Woolsey's findings was firmly established by Thompson (1960). Thompson made ablations similar to those employed by Meyer and Woolsey, and although these animals were also unable to perform Meyer and Woolsey's frequency discrimination procedure, the same animals showed no loss in frequency sensitivity when evaluated with the postoperative testing procedure used by Butler and colleagues. Therefore, frequency discrimination, like intensity discrimination, is not lost following ablation of auditory cortex.

As it turns out, a careful consideration of Thompson's (1960) data yields an important clue to the nature of the cortical deficit. Thompson discovered that his animals invariably made their errors by making an avoidance response when the safe signal was presented, and not by failing to avoid the warning signal. Thompson suggested that this deficit following removal of auditory cortex is not primarily sensory in nature. Rather, he argued, the deficit is more closely related to the ability to inhibit responses to the unshocked stimulus. In the years since Thompson's initial suggestion, numerous experiments have been conducted involving cortical lesions and frequency discrimination. In a 1972 review paper, Elliott and Trahiotis interpreted these experiments by rephrasing Thompson's original suggestion in terms of either symmetrical reinforcement (in which the animal is reinforced on safe and warning trials) or asymmetrical reinforcement (in which the animal is reinforced on only one type of trial) . Quite simply, following removal of auditory cortex, deficits in pitch perception are more likely to be found if asymmetrical reinforcement is used, whereas little or no loss in pitch sensitivity is found if symmetrical reinforcement is employed. This same conclusion holds for absolute as well as relative pitch discriminations (cf. Cranford *et al.*, 1976*a*). Thus the results of frequency discrimination experiments indicate that what deficits appear are more related to some sort of intellectual impairment than to a deficiency in perception itself.

The idea that the contribution of auditory cortex seems more closely related to the intellectual or nonsensory demands of the experiment than to pitch perception itself raises a major and still unanswered paradox about the organization of auditory cortex: if cortex is not involved in pitch perception, what then is the behavioral significance of the orderly, tonotopic projection from the cochlea to auditory cortex?

TEMPORAL PATTERNS. With the discovery by Butler *et al.* (1957) and Thompson (1960) that pitch perception is not dependent on auditory cortex, research was temporarily stymied. If the contribution of auditory cortex was not the ability to sense the occurrence of a sound, or to distinguish the chief physical parameters of tones such as intensity and frequency, what remained? Experimenters began to wonder if *any* sensory deficit could be demonstrated after destruction of auditory cortex. This frustrating period was marked by the emergence of a series of new concepts concerning the role of neocortex in hearing. Although at the time of their conception these ideas appeared disjunct and unrelated, their final impact leads to a reorganization of our understanding of neocortical contributions to hearing.

The first of these views is found in the final paragraphs of an article by Hallowell Davis in *Physiological Reviews* (1957). In his concluding remarks, Davis suggests that more attention should be given to auditory transients and to the temporal aspects of auditory excitation:

> In the classical preoccupation with steady tones and the problem of frequency discrimination, transients, and temporal relations including binaural localization, were largely overlooked. Hearing has a time dimension as well as a frequency dimension. (Davis, 1957, p.43)

Later in that same year Diamond and Neff contributed behavioral evidence that also served to emphasize the temporal aspect of hearing. They reported that cats deprived of auditory cortex are unable to discriminate between tonal patterns. More specifically, cats deprived of auditory cortex are able to perform the frequency discriminations, but these same animals are unable to discriminate patterns of tones. In a collateral series of experiments, Diamond *et al.* (1962) found that bilateral cortical ablation permanently impaired tasks requiring detection of the elimination of a frequency component. Since Butler and colleagues had already demonstrated that the discrimination of frequency is unaffected in such animals, the pattern deficit must include a change in the ability to make mental comparisons between two successive tonal sequences separated in time.

In recent years several additional lines of evidence have emerged which also point toward a contribution of auditory cortex to this temporal aspect of hearing. For example, ablation-behavior experiments have found deficits in discrimination of tone duration (Scharlock *et al.*, 1965), temporal discontinuity (Symmes, 1966), interaural order (Kass *et al.*, 1967; Whitfield *et al.*, 1972) and complex periodic stimuli (Stepien *et al.*, 1960; Dewson *et al.*, 1970). In contrast, this apparent breakdown in the ability to make temporal pattern comparisons following auditory cortex lesions does not extend to discriminations involving click rates (French, 1942; Cranford *et al.*, 1975; Heffner, 1976). When these facts are combined, the idea emerges that it may be fruitful to think of auditory cortex as the substrate for a variety of complex temporal processing abilities. Although the exact nature of this sort of deficit remains elusive, it is quite possible that this so-called temporal processing deficit may be a secondary symptom of a more basic neurological deficit, i.e., one involving some aspect of short-term but strictly auditory memory. That is, any experiment which requires the storage of the neural processes required for temporal analysis over time and results in a temporal deficit of some sort may be due to a breakdown in the storage process itself. Indeed, Neff touched on this possibility years ago when he argued that "the geniculocortical part of the auditory system appears to provide a mechanism for short-term 'memory' or storage" (Neff, 1961, p. 277).

SOUND LOCALIZATION. At about the same time that Diamond and Neff first reported that auditory cortex is involved in the temporal analysis of sound, Neff *et al.* (1956) showed that a cat's spatial localization of a sound source is dramatically disrupted by removal of auditory cortex. Previously, Neff *et al.* (1950) had noted

RICHARD J. RAVIZZA
AND SUSAN M.
BELMORE

that normal cats can discriminate angular separations of less than 5°, whereas cats with partial lesions of auditory cortex are unable to discriminate angular separations of less than 40°. Indeed, the animals were so completely disrupted that although they were capable of discriminating separations of greater than 40°, their performance was extremely unreliable, even when continuous sounds were separated by as much as 180°. However, with extensive retraining the operated cats were able to localize above a chance level.

In a later experiment, Riss (1959) demonstrated that animals without auditory cortex are *completely unable* to localize the source of a brief sound, while if the sound is continuous, the animals can localize the sound source above chance levels. Riss interpreted this residual capacity to localize continuous sounds as evidence of the cats' scanning for intensity cues which signal the direction of the sound source. Further insight into the nature of this deficit was provided when Thompson and Welker (1963) noted that the reflexive head turns of a cat to an unexpected sound were virtually normal without auditory cortex. The nature of the sound localization deficits and residual capacities following removal of auditory cortex revealed in these experiments has proved to be important.

On initial inspection, the sound localization deficits and tonal pattern deficits seemed quite unrelated. However, the fact that binaural time differences (Δt) serve as important cues for the localization of brief sounds seemed to suggest a simple common denominator: an insensitivity to temporal cues, the same parameter that had been suggested by Davis.

In an effort to evaluate this idea, Masterton and Diamond (1964) trained cats to discriminate the small binaural time differences (less than 500 μsec in cats) involved in sound localization. Cats deprived of auditory cortex were severely handicapped in this task. Heffner (1973) has also shown changes in Δt sensitivity in the monkey following auditory cortex damage. However, before accepting the conclusion that the role of auditory cortex in sound localization is limited to the analysis of Δt we should consider a second fact uncovered by the Masterton and Diamond experiment: the same animals which suffered the profound Δt deficit were apparently sensitive to binaural spectrum differences (Δfi) which also play an important role in localization. If cats without auditory cortex are indeed sensitive to binaural intensity differences when tested in the grill box, why then were Neff's and Riss's operated cats unable to localize sound at normal levels in the open field using binaural intensity differences alone? One possible answer is that there may be a second deficit following removal of auditory cortex which somehow disrupts the operated cat's ability to utilize its residual Δfi sensitivity to locate the source of a brief sound in an open field apparatus.

As in the earlier ablation-behavior experiments involving pitch discrimination, an important difference exists in the behavioral procedures involved in these experiments, and an analysis of these procedural differences provides a clue to the nature of the cortical deficit. Masterton and Diamond's procedure required the animals to detect a change in apparent sound lateralization which signaled an impending shock. The shock could be avoided by crossing to the opposite side of a double grill box. In contrast, in the Neff sound localization procedure the animal had to use the sound to guide its movements through space to the sound source itself—a much more natural use of sounds. There are several recent ablation-behavior experiments which indicate that these differences in the requirements of the behavioral task provide an important additional clue to the nature of the localization deficit following removal of auditory cortex.

In one set of experiments the sensitivity of opossums (Ravizza and Masterton, 1972) and monkeys (Heffer and Masterton, 1975) to localize sounds without auditory cortex was determined using the "conditioned suppression" technique (see Smith, 1970) or a simple lever-pressing task. For present purposes, the essential feature of these procedures is that the animals are able to indicate sound direction immediately. That is, they are not required to move toward the source of the sound or delay their response in any way. In these circumstances, both monkeys and opossums without auditory cortex suffer only slight losses in their ability to localize sounds. The Heffner and Masterton experiment with monkeys is particularly interesting because the very same animals were also tested in a second situation in which, like Neff's cats, they were required to move to the sound source in order to receive reward. The same monkeys which, the day before, performed almost normally in the conditioned suppression and lever-pressing procedures were now totally unable to indicate the direction of a sound. Taken together, these results indicate that the difficulty in localizing brief sounds may stem not only from the brevity of the sound as suggested by Riss (1959) but also from some other aspect of the test situation—perhaps the delay interposed between stimulus and response or an impairment to respond on the basis of sound locus alone.

Support for this notion is provided by a recent experiment involving auditory cortex lesions in hedgehogs and bushbabies (Ravizza and Diamond, 1974). In this experiment, the Neff procedure for testing sound localization was modified so that after release from the start box the animals were restrained by a wire enclosure for 5 sec while a continuous sound signaled the location of the reward. If the sound was turned off as the animal was released, the performance of the operated animals was still impaired, particularly if they failed to use body orientation as a mnemonic device.

These results indicate that the sound localization deficit may not be solely a deficit in the ability to utilize binaural time difference cues to localize sounds. Rather, the profound inability of mammals without auditory cortex to move to the source of a brief sound may also be related to an inability to use or perhaps even store the required spatial information long enough to guide the appropriate motor behavior. This entire series of sound localization experiments indicates that it may be fruitful to think of free-field sound localization tasks as consisting of two parts: (1) the ability to localize brief sounds (based on both ΔI and Δft cues and (2) the ability to use this information to move toward the sound source. If this line of reasoning is correct and if the sound localization impairment does reflect a dual deficit involving both the extremely short temporal dimension required for Δt analysis and the longer temporal dimensions involved in the utilization of spatial information to move to the sound source, then these two components of sound localization can be added to the list of known deficits which can be attributed to ablation of auditory cortex.

Assuming for a moment that the sound localization deficit is related to some sort of temporal disruption, then deficits resulting from auditory cortex ablation extend over a wide temporal range. On one hand, the analysis of very brief

RICHARD J. RAVIZZA
AND SUSAN M.
BELMORE

intervals, such as the 50–500 μsec range involved in the analysis of the binaural time differences used in sound localization, is affected. On the other hand, the utilization of auditory information over several seconds (the time required either to detect a change in the order of multiple sound sequences or perhaps even to reach the locus of sound in space) seems equally dependent on auditory cortex.

However, it should be emphasized that auditory cortex ablation does not result in a total collapse of auditory memory; many facets of auditory memory are unimpaired. For example, animals with auditory cortex lesions retain many previously learned responses to sound as well as normal animals do. They are even capable of absolute pitch discriminations in which they must make a response to one frequency and later a second response to another frequency. Indeed, Heffner has recently shown that dogs with auditory cortex lesions are readily able to solve the open-field Neff sound localization procedure when its solution is based on a 0.3-sec rate discrimination from a central speaker, but suffer severe impairments when required to locate these same brief stimuli (Heffner, 1976). Instead, the deficit seems more related to short- or intermediate-term storage of only some types of auditory information, and this includes information about spatial aspects of sound sources such as binaural time differences and the comparison of multiple sound sequences.

The idea that the role of auditory cortex is largely concerned with the utilization of certain types of sounds over a period of time provides a common factor for a wide variety of deficits known to result from auditory cortex ablation. Yet there are three aspects of the history of experimentation in the function of auditory forebrain that combine to suggest keeping an open mind toward other alternatives. The first is that, in almost every experiment, sequential stimuli have been employed. Unlike experimentation on visual cortex, simultaneous auditory discriminations have rarely, if ever, been required. (For example, there is little evidence available on the role of auditory cortex in auditory masking or critical band phenomenon, or, for that matter, in an animal's ability to act on the higher pitched of two simultaneous sounds, etc.)

Second, to date there have been few attempts to determine the possible modality-specificity of the deficits resulting from auditory cortex ablation. That is, is auditory cortex required for more than just analysis of auditory stimuli? One notable exception is a series of experiments by Colavita (1972) in which animals were required to discriminate temporal patterns of *visual* intensity sequences which were similar to the frequency pattern discriminations employed by Diamond and Neff (1957). After lesions of insular and temporal auditory cortex, the cats were severely disrupted on this visual discrimination, a result consistent with the idea that parts of auditory cortex may be involved in the temporal analysis of even nonauditory stimuli.

The third point evoking hesitation centers on the notion that the neocortex might indeed play very significant additional roles in mammalian hearing. One possibility is that neocortex may be involved with the extraction of more biologically relevant information from naturally occurring sounds. Because this approach stands in marked contrast to earlier emphases, the rationale underlying this idea will be described in the following section.

The idea of biological relevancy originated with the Darwinian concept that a biological structure is a part of a living organism solely because it is advantageous for the survival of the species. The significance of this idea lies in the notion that because all components of the auditory system are essential to the species' survival, their primary function must be their contribution in the extraction of information required for survival and reproduction. In other words, instead of considering the auditory system as primarily an analyzer of the physical parameters of pure tones or combinations of pure tones, it might prove useful to think of the auditory system as an important source of information about environmental events which change an animal's probability for survival and reproduction.

A central notion in this concept of auditory function is the idea that some sounds are more important to the survival of an organism than others and that some qualities of sound are more important than other qualities. In order to gain insight into the various kinds of sounds that are of greater or lesser importance to an organism, consideration of the natural environment in which animals exist is required. Natural sounds of low significance are those whose detection has rarely, if ever, played a pivotal role in survival or mating of a member of the species. For example, the steady background noise of wind or continuous rustling of leaves is a sound of low biological importance. Furthermore, it is on this background that sounds of high significance are superimposed.

Because the survival of an animal depends on the outcome of its competition with other animals, sounds which indicate the presence of other animals are certainly of high survival value. Whether the sound is the betraying snap of a twig by an unseen predator, the chirp of a fallen bird, or the vocalization of a potential mate, the ability of an animal to detect, to localize, and to identify the sources of these sounds constitutes a biological function of the greatest significance to the ultimate survival of the species.

On initial inspection, the snap of a twig and the chirp of a bird seem to have little in common. Yet a moment's reflection reveals that they, and indeed most biologically relevant sounds, are to a large extent composed of auditory transients. This fact suggests that auditory transients are one crucial common factor for all biologically relevant sounds. In a similar way, the fact that sounds of low survival value (such as the sound of the wind) are usually relatively free of auditory transients suggests that steadiness may be a common feature of sounds of low biological relevance.

The parallel between high and low biological significance on the one hand and transient and steady sounds on the other has begun to attract several investigators, and, of course, the entire literature on localization of brief sounds already described falls into this emphasis on the attributes of natural sounds (e.g., see Masterton and Diamond, 1973). In addition, Russian investigators have reported both absolute threhold shifts and frequency difference threshold shifts using brief sounds in dogs with large auditory cortex lesions (Gersuni, 1971; Gersuni *et al.*, 1968; Baru, 1967). Further evidence implicating a role of auditory cortex in the analysis of naturally occurring sounds comes from a series of studies by Dewson *et al.* (1969) and Dewson (1964). In these experiments, a severe deficit in discrimination of human vowel sounds (/i/ vs. /u/) was uncovered in both cat and monkey following even partial lesions of auditory cortex. Although human speech sounds are by no means crucial sounds for cats and monkeys, the fact that these same operated animals are readily able to perform pitch discriminations points toward the importance of auditory cortex in analyzing sounds more natural than continuous pure tones or their combinations.

Hupfer *et al.* (1977) pursued this idea further when they examined the role of squirrel monkey auditory cortex in the recognition of species-specific calls. Briefly, they found that the monkey's ability to discriminate species-specific sounds was permanently disrupted by auditory cortex ablation. Further, their subjects with large but less than complete lesions could discriminate species-specific calls from non-species-specific sounds, whereas their subjects with complete removal of auditory cortex could not discriminate these two classes of sounds. In contrast, Heffner (1977) found that dogs with complete auditory cortex lesions exhibited transient deficits in the discrimination of dog sounds from nondog sounds. Whether this difference between dog and squirrel monkey reflects methodological differences or some fundamental differences in the organization of auditory cortex in these two species must await further study. In the meantime, ablation-behavior experiments of this sort suggest that one potential area of cortical function which still remains unexplored is its role in the analysis of biological information, particularly the perception of species-specific sounds.

ABLATION-BEHAVIOR EVIDENCE FOR A LONGITUDINAL SUBDIVISION OF THE AUDITORY FOREBRAIN

So far, only the effects of bilateral ablation of the entire auditory cortex have been emphasized. In addition, there have been several behavioral experiments involving lesions of specific architectonic subdivisions of auditory cortex which conform to the concept of a three-way anatomical subdivision of auditory forebrain as outlined in the first section of this chapter.

In one line of experiments, Strominger (1969 and personal communication) investigated the role of subdivisions of auditory cortex in sound localization. Briefly, he found that partial lesions of AI produced slight deficits in localization while lesions in the other subdivisions had no effect. In one of his subjects (and several reported in earlier experiments by other workers) the lesions included the entire projection area of the ventral division of the medial geniculate (AI) with only slight damage to the immediately surrounding areas of AII and EP. When this core system was completely destroyed, the animals suffered a marked and prolonged deficit in their ability to move to the source of a brief sound. In contrast, large lesions of the projection area of the dorsal division of the medial geniculate had no measurable effect on the ability to move to the source of a sound. Similar results have been reported for the dog by Szwejkowska and Sychowa (1971). In particular, they found that lesions involving primarily the projection area of the ventral division of the medial geniculate resulted in lasting sound localization impairments, whereas lesions involving the projection area of the dorsal division did not. If the analysis of sound localization experiments developed earlier in this section is correct, and if such a deficit is more closely related to the analysis of the binaural cues and the utilization of spatial information over time, then one conclusion worth exploring is that the core system of auditory forebrain (the ventral division of the medial geniculate and its projection areas) is involved in the analysis and utilization of auditory spatial information while the dorsal and medial division systems are not.

In a second line of experiments the effect of partial lesions of auditory cortex on a frequency-pattern discrimination was examined by Diamond and Neff (1957). Their results indicate that a partial or complete removal of the cortex (AI) or even AI plus adjoining portions of AII and EP caused only slight amnesia for the discrimination. In contrast, when these lesions extended into the fringe region (I-T) or if the I-T area alone was removed, profound deficits occurred in the discrimination (Diamond and Neff, 1957; Goldberg *et al.*, 1957). Kelly (1973) reports a similar outcome for temporal sequences involving frequency-modulated signals.

Finally, Neff *et al.* (1972) and Scharlock *et al.* (1965) found that deficits in duration sensitivity occurred with large lesions of auditory cortex only when the rostral portion of SF was involved. Although sensitivity to sound duration has yet to be measured following ablation of SF alone, their conclusion suggests that unlike other portions of auditory forebrain the medial division system may form the substrate for auditory duration sensitivity.

Taken together, these results support the idea that the ventral system is primarily involved in sound localization while the surrounding systems are involved in the analysis of other temporal aspects of hearing. If the analysis of the abilities involved in the sound localization experiments described above is correct, and if that deficit is due either to a disruption of binaural cues or perhaps even to the utilization of spatial information over time, then one conclusion might be that the core portion of auditory forebrain is involved in the analysis and utilization of the spatial aspects of hearing whereas the fringe or surrounding systems are involved in the utilization or storage of temporal sequences.

SUMMARY OF BEHAVIORAL EXPERIMENTS

From the onset of the study of cortical function, the central idea has been that auditory cortex is directly involved in the conscious perception of sound. Thirty years of careful experimentation has now demonstrated that, whatever its role, auditory cortex is *not* involved in the direct analysis of the physical parameters of sound. That is, absolute threshold and frequency and intensity difference thresholds are essentially unchanged after removal of auditory cortex. Instead, the available facts indicate that auditory cortex plays a major role in the natural process of localizing sounds in space and in the temporal aspects of hearing, which embraces both the brief binaural time differences involved in sound localization and the process of sequential memory. However, before the early idea that cortex is directly involved in the analysis of simple sounds is abandoned, at least two further ideas might be tested. First, auditory cortex may be involved in the processing of simultaneous sounds. Along this line, the effects of auditory cortex ablation on masked band phenomena and on the localization of one of two simultaneous sounds might be studied. Second, auditory cortex may be directly involved in the analysis of sounds more natural than the pure tones typically used in laboratory experiments. For example, the role of auditory cortex in the analysis of transient sounds or even complex timbre differences such as those involved in vocalizations might be a starting point for this sort of analysis.

The idea proposed at the end of the previous section, that structurally the auditory forebrain can be subdivided into three systems, receives direct support from evidence based on partial lesions of auditory cortex. Briefly, these experiments suggest that the ventral division system is involved in the analysis and utilization of spatial information about the location of sound sources and that the dorsal and medial division systems are involved in the utilization or storage of temporal sound sequences.

Human Auditory Forebrain

The purpose of this section is to expand the present discussion to the contributions of auditory forebrain to human hearing. A major goal is to examine the possibility of separating certain uniquely human characteristics of auditory forebrain from those features man shares with other mammals. Several sources of evidence which shed light on the functions of human auditory cortex will first be examined. Whenever possible, attempts will be made to draw direct comparisons between the functions of human and nonhuman auditory forebrain. Two important assumptions underlie this discussion: (1) the essential continuity in evolutionary development of the auditory system in all mammals, including man, and (2) the possibility of qualitatively or quantitatively distinct auditory functions in man that may have been superimposed on phylogenetically older functions which man shares with other mammals.

Before proceeding, it is first necessary to place the human data in perspective by considering certain methodological considerations which stem from working with human subjects rather than nonhuman animals. The first issue concerns limitations arising from obvious ethical factors involved in examining the effects of brain damage in human subjects. The second explores the strategy of neuropsychological experimentation with normal human subjects as a source of information about human brain function.

Methodological Considerations in Human Research

The two primary means of investigating human brain-behavior relationships involve behavioral observations of either brain-damaged or normal subjects. Inferences about human cortical functioning may be drawn from either of these data sources or, preferably, from an integration of the two. Both approaches, however, have their own characteristic limitations. Direct investigation of human brain-behavior relationships in brain-damaged subjects is, of course, severely constrained by ethical considerations. Extensive postoperative behavioral observation is often precluded by clinical considerations. Further, adequate anatomical verification of lesions at autopsy is rarely possible. Still further, brain damage in human patients often follows the distribution of blood vessels, and thus is seldom limited to a single cortical area. Finally, the two problems identified earlier in connection with ablation-behavior studies on laboratory animals also exist with human subjects, often in a magnified form: that is, confusing purely "sensory" deficits with malfunctions of "higher mental processes," and allowing compensating abilities to mask existing deficits.

The use of normal subjects in neuropsychological experiments designed to illuminate cerebral processes represents a highly indirect means of investigation. One common use of such behavioral techniques is to examine asymmetries in auditory or visual perception which reveal functional differences between the two hemispheres. For instance, in the *dichotic listening* paradigm, different auditory stimuli are presented simultaneously, one to each ear. This technique depends on the fact that the contralateral or crossed pathways from ear to cortex have a greater number of fibers and faster transmission speed than the ipsilateral projections, in man as well as in other mammals (Majkowski *et al.*, 1971; Rosenzweig, 1951). Greater speed or accuracy in reporting material presented to a given ear is thus taken as indirect evidence that the contralateral hemisphere is relatively more efficient in processing that material. The interaction between ear of presentation and type of material presented is the object of interest in this paradigm. Typically, the complexity of cross-hemispheric neural interactions in the intact brain allows the observation of only small statistical differences in such tests with normal subjects. The usual finding in the dichotic listening paradigm is a small but significant right ear (left hemisphere) advantage in accuracy of performance if *verbal* material is used (Bryden, 1963; Kimura, 1967) and a left ear (right hemisphere) advantage for music, environmental sounds, or other *nonverbal* material (Curry, 1967; Kimura, 1964). Data of this sort are part of the evidence supporting the notion of cerebral dominance, i.e., the specialization of each hemisphere of the human brain for different forms of information processing. One hemisphere, usually the left in most right-handed individuals, is "dominant" for language and time-related processing, while the "minor" or "nondominant" hemisphere is believed to be specialized for nonverbal material and visuospatial analysis. The verbal vs. nonverbal distinction suggests that this behavioral phenomenon is cortical, and that it may be uniquely developed in man. Thus, it may be of fundamental importance in understanding the organization of human auditory forebrain and how it differs from nonhuman auditory forebrain. These functional asymmetries are believed to be linked to the sort of anatomical asymmetries described previously in the anatomical section.

The existence of cerebral dominance must be taken into account in research with both normal and brain-damaged patients. One goal of brain-behavior investigations is to differentiate bilateral abilities from predominantly unilateral (or lateralized) abilities. In neurological research, this information is provided by correlating a specific performance decrement with the hemispheric locus of a circumscribed lesion. In behavioral investigations using normal subjects, accuracy or speed of performance on a given task is compared for stimuli presented to first one hemisphere and then the other. Thus, although behavioral studies of this sort involving normal subjects do not yield direct information about localized brain mechanisms, they permit inferences about cerebral functioning which may be useful in two ways. First, they can provide clues to the sorts of auditory phenomena which might be processed at the cortical level. Second, they may also constitute an important source of information about the bilateral organization of the human brain, i.e., left hemisphere vs. right hemisphere functions.

For the present purpose, the phenomenon of cerebral dominance in man raises two issues concerning the organization of mammalian auditory forebrain: (1) the possibility that different forms of auditory processing may be preferentially performed by one or the other of the human hemispheres, and (2) the relationship of these lateralized capacities to aspects of hearing which are under bilateral control in nonhuman mammals.

In the next section, clinical and experimental data will be reviewed in an attempt to determine the degree of correspondence between cortical functions in man and other animals. Evidence for both bilateral and unilateral aspects of auditory function will be considered. The next section attempts to review several lines of evidence which, taken together, indicate that human neocortex is intimately involved in the temporal aspects of hearing. In addition, the possibility will be examined that during man's recent evolution a given hemisphere may have become singularly specialized for certain aspects of hearing which may be under bilateral control in nonhuman mammals.

Role of Auditory Cortex in Human Hearing

The classical identification of neocortex with the capacity for auditory sensation profoundly influenced early views of brain function in man as well as in other animals. With respect to the human auditory system, it was predicted that bilateral damage to temporal lobe cortex would result in "psychic deafness" (Munk, 1881) or "cortical deafness" (Bramwell, 1927; Le Gros Clark and Russell, 1938). However, more recent clinical data do not support this contention. Landau *et al.* (1960) reported only slight decreases in the pure-tone sensitivity of a young subject with anatomically verified bilateral temporal lobe lesions accompanied by almost complete medial geniculate degeneration bilaterally. In three exceptionally well-documented cases, subjects with successive lesions in both hemispheres showed only slight impairments on pure-tone audiograms (Jerger *et al.*, 1969, 1972; Lhermitte *et al.*, 1971).

As in the animal literature, the growing realization that cortical damage does not cause total deafness in the human led to a search for more subtle deficits. Initially, this search focused on specific physical parameters of sound, with results similar to those summarized in the last section. That is, there is little disruption of sensitivity to changes in frequency or intensity after either bilateral or unilateral auditory cortex lesions (Jerger *et al.*, 1969; Lhermitte *et al.*, 1971; Milner, 1962; Swisher, 1967).

However, human cortex does seem to be involved in certain types of complex auditory analysis. In the earlier discussion of cortical function in nonhuman mammals, it was suggested that while stable frequency and intensity parameters can be analyzed at subcortical levels if necessary, cortex seems to be essential for the analysis of many aspects of the temporal dimension of sound. In a similar way, convergent lines of evidence, reviewed below, suggest that human cortex also plays an important role in the temporal aspects of hearing.

The forms of temporal analysis which are known to be dependent on human auditory cortex can be roughly categorized into two classes: (1) "perceptual" processes of a relatively immediate nature and (2) "memory" processes involving storage of acoustic traces over time.

PERCEPTUAL CONTRIBUTIONS. Although the processing of simple acoustic parameters such as ongoing frequency and intensity may be accomplished after cortical damage in man, the processing of brief sounds, particularly those that change rapidly in relation to each other, is less efficient following cortical damage. For example, human cortex seems to be especially important for the perceptual analysis of *brief* sounds. Cortical lesions in either hemisphere have the effect of slightly elevating absolute detection thresholds for sounds of less than 14 msec duration in the contralateral ear (Baru and Karaseva, 1972; Gersuni *et al.*, 1968; Gersuni, 1971; Karaseva, 1972). These investigators found similar effects following cortical lesions in dogs (Baru, 1966, 1967; Gersuni, 1971). Further, Tallal and Piercy (1974) have reported that patients with left hemisphere lesions are significantly impaired in discriminating 43-msec sounds of changing frequency, but performed normally when the duration of these sounds was increased to 95 msec. Because Tallal and Piercy's study involved only subjects with left hemisphere damage, this study does not indicate whether either hemisphere is preferentially equipped for processing brief, frequency-modulated signals. However, a growing number of dichotic listening studies with normal subjects suggest that the hemisphere dominant for speech is also specialized for the analysis of brief sounds involving frequency transitions. Stimuli of unchanging frequency do not show similar evidence of lateralization, but a clear left hemisphere advantage appears for sounds which include a brief segment of changing frequency (Cutting, 1972; Darwin, 1971; Halperin *et al.*, 1973). Thus, on the basis of available data, it seems that both hemispheres are involved in threshold sensitivity to brief sounds but that the left hemisphere is more strongly involved than the right hemisphere in the analysis of brief sounds, especially brief sounds of rapidly changing frequency.

In a similar way, human cortex also seems to be involved in judgments of simultaneity of brief sounds, that is, the discrimination or segmentation of sounds. For example, human neurological data suggest that cortical lesions increase the time requirements for making segmentation discriminations and further that the hemispheres may be differentially specialized for segmentation. Both neurological and normal behavioral data suggest that this ability may be more highly developed in the left hemisphere. Lackner and Teuber (1973) reported that auditory (but not tactile) fusion thresholds are permanently lowered after left hemisphere lesions, while right hemisphere damage has no apparent effect. This same suggestion is related to Efron's (1963a) experiments with normal subjects. Efron observed that a tone in the ear contralateral to the nondominant hemisphere must be presented 2–6 msec before a similar stimulus presented to the dominant hemisphere in order for the two stimuli to be judged as simultaneous. Efron inferred from such data that input to the right hemisphere must be "transferred" across the corpus callosum to the left hemisphere before the temporal relationship of the two stimuli can be perceived. He speculated that a single "temporal comparator" mechanism may be lateralized in the left hemisphere.

Available evidence also indicates that human cortex plays a role in the judgment of temporal order (which presupposes accurate segmentation). Following cortical lesions, judgments of sequential order are less accurate and require longer interstimulus intervals to make. For normal subjects, two stimuli separated by 50–60 msec permit correct judgment of temporal order (Hirsh and Sherrick, 1961). In contrast, patients with left hemisphere cortical lesions may require as much as 500 msec or more to judge the temporal order of two brief nonverbal stimuli (Edwards and Auger, 1965; Efron, 1963b). That the left hemisphere may be preferentially involved in temporal order sensitivity was also suggested by Swisher and Hirsh (1972). They reported that temporal order judgments are significantly less accurate than normal following left but not right hemisphere damage.

Further experiments indicate that other aspects of hearing may be preferentially processed by the right rather than left cortex. For example, Milner (1962) reports deficits in duration, timbre, and intensity discriminations following right but not left lesions. This asymmetry is presumably related to the right hemisphere's superiority in processing complex nonverbal stimuli such as music and natural sounds in normal subjects (Curry, 1967; Kimura, 1964).

The above lines of evidence taken either from observations of brain-damaged patients or from neuropsychological experimentation with normal subjects indicate that human cortex is involved with the temporal aspects of hearing. While one major conclusion from these data is that man and other mammals are very much alike in the cortical processing of temporally patterned information, a second implication is that the neural organization of these capacities is in some ways fundamentally different in man. That is, although certain temporal discriminations in man seem to be performed equally well by either the left or the right cortex, other functions are lateralized to one side or the other. The analysis of some nonverbal sounds is most affected by right hemisphere damage, while discriminations involving brief transients and temporal order judgments seem to be most dependent on the left hemisphere.

MEMORY CONTRIBUTIONS. Deficits which are not based on faulty reception of stimuli but on faulty storage of perceptual traces over time constitute a second type of disruption of temporal processing following damage to human auditory cortex. Deficits of this sort fall into two classes: (1) the storage of a single sound until action utilizing that information is completed and (2) the storage of sequences of sounds.

As in animals, human neuropathology involves deficits in delayed-response single-sound localization tasks after cortical brain damage (Jerger et al., 1969;

Milner, 1967; Sanchez-Longo and Forster, 1958; Sanchez-Longo *et al.*, 1957; Teuber and Weinstein, 1956). In order to shed light on the nature of this deficit in man, Shankweiler (1961) explicitly compared performance in different sound localization paradigms: one involving a delayed response (indicating whether a second sound is to the left or right of a previous sound) and another requiring an immediate response (spatial pointing). A sound localization deficit after cerebral damage was apparent only with the delayed procedure. Shankweiler attributes subnormal performance to "defects in immediate memory and judgmental ability rather than to a specific auditory factor" (1961, p. 381).

The storage of discrete auditory information over time is thus another function which human auditory cortex shares with nonhuman mammalian cortex. Unlike other animals, however, the differential specialization of the human cortical hemispheres determines the precise nature of these memory disorders. Following unilateral damage, the type and degree of impairment on memory tasks depends on which hemisphere has been damaged. For example, although unilateral lesions in either hemisphere impair delayed-response sound localization performance, right hemisphere lesions are more disruptive than left (Shankweiler, 1961; Teuber and Weinstein, 1956). This finding may reflect the right hemisphere's specialization for nonverbal stimuli such as those used in sound localization tests. Short-term memory tasks involving verbal stimuli, on the other hand, are more impaired by left hemisphere damage (Milner, 1967). Thus the role of neocortex in short-term storage of auditory signals, which is common to all mammals, is augmented in man by the phenomenon of hemispheric asymmetry.

The second form of memory-processing deficits involves the retention of multiple stimuli rather than the persistence of a single stimulus trace as in a delayed sound localization task. In a set of animal ablation-behavior studies, described in the last section, Diamond and Neff (1957) reported deficits in discrimination of simple tonal patterns following cortical lesions in cats. These animals were not impaired, however, on frequency discrimination tests which involved the same tones. It seems, then, that they were impaired in their retention of the sequence of stimuli rather than in their perception of the stimuli themselves.

Parallel results may be seen in the human neurological data concerning sequential auditory memory. Short-term memory for auditory sequences is impaired by either unilateral or bilateral damage to the temporal lobes in humans (Kim, 1976; Lhermitte *et al.*, 1971; Milner, 1967; Shankweiler, 1966). Left hemisphere damage can be more detrimental than right hemisphere damage to short-term memory for either verbal or nonverbal stimuli, although both are inferior to normal individuals (Albert, 1976; Kim, 1976; Kimura, 1961; Milner, 1958). This is consonant with the fact that normal subjects show a left hemisphere advantage in short-term memory for dichotically presented rhythmic sequences, even for nonverbal material (Natale, 1977).

However, which hemisphere is damaged can also determine whether verbal or nonverbal sequences are most affected. Left temporal lobe damage is more disruptive than right hemisphere damage for memory of sequences of verbal material (Kimura, 1961; Milner, 1958). Albert (1976) has demonstrated that the deficit in auditory verbal short-term memory is specific to *order* information, rather than memory for the items themselves. It seems that the dominant hemisphere may be specialized for a general auditory sequencing mechanism; it is not known whether such a mechanism is a cause or an effect of the left hemisphere's specialization for language, although language processing is heavily dependent on sequential analyses. Right hemisphere lesions, on the other hand, can impair memory for sequences of certain complex nonverbal sounds more than left hemisphere lesions (Milner, 1962; Shankweiler, 1966). Milner used the Tonal Memory subtest of the Seashore Measures of Musical Talents. In this test two series of three to five notes each are played, and the subject must indicate which note is changed in the second pattern. This test represents an explicit analogue to the tone pattern discrimination studies with cats by Diamond and Neff (1957). Human subjects with right temporal lobectomies showed much greater deficits on this test than left hemisphere patients, whose perceptions were not significantly different from preoperative levels. These data led Milner (1967) to conclude that "in man the right hemisphere makes a greater contribution than the left to those aspects of auditory discrimination known to be affected by bilateral cortical lesions in the monkey" (p. 187), that is, temporal processing of nonspeech.

Before such a conclusion is accepted, the marked lack of parallels in human and animal auditory experimentation should be noted. For example, much of the clinical brain damage literature evaluates speech perception, whereas few attempts have been made to determine the role of nonhuman auditory cortex in the perception of its own species-specific vocalizations. Further, unlike the human clinical data, which contain much information about unilateral damage, the animal literature is based mostly on bilateral cortical damage.

The picture that emerges from these data for both humans and other mammals is that mammalian neocortex makes a fundamental contribution to temporal auditory functions of many sorts, embracing both perception and memory. However, only in man does there appear to be differential specialization of temporal capacities within the cerebral hemispheres. Specifically, the left or dominant hemisphere in man shows slightly greater efficiency in temporal parameters such as the discrimination of brief transient sounds and simultaneity, as well as the storage of verbal sequences. The right hemisphere, on the other hand, seems more directly involved in the storage of steady-state information and nonverbal sequences.

In addition to the above tasks which are more or less common to both man and other animals, auditory cortex may be involved in other functions which are much less apparent in other mammals and which are even more clearly lateralized in the human brain. In particular, the phonetic processing of human speech appears to be the auditory function most unique to man, and one which is strongly controlled by the left hemisphere. The final pages of this chapter will deal with human speech perception. Although it is not common to other mammals, human speech perception seems to be dependent on many of the same temporal analyses known to be performed by auditory cortex in nonhuman mammals. Those aspects of temporal processing shared by all mammals may have composed an evolutionary substrate on which the specific skills required for human speech perception were superimposed. The question at issue here is: which factors of speech perception involve purely acoustic processing and are therefore more likely to be shared by other mammals, and which are more nearly limited to man?

SPEECH PERCEPTION. Our approach to the study of human speech perception views it as an aspect of hearing which involves cortical auditory functions common to man and other mammals. For example, one major conclusion of the preceding pages is that common specializations of mammalian auditory cortex might include the perception of brief transient sounds and some aspects of auditory memory. As it turns out, both these capacities play a fundamental role in speech perception: brevity and transience are especially important features for discriminating human speech sounds, and the ability to store sound sequences until processing is completed is a prerequisite for decoding ongoing speech. Thus many of the capacities required for human speech perception are not only common to other mammals but probably also dependent on auditory forebrain.

Originally, each phoneme or unit of perceived speech was thought to be associated with a specific configuration of acoustic cues. An intensive effort was therefore made to identify the critical acoustic cues associated with each phoneme (Liberman and Cooper, 1970). The specification of acoustic cues in human speech perception was made possible by the development of computer-controlled speech synthesizers which mimic the action of the human vocal apparatus. Mechanical synthesis allows the systematic and independent variation of many possible acoustic dimensions in the speech signal, one at a time. In this way, those acoustic cues which are particularly associated with the perception of certain phonemes can be identified. If perception changes from one phoneme to another as the values of a single dimension change, then that dimension is defined as a critical acoustic cue for discrimination of those phonemes.

Through behavioral investigations of this sort with normal subjects, our understanding of speech perception has greatly increased (see Liberman *et al.*, 1967, for a review). Briefly, each minimal speech sound (or *phoneme*) is composed of several identifiable bands of acoustic energy of different frequencies which are called "formants." It has been found that most of the relevant information for simple speech perception is carried either by the steady portion of the formant or by a segment of rapidly changing frequencies leading into or out of the formants (called "formant transitions"). A visual representation of formants and formant transitions can be seen in the simplified speech spectrogram shown in Fig. 6.

There are two large classes of speech sounds: vowels and consonants. Of these two classes, consonants are the most important for speech perception; vowels carry relatively little information. With the use of speech synthesizers it has been determined that the critical acoustic cues are very different for vowels and consonants (Liberman *et al.*, 1967). The minimal acoustic cues for the perception of *vowels* are the frequency values of the steady-rate portions of the formants. Critical cues for *consonants*, on the other hand, most often involve characteristics associated with formant transitions. These include the direction and magnitude of these formant transitions, or the duration of intervals of noise or silence before a

RICHARD J. RAVIZZA
AND SUSAN M.
BELMORE

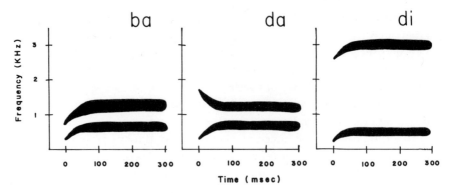

Fig. 6. Simplified spectrogram of the syllables /ba/, /da/, and /di/. Only the first two formants are shown for each syllable. Note that each formant shown here is composed of segments of steady and transitional frequency.

transition. These cues for consonants are rarely available for longer than 50 msec. On the other hand, the cues for vowels are relatively long; they may last up to 350 msec. Thus the critical acoustic cues for vowels and consonants differ in several ways. The cues for vowels are relatively long and unchanging, at least in synthetic speech, whereas those for consonants are brief and transitional.

Even after the critical acoustic characteristics of both vowels and consonants have been determined, the question of the nature of the relationship between these acoustic cues and the perceived units of speech remains. If each segment of the acoustic signal corresponds to a single phoneme, then the speech stream could be interpreted in strict sequential order into successive phonemes, syllables, and words. The result would be a straightforward "speech alphabet" with a one-to-one relationship between the acoustic stimulus and perceived speech. However, this does not seem to be the case. Liberman *et al.* (1967) have outlined several reasons why such a simple view of speech perception is not adequate. First, many of these cues (especially consonant cues) are not invariant, but are highly context dependent. A single acoustic event can be perceived as different phonemes and different acoustic cues may be perceived as the same phoneme, depending on context (Liberman *et al.*, 1952, 1967). Specific cues, therefore, cannot be automatically translated into specific speech sounds without additional analysis.

Second, it is now known that if the acoustic cues for successive phonemes were simply strung end-to-end along the speech signal, our normally high rates of processing speech would be impossible, because of limits on the temporal resolving power of the human ear. The great speed of human speech processing (Foulke and Sticht, 1969) is made possible by the fact that significant acoustic cues seem to be thoroughly intermixed and overlapping in the speech signal. Human speech is said to be characterized by *parallel transmission* of information: cues for a single phoneme may be scattered over several neighboring sound units, and cues for successive phonemes may be carried on the same sound segment. Parallel transmission thus eliminates the possibility of strict sequential processing. The listener must therefore utilize some sort of echoic (short-term) storage system which is able to hold information about several segments at once.

The third reason for the failure of a straightforward speech alphabet is that consonants seem to be perceived in a fundamentally different manner from vowels. The paradigm used to investigate these perceptual differences involves the identification and discrimination of synthetic speech sounds. A series of synthetic stimuli are constructed which vary in the value of a single critical acoustic dimension such as the direction and duration of a formant transition. The subject is then asked to identify which speech sound he hears for each stimulus in the series and to discriminate between pairs of such stimuli. For vowels, perception changes gradually from one speech sound to another as values of the critical acoustic cue are changed. Also, many stimuli which the subject identifies by the same category label can, in fact, be discriminated from one another when necessary. This response pattern is called "continuous perception," and is typical of vowels as well as most nonverbal auditory stimuli (Eimas, 1963; Fry *et al.,* 1962). Consonants, on the other hand, are perceived quite differently. Identification boundaries between one speech sound and another are very sharply defined. Furthermore, pairs of consonants can be accurately discriminated only at category boundaries; discrimination within categories occurs at chance levels (Liberman *et al.,* 1967). This pattern of performance is called "categorical perception."

Categorical perception is largely restricted to the perception of certain consonants. In contrast, continuous perception is the usual pattern for nonspeech sounds and most vowels. However, vowels are also categorically perceived under conditions of perceptual difficulty such as noise, confusability, or truncation (Godfrey, 1974; Pisoni, 1973). This finding suggests that categorical perception may be dependent on the brevity or transience of acoustic cues.

Thus there are three related reasons why a simple isomorphic model of speech perception is not adequate: contextual dependency, parallel transmission, and categorical perception. For these reasons, Liberman *et al.* (1967) have argued that the relation between acoustic input and perceived speech constitutes a complex "speech code" rather than a simple alphabet. Speech sounds vary in the degree to which they are encoded in the speech code. Sounds to which these three criteria apply (e.g., stop consonants) are said to be highly encoded in the speech code; sounds which do not meet these criteria (including vowels and most nonverbal sounds) are said to be relatively unencoded. The speech code seems to be especially dependent on the acoustic characteristics of brevity and transience.

To summarize, it has been argued that human speech perception is a highly complex phenomenon. For many speech sounds, perception from the acoustic signal is not straightforward, but involves an indirect code characterized by contextual dependency, parallel transmission, and categorical perception. It was seen that speech sounds vary in their degree of encodedness and that those sounds most representative of the speech code (the stop consonants) are identified with cues of a brief, transitional nature. It is already known that cortex is involved in processing brief, transient sounds, rather than continuous sounds; this fact sug-

RICHARD J. RAVIZZA
AND SUSAN M.
BELMORE

gests that the temporal processing abilities of mammalian cortex may be more heavily implicated in the perception of highly encoded consonants than the less encoded vowels. In order to shed light on this possibility, the final section of this chapter considers the question of the brain mechanisms underlying the speech code.

Speech Code and Cerebral Dominance

Little specific information is available about the cortical brain mechanisms involved in the complex process of human speech perception. The research summarized above has been interpreted as an indication that speech perception requires psychological processes which are distinct from all other forms of human perception (Liberman *et al.*, 1967) and physiological mechanisms which are not available to any nonhuman mammals (Mattingly and Liberman, 1969). This apparent uniqueness of the speech code suggests that it might be somehow related to the phenomenon of cerebral dominance, which also seems to be unique to man. In fact, both behavioral and neurological data reveal a close correlation between the speech code and hemispheric asymmetry.

It has been known for many years that speech is often severely disrupted following left hemisphere brain damage but is rarely affected by comparable damage to the right hemisphere (Milner *et al.*, 1966). The left hemisphere's importance is even more dramatically shown in the so-called split-brain subjects, whose hemispheres have been permanently separated by surgical section of the corpus callosum for therapeutic reasons (Sperry *et al.*, 1969). In behavioral tests with split-brain subjects, the right hemisphere is capable of only limited speech perception or production when acting in isolation, yet the left hemisphere can operate with normal efficiency under such conditions (Gazzaniga and Sperry, 1967).

As it turns out, the phenomenon of cerebral dominance has an important relationship to the speech code. In the normal brain, not all speech sounds are preferentially processed by the left hemisphere but only those which are highly encoded in the speech code. For example, a left hemisphere processing advantage is found to exist for precisely those phonemes which most reliably elicit the categorical pattern of perception—one characteristic of the speech code. In dichotic listening tests with normal subjects, highly encoded consonants exhibit a right ear (left hemisphere) advantage (Shankweiler and Studdert-Kennedy, 1967). Vowels, on the other hand, can be processed by either hemisphere, depending on experimental conditions (Spellacy and Blumstein, 1970). In brain-damaged subjects, perception of consonants is more impaired than perception of vowels following left hemisphere damage (Luria, 1966). Indeed, perception of any phonemes requiring analysis of spectral cues (e.g., frequency or intensity) seems to be less affected by left hemisphere damage than perception involving cues which are temporal in nature, such as frequency transitions and duration judgments (Carpenter and Rutherford, 1973).

Based on data of this sort, Studdert-Kennedy and Shankweiler (1970) identified the fact of cerebral dominance with the speech code. They propose that both human hemispheres can perceive and analyze critical acoustic cues but that only the dominant left hemisphere is capable of the identification of speech sounds.

Until recently, it seemed that an apparently unique structural aspect (cerebral dominance) of the human brain might be directly linked with an apparently unique functional aspect of human speech perception: the speech code. The strong form of the claim that these characteristics are unique to human speech perception cannot be maintained, however, for recent evidence indicates that neither categorical perception nor cerebral dominance is entirely unique to man. Consequently, the special status of human speech perception is currently undergoing serious reexamination. For example, it was recently proposed (Kuhn, 1975) that acoustic cues involving the resonant frequency of the mouth cavity may provide a more invariant relationship between the speech signal and speech perception than previously believed, thereby reducing the necessity for positing a complex speech code. Along this same line, Cutting has argued that there may be no unique behavior specific to the speech code at all. Indeed, he has demonstrated that all the auditory phenomena thought to define the speech code, including a right ear advantage in dichotic listening tasks, can be produced by certain non-speech sawtooth stimuli differing in rise time (Cutting, 1974; Cutting and Rosner, 1974, 1976). Even in man, categorical perception seems to be a more general phenomenon than first thought. The categorical pattern has been observed in other sensory modalities including color perception in infants (Bornstein *et al.,* 1976) and form perception in adults (Cooper and Shepard, 1973). Furthermore, preliminary evidence also indicates that categorical perception may be present in nonhuman animals. Rhesus monkeys (Morse and Snowdon, 1974) and even chinchillas (Kuhl and Miller, 1975) exhibit rudimentary forms of categorical perception when tested with human speech sounds. The crucial tests for the presence of categorical perception in the auditory behavior of other mammals, which have not yet been performed, would of course involve animals' perception of their own species-specific communication signals, rather than human speech stimuli. If it turns out that nonhuman mammals use categorical perception in the interpretation of species-specific sounds as well as the above instances, then this form of perception can hardly be unique to man. For our understanding of brain mechanisms, this implies that the neural substrate underlying this phenomenon may be formed in part by those parts of auditory forebrain which man shares with nonhuman mammals.

Evidence which contradicts the notion that cerebral dominance is unique to man has likewise been accumulating from a variety of sources, including the presence of anatomical asymmetries of auditory cortex in other primates and ablation-behavior techniques with laboratory animals. For example, recent investigations have revealed the presence of anatomical asymmetries between the left and right hemispheres of nonhuman primates (Groves and Humphrey, 1973; LeMay, 1976; LeMay and Geschwind, 1975; Yeni-Komshian and Benson, 1976).

RICHARD J. RAVIZZA
AND SUSAN M.
BELMORE

These asymmetries involve the auditory areas surrounding the sylvian fissure, and are presumed analogous to those seen in the human brain (Geschwind and Levitsky, 1968). Further, Dewson and his colleagues (Dewson, 1976; Dewson *et al.*, 1975) have reported preliminary evidence showing permanent deficits in auditory memory in rhesus monkey following unilateral ablation of auditory association cortex in the left but not in the right hemisphere.

If, as these data indicate, rudimentary forms of the categorical pattern of perception and cerebral dominance are shared with nonhuman animals, then neither phenomenon can be considered uniquely human, but only uniquely developed in man.

SUMMARY OF HUMAN AUDITORY FOREBRAIN

A convergence of human and nonhuman data is becoming apparent. Certain acoustic parameters involving fine temporal perception (brevity, transience, and short-term acoustic storage) have been identified as primarily cortical functions that seem to be common to mammals. In man, however, these same parameters are precisely those which are known to be most important for perception of the human speech code, and those for which the human left hemisphere shows a preferential processing advantage. Thus it seems that those abilities which are most dependent on cortex in other mammals are similar to those which have become most lateralized in the left hemisphere of man, and which have come to constitute the critical cues for human speech perception. Consonants, the sounds most highly encoded in the speech code, are known to be preferentially processed in the left hemisphere and to be most dependent on time-related analyses. Vowels, on the other hand, which are more similar to nonspeech sounds, are dependent on relatively stable spectral cues whose processing can be subcortically executed, and which show no clear hemispheric advantage.

To return to the question raised at the very beginning of this section: is it possible to separate uniquely human characteristics of auditory forebrain from those features man shares with other mammals? If speech is viewed as the auditory manifestation of our conspecific communication system, it might be expected to involve a combination of some abilities common to all mammals and some abilities unique to man. Fine temporal processing and auditory storage over time are both fundamental to the perception of speech, and, to some extent, seem to be functions characteristic of cortex in other mammals. On the other hand, although recent studies of categorical perception and brain structure question the notion that a complex speech code and the physiological phenomenon of cerebral dominance are unique to man, the fact that categorical perception for speech sounds and at least some aspects of cerebral dominance may be shared with other mammals indicates that it might prove fruitful to characterize differences between auditory forebrain of man and other mammals along more quantitative rather than qualitative dimensions than was thought possible a few years ago. That is, those brain-behavior relationships involving speech perception and hemispheric differences, while they may not be unique to man, are at least much more highly developed in man than in other mammals.

Concluding Remarks: An Overview

In a brief chapter of this sort, it is possible to highlight only a few major issues that have attracted the attention of investigators interested in the function of auditory forebrain. Nevertheless, several anatomical and functional conclusions now seem reasonable that would have not been so even a few decades ago.

To begin with, the basic anatomical organization of auditory forebrain seems to be remarkably similar among all mammals including humans. Briefly, this basic plan is organized around a three-part subdivision of the auditory forebrain into ventral, dorsal, and medial divisions of the medial geniculate and their respective cortical projection areas. In the course of man's evolution, specializations which characterize the human auditory forebrain have been superimposed on this basic plan. First, compared to other mammals, man has extremely well-developed auditory koniocortex. Second, human auditory cortex may be unique in that it is structurally asymmetrical. That is, in most people, the left auditory cortex is somewhat larger than the right.

Functionally, notions of the role of auditory cortex in hearing have changed rapidly. Once it was assumed to include the conscious sensation and discrimination of sound itself. Ablation-behavior experiments over the past 30 years have repeatedly shown that this is simply not the case in man or in other mammals. Following removal of auditory cortex, auditory sensitivity is virtually unchanged for almost all primary attributes of sound. For example, absolute pure-tone sensitivity and pitch and loudness difference thresholds are virtually unchanged. Thus, several aspects of hearing simply do not depend on intact auditory cortex. However, before abandoning the idea that auditory cortex plays a role in the analysis of simple sounds, its role in analyzing natural sounds of high biological relevance remains to be examined.

In contrast to the lack of simple acoustic deficits resulting from auditory cortex ablations, auditory cortex seems to play an important role in temporal analysis and the storage of certain types of auditory information. Indeed, the evidence indicates that each division of the auditory system may be involved in different aspects of this process. The ventral division system seems to be essential to the analysis and perhaps the storage of spatial information, the dorsal system is required for the comparison of various sound sequences, and the medial system may play an important role in extracting information about sound duration.

Finally, evidence from brain-damaged patients and normal human subjects indicates that human auditory cortex is involved in many of the same aspects of hearing as it is in other mammals. For example, following auditory cortex lesions, deficits in transient sound analysis or in the storage of auditory information are observed in man and other mammals. The fact that human speech perception is also dependent on these abilities known to be controlled by auditory cortex is consistent with the idea that many abilities fundamental to human speech perception are present in rudimentary form in nonhuman mammals. In the past, it has been assumed that human auditory forebrain also formed the substrate for certain unique capacities involving the "speech code" and cerebral dominance. However, the possible existence in other mammals of one important aspect of the speech code—categorical perception—and the possibility of cerebral dominance in other mammals suggest that human auditory forebrain may be less different than was thought even a few years ago.

Acknowledgments

The authors are indebted to P. Cornwell, J. L. Cranford, W. C. Hall, R. S. Heffner, H. E. Heffner, D. L. Oliver, M. L. Schnitzer, and J. Winer for their many suggestions on an earlier draft. Special thanks are extended to Gloria Bathurst and Anna Mary Madden for typing the manuscript and to Anita Monyok for the artwork.

REFERENCES

Aitkin, L. M., and Webster, W. R. Tonotopic organization in the medial geniculate body of the cat. *Brain Res.,* 1971, *26*, 402–5.

Albert, M. L. Short-term memory and aphasia. *Brain Lang.* 1976, *3*, 28–33.

Altman, J. A., Syka, J., and Shmigidina, G. W. Neuronal activity in the medial geniculate body of the cat during monaural and binaural stimulation. *Exp. Brain Res.,* 1970, *10*, 81–93.

Bard, P., and Rioch, D. M. A study of four cats deprived of neocortex and additional portions of the forebrain. *Bull. Johns Hopkins Hosp.,* 1937, *60*, 73–147.

Baru, A. V. Role of the temporal cortex in the detection of acoustic stimuli of different duration. *Zh. Vyssh. Nerv Deyat.,* 1966, *16*, 655–665.

Baru, A. V. Differential thresholds of frequency in relation to duration of tonal series in animals after ablation of the auditory cortex. In *Mechanisms of Hearing.* Nauka, Leningrad, 1967.

Baru, A. V., and Karaseva, T. A. *The Brain and Hearing: Hearing Disturbances Associated with Local Brain Lesions.* Plenum, New York, 1972.

Boivie, J. The termination of the spinothalamic tract in the cat: An experimental study with silver impregnation methods. *Exp. Brain Res.,* 1971, *12*, 331–353.

Bornstein, M., Dessen, W., and Weiskopf S. Color vision and hue categorization in young human infants. *J. Exp. Psychol.,* 1976, *2*, 115–129.

Bramwell, E. A case of cortical deafness. *Brain,* 1927, *50*, 579–580.

Bremer, F., and Dow, R. S. The cerebral acoustic area of the cat: A combined oscillographic and cytoarchitectonic study. *J. Neurophysiol.,* 1939, *2*, 308–318.

Bryden, M. P. Ear preference in auditory perception. *J. Exp. Psychol.,* 1963, *65*, 103–105.

Burton, H., and Jones, E. G. The posterior thalamic region and its cortical projection in New World and Old World monkeys. *J. Comp. Neurol.,* 1976, *168*, 249–303.

Butler, R. A., Diamond, I. T., and Neff, W. D. Role of auditory cortex in discrimination of changes in frequency. *J. Neurophysiol.,* 1957, *20*, 108–120.

Carpenter, M. B. Experimental anatomical-physiological studies of the vertibular nerve and cerebellar connections. In G. L. Rasmussen & W. F. Windle (eds.), *Neural Mechanisms of the Auditory and Vestibular Systems.* Thomas, Springfield, Ill., 1960.

Carpenter, R L. and Rutherford, D. R. Acoustic cue discrimination in adult aphasia. *J. Speech and Hear. Res.,* 1973, *16*, 534–542.

Casseday, J. H., Diamond, I. T., and Harting, J. K. Auditory pathways to the cortex in *Tupaia glis. J. Comp. Neurol.*, 1976, *166*, 303–340.

Colavita, F. B. Auditory cortical lesions and visual pattern discrimination in the cat. *Brain Res.*, 1972, *39*, 437–447.

Cooper, F. S. Spectrum analysis. *J. Acoust. Soc. Am.*, 1950, *22*, 761–762.

Cooper, L. A., and Shepard, R. N. Chronometric studies of the rotation of mental images. In W. G. Chase (ed.), *Visual Information Processing*. Academic Press, New York, 1973.

Cowan, W. M. Gottlieb, D. I., Hendrickson, A. E., Price, J. L., and Woolsey, T. A. The autoradiographic demonstration of axonal connections in the central nervous system. *Brain Res.*, 1972, *37*, 21–51.

Cranford, J. L., Igarashi, M., and Stramler, J. Effect of auditory neocortex ablation on discrimination of click rates in the cat. *Neurosci. Abs.*, 1975, *1*, 27.

Cranford, J. L., Igarashi, M., and Stramler, J. H. Effect of auditory neocortex ablation on pitch perception in the cat. *J. Neurophysiol.*, 1976a, *39*, 143–153.

Cranford, J. L., Ladner, S. S., Campbell, C. B. G., and Neff, W. D. Efferent projections of the insular and temporal neocortex of the cat. *Brain Res.*, 1976b, *117*, 195–210.

Curry, F. K. W. A comparison of left-handed and right-handed subjects on verbal and non-verbal dichotic listening tasks. *Cortex*, 1967, *3*, 343–352.

Cutting, J. E. Perception of speech and nonspeech, with and without transitions. *Haskins Labs Stat. Rep. Speech Res.*, 1972, *29/30*, 61–68.

Cutting, J. E. Different speech-processing mechanisms can be reflected in the results of discrimination and dichotic listening tasks. *Brain Lang.*, 1974, *1*, 363–373.

Cutting, J. E. There may be nothing peculiar to perceiving in the speech mode. Paper presented to Annual Meeting of the Psychonomic Society, St. Louis, 1976.

Cutting, J. E., and Rosner, B. S. Categories and boundaries in speech and music. *Percept. Psychophys.*, 1974, *16*, 564–570.

Cutting, J. E., and Rosner, B. S. Discrimination functions predicted from categories in speech and music. *Percept. Psychophys.*, 1976, *20*, 87–88.

Darwin, C. J. Ear differences in the recall of fricatives and vowels. *J. Exp. Psychol.*, 1971, *23*, 46–62.

Davis, H. Biophysics and physiology of the inner ear. *Physiol. Rev.*, 1957, *37*, 1–49.

Dewson, J. H. Speech sound discrimination by cats. *Science*, 1964, *144*, 555–556.

Dewson, J. H. Preliminary evidence of hemispheric asymmetry of auditory function in monkeys. In S. R. Harnard, R. W. Doty, L. Goldstein, J. Jaynes, and G. Krauthamer (ed.), *Lateralization in the Nervous System*. Academic Press, New York, 1976.

Dewson, J. H., Pribram, K. H. and Lynch, J. C. Effects of temporal cortex ablation upon speech sound discrimination in the monkey. *Exp. Neurol.*, 1969, *24*, 579–591.

Dewson, J. H., Cowey, A., and Weiskrantz, L. Disruptions of auditory sequence discrimination by unilateral and bilateral cortical ablations of superior temporal gyrus in the monkey. *Exp. Neurol.*, 1970, *28*, 529–48.

Dewson, J. H., Burlingame, A., Kizer, K., Dewson, S., Kenney, P., and Pribram, K. H. Hemispheric asymmetry of auditory function in monkeys. *J. Acoust. Soc. Am.*, 1975, *58*, S66.

Diamond, I. T., and Neff, W. D. Ablation of temporal cortex and discrimination of auditory patterns. *J. Neurophysiol.*, 1957, *20*, 300–315.

Diamond, I. T., Chow, K. L., and Neff, W. D. Degeneration of caudal medial geniculate body following cortical lesions ventral to auditory area II in the cat. *J. Comp. Neurol.*, 1958, *109*, 349–362.

Diamond, I. T., Goldberg, J. M., and Neff, W. D. Tonal discrimination after ablation of auditory cortex. *J. Neurophysiol.*, 1962, *25*, 223–235.

Diamond, I. T., Jones, E. C., and Powell, T. P. S. Interhemispheric fiber connections of auditory cortex of cat. *Brain Res.*, 1968, *11*, 177–193.

Diamond, I. T., Jones, E. G., and Powell, T. P. S. The projection of the auditory cortex upon the diencephalon and brain stem in the cat. *Brain Res.*, 1969, *15*, 305–340.

Edwards, A. E., and Auger, R., The effect of aphasia on the perception of precedence. *Proc. of 73rd Annu. Meet. APA*, 1965, 207–208.

Efron, R. The effects of handedness on the perception of simultaneity and temporal order. *Brain*, 1963a, *86*, 261–284.

Efron, R. Temporal perception, aphasia, and deja vu. *Brain*, 1963b, *86*, 403–424.

Eimas, P. D. The relation between identification and discrimination along speech and non-speech continua. *Lang. Speech*, 1963, *6*, 206–217.

RICHARD J. RAVIZZA
AND SUSAN M.
BELMORE

Elliott, D. N., and Trahiotis, C. Cortical lesions and auditory discrimination. *Psychol. Bull.,* 1972, *77,* 198–222.

Ferrier, D. *The Functions of the Brain,* 2nd ed. Smith Elder, London, 1886, pp. 305–312.

Fink, R. P., and Heimer, L. Two methods for selective silver impregnation of degenerating axons and their synaptic endings in the central nervous system. *Brain Res.,* 1967, *4,* 369–374.

Foulke, E., and Sticht, T. G. Review of research on the intelligibility and comprehension of accelerated speech. *Psychol. Bull.,* 1969, *72,* 50–62.

French, R. L. The function of the cerebral cortex of the rat in the discrimination of simple auditory rhythms. *J. Comp. Psychol.,* 1942, *33,* 1–32.

Fry, D. B., Abramson, A. S., Eimas, P. D., and Liberman, A. M. The identification and discrimination of synthetic vowels. *Lang. Speech,* 1962, *5,* 171–189.

Galli, F., Lifschitz, W., and Adrain, H. Studies on the auditory cortex of rabbit. *Exp. Neurol.,* 1971, *30,* 324–35.

Gazzaniga, M. S., and Sperry, R. W. Language after section of the cerebral commissures. *Brain,* 1967, *90,* 131–148.

Gersuni, G. V. Temporal organization of the auditory forebrain. In G. V. Gersuni (ed.), *Sensory Processes at the Neuronal and Behavioral Levels.* Academic Press, New York, 1971.

Gersuni, G. V., Baru, A. V., and Karaseva, T. A. Role of auditory cortex in discrimination of acoustic stimuli. *Neural Sci. Transl.,* 1968, *4,* 370–383.

Geschwind, N., and Levitsky, W. Human brain: Left-right asymmetries in temporal speech region. *Science,* 1968, *161,* 186–187.

Girden, E. The acoustic mechanisms of the cerebral cortex. *Am. J. Psychol.,* 1942, *55,* 518–27.

Godfrey, J. J. Perceptual difficulty and the right ear advantage for vowels. *Brain Lang.,* 1974, *1,* 323–336.

Goldberg, J. M., Diamond, I. T., and Neff, W. D. Auditory discrimination after ablation of cortical projection areas of the auditory system. *Fed. Proc.,* 1957, *16,* 47.

Graybiel, A. M. Some thalamocortical projections of the pulvinar-posterior system of the thalamus in the cat. *Brain Res.,* 1970, *22,* 131–136.

Graybiel, A. M. The thalamocortical projection of the so-called posterior nuclear group: A study with anterograde degeneration methods in the cat. *Brain Res.,* 1973, *49,* 229–244.

Groves, C. P., and Humphrey, N. K. Asymmetry in gorilla skulls: Evidence of lateralized brain function? *Nature,* 1973, *244,* 53–54.

Halperin, Y., Nachshon, I., and Carmon, A. Shift of ear superiority in dichotic listening to temporally patterned nonverbal stimuli. *J. Acoust. Soc. Am.,* 1973, *53,* 46–50.

Hamilton, C. R. Investigations of perceptual and mnemonic lateralization in monkeys. In S. R. Harnad, R. W. Doty, L. Goldstein, J. Jaynes, and G. Krauthamer (eds.), *Lateralization in the Nervous System.* Academic Press, New York, 1976.

Hand, P. J., and Lui, C. N. Efferent projection of the gracilis nucleus. *Anat. Rec.,* 1966, *154,* 353.

Harrison, J. M., and Howe, M. E. Anatomy of the descending auditory system (mammalian). In W. D. Keidel and W. D. Neff (eds.), *Handbook of Sensory Physiology,* Vol. V/I, Chap. 11. Springer, New York, 1974a.

Harrison, J. M., and Howe, M. E. Anatomy of the afferent auditory nervous system of mammals. In W. D. Keidel and W. D. Neff (eds.), *Handbook of Sensory Physiology,* Vol. V/I, Chap. 9. Springer, New York, 1974b.

Harting, J. K., Hall, W. C., Diamond, I. T., and Martin, G. F. Anterograde degeneration study of the superior colliculus in *Tupaia glis:* Evidence for a subdivision between superficial and deep layers. *J. Comp. Neurol.,* 1973, *148,* 361–386.

Heath, C. J., and Jones, E. C. An experimental study of ascending connections from the posterior group of the thalamic nuclei in the cat. *J. Comp. Neurol.,* 1971, *141,* 397–426.

Heffner, H. E. The effect of auditory cortex ablation on sound localization in the monkey *(Macaca mulatta).* Doctoral dissertation, Florida State University, 1973.

Heffner, H. Effect of auditory cortex ablation on the localization and discrimination of brief sounds. Paper presented at Neuroscience Meeting, 1976.

Heffner, H. E. Effect of auditory cortex ablation on the perception of meaningful sounds. *Neuroscience,* 1977, *3,* 6.

Heffner, H., and Masterton, R. B. Contribution of auditory cortex to sound localization in the monkey *(Macaca mulatta).* *J. Neurophysiol.,* 1975, *38,* 1340–1359.

Herrick, C. J. *Neurological Foundations of Animal Behavior.* Holt, Rinehart and Winston, New York, 1924.

Hirsh, I. J., and Sherrick, C. E. Perceived order in different sense modalities. *J. Exp. Psychol.*, 1961, *62*, 423–432.

Hupfer, K., Jürgens, V., and Ploog, D. The effect of superior temporal lesions on the recognition of species-specific calls in the squirrel monkey. *Exp. Brain Res.*, 1977, *30*, 75–87.

Jerger, J., Weikers, N. J., Sharbrough, R. W., and Jerger, S. Bilateral lesions of the temporal lobe. *Acta Otol.*, 1969, Suppl. 258.

Jerger, J., Lovering, L., and Wertz, M. Auditory disorder following bilateral temporal lobe insult: Report of a case. *J. Speech Hear. Disorders*, 1972, *37*, 523–53.

Jones, E. G., and Burton, H. Areal differences in the laminar distribution of thalamic afferents in cortical fields of the insular, parietal, and temporal regions of primates. *J. Comp. Neurol.*, 1976, *168*, 197–249.

Jones, E. G., and Leavitt, R. Y. Demonstration of thalamocortical connectivity in the cat somato-sensory system by retrograde axonal transport of horseradish peroxidase. *Brain Res.*, 1973, *63*, 414–418.

Jones, E. G., and Powell, T. P. S. The projection of the somatic sensory cortex upon the thalamus in the cat. *Brain Res.*, 1968, *10*, 369–391.

Kaas, J., Axelrod, S., and Diamond, I. T. An ablation study of the auditory cortex in the cat using binaural tonal patterns. *J. Neurophysiol.*, 1967, *30*, 710–724.

Karaseva, T. A. The role of the temporal lobe in human auditory perception. *Neuropsychologia*, 1972, *10*, 227–231.

Kelly, J. B. The effects of insular and temporal lesions in cats on two types of auditory pattern discrimination. *Brain Res.*, 1973, *62*, 71–87.

Kemp, J. M., and Powell, T. P. S. The cortico-striate projection in the monkey. *Brain*, 1970, *93*, 525–546.

Killackey, H., and Ebner, F. Convergent projection of three separate thalamic nuclei on to a single cortical area. *Science*, 1973, *179*, 283–285.

Kim, Y. C. Deficits in temporal sequencing of verbal material: The effect of laterality of lesion. *Brain Lang.*, 1976, *4*, 507–515.

Kimura, D. Cerebral dominance and the perception of verbal stimuli. *Can. J. Psychol.*, 1961, *15*, 166–171.

Kimura, D. Left-right differences in the perception of melodies. *Q. J. Exp. Psychol.*, 1964, *16*, 355–358.

Kimura, D. Functional asymmetry of the brain in dichotic listening. *Cortex*, 1967, *3*, 163–178.

Kryter, K. D., and Ades, H. W. Studies on the function of the higher acoustic nervous centers in the cat. *Am. J. Psychol.*, 1943, *56*, 501–536.

Kuhl, P. K., and Miller, J. D. Discrimination of speech sounds by the chinchilla: /t/ vs. /d/ in CV syllables. *J. Acoust. Soc. Am.*, 1974, *56*, 552–553.

Kuhl, P. K., and Miller, J. D. Speech perception by the chinchilla: Voice-voiceless distinction in alveolar plosive consonants. *Science*, 1975, *190*, 69–72.

Kuhn, G. M. On the front cavity resonance, and its possible relevance in speech perception. *Haskins Lab. Status Rep. Speech Res.*, 1975, *41*, 105–116.

Kusma, T., Otani, E., and Kawana, E. Projections of the motor, somatic sensory, auditory and visual cortices in cats. In T. Tokizene and J. P. Schade (eds.), *Progr. Brain Res.*, 1966, *21a*, 292–322.

Lackner, J. R., and Teuber, H. L. Alternations in auditory fusion thresholds after cerebral injury in man. *Neuropsychologia*, 1973, *11*, 409–415.

Landau, W. M., Goldstein, R., and Kleffner, F. R. Congenital aphasia: A clinicopathologic study. *Neurology*, 1960, *10*, 915–921.

LaVail, J. H., and LaVail, M. M. The retrograde intra-axonal transport of horseradish peroxidase in the click visual system: A light and electron microscopic study. *J. Comp. Neurol.*, 1974, *157*, 303–357.

LeGros Clark, W. E., and Russell, L. M. R. Cortical deafness without aphasia. *Brain*, 1938, *61*, 375–383.

LeMay, M. Morphological cerebral asymmetries of modern man, fossil man, and nonhuman primate. In S. R. Harnad, H. D. Steklis, and J. Lancaster (eds.), *Origins and Evolution of Language and Speech*. New York Academy of Sciences, New York, 1976.

LeMay, M., and Geschwind, N. Hemispheric differences in the brains of great apes. *Brain Behav. Evol.*, 1975, *11*, 48–52.

Lhermitte, F., Chain, F., Escourolle, R., Ducarne, B., Pillon, B., and Chedru, G. Etudes troubles perceptifs auditifs dans les lesions temporales bilaterales. *Rev. Neurol.*, 1971, *124*, 329–351.

Liberman, A. M., and Cooper, F. S. In search of the acoustic cues. In A. Valdman (ed.), *Mélange à la Mémoire de Pierre Delattre*. Mouton, The Hague, 1970.

Liberman, A. M., Delattre, P. C., and Cooper, F. S. The role of selected stimulus variables in the perception of the unvoiced-stop consonants. *Am. J. Psychol.*, 1952, *65*, 497–516.

Liberman, A. M., Cooper, F. S., Shankweiler, D. P., and Studdert-Kennedy, M. Perception of the speech code. *Psychol. Rev.*, 1967, *74*, 431–461.

Liedgren, S. R. C., Milne, A. C., Rubin, A. M., Schwarz, D. W. F., and Tomlinson, R. D. Representation of vestibular afferents in somatosensory thalamic nuclei of the squirrel monkey (*Saimiri sciureus*). *J. Neurophysiol.*, 1976, *39*, 601–612.

Lippe, W. R., and Weinberger, N. W. The distribution of sensory evoked activity within the medial geniculate body of the anesthetized cat. *Exp. Neurol.*, 1973*a*, *40*, 431–44.

Lippe, W. R., and Weinberger, N. M. The distribution of click evoked activity within the medial geniculate body of the anesthetized cat. *Exp. Neurol.*, 1973*b*, *39*, 507–523.

Lisker, L., Cooper, F. S., and Liberman, A. M. The uses of experiment in language description. *Word*, 1962, *18*, 82–106.

Locke, S. The projection of the magnocellular medial geniculate body. *J. Comp. Neurol.*, 1961, *116*, 179–193.

Luria, A. R. *Higher Cortical Functions in Man.* Basic Books, New York, 1966.

Majkowski, J., Bochenek, Z., Bochenek, W., Knapik-Fijalkowska, D., and Kopec, J. Latency of averaged evoked potentials to contralateral and ipsilateral auditory stimulation in normal subjects. *Brain Res.*, 1971, *25*, 416–419.

Majorossy, K., and Réthelyi, M. Synaptic architecture in the medial geniculate body (ventral division). *Exp. Brain Res.*, 1968, *6*, 306–323.

Masterton, R. B., and Diamond, I. T. Effects of auditory cortex ablation on discrimination of small binaural time differences. *J. Neurophysiol.*, 1964, *27*, 15–36.

Masterton, R. B., and Diamond, I. T. Hearing: Central neural mechanisms. In E. C. Carterette and M. P. Friedman (eds.), *Handbook of Perception*, Vol. 3, Academic Press, New York, 1973, pp. 408–448.

Mattingly, I. G., and Liberman, A. M. The speech code in the physiology of language. In K. N. Leibovic (ed.), *Information Processing and the Nervous System.* Springer, Berlin, 1969.

Mehler, W. R. Some observations on the secondary ascending afferent systems in the CNS. In R. S. Knighton and P. R. Dumke (eds.), *Pain.* Little, Brown, Boston, 1966, p. 11–32.

Merzenich, M. M., Knight, P. L.,and Roth, G. L. Representation of cochlea within primary auditory cortex in the cat. *J. Neurophysiol.*, 1975, *38*, 231–249.

Mesulam, M. M., and Pandya, D. N. The projection of the medial geniculate complex within the sylvian fissure of the rhesus monkey. *Brain Res.*, 1973, *60*, 315–333.

Mettler, F. A., Finch, G., Girden, E., and Culler, E. A. Acoustic value of the several components of the auditory pathway. *Brain*, 1934, *57*, 475–84.

Meyer, D. R., and Woolsey, C. N. Effects of localized cortical destruction on auditory discrimination conditioning in the cat. *J. Neurophysiol.*, 1952, *15*, 149–162.

Milner, B. Psychological defects produced by temporal lobe excision. *Res. Pub. Assoc. Res. Nerv. Ment. Dis.*, 1958, *36*, 244–257.

Milner, B. Laterality effects in audition. In V. Mountcastle (ed.), *Interhemispheric Relations and Cerebral Dominance.* Johns Hopkins University Press, Baltimore, 1962.

Milner, B. Brain mechanisms suggested by studies of temporal lobes. In C. N. Millikan and F. L. Darley (ed.), *Brain Mechanisms Underlying Speech and Language.* Grune and Stratton, New York, 1967.

Milner, B., Branch, C., and Rasmussen, T. Evidence for bilateral speech representation in some non-right-handers. *Trans. Am. Neurol. Assoc.*, 1966, *91*, 306–308.

Moore, R. Y., and Goldberg, J. M. Ascending projections of the inferior colliculus in the cat. *J. Comp. Neurol.*, 1963, *121*, 109–135.

Morest, D. K. The neuronal architecture of the medial geniculate body of the cat. *J. Anat.*, 1964, *98*, 611–630.

Morest, D. K. The lateral tegmental system of the midbrain and the medial geniculate body: A study with Golgi and Nauta methods in the cat. *J. Anat.*, 1965, *99*, 611–634.

Morest, D. K. Synaptic relationships of Golgi type II cells in the medial geniculate body of the cat. *J. Comp. Neurol.*, 1975, *162*, 157–194.

Morrison, A. R., Hand, P. J., and O'Donoghue, J. Contrasting projections from the posterior and ventrobasal thalamic nuclear complexes to the anterior ectosylvian gyrus of the cat. *Brain Res.*, 1970, *21*, 115–121.

Morse, P. A., and Snowdon, C. T. Speech perception in monkeys: Implications for theories of human speech perception. Paper presented to Eastern Psychological Association Meeting, Philadelphia, April 1974.

Munk, H. *Über die Funktionen der Grobhirnrinde: Gesammelte Mitteilungen aus den Jahren, 1877–1880.* Hirschwald, Berlin, 1881.

Natale, M. Perception of nonlinguistic auditory rhythms by the speech hemisphere. *Brain Lang.,* 1977, *4*, 32–44.

Nauta, W. J. H., and Kuypers, H. G. J. M. Some ascending pathways in the brain stem reticular formation. In H. H. Jasper (ed.), *Reticular Formation of the Brain.* Little, Brown, Boston, 1958, p. 3.

Neff, W. D. Neural mechanisms of auditory discrimination. In W. A. Rosenblith (ed.), *Sensory Communication.* Wiley, New York, 1961, pp. 259–278.

Neff, W. D., Arnott, G. P., and Fisher, J. F. Functions of auditory cortex: Sound localization in space. *Am. J. Psychol.,* 1950, *163*, 738.

Neff, W. D., Diamond, I. T., Fisher, J. F., and Yela, M. Role of auditory cortex in discrimination requiring localization of sound in space. *Neurophysiology,* 1956, *19*, 500–512.

Neff, W. D., Casseday, J. H., and Cranford, J. L. The medial geniculate body and associated thalamic cell groups: Behavioral studies. *Brain Behav. Evol.,* 1972, *6*, 302–310.

Niimi, K., and Naito, F. Cortical projections of medial geniculate body in the cat. *Exp. Brain Res.,* 1974, *19*, 326–342.

Oesterreich, R. E., Strominger, N. L., and Neff, W. D. Neural structures mediating differential sound intensity discriminations in the cat. *Brain Res.,* 1971, *27*, 251–270.

Oliver, D. L., and Hall, W. C. Subdivisions of the medial geniculate body in the tree shrew *(Tupaia glis).* *Brain Res.,* 1975, *86*, 217–227.

Otellin, V. A. Projections of the auditory cortex to the enostriatum. *Neurosci. Behav. Physiol.,* 1972, *5*, 267–274.

Paula-Barbosa, M. M., and Sousa-Pinto, A. Auditory cortical projections to the superior colliculus in the cat. *Brain Res.,* 1973, *50*, 47–61.

Pisoni, D. B. Auditory and phonetic memory codes in the discrimination of consonants and vowels. *Percept. Psychophys.,* 1973, *13*, 253–260.

Poggio, G. F., and Mountcastle, V. B. A study of the functional contribution to the lemniscal and spinothalamic systems to somatic sensibility: Central nervous mechanisms in pain. *Bull. Johns Hopkins Hosp.,* 1960, *106*, 266–316.

Pontes, C., Reis, F. F., and Sousa-Pinto, A. The auditory cortical projections on to the medial geniculate body in the cat: An experimental anatomical study with silver and autoradiographic methods. *Brain Res.,* 1975, *91*, 43–63.

Raab, D. H., and Ades, H. W. Cortical and midbrain mediation of a conditioned discrimination of acoustic intensities. *Am. J. Psychol.,* 1946, *59*, 58–83.

Raczkowski, D., Diamond, I. T., and Winer, J. Organization of thalamocortical auditory system in the cat studied with horseradish peroxidase. *Brain Res.,* 1976, *101*, 345–354.

Ravizza, R. J., and Diamond, I. T. Projections from the auditory thalamus to neocortex in hedgehog *(Paraechinus hypomelas). Anat. Rec.,* 1972, *172*, 390–391.

Ravizza, R. J., and Diamond, I. T. Role of auditory cortex in sound localization: A comparative study of hedgehog and bushbaby. *Fed. Proc.,* 1974, *33*, 1917–1919.

Ravizza, R. J., and Masterton, R. B. Contribution of neocortex to sound localization in the opossum *(Didelphis virginiana). J. Neurophysiol.,* 1972, *35*, 344–356.

Ravizza, R. J., Straw, R. B., and Long, P. D. Efferent projections of auditory cortex in the golden Syrian hamster *(Mesocricetus auratus). Anat. Rec.,* 1976, *184*, 509–510.

Rinvik, E. The corticothalamic projection from the second somatosensory area in the cat: An experimental study with silver impregnation methods. *Exp. Brain Res.,* 1968, *5*, 153–172.

Riss, W. Effect of bilateral temporal cortical ablation on discrimination of sound direction. *J. Neurophysiol.,* 1959, *22*, 374–384.

Rockel, A. J., and Jones, E. G. The neuronal organization of the inferior colliculus of the adult cat. I. The central nucleus. *J. Comp. Neurol.,* 1973, *147*, 11–60.

Rose, J. E. The cellular structure of the auditory region of the cat. *J. Comp. Neurol.,* 1949, *91*, 409–440.

Rose, J. E., and Woolsey, C. N. The relations of thalamic connections, cellular structure and evocable electrical activity in the auditory region of the cat. *J. Comp. Neurol.,* 1949, *91*, 441–466.

Rosenzweig, M. R. Discrimination of auditory intensities in the cat. *Am. J. Psychol.,* 1946, *59*, 127–136.

Rosenzweig, M. R. Representation of the two ears at the auditory cortex. *Am. J. Physiol.,* 1951, *167*, 147–158.

Ryugo, D. K., and Killackey, H. P. Differential telencephalic projections of the medial and ventral divisions of the medial geniculate body of the cat. *Brain Res.,* 1974, *82*, 173–177.

RICHARD J. RAVIZZA
AND SUSAN M.
BELMORE

Sanchez-Longo, L. P., and Forster, F. M. Clinical significance of impairment of sound localization. *Neurology,* 1958, *8*, 119–125.

Sanchez-Longo, L. P., Forster, F. M., and Auth, T. L. A clinical test for sound localization and its applications. *Neurology,* 1957, 7, 655–663.

Sanides, F. Comparative architectonics of the neocortex of mammals and their evolutionary interpretation. *Ann. N. Y. Acad. Sci.,* 1969, *167*, 404–423.

Sanides, F. Functional architecture of motor and sensory cortices in primates in the light of a new concept of neocortex evolution. In C. R. Noback and W. Montagna (eds.), *The Primate Brain.* Appleton-Century-Crofts, New York, 1970.

Sanides, F. Comparative neurology of the temporal lobe in primates including man with reference to speech. *Brain Lang.,* 1975, *2*, 396–419.

Scharlock, D. P., Neff, W. D., and Strominger, N. L. Discrimination of tone duration after bilateral ablation of cortical auditory areas. *J. Neurophysiol.,* 1965, *28*, 673–681.

Shankweiler, D. P. Performance of brain damaged patients on two tests of sound localization. *J. Comp. Physiol. Psychol.,* 1961, *54*, 375–381.

Shankweiler, D. Effects of temporal lobe damage on perception of dichotically presented melodies. *J. Comp. Physiol. Psychol.,* 1966, *62*, 115–119.

Shankweiler, D., and Studdert-Kennedy, M. Identification of consonants and vowels presented to left and right ears. *Q. J. Exp. Psychol.,* 1967, *19*, 59–63.

Smith, J. C. Conditioned suppression as an animal psychophysical technique. In W. C. Stebbins (ed.), *Animal Psychophysics: The Design and Conduct of Sensory Experiments.* Appleton-Century-Crofts, New York, 1970, pp. 125–161.

Sousa-Pinto, A. Cortical projections of the medial geniculate body in the cat. *Adv. Anat. Embryol. Cell Biol.,* 1973, *48(2)* , 1–42.

Spellacy, R., and Blumstein, S. Ear preference for language and nonlanguage sounds: A unilateral brain function. *J. Aud. Res.,* 1970, *10*, 349–355.

Sperry, R. W., Gazzaniga, M. S., and Bogen, J. E. Interhemispheric relationships: The neocortical commissures, syndromes of hemispheric disconnection. In P. Vinken and G. Bruyn (eds.), *Handbook of Clinical Neurology.* Vol. 4, North Holland, Amsterdam, 1969.

Stepien, L. S., Cordeau, J. P., and Rasmussen, T. The effects of temporal lobe and hippocampal lesions on auditory and visual recent memory in monkeys. *Brain,* 1960, *83*, 407–489.

Stoughton, G. S. The role of the cortex in retention of a conditioned response to auditory signals. Doctoral dissertation, University of Chicago, 1954.

Strominger, N. L. Subdivisions of auditory cortex and their role in localization of sound in space. *Exp. Neurol.,* 1969, *24*, 348–362.

Studdert-Kennedy, M., and Shankweiler, D. Hemispheric specialization for speech perception. *J. Acoust. Soc. Am.,* 1970, *48*, 579–594.

Swisher, L. Auditory intensity discrimination in patients with temporal-lobe damage. *Cortex,* 1967, *3*, 179–193.

Swisher, L., and Hirsh, I. J. Brain damage and the ordering of two temporally successive stimuli. *Neuropsychologia,* 1972, *10*, 137–152.

Symmes, D. Discrimination of intermittent noise by macaques following lesions of the temporal lobe. *Exp. Neurol.,* 1966, *16*, 201–214.

Szwejkowska, G., and Sychowa, B. The effects of lesions of auditory cortex on discrimination of sound localization in dog. *Acta Neurobiol. Exp.,* 1971, *31*, 237–250.

Tallal, P., and Piercy, M. Developmental aphasia: Rate of auditory processing and selective impairment of consonant perception. *Neuropsychologia,* 1974, *12*, 83–93.

Teuber, H. L., and Weinstein, S. Ability to discover hidden figures after cerebral lesions. *Arch. Neurol. Psychiat.,* 1956, *76*, 369–379.

Thompson, R. F. Function of auditory cortex of the cat in frequency discrimination. *J. Neurophysiol.,* 1960, *23*, 321–334.

Thompson, R. F., and Welker, W. I. Role of auditory cortex in reflex head orientation by cats to auditory stimuli. *J. Comp. Physiol. Psychol.,* 1963, *56*, 996–1002.

Wada, J. Interhemispheric sharing and shift of cerebral speech function. Paper presented at the 9th International Congress of Neurology, New York, September 1969.

Warren, J. M., and Nonneman, A. J. The search for cerebral dominance in monkeys. In S. R. Harnad, H. D. Steklis, and J. Lancaster (eds.), *Origins and Evolution of Language and Speech.* New York Academy of Sciences, New York, 1976.

Webster, K. E. The cortico-striatal projection in the cat. *J. Anat.,* 1965, *99*, 329–337.

Webster, W. G. Functional asymmetry between the cerebral hemispheres of the cat. *Neuropsychologia,* 1972, *10,* 75–87.

Wegener, J. G. The role of cerebral cortex and cerebellar systems in sensory discrimination. Doctoral dissertation, University of Chicago, 1954.

Whitfield, I. C., and Purser, D. Microelectrode study of the medial geniculate body in unanesthetized free-moving cats. *Brain Behav. Evol.,* 1972, *6,* 311–328.

Whitfield, I. C., Cranford, J. L., Ravizza, R. J., and Diamond, I. T. Effect of unilateral auditory cortex ablation on localization of complex sounds in the cat. *J. Neurophysiol.,* 1972, *35,* 713–731.

Wilson, M. E., and Cragg, B. G. Projections from the medial geniculate body to the cerebral cortex in the cat. *Brain Res.,* 1969, *13,* 462–475.

Winer, J. A., Diamond, I. T., and Raczkowski, D. Subdivisions of the auditory cortex of the cat: The retrograde transport of horseradish peroxidase to the medial geniculate body and posterior thalamic nuclei. *J. Comp. Neurol.,* 1977, *176,* 387–414.

Witelson, S., and Pallie, A. Left hemisphere specialization for language in the newborn. *Brain,* 1973, *96,* 641.

Woolsey, C. N. Organization of cortical auditory system: A review and a synthesis. In G. L. Rasmussen and W. F. Windle (eds.), *Neural Mechanisms of the Auditory and Vestibular Systems.* Thomas, Springfield, Ill., 1960.

Woolsey, C. N., and Walzl, E. M. Topical projection of nerve fibers from local regions of the cochlea to the cerebral cortex of the cat. *Bull. Johns Hopkins Hosp.,* 1942, *71,* 314–344.

Yeni-Komshian, G., and Benson, D. Anatomical study of cerebral asymmetry in the temporal lobe of humans, chimpanzees, and rhesus monkeys. *Science,* 1976, *192,* 387–389.

13

Gustatory System

LINDA M. BARTOSHUK

INTRODUCTION

Taste sensations do not have the complexity of auditory and visual sensations; rather, the most salient attributes of taste sensations are simply quality and intensity. The nature of taste quality has been debated by taste scientists for decades. Psychophysical studies of human taste have tended to emphasize the four basic taste qualities bequeathed to us by the nineteenth century, while electrophysiological studies of the neural coding of taste quality in other species have challenged this classical view. A large portion of this chapter is devoted to this apparent conflict and the information about taste quality that it has generated.

The last part of this chapter focuses on taste in nonhuman species. Although a species like the rat cannot describe the taste of a substance in the way a human subject can, animal psychophysicists have devised ingenious ways to ask taste questions that a rat can answer. Animal psychophysics coupled with neural recordings provides remarkable insight into the taste worlds of other species.

This chapter begins with a consideration of the anatomy and physiology of the neural structures that mediate taste sensations. Although much is unknown, particularly about the transduction process that permits chemical stimuli to produce neural signals, the information that is available is important to theories of the coding of taste quality.

LINDA M. BARTOSHUK   John B. Pierce Foundation and Yale University, New Haven, Connecticut 06519.

LINDA M. BARTOSHUK

PAPILLAE

Four kinds of projections, or papillae, can be identified on the human tongue. The filiform papillae, which contain no taste buds, give the tongue its rough, filelike appearance. The fungiform papillae, shaped like button mushrooms, appear primarily on the tip of the tongue and along the edges of the front of the tongue; taste buds are buried in the surface epithelium of these papillae. The foliate papillae consist of a set of three to eight parallel folds on the rear edges of the tongue, with taste buds buried in the sides of the folds. The circumvallate papillae, nine to ten in number, are shaped like flat mounds surrounded by a trench; they form an inverted V on the rear of the tongue. Taste buds lie in the sides of the papillae and in the wall of the surrounding trench. The human, between the ages of 20 and 70, has about 250 taste buds in each circumvallate papilla and a total of about 1300 taste buds in the foliate papillae (Bradley, 1971). A human fungiform papilla can contain up to eight taste buds (Bradley and Mistretta, 1975).

Taste buds are also found on the soft palate (the soft part of the roof of the mouth), the pharynx (throat), the larynx, the esophagus, and the epiglottis, which closes off the larynx to prevent the entrance of food and fluids during swallowing (Bradley, 1971).

TASTE BUDS

Murray (1973) has provided a detailed description of the taste bud in the foliate papilla of the rabbit. This taste bud is a globular cluster of cells arranged something like the segments of an orange (see Fig. 1). The taste bud is surrounded by epithelial or skin cells. The opening through these epithelial cells that links the taste bud to the tongue surface is called the "outer taste pore." The tops of one type of cell in the taste bud (type 3 in Fig. 1) taper to blunt pegs. Murray suggests that these cells are the actual taste receptor cells. The tops of two other kinds of cells (types 1 and 2 in Fig. 1) taper into small fingerlike projections called microvilli. The projections of the cells nearest the outside of the taste bud form a ring called the "inner taste pore." This area enlarges below into a space called the "taste pit," which is filled with a dense substance produced by the type 1 cells that completely covers the microvilli of the type 2 cells. However, the peglike projections of the type 3 cells as well as the microvilli of the taller type 1 cells rise above this dense substance in the pit.

It is unlikely that tastants contact nerves directly, because the cells are tightly joined to one another, effectively sealing the taste pit. This suggests that interactions between tastants and receptor cells occur at the membranes of the peglike projections of the type 3 cells. Electron microscopy shows synapses between type 3 cells and nerve fibers. Type 2 cells make extensive contact with nerves, but their role, if any, in the generation of nerve impulses is not understood. The taste buds in the circumvallate papillae resemble those of the foliate papillae; however, in the fungiform papillae, the substance found in the taste pit is different and the distinctions among cell types are less clear (Farbman, 1965a,b; Murray, 1973).

Individual cells in the taste buds have a remarkably short lifetime and must be continually replaced. The epithelial cells surrounding the taste bud are the source for the replacement cells. When the newly dividing epithelial cells of the rat taste bud were radioactively labeled, daughter cells were found to move into the taste bud at the rate of one every 10 hr. Periodic examination at various intervals showed that cells within the taste bud had a life span of about 10 days (Beidler and Smallman, 1965). During its life cycle, a cell moves from the edge to the center of the taste bud. Since the nerve fibers do not move, the receptor cells are presumably innervated by different nerve fibers as they change location. This poses a problem for stable quality perception. The sequence of receptor cells synapsing with a single fiber should presumably have the same sensitivities in order to ensure that particular neural signals always correlate with the same stimuli, but the sensitivities of such a sequence of cells are unknown.

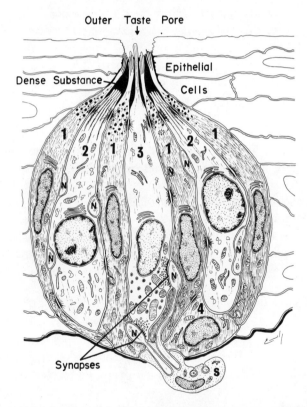

Fig. 1. Longitudinal section of a taste bud from a rabbit foliate papilla. Type 3 cells are believed to be taste cells and type 1 to be supportive cells. Type 2 cells do not form synapses but show extensive contact with nerve fibers (N) and may be involved with the generation of neural signals. The type 4 cell is believed to play a role in the replacement of cells in the taste bud. A Schwann cell (S) is shown surrounding the nerve fibers that synapse with the type 3 cell. Reprinted with permission of publisher and author from Murray, in *The Ultra Structure of Sensory Organs,* copyright, 1973 by Elsivier, North Holland.

The turnover of taste cells complicates the description of cell types given above. There is still disagreement over whether or not the observed cell types are actually different stages in the life cycle of one type of cell.

Mammalian and fish taste buds require intact innervation; if the peripheral taste nerve is cut or crushed, the taste buds will degenerate. As the nerve fibers regenerate, taste buds will reappear (Guth, 1971). In the gerbil, taste responses could be recorded in the peripheral nerve as early as 11 days after crushing (Oakley and Cheal, 1975). The chorda tympani nerve which innervates the front of the tongue and the glossopharyngeal nerve which innervates the back of the tongue can be cut and then crossed so that when each nerve regenerates it innervates the tongue area previously innervated by the other nerve. In the normal animal, these two nerves show characteristically different sensitivities to taste and temperature stimuli. After cross-regeneration was complete, the nerves had exchanged sensitivities; that is, the tongue area innervated seemed to control the characteristic sensitivities shown by the nerves (Oakley, 1967). This appears to rule out the possibility that the sensitivity of a taste receptor cell is determined by the fiber that innervates it. However, the sensitivities of all receptors innervated by a single fiber in the chorda tympani of the cat were remarkably similar (Oakley, 1975). This suggests that a fiber may essentially "select" receptor cells of homogeneous sensitivity from those present.

The sheep has been used to study the early development of the taste bud (Bradley and Mistretta, 1975). In sheep, as in the human, taste buds develop *in utero*. The early taste buds in sheep, called "presumptive taste buds," have a nerve supply on appearance at about 49 days, with one presumptive taste bud per papilla. At about 100 days, a taste pore appears. At this time a papilla may contain two taste buds, and by birth (about 147 days) three to four buds. Single-fiber responses from the chorda tympani of fetuses aged 109 days to term were similar to those of lambs and adult sheep. That is, as long as 5 weeks before birth, the responses appeared similar to those of the adult.

The early development of taste buds suggests that the fetus may taste substances in amniotic fluid. This is especially important for the evaluation of the effects of early experience on taste preferences. At birth, an organism already may have had a considerable amount of taste experience (Bradley and Mistretta, 1973).

INNERVATION OF TASTE BUDS

Taste nerve fibers branch before forming synapses with receptor cells. A picture of the nature of this branching is beginning to emerge thanks to a variety of anatomical and recording studies done primarily on the rat chorda tympani nerve.

There are about 1000 nerve fibers in the rat chorda tympani. The efferent fibers which supply salivary glands as well as other tongue structures (Hellekant, 1971) and lingual nerve afferents (e.g., fibers mediating touch sensations) account for about 50% of these (Farbman and Hellekant, 1976). Since there are, on the average, 89 fungiform papillae on one-half the rat tongue (Fish *et al.*, 1944), the 500 taste fibers should provide about six fibers per taste papilla. However, electron microscopy shows that the average papilla contains 224 nerve fibers at its base (Beidler, 1969). The number of these fibers that are taste fibers is not known but it is surely much greater than six. Thus the taste fibers in the chorda tympani of the rat must branch several times before innervating taste receptor cells. Histological examination shows that this branching occurs in the fiber bundles which carry the fibers to papillae and at the base of the papillae (Miller, 1974) as well as within the taste bud itself (Beidler, 1969). The receptor cells innervated by a single fiber can even be in separate taste buds (Miller, 1971; Oakley, 1972).

The funneling of the output of several receptor cells into each taste fiber is obviously important for the sensory coding of taste quality. It would be of great interest to know in addition whether or not a single receptor cell could be innervated by more than one nerve fiber. This seems likely in the light of histological evidence that some nerve fibers contact more than one receptor cell in a taste bud (Beidler, 1969); however, the contacts may not all have been functional, so the issue remains unresolved.

PERIPHERAL INTEGRATION IN TASTE

The taste system lacks the complex lateral connections that can be found in the visual system. Nonetheless, there are anatomical possibilities for the peripheral integration of taste information involving the branching patterns of taste fibers. When a taste receptor cell is stimulated, impulses travel toward the central nervous system. When neural impulses in one branch reach dividing points in a nerve fiber, the impulses can travel antidromically back along the other branches toward the other receptor cells served by that fiber (Rapuzzi and Casella, 1965; Filin and Esakov, 1968). A possible inhibitory function of antidromic activity was demonstrated in the frog (Taglietti et al., 1969). The neural response produced when several taste papillae were stimulated was smaller than the simple sums of the responses to each individual papilla. Antidromic activity was apparently responsible for the decreased responses from individual papillae. As concentration increased, the discrepancy between the response actually produced by several papillae and the simple sum of their individual responses increased. That is, it would appear that the degree of mutual inhibition increases with concentration. This suggests that antidromic inhibition might play a role in a very important phenomenon, compression. Compression is said to occur when successive concentration increments produce successively smaller increments in perceived intensity (Stevens, 1958). Compression occurs in a variety of sensory modalities (e.g., visual brightness and auditory intensity).

A second mechanism for peripheral integration in taste involves summation of generator potentials along unmyelinated terminals of single taste nerve fibers (Miller, 1971). This mechanism is supported by the observation that the neural response to an application of NaCl to a single rat papilla (which contains only a single taste bud) can be decreased by the application of potassium benzoate to an adjacent papilla. Antidromic inhibition cannot explain this observation because the concentration of potassium benzoate was below that necessary to produce action potentials. Miller's explanation is as follows. Taste responses are produced when a reaction between a taste stimulus and the receptor depolarizes the peripheral terminal of a taste nerve fiber. If the benzoate anion in potassium benzoate were to hyperpolarize one branch of a nerve fiber that joined another branch that was depolarized by NaCl, a decrement in the fiber's response to NaCl would be expected.

The functional significance of these two potential mechanisms for peripheral integration is still unclear. However, they have been mentioned in connection with quality coding (Miller, 1971), cross-adaptation and enhancement (Wang and Bernard, 1969; Bernard, 1971), and mixture interactions (Wang, 1973; Bartoshuk, 1975).

Ascending Taste System

The central projections of the taste system of the rat, the species in which they are best understood, are shown in Fig. 2.

Nerves Mediating Taste. Taste information is transmitted via three nerves: the chorda tympani (part of the facial or VIIth cranial nerve), the glossopharyngeal (IXth cranial nerve), and the vagus (Xth cranial nerve). The chorda tympani nerve innervates the fungiform papillae and the glossopharyngeal nerve innervates the foliate and circumvallate papillae. The innervation of the taste buds found on other oral structures is not as well established. Taste buds on the soft palate are innervated primarily by the greater superficial petrosal nerve (which is a branch of the facial nerve) although the glossopharyngeal and vagus nerves may also play a role (Cleaton-Jones, 1976). Taste buds on the laryngeal surface of the epiglottis are innervated by the superior laryngeal nerve (which is a branch of the vagus nerve). These receptors have been implicated in the chain of events leading to sudden infant death syndrome (Storey and Johnson, 1975).

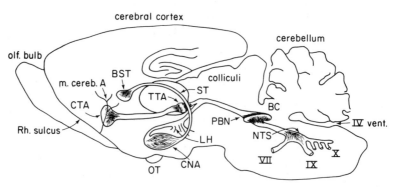

Fig. 2. Central projections of the taste system of the rat. NTS, Nucleus of solitary tract; PTA, pontine taste area; BC, brachium conjunctivum; TTA, thalamic taste area, CTA, cortical taste area; CNA, central nucleus of the amygdala; ST, stria terminalis; BST, bed nucleus of stria terminalis; OT, optic tract; IV vent, fourth ventricle; VII, IX, X, taste afferents of seventh, ninth, and tenth cranial nerves; Rh. sulcus, rhinal sulcus; m. cereb. A, middle cerebral artery. From Norgren (1978). Reprinted by permission.

MEDULLA. The three nerves mediating taste project ipsilaterally to the solitary nucleus of the medulla (NTS in Fig. 2). Although the areas to which they project overlap to some extent, the chorda tympani (VII) terminates in the rostral end of the nucleus, the vagus (X) in the caudal end, and the glossopharyngeal (IX) in an area between these two (Burton and Benjamin, 1971).

PONS. A taste relay in the pontine area (PTA in Fig. 2) of the rat receives ipsilateral projections from both rostral and caudal locations in the solitary nucleus. This suggests the interesting possibility that a particular pontine neuron may receive inputs from two different tongue areas (Norgren and Pfaffman, 1975). Some pontine neurons project to the dorsal thalamus (TTA in Fig. 2), but others project through the substantia inominata to the central nucleus of the amygdala (CNA in Fig. 2), an area that may be important for the regulation of feeding and drinking (Norgren, 1976). Neurons of a third group project to both areas (Norgren and Leonard, 1973; Norgren, 1974). Very little is known about the possibility of similar pontine projections in other species.

THALAMUS. Taste is located near the tongue portion of the somesthetic projections in the thalamus. The body surface is represented somatotopically in the somesthetic system with the tongue at the extreme anterior end; the thalamic taste area (TTA in Fig. 2) is located near the tip of the thalamic tongue area (Burton and Benjamin, 1971). The thalamic taste area receives bilateral projections from the pontine taste area in the rat (Norgren and Leonard, 1973).

CORTEX. Two cortical areas responsive to electrical stimulation of the chorda tympani and glossopharyngeal nerves have been identified in the squirrel monkey (Burton and Benjamin, 1971). One of these is in the tongue portion of the somatotopic projection of the body surface in somatic sensory area I. Spatial localization on the tongue is maintained in this area. The second area, located just rostral to the first, is in the anterior opercular-insular cortex. This second area is unresponsive to tactile stimulation, and chorda tympani and glossopharyngeal inputs overlap. Evidence for two cortical taste areas has also been found in the cat but not in the marmoset (Ganchrow and Erickson, 1972) or the rat (Burton and Benjamin, 1971; Norgren and Wolf, 1975). The cortical taste area for the rat is shown in Fig. 2 (CTA).

TRANSDUCTION

Taste "transduction" refers to the initial events in taste: the interactions of stimulus and receptor that ultimately give rise to a neural signal.

The nature of these interactions is elusive because they must be studied indirectly. Stimulus molecules are believed to interact with molecules in the membranes of the parts of the receptor cells that project into the inner taste pore; these reactive molecules are called "receptor sites." However, even the locus of the stimulus-receptor interaction has been questioned for some bitter stimuli.

The specificity of the stimulus-receptor interaction and the mechanism by which a neural response results from that interaction will be considered separately below (see Price and DeSimone, 1977, for a comprehensive review of transduction models).

SPECIFICITY OF STIMULUS-RECEPTOR INTERACTION

A variety of models have been proposed to explain the selectivity of receptors. Most of these models assume that taste stimuli interact with molecules in the membranes of the receptor cells. One of the main reasons for this belief is that many substances (e.g., strychnine, cyanide, and concentrated acids) that would be expected to do serious damage if they could cross the membrane and enter the receptor cells can be tasted without apparently damaging the taste system. In addition, some proteins (e.g., monellin and thaumatin) are sweet even though they are not believed to cross the taste membrane.

Models of the stimulus-receptor interaction tend to be based on physical or chemical characteristics that are common to stimuli with similar taste qualities. Since human taste experience is usually described as salty, sour, sweet, and bitter, most models have been constructed to deal with a class of substances which have one of these qualities in common.

SALTY. *Stimuli.* The salty taste is produced primarily by inorganic salts dissolved in water to produce a solution of positive ions (cations) and negative ions (anions). The salt with the purest salty taste is sodium chloride ($NaCl$). (See below for a discussion of the sweet taste of dilute $NaCl$.) Other salts taste sour, bitter, or sweet as well as salty. The tastes of a variety of these salts can be duplicated by a mixture of $NaCl$, quinine hydrochloride, tartaric acid, and glucose (von Skramlik, 1922). In general, as the anion and cation get larger, salts taste increasingly bitter (Moncrieff, 1967). One salt, monosodium glutamate, is sometimes said to have a taste quality that cannot be described by sweet, salty, sour, and bitter. However, salts of some amino acids (monosodium glutamate is the sodium salt of glutamic acid) as well as the amino acids themselves produce unusually persistent tastes as well as nontaste sensations (e.g., tactile sensations). Whether or not the taste quality itself is unique is unclear.

Models of Salt Receptors. Beidler suggested (1954, 1967) that cations are excitatory and anions are inhibitory in taste. His conclusion that the cation is the actual stimulus in a salt was based on the following observations: 0.1 M concentrations of $NaCl$, $NaBr$, and $NaNO_3$, have the Na^+ cation in common and produce neural responses of about the same magnitude, while 0.1 M concentrations of $NaCl$, $LiCl$, NH_4Cl, $RbCl$, KCl, and $CsCl$ have the Cl^- anion in common and produce responses of very different magnitudes (Beidler, 1953). His conclusion that the anion inhibits the action of the cation was based on the observation that the magnitudes of the neural responses to salts with a common cation tend to decrease as the size of the anion increases. Since the ability of anions to bind with proteins (long thought to be potential receptor molecules) tends to increase as the size of the anion increases, Beidler suggested that the binding of anions might inhibit the action of the cations. The neural response produced by any given salt would then depend on the relative numbers of sites available to bind cations and anions as well as on the ability of a given ion to bind to a site.

A physical model of the taste cell membrane was constructed by impregating phospholipids extracted from cow tongues into filter paper (Kamo *et al.,* 1974). The application of salts to the filter paper produced changes in potential that simulated receptor potentials. This suggests the possibility that salts might stimulate by binding to phospholipids in the receptor cell membrane.

A third model for salt receptors builds on the results with the phospholipid model to explain the effects of anions without assuming that they bind to particular sites and thereby inhibit the action of the cations (DeSimone and Price, 1976). According to the analysis presented for this third model, the phospholipid layer is basically a layer of negative charge that is neutralized when cations bind to it. This neutralization is seen to be the initial event that ultimately leads to taste action potentials. Anions, having the same negative charge as the phospholipid layer, would be repelled. The effects of anions on taste responses are then explained as follows. Certain anions form pairs with cations. These neutral pairs then compete with cations for the sites on the taste cell membrane. However, when the neutral pair binds, there is no reduction in the negative charge of the membrane. This means that the salts that produce smaller neural responses will be those with anions that have greater ability to form pairs with cations.

Anions can have tastes of their own in addition to any possible effects they may have on the action of cations. For example, the sweet taste of Na saccharin results from interactions between the saccharin anion and the sweet receptor site. Thus the taste of a salt depends on its ability to stimulate all taste receptors and not just those sensitive to cations.

Saltiness. The models of the salt receptor deal with the mechanism by which salts as a chemical class stimulate, but the determination of the origin of saltiness is a separate question. Psychophysical studies with human subjects have been oriented toward identifying the ions responsible for the salty taste quality. This work (see Dzendolet and Meiselman, 1967) seems to lead to the conclusion that the chloride (Cl^-) and to a lesser extent the sulfate (SO_4^{2-}) ions are responsible for saltiness. This conclusion is not consistent with the neural data. For example, the taste of NaCl, the only salt having a pure salty taste, is attributed to the Na^+ cation by the neural studies and to the Cl^- anion by the human psychophysical studies.

The results of the human studies can be reinterpreted. The salty taste was attributed to Cl^- ions because salts containing these ions tend to be the saltiest salts. However, possible inhibitory effects of the anions have been neglected in this argument. For example, Beidler's anionic inhibition theory would argue that the cations produce salty (as well as other) tastes and these tend to be more intense in salts containing Cl^- ions because these small ions produce less anionic inhibition.

The salty taste can thus be attributed to the binding of cations to certain sites (e.g., the sites binding Na). Cations bind to other sites as well, which partially explains the complex tastes of salts. For example, the K^+ cation in KCl appears to bind to two sites (Beidler, 1961). KCl tastes salty-bitter. Perhaps the saltiness is produced by the binding of K^+ to the sites binding Na^+ and the bitterness is produced by the binding of K^+ to other sites that somehow give rise to a bitter taste.

Sweet Taste of Dilute Salts. A variety of salts, including NaCl, taste sweet at low concentrations (Renqvist, 1919; Bartoshuk *et al.,.* 1964; Dzendolet and Meiselman, 1967; Bartoshuk, 1974*b*). This sweet taste may be produced because the water shells that form around the cation of dilute salts (Dzendolet, 1968; Anderson, 1971; Shallenberger and Acree, 1971) may be able to bind to the same receptor sites that bind sugars. This is supported by the observation that adaptation to sucrose completely cross-adapts the sweet taste of dilute NaCl (Bartoshuk, Murphy and Cleveland, unpublished data).

SOUR. *Stimuli.* The sour taste is believed to result from the dissociated hydrogen (H^+) in acids. Acids do not all dissociate to an equal extent into hydrogen ions and anions when in solution. If hydrogen ions alone were responsible for the sour taste, then the H^+ concentration (i.e., pH) would predict sourness; however, weak organic acids (e.g., acetic acid) tend to taste more sour than strong acids (e.g., HCl) of the same pH. Research with acetic acid suggests that the anions rather than the undissociated molecules of the acid are responsible for the strong sour taste of organic acids (Beidler, 1967).

Not all acids are predominantly sour; for example, picric acid is bitter. This probably results from the presence of NO_2 groups in the anion of picric acid that produce a bitter taste intense enough to suppress the sour taste of the H^+ ions (Moncrieff, 1967).

Models of Acid Receptors. Beidler's model of acid receptors is very similar to his model of salt receptors. Both the hydrogen ions and the anions bind to specific sites, but the binding of the hydrogen ions produces the neural response and the anions merely inhibit the action of the hydrogen ions. At this point, the model would seem to predict that organic acids with large, inhibitory anions should produce smaller taste responses than inorganic acids, when just the opposite is true. However, there is an additional factor operating with acids. The binding of the anions decreases the net positive surface charge so that more H^+ ions can bind. The additional binding of H^+ overcomes the inhibition produced by the anions.

The anions of acids and/or the undissociated molecules can apparently stimulate sweet and bitter tastes just as the anions of salts can. For example, saccharin is available in "soluble" or "insoluble" form. The "soluble" saccharin is the sodium salt of saccharin and the "insoluble" saccharin is the acid containing the saccharin anion. In both cases, the anion is sweet.

SWEET. *Stimuli.* Although sugars are the prototypical sweet stimuli, a few inorganic compounds and a variety of organic compounds taste sweet, as evidenced by the many substances considered to have potential as nonnutritive sweeteners. There have been many attempts to find structural similarities among sweet substances, but only one such attempt has proved successful. Shallenberger identified an AH, B system common to a large variety of sweet substances (Shallenberger and Acree, 1967). "AH" refers to an electronegative atom A, like oxygen or nitrogen, covalently bonded to a hydrogen atom, H, and "B" refers to a second electronegative atom (or an electronegative center; see Shallenberger and Acree, 1971, for details). AH and B must be separated by about 3 Å. For sugars, the AH, B system consists of two OH units positioned so that one OH could be the AH group and the oxygen atom of the other OH group could be B.

This system has been extended (Kier, 1972; Shallenberger and Lindley, 1977) by adding a third binding group. This transforms the bipartite AH, B system into a tripartite AH, B, γ system. The γ binding point makes the saporous unit (i.e., the AH, B, γ system) asymmetrical, which can account for the unequal sweetnesses of enantiomers (i.e., D and L forms of compounds).

The AH, B, γ system resulted from the search for common structures among sweet compounds. Now that this suggestion concerning the identity of the sweet taste unit exists, it can be utilized to study groups of related compounds to locate the exact source of sweetness in each substance (Birch, 1976).

Models of Sweet Receptors. The success of Shallenberger in identifying a molecular configuration common to sweet-tasting substances suggests that the sweet receptor site has a configuration complementary to that of the sweet tasting unit.

Neural recordings from gerbil have been used to provide a detailed description of the "sucrose site" in that species. In the gerbil, each of a series of sugars and sugar alcohols appears to interact with a single receptor site (Jakinovitch, 1976; Jakinovitch and Goldstein, 1976; Jakinovitch and Oakley, 1976). This was determined with the aid of Beidler's theory (the theory predicts one kind of relation between neural response and concentration for substances that interact with a single kind of receptor site and predicts a different relation for substances interacting with more than one kind of receptor site, Beidler, 1961). Assuming that all the sugars and sugar alcohols interact with the same sites, the maximum neural response to each substance determines how well that substance "fits" the common site and permits the construction of a model of the site.

The modeling of the sweet receptors contains a potentially serious logical flaw: the relative effectiveness of sweet substances is assumed to reflect how well it "fits" *the* sweet receptor site. However, recordings from single fibers show that the relative effectiveness of sweet substances varies across individual fibers (Bartoshuk, cited in Pfaffmann, 1969; Pfaffmann *et al.*, 1976). Thus receptor sites binding sweet substances do not all appear to have identical characteristics. This complicates the task of the investigators who infer the structural characteristics of receptors from the relative effectiveness of a variety of compounds. The accuracy of the inferences is limited unless there is reason to believe that all of the sweet substances in question interact with one common receptor structure and no others. Single-fiber studies would provide better ranking of the effectiveness of sweeteners, but even these cannot be assumed to reflect the responses of receptor binding sites with identical structures. Despite the difficulties, this approach is a creative one that deserves further study.

Experimental isolation of the receptor molecules that interact with sweet substances would provide a different way to discover their binding characteristics. The earliest attempt (Dastoli and Price, 1966) produced a protein fraction from cow tongues that complexed with sugars. The possibility that the proteins found in this and similar studies (Hiji and Sato, 1973) are receptor proteins has been questioned, in part because the yields of this protein seem very high given the small proportion of tongue epithelium that is part of receptor cell membranes (Price and Hogan, 1969); however, the receptor molecules that interact with tastants might not be restricted to receptor cells. Since potentials that resemble taste receptor potentials have been recorded from nontaste cells in toad (Eyzaguirre, 1972) and catfish (Teeter and Kare, 1974), the possibility exists that taste receptor molecules may be present in nontaste cells.

A variety of biochemical and biophysical techniques are beginning to be applied to the study of the properties of sweet receptor molecules as well as other receptor molecules. For example, radioactively labeled sugars have been shown to bind more to tissue from cow papillae containing taste buds than to control tissue containing no taste buds (Cagan, 1971) and radioactively labeled alanine has been shown to bind more to catfish barbels than to tissue from another area containing fewer taste buds (Krueger and Cagan, 1976).

Bitter. *Stimuli.* Bitterness, like sweetness, is produced by some inorganic and a variety of organic compounds. There is no single generalization for bitter substances as inclusive as the AH, B, γ system for sweet substances; however, some observations about the relation between structure and taste are possible.

Alkaloids are found naturally in plants; some examples are caffeine, nicotine, solanine, cocaine, strychnine, and frucine (Shallenberger and Acree, 1971). The toxicity of these substances is often cited as an environmental pressure that may have promoted the evolution of the aversion to bitterness found in so many species. Species that avoided alkaloids would have had a selective advantage over those that did not.

Glycosides are derived from certain sugars and are also found in plants (Shallenberger and Acree, 1971). Some of the glycosides have been studied in detail to determine the effect of substitutions at various sites on the molecules (Horowitz and Gentili, 1969). These studies are very important to the development of any comprehensive theory of bitterness; however, they have also had a more practical impact. Certain substitutions produce compounds that can produce strong sweet tastes at low concentrations: neohespridine and naringin dehydrochalcone. These compounds may be useful as nonnutritive sweeteners.

Another group of organic compounds found in plants, diterpenes, have also been analyzed for structure-bitterness relations (Kubota and Kubo, 1969). An AH, B system similar to that of Shallenberg was suggested as the common link. However, in this case the AH and B are separated by 1.5 Å instead of 3 Å, which produces an intramolecular hydrogen bond between AH and B.

PTC (phenylthiocarbamide or phenylthiourea) and other compounds containing the H—N—C≡S grouping are of special interest because sensitivity to their bitter taste is genetically mediated by a single Mendelian dominant gene. That is, an individual with two recessive genes has a high threshold leading to the classification "nontaster" or "taste blind" while an individual with one or both dominant genes has a low threshold leading to the classification "taster." Saliva is often related to PTC tasting because a very early study (Cohen and Ogden, 1949) seemed to show that a taster had to have his/her saliva present in order to taste PTC. This is not supported by modern data (Hall *et al.,* 1975).

The exact requirements for the molecular grouping responsible for the taste of PTC have been questioned (Fischer, 1971). Two other molecules that do not contain the H—N—C$\equiv$S grouping, anetholtrithione and caffeine, have been found to produce a bimodal threshold distribution that is essentially the PTC distribution (Kalmus, 1971; Hall *et al.,* 1975). The other molecules do contain groupings that are isosteric with H—N—C$\equiv$S; that is, the other molecules contain groupings in which atoms have been substituted that contain the same numbers of electrons in the outer shell (Fischer, 1971). This may mean that sensitivity to the bitter taste of a variety of compounds will be related to sensitivity to PTC. It is important to note that a compound that contains H—N—C$\equiv$S or a related group may also contain some other bitter-tasting group that does not show a bimodal distribution. This may be the case with caffeine (Hall *et al.,* 1975).

A variety of additional structure-bitterness generalizations have been suggested (Moncrieff, 1967). It is still too early to tell whether or not all of these can be related; however, no synthesis appears likely to occur soon.

Models of Bitter Receptors. Since there is no overall generalization about properties common to all bitter substances, there can be no general model of the bitter receptor. The AH, B system proposed for the bitterness of diterpenes (Kubota and Kubo, 1969) suggests a complementary receptor structure for this group of compounds.

There have been attempts to isolate a bitter receptor protein (Dastoli *et al.,* 1968), but the protein found does not appear to have the right properties (Price and DeSimone, 1977).

One suggestion for a bitter mechanism is especially interesting because it departs from the conventional view that taste receptor sites are located in the receptor membrane. Rather, bitter substances are seen as entering the receptor cell and affecting intracellular processes (Price, 1973, 1974; Kurihara and Koyama, 1972). The ease with which a compound can enter the cell is suggested to be related to its lipid solubility so that those compounds of the greatest lipid solubility would be the most bitter (Kurihara and Koyama, 1972).

PRODUCTION OF NEURAL RESPONSES

Stimuli of different taste qualities are believed to differ in the precise way in which they bind to receptor molecules, as discussed above. There are two theories that deal with binding properties common to all stimuli. These theories, occupation theory (Beidler, 1954) and rate theory (Paton, 1961; Heck and Erickson, 1973), are concerned with the part of the binding process that initiates neural responses. Since these theories are based on the temporal properties of receptor potentials and responses from the peripheral nerves, these are discussed below.

RECEPTOR POTENTIALS. Although these experiments are technically very difficult, potentials believed to be receptor potentials have been recorded from rat

(Tateda and Beidler, 1964; Kimura and Beidler, 1961; Ozeki and Sato, 1972), hamster (Kumira and Beidler, 1961), and frog (Sato, 1969). Microelectrodes were inserted into a taste papilla until a sudden negative potential suggested that a receptor cell had been pierced. The application of taste substances to the tongue then caused slow positive deflections of the negative resting potential of the cells. The response of a typical hamster cell to a variety of tastants is shown in Fig. 3. The receptor potential rises slowly with time and finally levels off at a level of response which appears to remain relatively unchanged as long as the taste stimulus remains on the tongue.

The size of the receptor potential increases as concentration increases; however, in general, for the higher concentrations, doubling the concentration does not double the response. That is, the functions show compression. Assuming that this compression is transferred across the synapse, any compression produced by antidromic inhibition (discussed above) would add to the compression already present in the receptor potential function.

The responses of single receptor cells are not specific to a single stimulus. Rather, the cells tend to respond to a variety of tastants.

ACTION POTENTIALS IN THE PERIPHERAL NERVE. Action potentials have been recorded from individual neurons as well as from the whole chorda tympani nerve in a variety of species. Whole nerve recordings are even available from human subjects thanks to the fact that the chorda tympani nerve, on its way to the medulla, crosses the eardrum, where it is occasionally exposed during ear surgery (Borg *et al.*, 1967).

Single neurons typically respond to salts and acids with an initial high frequency (transient response) that declines rapidly to a relatively constant frequency (steady state) that may also decline more slowly over time (Smith *et al.*, 1975). Responses to sugars and bitter substances often show a slower onset and build to a peak response before declining. Figure 4 shows the responses of a single neuron in the rat to applications of NaCl.

Recordings from whole nerves look much like many superimposed single neuron recordings; whole chorda tympani responses are usually processed through electronic circuitry (Beidler, 1953) that provides a running average of the frequency of impulses in the whole nerve. The processed whole nerve responses in Fig. 5 show the same initial transient to NaCl shown in the single-fiber responses

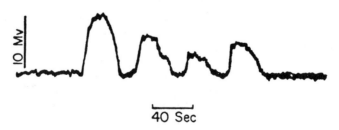

Fig. 3. Receptor potential recorded from a hamster taste receptor cell to 0.1 M NaCl, 0.02 M quinine hydrochloride, 0.5 M sucrose, and 0.01 M HCl applied to the tongue with water rinses between stimuli. From Kimura and Beidler (1961).

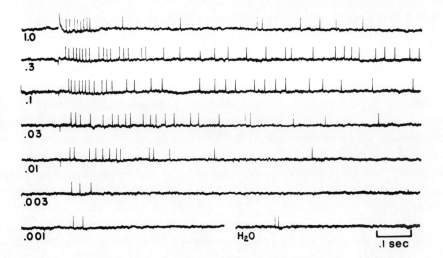

Fig. 4. Action potentials recorded from a single neuron in the chorda tympani of the rat to various concentrations of NaCl. From Pfaffmann (1955). Reprinted with permission of the American Physiological Society.

in Fig. 4. Some processed whole nerve responses do not show such transients (Beidler, 1953) because the electronic circuits used to process the whole nerve responses can be set to average over various time periods and the short time periods show the transient responses while the longer time periods do not.

Neural responses to taste substances are reversible. Transient responses reflect the difference in concentration between the stimulus solution and the

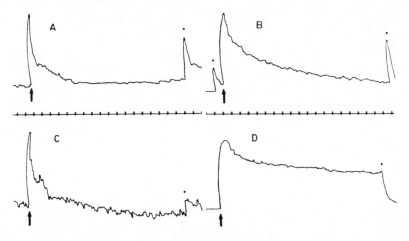

Fig. 5. Ink tracings of whole chorda tympani responses processed through an electronic summator. The height of the ink tracing is approximately proportional to the frequency of the action potentials in the whole nerve response. Records reading from left to right show whole chorda tympani responses to a 3-min flow of 0.2 M NaCl in human patients (A, B, and C) as well as in a rat (D). Arrows indicate NaCl application and dots indicate water application. Since the water was cooler than the NaCl solution for the patients, the responses to water may actually represent cooling and touch rather than taste. From Borg *et al.* (1967). Copyright 1967 by Pergamon Press, Inc. Reprinted by permission.

solution that just preceded it on the tongue, while steady-state responses depend only on the concentration of the stimulus. For example, Fig. 6 shows responses from the rat chorda tympani to 0.03 M NaCl following 0.1 M NaCl and following water. The steady-state response to 0.03 M NaCl is the same in both cases but the transient response is different; after 0.1 M NaCl, 0.03 M produces a transient decrement and after water, 0.03 M produces a transient increment. In general, when the stimulus is more concentrated than the adapting solution, the stimulus will produce a transient increase in the neural response followed by a decrease to the steady-state response characteristic of the stimulus concentration but when the stimulus is less concentrated, it will produce a transient decrease in the neural response followed by an increase to the steady-state characteristic of the stimulus concentration.

Single neurons typically respond to more than one of the four basic tastes. This could result from the innervation of several receptor cells by a single neuron or it also could simply reflect the nonspecificity already at the receptor cell.

ORIGIN OF THE TRANSIENT RESPONSE IN THE PERIPHERAL NERVE. The receptor potential lacks the transient response shown by the recordings in the peripheral nerve. The origin of the transient is important to theories about the generation of the receptor potential.

The lack of the transient in the receptor potential could be the result of the very slow application of stimuli. Since the recording electrode is inserted into the cell which must be stimulated, taste stimuli are not usually flowed across the tongue at rates as high as those used for the nerve recordings. Instead, the stimuli are applied at a distance from the electrode and are allowed to slowly diffuse over the tongue area into which the electrode is inserted. Perhaps if stimuli were applied this slowly in experiments recording from the peripheral nerves the neural transient would disappear. This possibility is supported by whole chorda

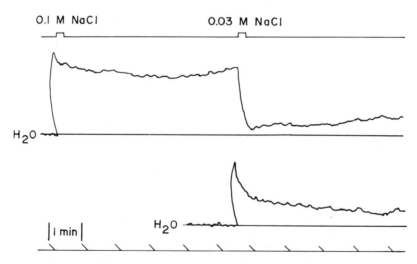

Fig. 6. Ink tracings similar to those in Fig. 5. Records show whole chorda tympani responses to 0.03 M NaCl following 0.1 M NaCl (upper tracing) and following water (lower tracing) in the rat. Stimulus onset is shown at the top of the figure. Modified from Pfaffmann and Powers (1964).

tympani responses to stimulation of the tongue with anodal current (Smith and Bealer, 1975). Although not conclusively proved, this current appears to stimulate taste receptors by causing cations to flow toward receptor sites so that varying the rise time of the current amounts to varying the "flow" rate of cations. When the "flow" rate was high, transients occurred, but when the "flow" rate was successively decreased, the transient decreased until it had disappeared and the peripheral nerve response resembled the receptor potentials.

On the other hand, the peripheral nerve responses might not be proportional to the receptor potentials. The transient response in the nerve might be produced at the synapse between the receptor cell and the peripheral neurons (Sato, 1971). This view is supported by recordings of receptor potentials and whole glossopharyngeal nerve responses from the frog obtained with the same flow rates of the NaCl stimulus (Sato, 1976). Although the flow rates used were quite low, the whole nerve response showed transients while the receptor potentials did not.

The transient may be proportional to the rate of rise of the receptor potential (Sato and Beidler, 1975; Sato, 1976). However, this would not explain the steady-state response recorded from the peripheral nerve of some species (e.g., rat) when the receptor potential is not changing.

OCCUPATION THEORY. The earliest information about the nature of the stimulus-receptor interaction came from Beidler (1954). He assumed that the interaction between stimulus and receptor could be considered to be a physical process at equilibrium and that the magnitude of the neural response was proportional to the number of ions or molecules in the stimulus that had interacted with the receptor sites. An analysis of neural responses in the rat based on these assumptions permitted calculations of the binding strengths for different taste stimuli. The weak forces involved led to the conclusion that taste molecules adsorb to rather than chemically react with the molecules of the receptor.

The assumption that the neural response reflects the number of receptor sites occupied produces a slowly rising receptor potential with no transient since relatively few molecules adsorb initially but, with time, the number of occupied sites increases. At equilibrium, just as many molecules are adsorbing as are desorbing so the same number of sites are always occupied and the receptor potential remains constant.

RATE THEORY. Rate theory (Paton, 1961; Heck and Erickson, 1973) changes one assumption in occupation theory. The neural response is assumed to be proportional to the rate of adsorption rather than the number of occupied sites. The actual adsorbing and desorbing of molecules to receptors are viewed the same in both theories. Rate theory requires a receptor potential with an initial transient.

TASTE QUALITY

Introspection originally led to the concept of four basic tastes. But before the power of four basic tastes was realized, lists of taste qualities were generally quite long. For example, in the eighteenth century Haller listed taste sensations as sour, sweet, rough, bitter, saline, urinous, spirituous, aromatic or pungent, acrid, insipid, and putrid in what is considered to be the first modern textbook of physiology. Lists provided by other investigators varied, but sweet, sour, salty, and bitter were usually present. Some limited information from primitive societies shows this same pattern (Chamberlin, 1903; Myers, 1904). When fewer than these four qualities are used to describe taste experience, as happens with some primitive societies (Myers, 1904), there seems to have been a collapse of sensory categories into hedonic categories, i.e., good vs. bad tasting.

Some of the reasons for the longer lists are clear. Horn (1825) argued that some of the terms used included sensations other than tastes. For example, pungent appears to be partly olfactory, and rough appears to be partly tactile. Horn narrowed the basic tastes to five: sweet, sour, bitter, salty, and alkaline. Alkaline was later concluded to be a mixture of taste and tactile sensations (Öhrwall, 1901), which left the four basic tastes. These were viewed as the irreducible units of taste experience.

Taste quality categories differ dramatically from those for olfactory qualities. Names of taste qualities are abstractions while names of odor qualities are usually related to the object that produces the odor (e.g., fruity, minty, etc.). In addition, taste names, at least in English, also have evaluative connotations (e.g., a sweet personality or salty language).

Henning (1927) is usually credited with formalizing the four basic tastes with his "taste tetrahedron." He placed the four basic tastes at the four corners of the tetrahedron, complex tastes containing two qualities along the appropriate edge, and those containing three tastes on a face. Henning left the tetrahedron hollow. He meant to represent only what he considered to be naturally occurring complex tastes on the tetrahedron and he did not believe that there were any that had all four basic tastes. The tetrahedron was not meant to represent the tastes of mixtures. For example, KCl would be located on the edge between salty and bitter, but Henning did not believe that its taste was equivalent to that of a mixture of a salty tasting substance with a bitter tasting substance. Von Skramlik (1922) proved Henning wrong by showing that the complex tastes of a variety of salts could be duplicated by mixtures of the four basic tastes. Although von Skramlik felt that the tetrahedron was not very useful, it is his interpretation of it that is usually cited. He meant it to reflect the analytical nature of taste quality. He believed that complex tastes can be analyzed into their constituent qualities by introspection and that complex tastes can be constructed by mixing simple tastes.

The emergence of the four basic tastes occurred within the context of important developments in the physiology and psychology of the senses. Johannes Müller's doctrine of specific nerve energies (1838) stated that a particular nerve mediates only one kind of sensory modality (e.g., vision or taste). Extensions of this doctrine stated that individual nerve fibers would mediate primary qualities within a modality (Natanson, 1844). Müller's student, Hermann Helmholtz, attempted to clarify "modality" and "quality" used as psychological terms. He argued that, if sensations are so different that there are no transitions between them and they cannot be viewed as more or less similar to one another, then they belong to different modalities (e.g., blue, sweet, warm, and high pitched). On the other hand, when there are transitions between sensations such that some sensations can be described as more similar than others (e.g., red and orange are more similar than red and blue), then these sensations represent different qualities within one modality (Helmholtz, 1879).

Some of the most important work done in the nineteenth century on the psychophysics of taste followed directly from the contributions of Müller and Helmholtz. Wundt, who founded the first laboratory of experimental psychology in Leipzig, and Holmgren, a physiologist mainly interested in color vision, were both students of Helmholtz, and in turn produced students who were two of the most important taste investigators of the late nineteenth century. Öhrwall, who studied with Holmgren, applied Helmholtz's distinction to taste and concluded that there are no transitions between taste qualities, and thus there are really four modalities of taste: sweet, salty, sour, and bitter (Öhrwall, 1891, 1901). Kiesow, who studied with Wundt, took a different approach leading to the view that the four basic tastes are qualities within a single modality. Kiesow looked for taste phenomena analogous to some found in color vision (Kiesow, 1894a,b, 1896). Colored afterimages and color mixing were well known at that time. Kiesow reported that exposing the tongue to a solution of one quality caused solutions of certain other qualities to taste stronger. He believed that this phenomenon was analogous to colored afterimages. He also showed that a mixture of weak sucrose and salt lacked both sweetness and saltiness and tasted flat. This he believed was analogous to the gray produced by mixing colors opposite to one another on the color circle. Öhrwall criticized Kiesow's interpretations of these studies and argued further that the independence of the four tastes could be compared to the independence of the touch, temperature, and pain senses in the skin. Kiesow's research has been widely cited in U.S. texts, perhaps in part because Wundt trained a number of American psychologists who, with their students, then wrote some of the early textbooks.

Taste research continued to flourish in the late nineteenth and early twentieth centuries, particularly in the German psychophysical labs. The methods were primarily the classic threshold procedures provided by Fechner's *Elemente der Psychophysik* (1860). However, during and between the two world wars taste psychophysics fell into decline. Some influence from the original German traditions was retained in the teaching and research of several U.S. psychologists trained in Wundt's laboratory at Leipzig. Although a new interest in taste psychophysics began to develop within food technology and gave rise to a considerable body of important research (Pangborn, 1964), the point of view developed by Kiesow in the nineteenth century was essentially unchanged.

A dramatic experiment on the physiology of taste challenged Kiesow's point of view. For the first time, Pfaffmann (1941) recorded from single fibers of the chorda tympani taste nerve of the cat. A single fiber responded to more than one of the four basic tastes. The nineteenth-century expectation that single nerve fibers would mediate primary qualities was not confirmed. This exciting finding played a major role in shifting the emphasis from human taste psychophysics to electrophysiological studies with other species.

Taste psychophysics reemerged during the 1960s partly as a result of the development of direct scaling techniques by S. S. Stevens and his colleagues at

Harvard. In one of the most widely used of Stevens's methods, direct magnitude estimation, subjects simply assign numbers to the intensity of the sensation evoked by a stimulus. The subjects are instructed to make their assigned numbers proportional to the perceived sensations, so that a stimulus that produces a sensation judged twice as large as the preceding sensation should be given a number twice as large. This procedure can produce a reliable scale for a single taste substance from an individual subject in half an hour. Using the indirect Fechnerian psychophysical techniques of the nineteenth century, a half hour was required to obtain a single threshold value. The direct methods of Stevens and his colleagues did more than just make taste psychophysics more practical. They focused attention on suprathreshold phenomena which relate more directly to experience.

MODERN TASTE PSYCHOPHYSICS AND THE FOUR BASIC TASTES

Modern psychophysical studies challenge many of the widely cited results of the nineteenth century but retain one central concept: the four basic tastes. The trend in the modern work is toward simplicity. The complex taste interactions, viewed by Kiesow to be analogous to phenomena of color vision, have been discarded in favor of the independence of the four basic tastes espoused by Öhrwall. Many operations (e.g., adapting and mixing) can change the perceived intensity of taste experience but that experience is still analyzable into the same four qualities. Tastes not easily described in terms of the four basic tastes are, if they exist at all, the exceptions, not the rule.

There is one crucial difference between the modern and the classic use of the "four basic tastes." In the nineteenth century, the basic tastes were believed to be the irreducible units of taste experience; that status carried with it the assumption that each taste quality was mediated by nerve fibers sensitive only to stimuli of one quality. The modern "four basic tastes" are less weighty. The categories are useful, indeed essential for the description of taste experience; but the jury is still out concerning the mechanisms underlying taste quality.

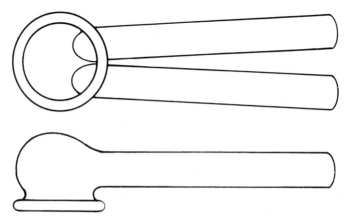

Fig. 7. Hahn's Geschmacksluppe. The circular opening is 1.5 cm in diameter. The opening is placed over the tongue area to be stimulated. Stimuli flow in one tube and out the other. From Hahn (1949).

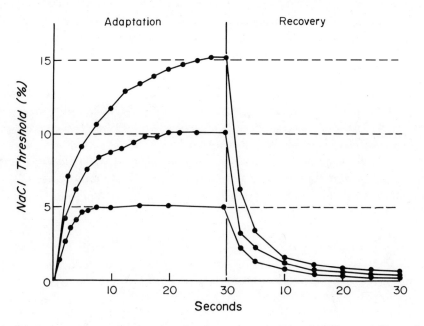

Fig. 8. Adaptation and recovery functions for three concentrations of NaCl. As NaCl was flowed through the Geschmacksluppe, the threshold (probably detection rather than recognition) increased until it reached a point just above the adapting concentration. When water was substituted for the NaCl, the threshold decreased again. From Hahn (1934).

The topics that follow are a selection of some of the results that have led to the modern four-quality view of taste.

ADAPTATION. *The Basic Phenomenon.* "Adaptation" refers to the diminished sensitivity that results from prolonged taste stimulation. Helmut Hahn, a German psychophysicist, depended exclusively on the Fechnerian threshold methods to study taste adaptation. He measured absolute thresholds before and after adaptation. In a decade of research spanning the 1930s and 1940s, Hahn and his colleagues measured nearly 15,000 thresholds for 108 taste substances on 43 subjects (Hahn and Ulbrich, 1948). Hahn stimulated the tongue through a "Geschmacksluppe" (shown in Fig. 7). This permitted a flowing solution to stimulate an area 1.5 cm in diameter. Hahn found that taste adaptation was usually complete; that is, if a solution was flowed across the tongue, its taste intensity decreased over time until it had no taste at all. After adaptation, the concentration that could barely be detected (i.e., the absolute threshold) was just above that of the adapting solution (Hahn, 1934; Hahn *et al.*, 1938). Hahn's results for NaCl are shown in Fig. 8.

Adaptation turns out to be of special importance in experience because the taste system is normally adapted to the NaCl in saliva. If saliva is removed with a water rinse, the NaCl threshold drops. A human subject can detect about 0.0001 M NaCl after a water rinse whereas thresholds in the presence of saliva are around 0.01 M NaCl (McBurney and Pfaffmann, 1963). The completeness of adaptation in the laboratory contrasts with ordinary experience. The tastes of foods and beverages do not fade as a meal progresses. This is usually attributed to changes in stimulus concentration caused by dilution with saliva and changes in the area stimulated caused by tongue movements. The taste system is extemely sensitive to very small changes in concentration (McBurney, 1977). Even under most laboratory conditions, taste adaptation does not proceed to completion (Meiselman, 1975), but with particularly rigorous control, taste adaptation is complete (McBurney, 1977).

The Taste of Water. We now know that a longstanding controversy over the "intrinsic' taste of water is related to adaptation. Water was initially considered to be a tasteless solvent, but by the nineteenth century several authors had expressed doubts about the tastelessness of distilled water. Öhrwall (1891) and Henle (1880)

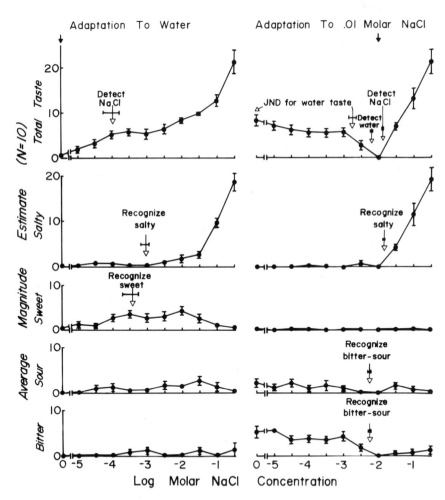

Fig. 9. Taste of water and NaCl under two adaptation conditions: water and 0.01 M NaCl (approximately equivalent to the Na and Cl content of saliva). The top functions show the total taste intensity and the lower functions show how the total is divided into salty, sweet, sour, and bitter components. All points are shown ± SEM. From Bartoshuk (1974b). Copyright 1974 by the American Psychological Association. Reprinted by permission.

argued that distilled water is flat rather than tasteless. Several investigators (Camerer, 1870; Kiesow, 1894*b;* von Skramlik, 1922) reported individual subjects who found distilled water to taste bitter. In 1914, Brown recorded evaluations of the taste of water from 100 subjects; he concluded that "The upshot of all these observations seems to be that water is not tasteless (in the broader sense of the word), that it tastes more like bitter than anything else, and that its taste can be neutralized by salt. . . . Furthermore there is evidence that some of the weakest solutions of salt in water give a substance which is as nearly tasteless as any which can be produced" (pp. 253, 254). Brown's comments proved prophetic. The amount of salt he recommended adding to "remove" the bitter taste of water bracketed the normal concentration of NaCl in saliva, the solution to which one is normally adapted.

As it turns out, the taste of water varies depending on what precedes it on the tongue. Figure 9 shows the relation between adaptation to NaCl and the taste of water. The top curves show the total intensity of the taste and the curves below break that into the perceived qualities. The left part of Fig. 9 shows the taste of water and NaCl after adaptation to water. Note that water after water is virtually tasteless. Weak NaCl after water tastes sweet, an observation made first by Renqvist (1919), and stronger NaCl tastes salty. The right part of Fig. 9 shows the same solutions tasted after adaptation to 0.01 M NaCl (about the concentration of NaCl in saliva) rather than water. Note that now the 0.01 M NaCl is virtually tasteless. Solutions more concentrated than 0.01 M taste salty, solutions less concentrated taste bitter-sour, and water produces the strongest bitter-sour taste. The relevant detection thresholds (the concentration at which a taste is detected) and recognition thresholds (the concentration at which a particular quality is recognized) are shown by arrows. The different descriptions of the taste of water can now be related at least in part to the normal variation in salivary electrolytes. High electrolyte content would be expected to produce the bitter-sour reports, low electrolyte content to produce the tasteless reports. "Flat" might result when an individual can detect some taste but cannot recognize the quality.

Figure 10 shows another water taste: the sweet taste of water following adaptation to various concentrations of the potassium salts of chlorogenic acid and cynarin, substances found in the globe artichoke. The sweetness of sucrose is shown on the same function for purposes of comparison. This effect is particularly interesting because not all individuals are equally sensitive to it.

All four basic taste qualities can be produced with a water stimulus by adapting to appropriate substances, but the most common water taste is sweet. Table I lists the tastes of water evoked by a variety of compounds. The taste of an adapting substance seems to predict the water taste quality better than does the chemical nature of the adapting substance (McBurney and Shick, 1971).

Cross-Adaptation among Substances with Similar Tastes. If adaptation to one substance decreases sensitivity to another substance, we say that cross-adaptation has occurred. Once again, Hahn *et al.* (1940) did the early systematic research on cross-adaptation. Adapting to one acid raised the thresholds for all other acids tested. However, the results for the other taste qualities were startling. For sweet, bitter, and alkaline stimuli, adapting to one substance did not always elevate the threshold for other substances of the same quality. The results for salts were the most bizarre. Among 24 salts tested, no cross-adaptation occurred. These results have been interpreted to mean that, except for sour, each taste quality is mediated by many separate mechanisms.

One of the first taste studies done with the new psychophysical methods of Stevens produced very different conclusions about cross-adaptation. McBurney and his students (McBurney and Lucas, 1966; Smith and McBurney, 1969; McBurney *et al.*, 1972; McBurney, 1972) measured suprathreshold rather than threshold sensations. They modified Stevens's procedures so that subjects gave magnitude estimates of individual qualities as well as total sensation magnitude which permitted them to monitor the effects of adaptation on individual qualities. McBurney's results were as startling in their simplicity as Hahn's were in their complexity. Adaptation to a salty substance decreased the salty taste of all salts tested (see Fig. 11). Results for sweet, sour, and bitter were similar, with one exception: some bitter substances did not cross-adapt (see later section).

Why Hahn failed to discover this simplicity is unknown since no one to date has attempted to replicate his Herculean feat, but suppose that Hahn actually measured detection thresholds rather than recognition thresholds. For detection thresholds, a subject need only detect the presence of any taste. For recognition

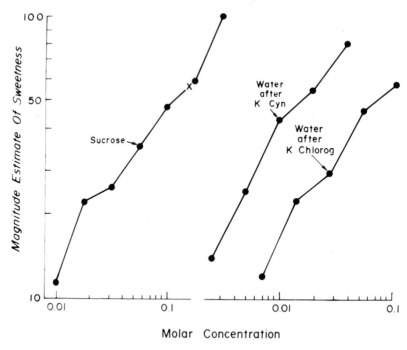

Fig. 10. Sweet taste of water following two of the active components in globe artichoke, the potassium salts of chlorogenic acid (K Chlorog) and cynarin (K Cyn) compared to the sweet taste of sucrose. The *x* on the sucrose function represents 2 tsp of sugar in 6 oz of water (0.16 M sucrose). The concentration of sucrose refers to the concentration tasted. The concentration of the salts refers to the concentration of the adapting solution that preceded the water. From Bartoshuk *et al.* (1972).

Stimulus	Taste of stimulus	Taste of water following stimulus
NaCl	Salty	Bitter
KCl	Salty-bitter	Sour
KBr	Salty	
Saccharin	Sweet	
KNO₃	Bitter	
Urea	Bitter	Salty
NaNO₃	Salty-sour-bitter	Sweet
Na₂SO₄	Salty-bitter	
NH₄Br	Salty-bitter	
CaBr₂	Bitter	
KNO₃	Bitter	
MgSO₄	Bitter	
Urea	Bitter	
Quinine hydrochloride	Bitter	
Quinine sulfate	Bitter	
Caffeine	Bitter	
Acetic acid	Sour	
Citric acid	Sour	
Lactic acid	Sour	

[a]Qualities listed were those reported on at least half the trials with that particular stimulus. Modified from McBurney and Shick (1971).

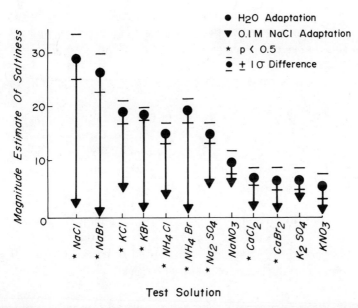

Fig. 11. Saltiness of 12 salts after adaptation to water (●) and after adaptation to 0.1 M NaCl (▼). The decrease in saltiness was statistically significant ($p < 0.05$) for the starred salts. From Smith and McBurney (1969).

thresholds, a subject must recognize the quality of the stimulus. Only the taste qualities in common between two substances would be expected to cross-adapt, yet in Hahn's experiments each of the two substances tested for cross-adaptation often had at least two taste qualities. For example, NaCl is salty and sweet and KCl is salty and bitter. Adapting to NaCl would reduce the saltiness of KCl but not the bitterness. Hahn might have measured the threshold for the detection of bitterness of KCl after adaptation to NaCl. All this shows how important it is to distinguish between detection and recognition thresholds.

There is an interesting historical footnote to add to a discussion of Hahn's cross-adaptation work. His data seem to argue against the four basic taste position prominent at that time. Yet, in a paper published later (Hahn and Ulbrich, 1948), Hahn discussed a new set of experiments that he believed proved the independence of the five basic tastes (Hahn added alkaline to the conventional four tastes). He reported that subthreshold concentrations of substances of similar quality could be combined to produce a threshold sensation while subthreshold concentrations of substances with different qualities could not. That is, despite failures to get cross-adaptation, Hahn believed in primary tastes. Hahn's last experiments have yet to be evaluated with modern methods. They may prove as provocative as those on cross-adaptation.

Cross-Adaptation among Substances with Different Tastes. Hahn studied adaptation across taste qualities as well as within taste qualities. He found that adapting to a substance of one taste quality did not affect the thresholds of other taste qualities, that is, there was no cross-adaptation among qualities. These results contradicted the taste contrast studied in the nineteenth century. Kiesow reported successive contrast between pairs of qualities (Kiesow, 1894*b;* Henning, 1927). This meant that exposing the tongue to a substance of one quality (e.g., sour) would intensify the taste of a substance of another quality (e.g., sweet). This phenomenon was considered to be analogous to colored afterimages. Since the contrast of the nineteenth century is really the psychophysical opposite of cross-adaptation, we now refer to it as "cross-enhancement." Cross-enhancement was also reported by others (Mayer, 1927; Dallenbach and Dallenbach, 1943; Meiselman, 1968).

The observations of cross-enhancement preceded much of the work on water tastes, so controls for water taste are absent in these studies. As already noted, adaptation can cause a water taste to be added to a solute taste. Properly controlled experiments suggest that the apparent cross-enhancement actually results from the addition of a water taste (McBurney and Bartoshuk, 1973).

Hahn's failure to observe cross-enhancement is consistent with the water taste explanation. Hahn dissolved his test solutions in his adapting solution rather than in water in order to shorten the time required to readapt for successive trials; however, this procedure would have prevented water tastes since it effectively prevented removal of the adapting solution. With no water tastes, Hahn found no cross-enhancement.

Recently the sourness of citric acid applied to single taste papillae was reported to be enhanced by adaptation to sucrose. This study included water taste controls and so may be the first case of true cross-enhancement (McCutcheon and Kuznicki, 1975). Similar cross-enhancement between other pairs of stimuli did not occur; however, the result with sucrose and acid suggests that additional work on this phenomenon is needed.

BITTERNESS: MORE THAN ONE KIND? *Cross-Adaptation.* The failures of some bitter substances to cross-adapt is the only currently known exception to the rule that substances of similar taste quality cross-adapt one another (Smith and McBurney, 1969; McBurney *et al.*, 1972; McBurney, 1972; McBurney and Barto-shuk, 1973). Some of the failures are symmetrical (e.g. adaptation to urea does not reduce the bitterness of caffeine and *vice versa*) while some may not be (e.g., adaptation to quinine hydrochloride does not reduce the bitterness of urea but adaptation to urea partially reduces the bitterness of quinine hydrochloride). In some cases, adaptation has been tested only in one direction (e.g., adaptation to quinine hydrochloride does not reduce the bitterness of PTC but partially reduces the bitterness of caffeine; the effects of adaptation to caffeine or PTC on the bitterness of quinine have not been tested).

Genetic Variation in Taste Thresholds for the Bitter Compound PTC. The bimodal threshold distribution for PTC and related compounds was discussed above under bitter stimuli. If molecular configurations that produce a bimodal threshold distribution stimulate a different receptor mechanism than those that produce a unimodal distribution, then these groups of stimuli should not show cross-adaptation. As the data above show, adaptation to QHCl does not cross-adapt PTC just as would be predicted.

Cross-adaptation tests are complicated by the possibility that a single stimulus molecule might contain both kinds of molecular configurations. Figure 12 shows a possible example. Note that QHCl is equally bitter for tasters and nontaster of PTC while caffeine is clearly less bitter for nontasters over part of the concentration range tested. If caffeine contained both groupings, then nontasters might be expected to taste caffeine as less bitter because fewer receptor sites would be stimulated in these individuals. The fact that the bitterness of caffeine is partially cross-adapted by QHCl supports this interpretation.

This is a very simplistic interpretation of what may be very complex receptor events. Nonetheless, cross-adaptation experiments offer the opportunity to organize the psychophysical data, and that organization may be useful to the physiologist as well as the psychophysicist.

How Many Bitters? The evidence discussed above is relevant to receptor mechanisms but does not necessarily imply that there are qualitative distinctions within bitterness. The different bitter receptor mechanisms may produce neural signals that are equivalent as far as the code for bitterness is concerned.

PSYCHOPHYSICAL SCALES. S. S. Stevens and his colleagues (Stevens, 1975) have shown that for a variety of sensory continua, perceived intensity (ψ) is a power function of stimulus (ϕ). That is,

$$\psi = \phi^\beta$$

If we take the logarithm of both sides of this equation, we see that

$$\log \psi = \beta \log \phi$$

which is the equation for a straight line of slope β. This equation suggests a particularly convenient means of plotting psychophysical data. The log of the perceived intensity plotted against the log of the concentration will yield a straight line with slope equal to β, the exponent of the power function relating ψ and ϕ.

Because of its convenience, the method of magnitude estimation has been widely used to generate psychophysical functions in taste. The resulting exponents have proved to be extremely variable. Meiselman (1971) demonstrated that some of the variation relates to the way in which stimuli are tasted. For example, a common procedure is that of "sip and spit." Typically, subjects simply sip substances at room temperature from a cup, judge the taste, and then spit them out. Stimuli can also be flowed across the tongue (McBurney and Pfaffmann, 1963). In general, NaCl, quinine and sucrose produce higher exponents when the solutions are sipped, but the situation is less clear for acids. The higher exponents for quinine may be related to the fact that the sip procedure stimulates the back of the tongue as well as the front while the flow procedure stimulates only the front (see discussion below on regional sensitivity). The reasons for the other differences are less clear but may relate to the effects of flow rate (Meiselman *et al.*, 1972) and temperature (Moskowitz, 1973) on perceived intensity.

If the stimulating conditions are held constant, substances with similar taste qualities appear to produce similar exponents. For example, when 16 sugars and

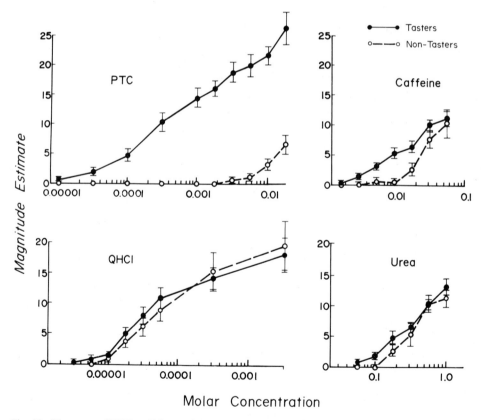

Fig. 12. Bitterness of PTC, caffeine, quinine hydrochloride (QHCl), and urea for tasters and nontasters. Each point is shown ± 1 SEM. From Hall *et al.* (1975).

24 acids were tested with the sip procedure, the sugars produced exponents around 1.3 and the acids produced exponents around 0.85 (Moskowitz, 1970, 1971). There are exceptions to this generalization, but the exceptions may reflect the effects of other qualities. For example, the sweetness of saccharin produces a lower exponent than that of sucrose, but this may be due to the presence of bitterness in saccharin.

Psychophysical functions have been compared to functions resulting from the neural recordings available from patients undergoing ear surgery (Diamant *et al.*, 1965; Zotterman, 1971). The psychophysical and neural functions obtained for each patient were remarkably similar. This is important because it suggests that there is no important transformation of the slope from the periphery to the central nervous system. Unfortunately, this work preceded recognition of the effects of the tasting procedure on psychophysical functions. During the neural recordings stimuli were flowed over the tongue, but for the psychophysical tests the stimuli were usually sipped (Diamant *et al.*, 1965). This means that the similarity between psychophysical and neural data may be fortuitous. Without further experiments there is no way to determine whether or not the psychophysical and neural functions have similar shapes.

REGIONAL SENSITIVITY OF THE TONGUE. The variation in sensitivity to sweet, sour, salty, and bitter with tongue locus is one of the most widely cited "facts" about the sense of taste. The familiar statement that sweet sensitivity is greatest on the tip, sour on the sides, and bitter on the back of the tongue (Hänig, 1901) was believed to be evidence for four specific receptors distributed differentially on the tongue.

Collings (1974) reexamined regional sensitivity with improved methods. She essentially confirmed Hänig but pointed out that a careful reading of Hänig shows that the differences that he originally reported were small and have been exaggerated in secondary sources. Regional differences did occur but were not pronounced (see Fig. 13). The one difference that did occur between the studies was that Collings found that the bitter threshold was actually slightly lower on the front than the back of the tongue. She noted that Hänig may have inadvertently touched the palate when he applied bitter stimuli to the back of the tongue; the palate is known to give low bitter thresholds (Henkin and Christiansen, 1967).

Variation of the shapes of the psychophysical functions for taste stimuli on different tongue loci is functionally more important than variation of thresholds across different loci. Regional differences for citric acid, quinine, and NaCl suggest that these stimuli may taste stronger on some tongue loci than others (Collings, 1974). For example, the bitterness of quinine increased with concentration faster on the back of the tongue than it did on any other locus. Most individuals have probably observed that bitter medicines taste particularly unpleasant at the back of the tongue. Figure 14 shows that for the higher concentrations, as a bitter stimulus moves from the front to the rear of the tongue, its bitterness increases.

Taste thresholds increase as the area of the tongue stimulated decreases (McBurney, 1969). However, the psychophysical functions for suprathreshold stimuli do not change shape as the area of the tongue stimulated decreases (Smith,

1971). This is important because it means that variation in the shape of the psychophysical function for various tongue loci is not due simply to variation in the number of receptors stimulated.

The source of the locus effect is unclear. In the case of bitter, there is already evidence for at least two receptor mechanisms. The locus effect might reflect differential distribution of these. In the cases of sour and salt, the locus effect remains unexplained.

MIXTURES. When substances are mixed, the taste qualities of the components can still be identified but the perceived intensities of those qualities are usually changed. The early work on taste mixtures was motivated by a desire to find analogies with color mixtures. Since the color of a two-component mixture can be predicted from the colors of the components, attempts were made to predict the taste of a two-component mixture from the taste qualities of the components (Kiesow, 1896). These attempts were largely unsuccessful. Experiments with the same pairs of qualities produced conflicting results, although, on the whole,

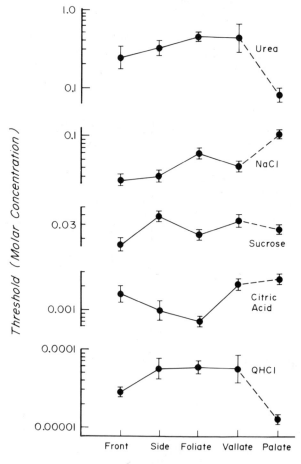

Fig. 13. Log taste thresholds (± 1 SEM) for four tongue loci and the soft palate, for urea, NaCl, sucrose, citric acid, and quinine hydrochloride. Modified from Collings (1974).

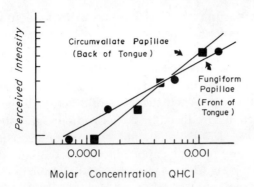

Fig. 14. Bitterness of quinine hydrochloride as a function of concentration for the front and the back of the tongue. Modified from Collings (1974).

mixtures of substances with different tastes tend to be less intense than the simple sum of the components (Pangborn, 1960; Moskowitz, 1972).

Other experiments concerned mixtures of substances with similar taste qualities, usually sweet (Cameron, 1947; Stone and Oliver, 1969; Yamaguchi *et al.,* 1970). In some cases the perceived intensity of the mixture was actually greater than the simple sum of the components (synergism) and in others the mixture was about equal to the simple sum (Moskowitz, 1974*a,b*).

Moskowitz proposed that in mixtures of substances with the same taste quality, the perceived intensity of the mixture either is equal to the simple sum of the perceived intensities of the components or is greater. However, in mixtures of substances with different taste qualities, suppression occurs that is proportional to the difference between the qualities: the greater the difference, the greater the suppression. This proposal retains the idea borrowed from color vision: that mixture interactions depend on the qualities of the components.

Figure 15 illustrates the logic underlying a different point of view. Figure 15 shows three power functions that represent the kinds of functions found for taste. The simplest kind of addition of two substances of similar taste is the addition of a substance to itself. Consider adding concentration 1.0 of A to itself. The perceived intensity of the sum, that is, of concentration 2.0, is 1.4. The same operation on B and C would produce perceived intensities of 2.0 and 2.8, respectively. The function for A is said to show "compression" and that for C is said to show "expansion" (Stevens, 1958). The only time a substance would add to itself such that the "mixture" is equal to the simple sum of the components would be when its perceived intensity is directly proportional to its concentration (e.g., the power function with an exponent equal to one in Fig. 15).

The logic of this argument was appreciated very early by Pfaffmann (1959) and Beidler (1961) in connection with their electrophysiological studies. Magnitude of neural response did not usually increase in direct proportion to concentration; rather, some functions showed compression while others showed expansion. If substances with similar tastes affect the same receptor sites, then the neural responses to these substances would obviously add along the concentration function typical of those receptor sites. If it were a compression function, then the mixture would show suppression; if it were an expansion function, then the mixture would show synergism.

A psychophysical analysis of mixtures of substances with similar tastes can take advantage of the fact that the shapes of the psychophysical functions can be manipulated by the choice of the method of tasting (e.g., sipping vs. flowing solutions over the tongue). When sugars were tasted with the flow method, the psychophysical functions produced by the individual sugars showed compression (exponents were about 0.7–0.8) and a mixture of four sugars tasted only 0.75 as sweet as the simple sum of the components. When the same sugars were tasted with the sip and spit method, the psychophysical functions produced by the individual sugars showed expansion (exponents were about 1.5–2.0) and the same mixture of four sugars tasted 3 times as sweet as the sum of the components (Bartoshuk and Cleveland, 1977).

Suppose the same logic were extended to mixtures of substances with differ-ent taste qualities. In this case, the intensities of the individual components in a mixture could be distinguished because the taste qualities are not identical. Tasted with the flow method, HCl will show the least compression (exponent 0.9) and QHCl the most (exponent 0.3). Sucrose and NaCl will fall between these extremes (Bartoshuk, 1968). Thus in mixtures where the components are about equally strong when unmixed, HCl should taste the most intense and QHCl the least, with sucrose and NaCl falling between them. Figure 16 shows the sourness, sweetness, saltiness, and bitterness of mixtures of from one to four components tasted with the flow method. Consider the bitterness function. The bitterness of the one-component "mixture" is the bitterness of QHCl alone. The bitterness of the two-

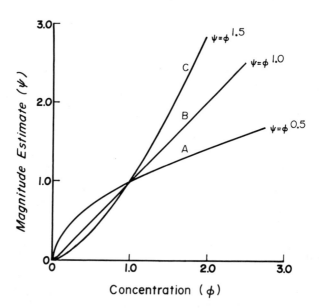

Fig. 15. Three hypothetical psychophysical functions for taste. Function C is said to show expansion while function A is said to show compression. From Bartoshuk (1975).

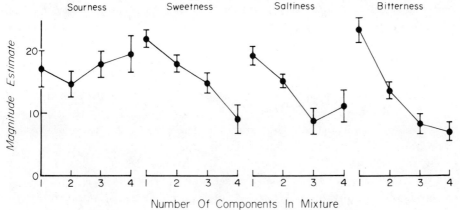

Fig. 16. Perceived intensity ± 1 SEM of each of the four classic taste qualities in mixtures of one, two, three, and four components. The bitterness function contains values only from mixtures containing QHCl, the sweetness function contains values only from mixtures containing sucrose, etc. From Bartoshuk (1975).

component mixture is the average bitterness of all of the possible two-component mixtures containing QHCl and so forth. Note that as the number of components goes up, the perceived bitterness goes down. Contrast this with the sourness function. Perceived sourness does not decrease as the number of components increases. That is, the greater the compression in the unmixed psychophysical function, the more that substance is suppressed in a mixture.

The shapes of psychophysical functions in taste can vary widely as the stimulating conditions vary, as noted above. Since mixture interactions depend on the shapes of the psychophysical functions produced by the components, mixture interactions should depend on the stimulating conditions. When most of the mixture studies were done, the importance of the stimulating conditions was not appreciated. This may explain the contradictions in the mixture literature. Particular taste quality pairs should not produce the same mixture interactions if the stimulating conditions are not identical across experiments.

Taste mixtures appear to be very different from color mixtures. When colors are mixed, they fuse into a new color that cannot be analyzed into its components, but the new color can be predicted from the component colors. When taste qualities are mixed, they do not seem to fuse into a new taste quality; rather, the qualities of the components can still be recognized but their intensities change. The changes in intensity can be predicted from the psychophysical functions of the components better than from the qualities of the components. This is another source of evidence for the independence of the four basic tastes. A taste quality is not modified by the presence of other qualities, and changes in the perceived intensity of that taste quality depend on factors other than the nature of the other qualities present.

TASTE MODIFIERS. Substances that can modify taste quality were of great interest in the nineteenth century and continue to fascinate investigators today.

Gymnema sylvestre was of special importance in the nineteenth century because it suppressed some qualities (particularly sweetness) and not others, which was considered to be evidence for separate receptor mechanisms.

Gymnema Sylvestre. *Gymnema sylvestre* is a woody climbing plant that runs over the tops of high trees in southern India, Ceylon, and tropical West Africa. It has been known as a taste modifier in the Western literature for more than a century, ever since a British officer stationed in India reported that after chewing the leaves of this plant he could not taste the sugar in his tea. The studies of *Gymnema sylvestre* in the nineteenth century concluded that it suppressed sweetness and to a lesser extent bitterness (Hooper, 1887; Shore, 1892; Kiesow, 1894c), but the effects on bitterness are now thought to be an artifact. The leaves themselves taste bitter and can cross-adapt bitter stimuli. When the bitter taste of *Gymnema sylvestre* is removed with a rinse, the taste of sucrose is suppressed but that of QHCl as well as NaCl, citric acid, and HCl is unaffected (Bartoshuk *et al.*, 1969, 1974; Bartoshuk, 1974a) (see Fig. 17).

Gymnema sylvestre has been tested on a variety of sweet substances and suppresses all of them, with the possible exception of chloroform (Kurihara, 1969). Although *Gymnema sylvestre* does not affect the saltiness and bitterness of stimuli

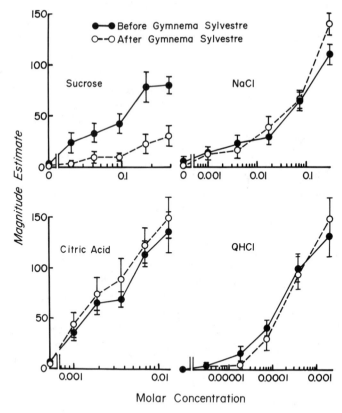

Fig. 17. Effects of *Gymnema sylvestre* on the tastes of sucrose, NaCl, citric acid, and QHCl. Taste intensities are shown ± 1 SEM. From Bartoshuk (1974a).

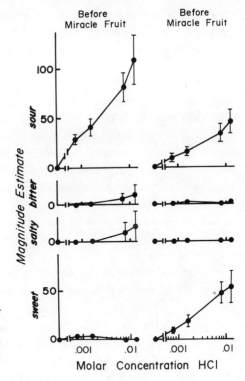

Fig. 18. Effects of miracle fruit on the taste of HCl. Total taste is divided into sweet, salty, bitter, and sour components (± 1 SEM). From Bartoshuk *et al.* (1974). Reprinted by permission.

like NaCl and quinine (Bartoshuk *et al.*, 1969), it does affect the saltiness and bitterness of some stimuli like alanine which are sweet as well as salty and bitter (Meiselman and Halpern, 1970). This may simply reflect the effects of mixture interactions. That is, when the sweetness of alanine is removed, its effects on the other taste qualities may be removed as well (Meiselman and Halpern, 1970).

It is important to be very cautious about drawing conclusions about the nature of the sweet receptor site from studies of the effects of *Gymnema sylvestre*. This substance may not actually complex with the sweet receptor molecules but might prevent sweet molecules from binding in some other way (e.g., by physically blocking them).

Miracle Fruit. Synsepalum dulcificum has been known by several names including *Bumelia dulcifica, Sideroxylon dulcificum, Bakeriella dulcifica,* and *Richardella dulcifica* (Bartoshuk *et al.*, 1974). The name "miracle fruit" was applied by Europeans who experienced its taste-modifying effects while traveling in tropical West Africa more than 100 years ago. After berries from this plant are eaten, sour substances taste sweetened and less sour than normal. The effect is dramatic. Lemons taste like lemonade and can be eaten like oranges. Figure 18 shows the sweet taste induced in HCl after miracle fruit.

An explorer working for the U.S. Department of Agriculture, David Fairchild, was responsible for introducing this plant to Americans. He suggested that miracle fruit inhibits sourness, thus permitting any sweet taste present to be more noticeable. He based this explanation on the observation that sourness is reduced when acids are sweetened by miracle fruit (see Fig. 18). An experiment with *Gymnema sylvestre* proves that this explanation is wrong. Sourness returns to normal when the sweetness induced by miracle fruit is removed with *Gymnema sylvestre* (Bartoshuk *et al.,* 1969, 1974). The reduction in the sourness of acids caused by miracle fruit appears to be a mixture effect; that is, adding sugar to acid will reduce the sourness of the acid in the same way that miracle fruit does (Bartoshuk *et al.,* 1974).

The mechanism by which miracle fruit adds sweetness to the sourness of acids is not clear, but Kurihara and Beidler (1969) have suggested that the glycoprotein that is the active component in miracle fruit might have two binding sites. One of these binds to the receptor membrane, and the other is actually a sugar molecule that can bind to the sweet receptor site in the usual fashion. Normally, the sugar molecule is held in a position that prevents its binding. Acid is assumed to change the conformation of the sweet receptor site so that it can come into contact with the sugar molecule.

Taste modifiers have practical importance. For example, miracle fruit has potential as a nonnutritive sweetener. Modifiers are also of use in the laboratory in the study of taste; however, this use is limited because the effects appear to be quite species specific. This will be discussed in a later section.

Temporal Properties of the Taste System. McBurney (1974, 1977) has suggested another experimental operation that differentiates the four basic tastes. Taste stimuli are applied such that the stimulus fluctuates between two concentrations of a tastant. The ability to detect fluctuation depends on the frequency of the fluctuation and the difference between the concentrations. The shape of the function showing this relation depends on the taste quality of the stimulus. That is, one particular characteristic function occurs for sweet substances, another for sour substances and so forth (see Fig. 19). This general approach, known as "linear systems analysis," has been used effectively in vision and offers another psychophysical tool for the study of taste quality.

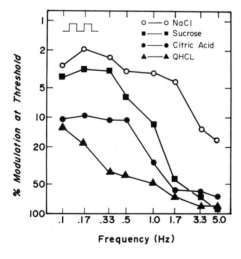

Fig. 19. Effects of temporal modulations on taste. For each point on the graph, two concentrations of a taste substance alternating on the tongue fused into a single sensation; that is, the point marks the threshold for flicker. The average of the two concentrations was always the same, but the smaller the percent modulation, the closer the two concentrations. From McBurney (1977).

TABLE II. TYPES OF FIBERS FOUND IN THE CAT CHORDA TYMPANI BY COHEN *et al.* (1955)

Stimulus	"Water" fiber	"Salt" fiber	"Acid" fiber	"Quinine" fiber	Sensation evoked
H_2O (salt <0.03 M)	+	0	0	0	Water
NaCl (>0.05 M)	0	+	0	0	Salt
HCl (pH 2.5)	+	+	+	0	Sour
Quinine	+	0	0	+	Bitter

ELECTROPHYSIOLOGY AND THE FOUR BASIC TASTES

ACROSS-FIBER PATTERNING CODE FOR QUALITY. *Early Single-Fiber Recordings and "Fiber Types."* Pfaffmann's (1941) discovery that single fibers in the cat chorda tympani were not specific to the four basic tastes required new thinking about the neural coding of taste quality. The sensitivities of the fibers seemed to classify them into a few simple types: acid, acid and NaCl, and acid and quinine. Pfaffmann concluded, "In such a system, sensory quality does not depend simply on the 'all or nothing' activation of some particular fiber group alone, but on the pattern of other fibers active" (p. 255). Acid would stimulate all fibers, NaCl would stimulate the acid-NaCl fibers but not the others, and quinine would stimulate the acid-quinine fibers but not the others.

Cohen *et al.* (1955) accepted the same logic for the sensory coding of taste quality but proposed somewhat different fiber types. Table II shows the stimuli exciting each type and the sensation resulting from each pattern of activity across fibers. Two of the fiber types are the same in both studies: the type responsive to HCl and NaCl and the type responsive to HCl. The fiber type that was specific to quinine was not observed in Pfaffmann's study. However, the most dramatic difference between the studies concerned the "water" fibers. These will be discussed more fully in a later section.

Later Single-Fiber Studies and the Nonspecificity of Taste Neurons. The early studies included relatively few fibers because of the difficulty of the dissection. As Pfaffmann (1955) accumulated more data he began to question the idea of fiber types. Each taste fiber seemed to be unique. This posed no problem for quality coding because if a particular quality is produced by the pattern of activity across a population of neurons it does not matter whether or not those neurons belong to classes.

Erickson (1963), a student of Pfaffmann, extended the idea of across-fiber patterning in taste. He reasoned that a plot of the patterns of activity across neurons for different tastants might predict which would taste most similar. He recorded responses to ammonium chloride (NH_4Cl), potassium chloride (KCl), and sodium chloride (NaCl) in 13 single fibers of the rat chorda tympani and plotted the across-fiber patterns that resulted (see Fig. 20). The patterns for KCl and NH_4Cl were similar but both were very different from that for NaCl. Erickson then tested these three salts behaviorally using generalization of shock avoidance. Rats shocked for drinking KCl avoided NH_4Cl and *vice versa*. Neither group

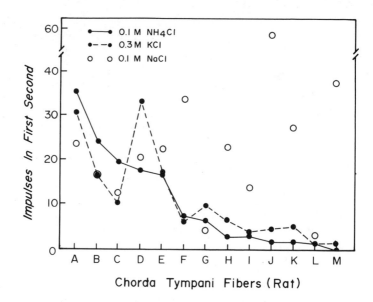

Fig. 20. Across-fiber patterns for three salts. Single fibers are arranged along the baseline in order of responsiveness to NH₄Cl. The KCl pattern is similar to the NH₄Cl pattern. Neither of these patterns is similar to the NaCl pattern. From Erickson (1963).

generalized as much to NaCl, and rats shocked for drinking NaCl generalized slightly but equally to KCl and NH₄Cl. This implies that the salts with similar neural patterns taste similar to the rat.

The neural similarities of tastants were then used to locate those tastants in a space such that the distance between any two tastants was assumed to reflect the qualitative similarity of the two to the rat (Erickson *et al.*, 1965). The cation turned out to be of primary importance in the location of salts. This agrees with the models of salt receptors that consider the binding of cations to particular sites to be the stimulus for salt tastes.

Frank's Classification of Taste Fiber Types. The typing of taste fibers, which was rejected largely on the basis of rat studies, reemerged with an analysis based on the hamster (Frank, 1973). The hamster fibers were classified according to the stimulus that produced the largest response. Figure 21 shows the profile of sensitivity shown by each type of fiber to stimuli representing the four basic tastes. The sucrose-best, NaCl-best, and HCl-best types stand out clearly. A quinine-best fiber type did not emerge, but the hamster chorda tympani is quite insensitive to stimuli that taste bitter to man. Frank subsequently studied single fibers in the rat glossopharyngeal nerve, which is known to show sensitivity to quinine, and Fig. 22 shows that a quinine-best type resulted.

This classification is reminiscent of that of Cohen *et al.* (1955), but there are two important differences. The types suggested by Cohen *et al.* are much more specific to certain stimuli than those of Frank. Her fiber types are broadly tuned neurons that peak at particular stimuli. In addition, her fiber types overlap systematically if the stimuli are ordered: sucrose, NaCl, HCl, and QHCl.

Another approach to the classification of taste fibers (Boudreau and Alev, 1973; Boudreau, 1974) utilizing stimuli chosen from substances commonly found in foods and also using measures of latency and spontaneous activity as well as chemical sensitivity appears to produce types that look similar to those described by Frank. Boudreau and his colleagues recorded from the geniculate ganglion (the cell bodies of the axons in the chorda tympani nerve) of the cat and classified fibers into types I, II, and III. Type I may correspond to Frank's acid-best fiber, and type II to her salt-best fiber. Type III units may not be a homogeneous group (Boudreau, 1974) but may include some QHCl-best fibers. The lack of a type corresponding to Frank's sucrose-best fibers probably reflects the cat's well-known insensitivity to this stimulus. The lack of a clear group of QHCl-best fibers may have resulted simply because recordings from the geniculate ganglion do not reflect the sensitivities of the rear of the tongue, which tends to be innervated by more QHCl-sensitive fibers than the front. Although Boudreau's fiber types cannot at present be distinguished from those described by Frank, his use of unconventional stimuli is provocative. In addition, recording from the geniculate

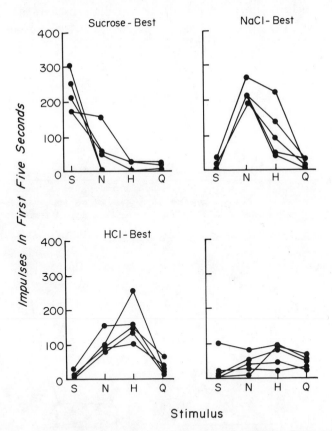

Fig. 21. Response profiles across the basic tastes: 0.1 M sucrose (S), 0.03 M NaCl (N), 0.003 M HCl (H), and 0.001 M quinine hydrochloride (Q) of 20 hamster chorda tympani fibers. These profiles are for the five fibers which respond most to NaCl (A), HCl (B), sucrose (C), or quinine (D). The response measure is the number of impulses in the first 5 sec of the response. From Frank (1973).

ganglion rather than nerve fibers may offer advantages in data collection. His approach applied to a species like the hamster for which there are good single-fiber data would permit a more definitive comparison of the Boudreau and Frank fiber types.

Frank's fiber types are compatible with across-fiber coding. The code for a quality simply becomes the profile of activity across the four fiber types rather than across a population of unique fibers.

CNS Studies. The sensitivities of taste neurons in the central nervous system (CNS) appear to be similar to those of peripheral fibers in that some neurons are quite specific to a single taste substance and others respond to several. In addition, just as in the periphery (Sato, 1963), some CNS neurons respond to temperature and/or touch as well as taste (Pfaffmann *et al.*, 1961). It is unknown whether or not the CNS neurons can be classified into types.

Erickson and his students have looked for possible changes in the across-fiber patterns generated for specific tastants at different levels of the nervous system. Neurons in the medulla had average firing frequencies of 4–5 times those found in the chorda tympani, but the across-fiber patterns were essentially the same for both levels (Ganchrow and Erickson, 1970). The patterns were altered somewhat at the thalamus. Transient responses appeared to be less prominent, tastants

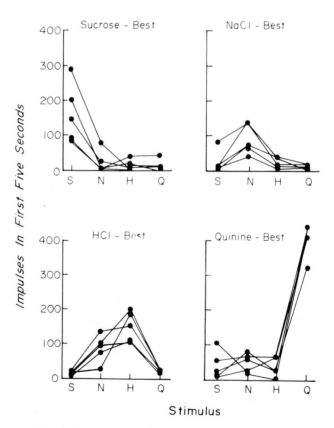

Fig. 22. Response profiles similar to those of Fig. 16 for the rat glossopharyngeal nerve. From Frank (1975).

closely grouped by similarity of across-fiber pattern in the periphery and medulla were less closely grouped in the thalamus, and the groups were not so strictly separated (Scott and Erickson, 1971). Pontine units appeared to be intermediate in function between those of the medulla and those of the thalamus (Scott and Perrotto, 1975).

Possible spatial separation of taste qualities in the CNS (i.e., chemotopic mapping) is of special interest because spatial codes are important in some other modalities (e.g., touch and audition). Evidence that taste qualities are spatially separated has been found in the medulla of the rat (Halpern, 1967), the thalamus of the cat (Ishiko *et al.*, 1967), and the cortex of the dog, rat (Funakoshi *et al.*, 1972), and cat (Ishiko and Akagi, 1972). However, some, and possibly all, of the apparent chemotopic mapping could result from the existence of some differential sensitivity to qualities on the tongue and faithful topographical projection of this distribution to higher levels of the nervous system.

RESOLUTIONS OF THE APPARENT CONFLICT BETWEEN THE FOUR BASIC TASTES AND ACROSS-FIBER CODING

The across-fiber patterning theory does not require the existence of "primary" or "basic" taste categories and yet modern taste psychophysics relies heavily on them. Three resolutions of this apparent conflict have been proposed. Von Békésy rejected the across-fiber code, Schiffman and Erickson rejected the four basic tastes, and Pfaffmann suggested a new neural coding theory in which the four basic tastes play an important role.

VON BÉKÉSY: TASTE PAPILLAE SPECIFIC TO THE FOUR BASIC TASTES. Von Békésy, who received the Nobel Prize for work in audition, rejected across-fiber patterning and much of the neural data that gave rise to it. He based his support of the four basic tastes on a reexamination of an old issue: the specificity of taste papillae.

In the nineteenth century, the taste papillae looked like promising candidates for receptors sensitive to one of the four tastes, but when individual fungiform papillae were stimulated with small brushes trimmed to fine points most papillae were not specific to one of the four. These results were taken to mean that any specific receptor would have to be smaller than a whole papilla. Von Békésy (1964, 1966) obtained some dramatically different results. He first stimulated individual papillae electrically and then later with conventional taste stimuli. In both cases, stimulation of a single papilla generally produced only one of the four basic tastes. Von Békésy felt that with practice his experimenters could even learn visually to recognize the four different types of taste papillae. He concluded that the four basic tastes are coded by specific papillae.

Von Békésy's results aroused enormous interest coming as they did after two decades of electrophysiological results that stressed the lack of specificity of taste neurons to the four basic tastes. Additional studies on the specificity of taste papillae have now appeared, using electrical stimulation (Plattig, 1972; Dzendolet and Murphy, 1974) and chemical stimulation (Harper *et al.*, 1966; McCutcheon and Saunders, 1972; Bealer and Smith, 1975). The study by Dzendolet and

Murphy confirmed von Békésy's observation that a given papilla generally produced only one taste quality when stimulated electrically, while the study by Plattig failed to confirm this result. All three studies using chemical stimulation failed to confirm von Békésy's finding of papillae sensitive to only one quality.

One peculiarity of von Békésy's work suggests a possible resolution of the conflict over the sensitivities of single papillae to the four basic tastes. Von Békésy used very weak stimuli. All others who have worked on the problem were unable to evoke any sensations at all unless the stimuli were quite strong. This is believed to result from the known fact that the threshold for a taste substance increases as the area stimulated decreases. The use of weak concentrations would tend to produce more specificity because individual papillae might well be more sensitive to some taste substances than to others. In any case, von Békésy's conclusion, that each taste papilla is specific to one of the four basic tastes, cannot be accepted in the face of the failures to replicate his results.

MULTIDIMENSIONAL SCALING: A POSSIBLE SOURCE FOR ALTERNATIVES TO THE FOUR BASIC TASTES. Schiffman and Erickson (1971) suggested a way to organize taste experience that did not make use of the four basic tastes but rather, much as Erickson had done with his neural data, emphasized a search for dimensions underlying taste. They used multidimensional scaling techniques to construct a similarity space such that the distance between any two taste stimuli was proportional to their perceived similarity. When a variety of dimensions were tested to see if they might "fit" the space well enough to be axes of the space, three dimensions emerged: molecular weight, pH, and hedonic value.

Since the location of any stimulus in the taste space can be specified by giving its coordinates in terms of these three axes, its taste can be said to be "described" by these coordinates. However, this is not a psychological description since "molecular weight," "pH," and "hedonic value" cannot be used to describe qualitative taste experiences.

Although the axes of this space did not provide an alternative to the four basic tastes, the location of some tastants challenged the four basic tastes in another way (see also Yoshida and Saito, 1969). Figure 23, a similarity space with a taste tetrahedron drawn in, shows that some tastants are located away from the sides of the tetrahedron. This means that these tastants differ from those in the tetrahedron in some way that the four basic tastes cannot describe. This difference may represent a failure of the four basic tastes to adequately describe taste quality; however, it may also simply reflect the effects of modalities other than taste (e.g., the "fatty" quality of oleic acid, tocopherol, and glutamine).

LABELED-LINE CODING OF QUALITY. Pfaffmann did not reject either the existing neural data or the four basic tastes. Instead, he reinterpreted the neural data and proposed a new theory of quality coding in which the four basic tastes play a role (Pfaffmann, 1974; Pfaffmann *et al.*, 1976). Pfaffmann's theory, known as the "labeled-line theory," was stimulated by the fiber types found in the hamster. Similar types were found in the squirrel monkey as well (Frank, 1974), and two of the types, both sensitive to sugars, turned out to be particularly provocative (Pfaffmann, 1974). Figure 24 shows that fibers more sensitive to sucrose than to salts, HCl, or quinine (i.e., sucrose-best fibers) responded more to sucrose than fructose while fibers more sensitive to salts than to sugars, HCl, or quinine (i.e., salt-best fibers) responded more to fructose than to sucrose. Pfaffmann related these results to a curious preference phenomenon that had puzzled investigators for some time. Whole nerve recordings showed that equimolar solutions of sugar were not equally effective. Fructose produced the largest response, sucrose was intermediate, and glucose produced the smallest response of the three. Yet, behavioral preference experiments showed that sucrose was the most preferred sugar followed by fructose and then glucose. However, if the sucrose-best fibers code sweetness and the NaCl-best fibers code saltiness, then the dilemma is resolved. Fructose produces a large whole nerve response because it stimulates two sets of fibers: sucrose-best and NaCl-best. However, fructose is not the most preferred sugar because it produces a complex taste, sweet and salty, and the sweetness in the complex taste is less intense than the sweetness of sucrose (note that the sucrose must also produce a complex sweet-salty taste but it would be more sweet and less salty).

The idea that each fiber carries only a single quality, that associated with the best stimulus for that fiber, has very interesting implications. For example, in Fig. 24 the fibers responding best to sucrose also responded to NH$_4$Cl. The labeled-line theory says that when NH$_4$Cl stimulates these fibers the taste quality evoked is

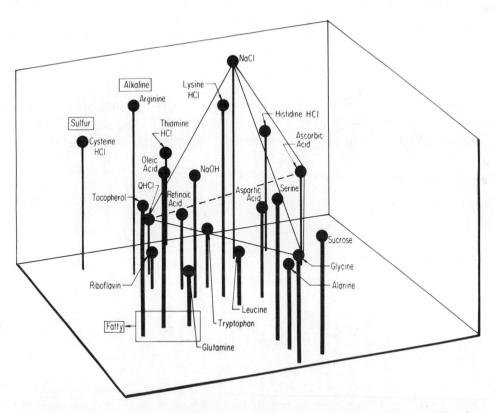

Fig. 23. A similarity space resulting from multidimensional scaling of a variety of tastants. A Henning taste tetrahedron is added to show that some tastants fall outside. From Schiffmann and Dackis (1975).

sweet. The complete taste of a particular stimulus is determined by the responses of all four types to that stimulus. For example, the taste of NaCl on the back of the rat tongue can be derived from Fig. 20 by noting the responses to NaCl from each fiber type. NaCl evokes a modest salty taste from the NaCl-best fibers, a sour taste of similar magnitude from the HCl-best fibers, a small sweet taste from the sucrose-best fibers, and a small bitter-taste from the quinine-best fibers. This as well as other similar derivations predict complex tastes for a variety of "simple" chemicals. In fact, these chemicals do have complex tastes. In particular, salts tend to taste sour, and acids tend to taste salty just as the labeled-line theory predicts.

WHICH RESOLUTION OF THE CONFLICT BETWEEN ACROSS-FIBER CODING AND THE FOUR BASIC TASTES IS CORRECT? *Taste Primaries.* The four basic or primary tastes seem somehow more legitimate if they are mediated by four fiber types; however, this contains echoes of the simplistic Müllerian view of the nineteenth century. The validity of psychophysical primaries does not depend on the complexity of the underlying physiological mechanisms. The justification for psychophysical primaries is their utility in describing experience.

A single modality can give rise to more than one set of primaries depending on the use to which they will be put. For example, color-naming experiments yield the primaries red, green, yellow, and blue as the colors that are psychologically pure (Boynton *et al.,* 1964). However, color mixture laws are stated in terms of three primaries. Any three colors chosen such that any one of them cannot be derived from the other two can be used to produce all other colors. The fact that certain sets of primaries are useful may very well be related to the nature of the underlying mechanisms, but the relationship must be demonstrated.

The four basic tastes are useful for describing taste experience. They are also useful for organizing psychophysical data. For example, the laws of cross-adaptation are simple when expressed in terms of the four basic tastes. Another set of primaries might generate equally useful results or dispensing with primaries altogether might be useful in some contexts; however, the four basic tastes will

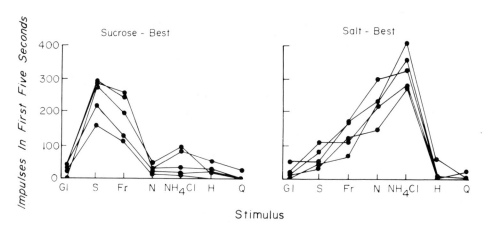

Fig. 24. Responses of five best sucrose fibers and five best salt-sucrose fibers to glucose (Gl), sucrose (Suc), fructose (Fr), sodium chloride (N). ammonium chloride (NH₄Cl), hydrochloric acid (H), and quinine hydrochloride (Q). From Pfaffmann (1974).

continue to dominate taste psychophysics unless a more useful system comes along no matter what the underlying physiological mechanisms turn out to be.

What Is the Relation between Taste Physiology and Taste Psychophysics? The psychophysical and physiological domains are logically independent of one another; however, if some connections between them are asserted, then others must follow. The two theories of quality coding in taste assert that perceived taste qualities are mediated by particular physiological mechanisms. Once this assertion is made, then relationships among the qualities in the psychophysical domain require isomorphic relationships among the mechanisms proposed as mediators of the qualities. For example, the sweet taste of a sugar is unaffected by adaptation to a bitter substance. If the neural message assigned to sweet were disrupted by adaptation to a bitter substance, then the assignment would be wrong. A theory of quality coding can be disproved by the discovery of physiological or psychophysical facts that violate the required isomorphism. However, the absence of such violations does not prove that a coding theory is correct because violations might still be discovered.

In practice, certain relations between physiology and psychophysics are accepted because they seem obvious even if they cannot be proved. For example, a famous visual psychophysicist proposed a rule that he believed permitted the drawing of physiological inferences from psychophysical data (Brindley, 1970). The rule was simply that "whenever two stimuli cause physically indistinguishable signals to be sent from the sense organs to the brain, the sensations produced by these stimuli, as reported by the subject in words, symbols, or actions, must also be indistinguishable" (p. 133). To others, less restrictive connections between physiology and psychophysics seem reasonable. For the most part, philosophical considerations like these do not arise; however, it is wise to remember how precarious some "scientific" conclusions can be.

Which Coding Theory: Cross-Fiber Patterning or Labeled Lines? Both coding theories are consistent with most of the known psychophysical data, but one phenomenon, that of taste mixtures, deserves special comment. First, consider the neural codes for the four taste qualities. According to the labeled-line theory, the four primary tastes are mediated by four types of fibers. The across-fiber patterning theory does not require primaries, nor does it exclude them. Each quality is mediated by a unique pattern of activity across neurons; therefore, each of the four taste qualities has its own unique profile.

What do the known facts about taste mixtures require of these theories? There is general agreement that in taste mixtures the identity of the components is not lost. For example, a mixture of sugar and acid tastes sweet and sour even though the perceived intensity of the components may be altered. Taste mixtures appear to be analytic as contrasted with color mixtures which are called synthetic because the colors in a mixture fuse into a new quality (e.g., a mixture of red and green can fuse to produce yellow). Erickson (1968, 1975) has suggested that analytic mixtures occur in sensory systems like audition in which individual qualities are coded by neurons that respond to a relatively narrow part of the stimulus range, while synthetic mixtures occur in sensory systems like color vision where the code for quality is a pattern generated across neurons such that the same neurons participate in the codes for more than one quality. The fusion in synthetic mixtures occurs because the across-fiber pattern generated by the mixture differs in shape from the across-fiber pattern produced by the components.

The labeled-line theory explains analytic taste easily. Quality depends on the particular fiber stimulated and this is not changed in a mixture. The problem with using the analytic nature of taste mixtures to support the labeled-line theory is that Erickson's assertion, that across-fiber patterns produce synthetic mixtures, is an assumption that may or may not prove to be true. That is, one can imagine mechanisms which would permit analytic mixtures even if the code for quality were the pattern of neural responses across fibers.

This discussion has been based on the classification of taste as an analytical sense. This seems appropriate to this author, but would be hotly debated by others. Erickson (1968, 1975) argues that taste is synthetic such that the tastes of sugar and acid fuse to a new taste when mixed that there is no name for. He believes that this new taste is described as sweet-sour in the same way one might describe orange as red-yellow if there were no name for the color orange. Unfortunately, the terms "analytic" and "synthetic" are not defined with enough precision to settle the argument. For the present, this debate as well as the larger debate over coding theories will have to continue (cf. Chapter 3).

Taste Worlds of Other Species

Sensitivity and Quality

The question of whether or not substances taste the same to other species as they do to man obviously must be approached indirectly. Neural and behavioral thresholds provided the earliest glimpse into the taste worlds of other species, particularly the rat, and suprathreshold functions added perspective about the relative sensitivity of a variety of species to common tastants. Ingenious psychophysical and neural studies have even led to some guarded conclusions about taste quality experience in other species.

Taste Thresholds: The Adrenalectomy Controversy The earliest rat threshold experiments were designed to resolve a controversy over the role of taste in the specific hunger for sodium induced by removal of the adrenal glands (adrenalectomy), but the value of the techniques developed goes far beyond this one problem. Richter (1936, 1939) demonstrated that adrenalectomy, which causes a loss of body sodium, dramatically increased the consumption of suprathreshold NaCl and also decreased the preference threshold for NaCl in the rat. He concluded (Richter, 1939) that "rats ingest more salt . . . because of chemical changes in the taste mechanisms in the oral cavity, giving rise to an enhanced salt discrimination" (p. 371). Richter's suggestion was tested directly with recordings from the chorda tympani taste nerves of adrenalectomized and normal rats (Pfaffmann and Bare, 1950). The neural thresholds were the same, about 0.001 M NaCl. This agreed with the preference threshold of adrenalectomized rats (about 0.001 M NaCl) but did not agree with the preference threshold of normal rats (about 0.01 M NaCl). The obvious conclusion seemed to be that normal rats were able to taste NaCl at 0.001 M but were indifferent to the concentrations between 0.001 and 0.01 M while the adrenalectomized rats, because of increased preference for NaCl, were not indifferent to these concentrations.

The "two-bottle" preference technique that Richter devised to demonstrate lowered preference thresholds for NaCl in adrenalectomized rats is extremely simple. An animal is given access to two solutions: water and a tastant dissolved in water. The concentration of the tastant is varied and the concentration at which preference or rejection fails is the threshold. Figure 25 shows preference and rejection functions for adrenalectomized and normal rats as well as for normal rats with extra NaCl added to the diet, and Fig. 26 shows preference and rejection functions for additional tastants. The two-bottle procedure has been widely used with suitable modifications for other species (e.g., see Bell, 1959, for the "two-bucket" procedure used with cattle). Its one major drawback led to the adrenalectomy controversy: the hedonic properties of the tastant provide the motivation for the behavior that generates the threshold. The preference threshold is not a true sensory threshold if an animal can taste a weak tastant but is indifferent to it.

To avoid this dilemma, new threshold procedures were designed to motivate the animals in other ways. The earliest of these studies used shock avoidance. Deprived rats were shocked for drinking NaCl (Harriman and MacLeod, 1953) or water (Carr, 1952) and subsequently avoided that substance. The concentration of NaCl was decreased until discrimination failed. The resulting thresholds were as low as (or even lower than) the neural threshold (see Table III), which confirmed the suggestion that the preference threshold for normal rats was not a true sensory threshold.

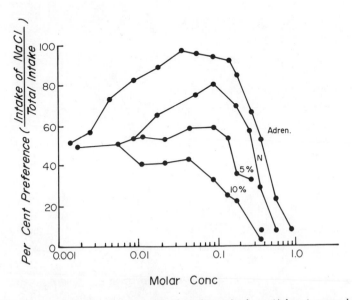

Fig. 25. NaCl preference-rejection functions for adrenalectomized rats (Adren.), normal rats (N), and rats with extra NaCl added to the diet (5% and 10% added). From Pfaffmann (1957).

Later threshold studies (Koh and Teitelbaum, 1961; Morrison and Norrison, 1966; Shaber *et al.,* 1970) have been less specifically aimed at the adrenalectomy controversy and more oriented toward comparing behavioral thresholds not based on preference with the preference and neural thresholds for a variety of tastants. For sucrose, hydrochloric acid, and quinine hydrochloride these values are quite similar (see Table III). NaCl seems to be the only substance for which the preference threshold is higher than the other thresholds.

If the NaCl in rat saliva is taken into consideration, then the various NaCl thresholds can be reinterpreted (Bartoshuk, 1974*b*). Rat saliva contains 0.005–0.01 M sodium (Hainsworth and Stricker, 1971). Since the absolute threshold for the taste of a salt is determined by the concentration of its cation in the adapting solution, experiments in which the rat is adapted to its saliva cannot produce NaCl thresholds lower than 0.005–0.01 M because that is the concentration of the sodium cation. The preference threshold (0.01 M NaCl) is probably a true sensory threshold based on adaptation to saliva. The neural thresholds were obtained with water rinses between stimuli so the low values are to be expected. The puzzling results are the low behavioral thresholds. They appear to be lower than the salivary sodium level, which is impossible. The answer to this dilemma comes from an analysis of what must actually be on the rat's tongue. When a single tastant is presented, then the rat is adapted to saliva, so an NaCl threshold below 0.005–0.01 (reference *m* in Table III) probably means that the rat tasted the water instead of the NaCl. The analogous threshold in human subjects is shown in the top function on the right side of Fig. 9. When saliva is removed with water, an NaCl threshold below 0.005–0.01 M (reference *w* in Table III) is a true NaCl threshold comparable to the neural threshold. Analysis of the probable adaptation state of the tongue suggests that the relatively high detection thresholds (references *n* and *l* in Table

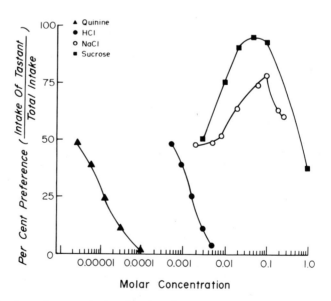

Fig. 26. Two-bottle preference-rejection functions for sucrose, NaCl, hydrochloric acid (HCl), and quinine for the rat. From Pfaffmann (1957).

TABLE III. RAT THRESHOLDS ARRANGED BY RINSE CONDITION ACCORDING TO BARTOSHUK (1974*b*)

	NaCl				Sucrose				HCl				Quinine HC1			
	Threshold				Threshold				Threshold				Threshold			
Adaptation condition	Neural	Detection	Preference	Reference	Neural	Detection	Preference	Reference	Neural	Detection	Preference	Reference	Neural	Detection	Preference	Reference
Saliva (0.005–0.01 M Na)	>0.003			*n*		0.005–0.02		*x*								
		0.05		*l*		0.00009–0.0009		*m*								
		0.001–0.01		*x*												
		0.00017–0.00054		*m*												
			0.0086	*y*												
No experimental rinse (Richter two-stimulus procedure)														0.000012		*j*
		0.0015		*d*		0.0099		*j*		0.00046		*j*			0.00024	*z*
		0.00074		*j*			0.017	*v*			0.0006	*r*			0.000003	*q,r*
		0.000067		*g*			0.01	*c,i*							0.000021	*b*
			0.01	*a,h,p,r,s,u*			0.003	*o,r*							0.00001	*k*
HOH	0.001			*f,n,q,r,s,aa*	0.01			*e,f,i,o,r*	0.0001			*t*	0.000003			*t*
	0.0002			*p*						0.00027		*w*		0.000003		*w*
		0.00034		*w*												

[a]Bare (1949).
[b]Benjamin (1955).
[c]Burright and Kappauf (1963).
[d]Carr (1952).
[e]Hagstrom and Pfaffmann (1959).
[f]Hardiman (1964).
[g]Harriman and MacLeod (1953).
[h]Hiji (1967).
[i]Hiji (1969).
[j]Koh and Teitelbaum (1961).
[k]Mook and Blass (1968).
[l]Morrison (1969).
[m]Morrison and Norrison (1966).
[n]Nachman and Pfaffmann (1963).
[o]Noma *et al.* (1971).
[p]Oakley (1962).
[q]Pfaffmann (1955).
[r]Pfaffmann (1957).
[s]Pfaffmann and Bare (1950).
[t]Pfaffmann *et al.* (1967).
[u]Richter (1939).
[v]Richter and Campbell (1940).
[w]Shaber *et al.* (1970).
[x]Tapper and Halpern (1968).
[y]Weiner and Stellar (1951).
[z]Young *et al.* (1963).
[aa]Zawalich (1971).

III) are true NaCl thresholds based on adaptation to saliva while the low thresholds not yet discussed (references *d*, *j*, and *g* in Table III) may represent either water taste thresholds or NaCl thresholds depending on the way the rat sampled the two bottles.

The low preference threshold for adrenalectomized rats remains a puzzle. Recent work has even added some new complexities. The saliva of adrenalectomized rats contains more sodium than normal but flows slower than normal (Sweeney and Catalanotto, 1976). Single fibers in the chorda tympani nerves of sodium-deprived rats tend to respond less than normal to 0.1 M NaCl (Contreras, 1976). Would this hold true for adrenalectomized rats too? Does the low preference threshold actually reflect a rejection of water, or does it reflect the rat's ability to learn to sample such that it can rinse saliva and thus taste weak NaCl? At present, the puzzle is unsolved.

As if the confusion over the sensory effects of adrenalectomy were not enough, a careful look at the adrenalectomized rat's consumption of suprathreshold concentrations of NaCl suggests a hedonic as well as a sensory effect. Figure 25 shows that the adrenalectomized rat consumes more at all concentrations of NaCl. If adrenalectomy simply made the rat more sensitive to the taste of NaCl, then 0.1 M NaCl would taste saltier than normal and the intake of it should go down. If adrenalectomy simply made the rat less sensitive to the taste of NaCl, then 0.1 M NaCl would taste less salty than normal and the intake of it should still go down. In sum, a simple change of taste sensitivity does not predict increased intake above the peak intake observed in a normal rat; rather, it predicts a shift in the position of the preference curve along the concentration dimension. The increased intake across concentration of the adrenalectomized animal is more consistent with increased preference for the taste of NaCl than it is with a change in taste sensitivity to NaCl.

Nearly four decades after the problem was introduced, the sensory contribution to the specific hunger for sodium shown by adrenalectomized rats is still unclear; there is one consolation, however. The two-bottle preference technique, interpreted with caution, has emerged as a simple and convenient way to obtain thresholds for a variety of tastants.

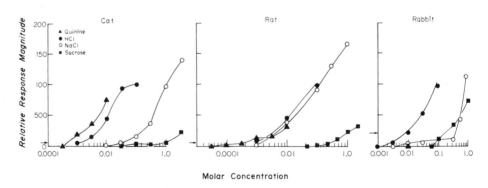

Fig. 27. Whole chorda tympanic nerve responses from the cat, rat, and rabbit to several tastants. Modified from Pfaffmann (1955).

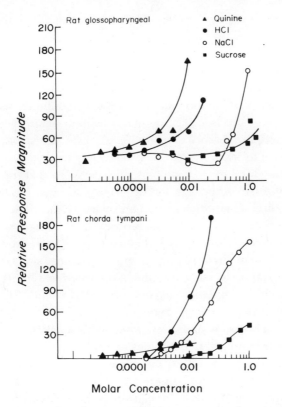

Fig. 28. Whole chorda tympani and glossopharyngeal nerve responses from the rat to several tastants. The fact that the functions in the upper figure do not start from zero reflects the responses to water (magnitude about 30) found in the glossopharyngeal nerve. From Pfaffmann *et al.* (1967).

SUPRATHRESHOLD FUNCTIONS. Thresholds are not the best indicators of relative sensitivity. A function relating magnitude of response (neural or behavioral) to concentration conveys more information. For example, Fig. 27 shows the magnitude of the chorda tympani nerve responses of the cat, rat, and rabbit to a variety of tastants, and Fig. 28 shows responses to the same tastants from the chorda tympani and glossopharyngeal nerves of the rat. The responses were obtained by placing the whole nerve on the recording electrode and electronically summating the electrical activity (Beidler, 1953). Figure 27 shows that the threshold for QHCl in the rat chorda tympani is lower than that in the cat chorda tympani; however, a comparison of the slopes of the functions suggests that QHCl is actually a less effective stimulus in the rat. Similarly, Fig. 28 shows that the thresholds for HCl in the chorda tympani and glossopharyngeal nerves do not convey an accurate picture of the relative sensitivity to HCl in those nerves.

Preference functions show the range of hedonically meaningful concentrations, but this range is sometimes smaller than the dynamic range of the taste nerves. For example, the threshold for rejection of QHCl (see Fig. 26) corresponds to the threshold for QHCl in the glossopharyngeal nerve (see Fig. 28), but rejection is total at a concentration producing only a moderate neural response. Rejection of HCl is also total at a concentration still within the dynamic range of the taste nerves; however, the preference functions for NaCl and sucrose cover almost the same range of concentrations as those that produce differential responding in the taste nerves.

QUALITY DISCRIMINATION. Although there is no way to find out if a substance tastes salty to the rat, it is possible to find out if a substance tastes similar to NaCl. The measurement of the similarity of two tastants is basic to both the behavioral and neural analyses of taste quality in nonhuman species.

One simple way to measure similarity is to make animals avoid a particular tastant and then see to what others the avoidance generalizes. For example, rats made ill by ingesting lithium chloride subsequently avoided lithium chloride. This avoidance generalized to other salts, the best so to NaCl, which is the salt judged to be most similar to lithium chloride by human subjects (Nachman, 1963). Similarly, rats made ill by exposure to radiation paired with the tasting of saccharin avoided DL-alanine and glycine but did not avoid glucose to the same extent (Tapper and Halpern, 1968). Human subjects find all four substances sweet but only glucose has a pure sweet taste. In an experiment discussed earlier (Erickson, 1963), generalization of shock avoidance suggested that NH_4Cl and KCl taste similar to each other and different from NaCl to the rat, just as they do to human subjects.

Similarity has also been measured with operant procedures using positive reinforcement. In a complex but ingenious design using a food reward, rats were trained to "compare" the taste of test substances to a series of standard substances consisting of NaCl, HCl, sucrose, and quinine sulfate (Morrison, 1967). This was done in the following way. Each of three groups of rats was given a discrimination problem. In the first group, a solution of either NaCl or quinine was presented; the rats were rewarded for pressing bar 1 when the solution was NaCl and for pressing bar 2 when the solution was quinine. After this training, a substance that produced responses on bar 1 could be presumed to taste like NaCl and a substance that produced responses on bar 2 could be presumed to taste like quinine. A second group of rats was trained with NaCl and sucrose, and a third group was trained with NaCl and HCl. The results suggested a number of similarities between the taste worlds of rat and man. Lithium chloride tasted the most like NaCl, the similarities among the salts were primarily determined by the cation with most salts tasting similar to quinine as well as NaCl, and water was not tasteless but rather tasted like quinine.

Neural analyses of qualitative similarities among tastants lead to essentially the same conclusion as the behavioral analyses: tastants are qualitatively "described" by other species much the same way human subjects describe them. For example, in the hamster, Frank's fiber-type analysis shows that sucrose-best fibers respond to fructose and saccharin, HCl-best fibers respond to other acids, and QHCl-best fibers respond to other compounds that taste bitter to man. Just as in the behavioral studies, the salts appear to evoke complex tastes. KCl stimulates the fibers responsive to HCl and QHCl as well as those responsive to NaCl (Frank, 1973).

The changes in quality that can occur with concentration were analyzed in another electrophysiological study (Ganchrow and Erickson, 1970). For example, as the concentration of saccharin was increased, the correlation between responses to saccharin and to QHCl increased while the correlation between saccharin and sucrose remained relatively constant. This parallels the familiar increase in bitterness experienced by human subjects when tasting increasing concentrations of saccharin.

An analysis of across-species comparisons of preferences for saccharin also supports qualitative similarities across species. Saccharin is rejected by some species but accepted by others even though all of those species accept sucrose. The variation in sensitivity to tastants suggests a reason for this. Human subjects describe saccharin as tasting sweet and bitter. If we think of saccharin as a mixture of sweet and bitter, then the animal preference data can be explained by looking at a given species' sensitivity to sweet substances and bitter substances (Bartoshuk *et al.*, 1975). For example, the cat chorda tympani is relatively insensitive to sucrose but is very sensitive to quinine. The cat rejects saccharin (Carpenter, 1956; Bartoshuk *et al.*, 1975). The chorda tympani responses of the rat and the rabbit are much more sensitive to sucrose than those of the cat and relatively less sensitive to quinine. The rat and the rabbit accept saccharin (Fisher *et al.*, 1965; Carpenter, 1956).

Although there are important differences across species, the similarities across species are more impressive. The behavioral and neurophysiological studies of taste quality suggest that the major differences across species are quantitative rather than qualitative.

Adaptation

The Basic Phenomenon. The term "adaptation" is not always used consistently even when applied to human taste phenomena, but it can be particularly confusing when its use is extended to neural responses in other species. For example, an application of NaCl to the tongue of a rat produces an initial sharp rise in neural activity (transient response) which then declines to a relatively stable level (steady-state response). Does this mean that the rat tastes NaCl as long as the NaCl stays on its tongue? Is there a central mechanism that causes sensation to diminish even with a continuing neural response? Is sensation produced only by transient responses so that no sensation occurs when the neural response is constant? Obviously neural data cannot show whether or not taste sensations in the rat change with constant stimulation the same way they do in man. As a result, with species other than man, the term "adaptation" is simply used to describe a decrement in neural response or to describe the operation of prolonged stimulation.

Insights about adaptation in the rat have resulted from comparisons of rat and human neural data, comparisons of rat neural data and human psychophysical data, and comparisons of rat neural data and rat behavioral data.

Human and rat chorda tympani responses to NaCl are compared in Fig. 5. Human neural responses to NaCl appear to be predominantly transients and do not include the prominent steady states so typical of rat responses to NaCl. The time course of the transient responses in both rat and man shown in Fig. 5 are about the same as that of psychophysical adaptation in man.

As discussed earlier, the transient part of the rat neural response to NaCl is dependent on the adapting solution just as the taste of NaCl in man is dependent on the adapting solution (Pfaffmann and Powers, 1964). Figure 6 illustrates this dependence. Note that the transient response to 0.03 M NaCl depends on whether it follows 0.1 M NaCl or water while the steady-state response to 0.03 M NaCl remains the same in both cases. In general, the transient response depends on the relation of the stimulus concentration to the concentration previously on the tongue (i.e., the adapting concentration). When the stimulus is more concentrated than the adapting solution, the stimulus will produce a transient increase in the neural response that is followed by a decrease to the steady-state response characteristic of the stimulus concentration. When the stimulus is less concentrated, it will produce a transient decrease in the neural response that is followed by an increase to the steady-state characteristic of the stimulus concentration.

When the adapting solution was experimentally altered in normal, behaving rats, then the rats' preferences were altered as well. In one experiment, rats were trained to lick one solution and then switch to a second (McCutcheon, 1971). With this procedure, the first solution presumably replaced the saliva usually bathing the tongue. The number of times a rat licked 0.10 M NaCl (the second solution) decreased as the concentration of the first solution was increased, just as would be expected if exposure to the first solution were lowering the perceived intensity of the 0.10 M NaCl. Other experiments, in which solutions were infused into the rat's mouth through tubing (Vance, 1970; Wilcove, 1973), produced similar results for saccharin and sucrose.

Although these experiments are complex and some of the results are open to alternate interpretations, the data so far available are consistent with the idea that the transient responses in rats are responsible for taste sensation. Whether or not the steady-state responses also play a role in sensation, whether they are removed by central mechanisms, or whether sensation is produced by change *per se* is unknown.

CROSS-ADAPTATION. Just as with adaptation, neural phenomena that correspond to cross-adaptation in man involve transient responses. That is, after the application of a particular adaptating substance, some stimuli will still produce transient responses and some will not. Those that do not are said to have been cross-adapted by the adapting solution.

Qualitative similarity may be important for predicting cross-adaptation in rats just as it is in man. This conclusion results from an extensive electrophysiological study of cross-adaptation among a variety of salts as well as QHCl, HCl, and sucrose in the rat (Smith and Frank, 1972). Cross-adaptation is best among salts with the same cation, and qualitative similarity in the rat (Morrison, 1967) is also greatest among salts with the same cation.

NEURAL RESPONSES TO WATER. Since water is the solvent for taste substances, Zotterman's (1949) discovery that it could be a taste stimulus itself in the frog was dramatic. The further discovery that man did not have the "water fibers" (Borg *et al.*, 1967) found in a variety of species like cat, dog, pig, and monkey (Liljestrand and Zotterman, 1954; Zotterman, 1956; Gordon *et al.*, 1959) seems to suggest that "water taste" might be a category of taste quality important in the taste worlds of some other species but lacking in man's.

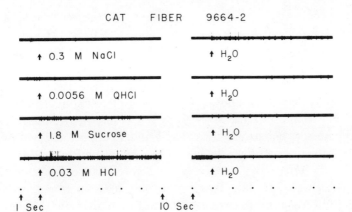

Fig. 29. Responses to water that are contingent on the nature of the preceding stimulus. Stimuli were flowed across the tongue in the order indicated from left to right and top to bottom. From Bartoshuk *et al.* (1971). Copyright 1971 by the American Association for the Advancement of Science. Reprinted by permission.

Later experiments (Bartoshuk and Pfaffmann, 1965; Bartoshuk *et al.*, 1971; Smith and Frank, 1972; Ogawa *et al.*, 1972; Yamamoto and Kawamura, 1974; Pfaffmann *et al.*, 1976) suggest a very different conclusion. Many taste neurons will respond to water but only if the water follows certain other substances. For example, Fig. 29 shows the responses of a fiber that was sensitive to water following NaCl. Some fibers are sensitive to water following sucrose, some to water following HCl, some to combinations of these adaptation conditions, and so forth. Neural responses to water depend on the nature of the adapting solution just as the taste of water to human subjects depends on the nature of the adapting solution. The original experiments on "water fibers" did not test a variety of adapting solutions but rather used Ringer's solution (a solution of approximately 0.15 M NaCl) as a rinse between stimuli. The responses to water probably were actually responses to water following NaCl.

In other species, water appears to take on various qualities depending on the adapting solution much as it does in man. In the rat, when the tongue is adapted to saliva, water tastes similar to quinine and HCl (Morrison, 1967), which corresponds to the bitter-sour taste of water to human subjects adapted to saliva. The neurons that respond to water following NaCl also tend to respond to quinine and HCl (Cohen *et al.*, 1955). This suggests the possibility that water takes on various qualities under different adaptation contingencies because the neural responses to water mimic the neural responses ordinarily associated with more conventional tastants.

Taste Modifiers

The effects of the two modifiers most studied with human subjects, *Gymnema sylvestre* and *Synsepalum dulcificum*, do not generalize widely to other species.

Gymnema Sylvestre. Extracts from the leaves of *Gymnema sylvestre* selectively suppressed both neural (Borg *et al.*, 1967) and psychophysical (Bartoshuk *et al.*, 1969) responses to sweet substances in man. *Gymnema sylvestre* suppressed neural responses to sugar in the dog (Andersson, 1950) and the hamster (Pfaffmann and Hagstrom, 1955; Hagstrom, 1957, Yackzan, 1969; Pfaffmann, 1969) but failed to do so in the squirrel monkey (Snell, 1965) and the African green monkey (*Cercopithecus aethiops*) (Hellekant *et al.*, 1974). In the rat *Gymnema sylvestre* depressed responses to several tastants (Oakley, 1962; Makous *et al.*, 1963), and in the housefly it affected responses to NaCl as well as sucrose (Kennedy *et al.*, 1975).

In the hamster, behavioral tests (Faull and Halpern, 1971) confirmed the suppression of the taste of sugar that was shown by the neural data; however, even in this species the effects of *Gymnema sylvestre* were not identical to the effects in man. The effects wore off much faster in the hamster than in man and equivalent concentrations were less effective in hamster than in man (Hagstrom, 1957; Yackzan, 1969; Pfaffmann, 1969; Faull and Halpern, 1971).

The specificity of the effect of *Gymnema sylvestre* on sweetness in the hamster is hard to evaluate. In one study (Yackzan, 1969) neural responses to NaCl, HCl, and QHCl as well as those to sucrose were suppressed, but in others (Hagstrom, 1957; Pfaffmann, 1969) the suppression was specific to sucrose.

MIRACLE FRUIT. Miracle fruit adds a sweet taste to the taste of acids in man and may have similar effects in certain species of monkeys (Diamant *et al.*, 1972; Hellekant *et al.*, 1974) but not in rats (Diamant *et al.*, 1972), guinea pigs, pigs, rabbits (Hellekant *et al.*, 1974), or hamsters (Harvey, 1970).

The failure of these taste modifiers to work across species does not imply that the sweet receptor sites in other species differ from those in man because there is no proof that either miracle fruit or *Gymnema sylvestre* complexes with sweet receptor molecules. For example, miracle fruit may sweeten by binding near a sweet receptor site and delivering a sugar molecule to that site when acid enters the mouth (Kurihara and Beidler, 1969). Its failure to work in another species could simply reflect a failure of the initial binding which would have no implications at all for taste quality.

SIMILARITIES ACROSS SPECIES

The taste experiences of other species (just as those of other individuals) cannot be shared, but the attributes of taste function revealed by behavioral and neurophysiological studies can be compared across species. That such a comparison emphasizes the similarities for species as diverse as man and rat is fortunate since research in nonhuman species often has a dual purpose. The results provide information about the species under investigation, but they are also intended to serve as a model for human taste. The animal studies discussed in the earlier sections of this chapter generally serve as such models.

CONCLUSIONS

The bulk of this chapter has been concerned with taste quality. Although far from clear, a picture of the way that taste quality is coded has been taking shape from experiments with various techniques at various levels of the nervous system.

The parts of molecules that have been identified as the taste stimuli for some salty, sour, sweet, and bitter substances suggest that the interactions between stimuli and receptors probably fall into four relatively discrete categories. This stimulus-receptor specificity is probably lost to some extent both because individual receptor cells can bind more than one kind of stimulus and because several receptor cells funnel into a single taste nerve fiber. However, sensitivities to different stimuli do not combine at random. Even though single fibers do not respond exclusively to stimuli of a single quality, the fibers tend to fall into four fiber types, each one optimally sensitive to stimuli having one of the four basic tastes. Each fiber might code only a single quality, that associated with the most effective stimulus. On the other hand, the relative activity across the fiber types might code quality. Either of these two theories, the labeled-line theory or the across-fiber pattern theory, can account for the known facts about taste including the important role that the four basic tastes play in human experience; however, the labeled-line theory has the advantage of offering the simpler explanation for the ability of human subjects to analyze complex taste sensations into the four basic tastes.

Studies on a variety of mammalian species suggest that the taste worlds of man and other mammals are probably qualitatively similar. Species show varying degrees of sensitivity to particular tastants but, on the whole, group substances by similarity of taste quality in the same way that a human subject does.

Sweet, sour, salty, and bitter seem to be ubiquitous in taste, yet there has been widespread ambivalence about their proper roles. The 19th century view that they are the irreducible units of taste experience is not popular today. The four basic tastes are now used more pragmatically. Modern taste psychophysics is devoted largely to a study of the functional characteristics of these taste qualities rather than to debate over whether they are exhaustive or unique.

REFERENCES

Andersen, H. T. Problems of taste specificity. In G. E. W. Wolstenholme and J. Knight (eds.), *Taste and Smell in Vertebrates.* J. and A. Churchill, London, 1970, pp. 71–82.
Andersson, B., Langren, S., Olsson, L., and Zotterman, Y. The sweet taste fibres of the dog. *Acta Physiol. Scand.,* 1950, *21*, 105–119.
Bare, J. K. The specific hunger for sodium chloride in normal and adrenalectomized rats. *J. Comp. Physiol. Psychol.,* 1949, *42*, 242–253.
Bartoshuk, L. M. Water taste in man. Percept. Psychophys., 1968, *3*, 69–72.
Bartoshuk, L. M. Taste illusions: Some demonstrations. *Ann. N.Y. Acad. Sci.,* 1974a, *237*, 279–285.
Bartoshuk, L. M. NaCl thresholds in man: Thresholds for water taste or NaCl taste? *J. Comp. Physiol. Psychol.,* 1974b, *87*, 310–325.
Bartoshuk, L. M. Taste mixtures: Is mixture suppression related to compression? *Physiol. Behav.,* 1975, *14*, 643–649.
Bartoshuk, L. M., and Cleveland, C. T. Mixtures of substances with similar tastes: A test of a new model of taste mixture interactions. *Sensory Processes,* 1977, *1*, 177–186.
Bartoshuk, L. M., and Pfaffmann, C. Effects of pre-treatment on the water taste response in cat and rat. *Fed. Proc.,* 1965, *24*, 207.
Bartoshuk, L. M., McBurney, D. H., and Pfaffmann, C. Taste of sodium chloride solutions after adaptation to sodium chloride: Implications for the "water taste." *Science,* 1964, *143*, 967–968.
Bartoshuk, L. M., Dateo, G. P., Vandenbelt, D. J., Buttrick, R. D., and Long, L. Effects of *Gymnema sylvestre* and *Synsepalum dulcificum* on taste in man. In C. Pfaffmann (ed.), *Olfaction and Taste III.* Rockefeller University Press, New York, 1969, pp. 436–444.

560

LINDA M. BARTOSHUK

Bartoshuk, L. M., Harned, M. A., and Parks, L. H. Taste of water in the cat: Effects on sucrose preference. *Science,* 1971, *171,* 699–701.

Bartoshuk, L. M., Lee, C. H., and Scarpellino, R. Sweet taste of water induced by artichoke *(Cynara scolymus). Science,* 1972, *178,* 988–990.

Bartoshuk, L. M., Gentile, R. L., Moskowitz, H. R., and Meiselman, H. L. Sweet taste induced by miracle fruit *(Synsepalum dulcificum). Physiol. Behav.,* 1974, *12,* 449–456.

Bartoshuk, L. M., Jacobs, H. L., Nichols, T. L., Hoff, L. A., and Ryckman, J. J. Taste rejection of nonnutritive sweeteners in cats. *J. Comp. Physiol. Psychol.,* 1975, *89,* 971–975.

Bealer, S. L., and Smith, D. V. Multiple sensitivity to chemical stimuli in single human taste papillae. *Physiol. Behav.,* 1975, *14,* 795–799.

Beidler, L. M. Properties of chemoreceptors of tongue of rat. *J. Neurophysiol.,* 1953, *16,* 595–607.

Beidler, L. M. A theory of taste stimulation. *J. Gen. Physiol.,* 1954, *38,* 133–139.

Beidler, L. M. Taste receptor stimulation. In *Progress in Biophysics and Biophysical Chemistry.* Pergamon Press, New York, 1961, pp. 107–151.

Beidler, L. M. Anion influences on taste receptor response. In T. Hayashi (ed.), *Olfaction and Taste II.* Pergamon Press, New York, 1967, pp. 509–534.

Beidler, L. M. Innervation of rat fungiform papilla. In C. Pfaffmann (ed.), *Olfaction and Taste III.* Rockefeller University Press, New York, 1969, pp. 352–369.

Beidler, L. M., and Gross, G. W. The nature of taste receptor sites. In W. D. Neff (ed.), *Contributions to Sensory Physiology.* Academic Press, New York, 1971, pp. 97–127.

Beidler, L. M., and Smallman, R. L. Renewal of cells within taste of buds. *J. Cell Biol.,* 1965, *27,* 263–272.

Bell, F. R. The sense of taste in domesticated animals. *Vet. Rec.,* 1959, *71,* 1071–1079.

Benjamin, R. M. Cortical taste mechanisms studied by two different test procedures. *J. Comp. Physiol. Psychol.,* 1955, *48,* 119–122.

Bernard, R. A. Antidromic inhibition: A new theory to account for taste interactions. In F. F. Kao, K. Koizumi, and M. Vassalle (eds.), *Research in Physiology.* Aulo Gaggi, Bologna, 1971, pp. 431–439.

Birch, G. G. Structural relationships of sugars to taste. *Crit. Rev. Food Sci. Nutr.,* 1976, *8,* 57–95.

Borg, G., Diamant, H., Oakley, B., Ström, L., and Zotterman, Y. A comparative study of neural and psychophysical responses to gustatory stimuli. In T. Hayashi (ed.), *Olfaction and Taste II.* Pergamon Press, New York, 1967, pp. 253–264.

Boudreau, J. C. Neural encoding in cat geniculate ganglion tongue units. *Chemical Senses Flavor,* 1974, *1,* 41–51.

Boudreau, J. C., and Alev, N. Classification of chemoresponsive tongue units of the cat geniculate ganglion. *Brain Res.,* 1973, *54,* 157–175.

Boynton, R. M., Schafer, W., and Neun, M. E. Hue-wavelength relation measured by color-naming method for three retinal locations. *Science,* 1964, *146,* 666–668.

Bradley, R. M. Tongue topography. In L. M. Beidler (ed.), *Handbook of Sensory Physiology,* Vol. IV: *Chemical Senses,* Section 2: *Taste.* Springer-Verlag, New York, 1971, pp. 1–30.

Bradley, R. M., and Mistretta, C. M. Investigations of taste function and swallowing in fetal sheep. In J. F. Bosma (ed.), *Oral Sensation and Perception,* Vol. 4. U.S. DHEW, Bethesda, Md., 1973, pp. 185–205.

Bradley, R. M., and Mistretta, C. M. The developing sense of taste. In D. A. Denton and J. P. Coghlan (eds.), *Olfaction and Taste V.* Academic Press, New York 1975, pp. 91–98.

Brindley, G. S. *Physiology of the Retina and Visual Pathology.* Williams and Wilkins: Baltimore, 1970.

Brown, W. The judgment of very weak sensory stimuli. *U. Calif. Publ.,* 1914, *1,* 199–268.

Burright, R. C., and Kappauf, W. E. Preference threshold of the white rat for sucrose. *J. Comp. Physiol. Psychol.,* 1963, *56,* 171–173.

Burton, H., and Benjamin, R. M. Central projections of the gustatory system. In L. M. Beidler (ed.), *Handbook of Sensory Physiology,* Vol. IV: *Chemical Senses,* Section 2: *Taste.* Springer-Verlag, New York, 1971, pp. 148–164.

Cagan, R. H. Biochemical studies of taste sensation. I. Binding of ^{14}C-labeled sugars to bovine taste papillae. *Biochim. Biophys. Acta,* 1971, *252,* 199–206.

Camerer, W. Ueber die Abhängigkeit des Geschmacksinns von der gereizten stelle der Mundhöhle. *Ztschr. Biolog.,* 1870, *6,* 440–452.

Cameron, A. T. The taste sense and the relative sweetness of sugars and other sweet substances. *Scientific Reports of the Sugar Research Foundation,* No. 9, New York, 1947.

Carpenter, J. A. Species differences in taste preferences. *J. Comp. Physiol. Psychol.,* 1956, *49,* 139–144.

Carr, W. J. The effect of adrenalectomy upon the NaCl taste threshold in rat. *J. Comp. Physiol. Psychol.,* 1952, *45,* 377–380.

Chamberlin, F. Primitive taste-words. *Am. J. Psychol.*, 1903, *14*, 146–153.

Cleaton-Jones, P. A denervation study of taste buds in the soft palate of the albino rat. *Arch. Oral Biol.*, 1976, *21*, 79–82.

Cohen, J., and Ogden, D. P. Taste blindness to phenyl-thio-carbamide as a function of saliva. *Science*, 1949, *110*, 532–533.

Cohen, M. J., Hagiwara, S., and Zotterman, Y. The response spectrum of taste fibers in the cat: A single fibre analysis. *Acta Physiol. Scand.*, 1955, *33*, 316–332.

Collings, V. B. Human taste response as a function of locus of stimulation on the tongue and soft palate. *Percept. Psychophys.*, 1974, *16*, 169–174.

Contreras, R. J. Changes in gustatory nerve discharges with sodium deficiency: A single unit analysis. Paper delivered at the Eastern Psychological Association, New York, 1976.

Dallenbach, J. W., and Dallenbach, K. M. The effects of bitter-adaptation on sensitivity to other taste qualities. *Am. J. Psychol.*, 1943, *56*, 21–31.

Dastoli, F. R., and Price, S. Sweet-sensitive protein from bovine taste buds: Isolation and assay. *Science*, 1966, *154*, 905–907.

Dastoli, F. R., Lopiekes, D. V., and Doig, A. R. Bitter-sensitive protein from porcine taste buds: Purification and partial characterization. *Biochemistry*, 1968, *7*, 1160–1164.

DeSimone, J. A., and Price, S. A model for the stimulation of taste receptor cells by salt. *Biophys. J.*, 1976, *16*, 869–880.

Diamant, H., Oakley, B., Ström, L., Wells, C., and Zotterman, Y. A comparison of neural and psychophysical responses to taste stimuli in man. *Acta Physiol. Scand.*, 1965, *64*, 67–74.

Diamant, H., Hellekant, G., and Zotterman, Y. The effect of miraculin on the taste buds of man, monkey, and rat. In D. Schneider (ed.), *Olfaction and Taste IV*. Wissenschaftliche Verlagsgesellschaft MBH, Stuttgart, 1972, pp. 241–251.

Dzendolet, E., and Meiselman, H. L. Cation and anion contributions to gustatory quality of simple salts. *Percept. Psychophys.*, 1967, *2*, 601–604.

Dzendolet, E., and Murphy, C. Electrical stimulation of human fungiform papillae. *Chem. Senses Flavor*, 1974, *1*, 9–15.

Erickson, R. P. Sensory neural patterns and gustation. In Y. Zotterman (ed.), *Olfaction and Taste I*. Pergamon Press, New York, 1963, 205–213.

Erickson, R. P. Stimulus coding in topographic and nontopographic afferent modalities: On the significance of the activity of individual sensory neurons. *Psychol. Rev.*, 1968, *75*, 447–465.

Erickson, R. P. Parallel "population" neural coding in feature extraction. In G. Warner (ed.), *Feature Extraction by Neurons and Behavior*. MIT Press, Cambridge, Mass., 1975, pp. 155–169.

Erickson, R. P., Doetsch, G. S., and Marshall, D. A. The gustatory neural response function. *J. Gen. Physiol.*, 1965, *49*, 247–263.

Eyzaguirre, C., Fidone, S., and Zapata, P. Membrane potentials recorded from the mucosa of the toad's tongue during chemical stimulation. *J. Physiol. (London)*, 1972, *221*, 515–532.

Farbman, A. I. Electron microscope study of the developing taste bud in rat fungiform papillae. *Dev. Biol.*, 1965a, *11*, 110–135.

Farbman, A. I. Fine structure of taste bud. *J. Ultrastruct. Res.*, 1965b, *12*, 238–350.

Farbman, A. I., and Hellekant, G. Efferent chorda tympani fibers to fungiform papillae of tongue. *Anat. Rec.*, 1976, *184*, 400.

Faull, J., and Halpern, B. P. Reduction of sucrose preference in the hamster by gymnemic acid. *Physiol. Behav.*, 1971, *1*, 903–907.

Fechner, G. T. *Elemente der Psychophysik*. Breitkopf und Härtel, Leipzig, 1860.

Filin, V. A., and Esakov, A. I. Interaction between taste receptors. *Byull. Eksp. Biol. Med.*, 1968, *65*, 12–15 (in English).

Fischer, R. Gustatory, behavioral and pharmacological manifestations of chemoreception in man. In G. Ohloff and A. F. Thomas (eds.), *Gustation and Olfaction*. Academic Press, New York, 1971, pp. 187–237.

Fish, H. S., Malone, P. D., and Richter, C. P. The anatomy of the tongue of the domestic Norway rat. *Anat. Rec.*, 1944, *89*, 429–440.

Fisher, G. L. Pfaffmann, C., and Brown, E. Dulcin and saccharin taste in squirrel monkeys, rats, and men. *Science*, 1965, *150*, 506–507.

Frank, M. An analysis of hamster afferent taste nerve response functions. *J. Gen. Physiol.*, 1973, *61*, 588–618.

Frank, M. The classification of mammalian afferent taste nerve fibers. *Chem. Senses Flavor*, 1974, *1*, 53–60.

Frank, M. Response patterns of rat glossopharyngeal taste. In D. A. Denton and J. P. Coghlan (eds.), *Olfaction and Taste V*. Academic Press, New York, 1975, pp. 59–64.

Funakoshi, M., Kasahara, Y., Yamamoto, T., and Kawamura, Y. Taste coding and central perception. In D. Schneider (ed.), *Olfaction and Taste IV*. Wissenschaftliche Verlagsgesellschaft MBH, Stuttgart, 1972, pp. 336–342.

Ganchrow, D., and Erickson, R. P. Thalamocortical relations in gustation. *Brain Res.*, 1972, *36*, 289–305.

Ganchrow, J. R., and Erickson, R. P. Neural correlates of gustatory intensity and quality. *J. Neurophysiol.*, 1970, *33*, 768–783.

Gordon, G., Kitchell, R., Ström, L., and Zotterman, Y. The response pattern of taste fibres in the chorda tympani of the monkey. *Acta Physiol. Scand.*, 1959, *46*, 119–132.

Guth, L. Degeneration and regeneration of taste buds. In L. M. Beidler (ed.), *Handbook of Sensory Physiology*, Vol. IV: *Chemical Senses*, Section 2: *Taste*. Springer-Verlag, New York, 1971, pp. 63–74.

Hagstrom, E. C. Nature of taste stimulation by sugar. Unpublished Ph.D. thesis, Brown University, 1957.

Hagstrom, E. C., and Pfaffmann, C. The relative taste effectiveness of different sugars for the rat. *J. Comp. Physiol. Psychol.*, 1959, *52*, 259–262.

Hahn, H. Die Adaptation des Geschmackssinnes. *Ztschr. Sinnesphysiol.*, 1934, *65*, 105–145.

Hahn, H. *Beiträge zur Reizphysiologie*. Scherer, Heideldberg, 1949.

Hahn, H., and Ulbrich, L. Eine systematische Untersuchung der Geschmacksschwellen. *Pflügers Arch.*, 1948, *250*, 357–384.

Hahn, H., Kuckulies, G., and Taeger, H. Eine systematische Untersuchung der Geschmacksschwellen. *Ztschr. Sinnesphysiol.*, 1938, *67*, 259–306.

Hahn, H. Kuckulies, G., and Bissar, A. Eine systematische Untersuchung der Geschmacksschwellen. *Ztschr. Sinnesphysiol.*, 1940, *68*, 185–260.

Hainsworth, F. R., and Stricker, E. M. Evaporation cooling in the rat: Differences between salivary glands as thermoregulatory effectors. *Can. J. Physiol. Pharmacol.*, 1971, *49*, 573–580.

Hall, M. J., Bartoshuk, L. M., Cain, W. S., and Stevens, J. C. PTC taste blindness and the taste of caffeine. *Nature (London)*, 1975, *253*, 442–443.

von Haller, A. *First Lines of Physiology*. Charles Elliot, Edinburgh, 1786 (Johnson Reprint Corp., New York, 1966).

Halpern, B. P. Chemotopic coding for sucrose and quinine hydrochloride in the nucleus of the fasciculus solitarius. In T. Hayashi (ed.), *Olfaction and Taste III*. Pergamon Press, New York, 1967, pp. 549–562.

Hänig, D. P. Zur Psychophysik des Geschmackssinnes. *Philos. Stud.*, 1901, *17*, 576–623.

Hardiman, C. W. Rat and hamster chemoreceptor responses to a large number of compounds and the formulation of a generalized chemosensory equation. Doctoral dissertation, Florida State University. University Microfilms, Ann Arbor, Mich., 1964, No. 64-10, 585.

Harper, H. W., Jay, J. R., and Erickson, R. P. Chemically evoked sensations from single human taste papillae. *Physiol. Behav.*, 1966, *1*, 391–325.

Harriman, A. E., and MacLeod, R. B. Discriminative thresholds of salt for normal and adrenalectomized rats. *Am. J. Psychol.*, 1953, *66*, 465–471.

Harvey, R. J. Gustatory studies relating to *Synsepalum dulcificum* (miracle fruit) and neural coding. Unpublished Ph.D. thesis, Worcester Polytechnic Insititute, 1970.

Heck, G. L., and Erickson, R. P. A rate theory of gustatory stimulation. *Behav. Biol.*, 1973, *8*, 687–712.

Hellekant, G. Efferent impulses in the chorda tympani nerve of the rat. *Acta Physiol. Scand.*, 1971, *83*, 203–209.

Hellekant, G., Hagstrom, E. C., Kasahara, Y., and Zotterman, Y. On the gustatory effects of miraculin and gymnemic acid in the monkey. *Chem. Senses Flavor*, 1974, *1*, 137–145.

Helmholtz, H. Die Thatsachen in der Wahrnehmung (1879) (the facts of perception). In R. M. Warren and R. P. Warren (transl.), *Helmholtz on Perception: Its Physiology and Development*. Wiley, New York, 1968, p. 210.

Henkin, R. I., and Christiansen, R. L. Taste localization on the tongue palate and pharynx of normal man. *J. Appl. Physiol.*, 1967, *27*, 316–320.

Henle, J. Ueber den Geschmackssinn. *Anthropol. Vortr.*, 1880, *2*, 3–24.

Henning, H. Psychologische Studien am Geschmackssinn. In E. Aberholden (ed.), *Handbuch der biologischen Arbeitsmethoden*. Urban and Schwarzenberg, Berlin, 1927, pp. 627–740.

Hiji, Y. Preference for and neural gustatory response to sodium salts in rats. *Kumamoto Med. J.*, 1967, *20*, 129–138.

Hiji, Y. Gustatory response and preference behavior in alloxan diabetic rats. *Kumamoto Med. J.*, 1969, *22*, 109–118.

Hiji, Y., and Sato, M. Isolation of the sugar-binding protein from rat taste buds. *Nature (London) New Biol.*, 1973, *244*, 91–93.

Hooper, D. An examination of the leaves of *Gymnema sylvestre*. *Nature (London)*, 1887, *35*, 565–567.

Horn, W. *Ueber den Geschmackssinn des Menschen*. Karl Groos, Heidelberg, 1825.

Horowitz, R. M., and Gentili, B. Taste and structure in phenolic glycosides. *Agr. Food Chem.*, 1969, *17*, 696–700.

Ishiko, N., and Akagi, T. Topographical organization of gustatory nervous system. In D. Schneider (ed.), *Olfaction and Taste IV*. Wissenschaftliche Verlagsgesellschaft MBH, Stuttgart, 1972, pp. 343–349.

Ishiko, N., Amatsu, M., and Sato, Y. Thalamic representation of taste qualities and temperature change in the cat. In T. Hayashi (ed.), *Olfaction and Taste II*. Pergamon Press, New York, 1967, pp. 563–572.

Jakinovitch, W. Stimulation of the gerbil's gustatory receptors by disaccharides. *Brain Res.*, 1976, *110*, 481–490.

Jakinovitch, W., and Goldstein, I. J. Stimulation of the gerbil's gustatory receptors by monosaccharides. *Brain Res.*, 1976, *110*, 491–504.

Jakinovitch, W., and Oakley, B. Stimulation of the gerbil's gustatory receptors by polyols. *Brain Res.*, 1976, *110*, 505–513.

Kalmus, H. The genetics of taste. In L. M. Beidler (ed.), *Handbook of Sensory Physiology, Vol. IV: Chemical Senses, Section 2: Taste*. Springer-Verlag, New York, 1971, pp. 165–179.

Kamo, N., Miyake, M., Kurihara, K., and Kobatake, Y. Physicochemical studies of taste reception. I. Model membrane simulating taste receptor potential in response to stimuli of salts, acids and distilled water. *Biochim. Biophys. Acta*, 1974, *367*, 1–10.

Kennedy, L. M., Sturckow, B., and Waller, F. J. Effect of gymnemic acid on single taste hairs of the housefly, *Musca domestica*. *Physiol. Behav.*, 1975, *14*, 755–765.

Kier, C. B. A molecular theory of sweet taste. *J. Pharm. Sci.*, 1972, *61*, 1394–1397.

Kiesow, F. Beiträge zur physiologischen Psychologie des Geschmackssinnes. *Philos. Stud.*, 1894a, *10*, 329–368.

Kiesow, F. Beiträge zur physiologischen Psychologie des Geschmackssinnes. *Philos. Stud.*, 1894b, *10*, 523–561.

Kiesow, F. Über die Wirkung des Cocain und der Gymnemasäure auf die Schleimhaut der Zunge und des Mundraums. *Philos. Stud.*, 1894c, *9*, 510–527.

Kiesow, F. Beiträge zue physiologischen Psychologie des Geschmackssinnes. *Philos. Stud.*, 1896, *12*, 255–278.

Kiesow, F. Schmeckversuche an einzelnen Papillen. *Philos. Stud.*, 1898, *14*, 591–615.

Kimura, K., and Beidler, L. M. Microelectrode study of taste receptors of rat and hamster. *J. Cell. Comp. Physiol.*, 1961, *58*, 131–140.

Koh, S. D., and Teitelbaum, P. Absolute behavioral taste thresholds in the rat. *J. Comp. Physiol. Psychol.*, 1961, *54*, 223–229.

Krueger, J. M., and Cagan, R. H. Biochemical studies of taste sensation. *J. Biol. Chem.*, 1976, *10*, 88–97.

Kubota, T., and Kubo, I. Bitterness and chemical structure. *Nature (London)*, 1969, *223*, 97–99.

Kurihara, Y. Antisweet activity of gymnemic acid A_1 and its derivatives. *Life Sci.*, 1969, *8*, 537–543.

Kurihara, K., and Beidler, L. M. Mechanism of the action of taste-modifying protein. *Nature (London)*, 1969, *222*, 1176–1179.

Kurihara, K., and Koyama, N. High activity of adenyl cyclase in olfactory and gustatory organs. *Biochem. Biophys. Res. Commun.*, 1972, *48*, 30–34.

Liljestrand, G., and Zotterman, Y. The water taste in mammals. *Acta Physiol. Scand.*, 1954, *32*, 291–303.

Makous, W., Nord, S., Oakley, B., and Pfaffmann, C. The gustatory relay in the medulla. In Y. Zotterman (ed.), *Olfaction and Taste I*. Pergamon Press, New York, 1963, pp. 381–393.

Mayer, B. Messende Untersuchungen über die Umstimmung des Geschmackswerkzeugs. *Ztschr. Sinnesphysiol.*, 1927, *58*, 133–152.

McBurney, D. H. A note on the relation between area and intensity in taste. *Percept. Psychophys.*, 1969, *6*, 250.

McBurney, D. H. Gustatory cross-adaptation between sweet tasting compounds. *Percept. Psychophys.*, 1972, *11*, 225–227.

McBurney, D. H. Are there primary tastes for man? *Chem. Senses Flavor*, 1974, *1*, 17–28.

McBurney, D. H. Temporal properties of the human taste system. *Sensory Processes*, 1977, *1*, 150–162.

McBurney, D. H., and Bartoshuk, L. M. Interaction between stimuli with different taste qualities. *Physiol. Behav.,* 1973, *10,* 1101–1106.

McBurney, D. H., and Lucas, J. A. Gustatory cross adaptation between salts. *Psychon. Sci.,* 1966, *4,* 301–302.

McBurney, D. H., and Pfaffmann, C. Gustatory adaptation to saliva and sodium chloride. *J. Exp. Psychol.,* 1963, *65,* 523–529.

McBurney, D. H., and Shick, T. R. Taste and water taste of twenty-six compounds for man. *Percept. Psychophys.,* 1971, *10,* 249–252.

McBurney, D. H., Smith, D. V., and Shick, T. R. Gustatory cross adaptation: Sourness and bitterness. *Percept. Psychophys.,* 1972, *11,* 228–232.

McCutcheon, N. B. Sensory adaptation and incentive contrast as factors affecting NaCl preference. *Physiol. Behav.,* 1971, *6,* 675–680.

McCutcheon B., and Kuznicki, J. Chemical interactions in single human papillae. Talk given at the Chemical Senses Meeting, Society for Neuroscience, 1975.

McCutcheon, N. B., and Saunders, J. Human taste papilla stimulation: Stability of quality judgments over time. *Science,* 1972, *175,* 214–216.

Meiselman, H. L. Adaptation and cross-adaptation of the four gustatory qualities. *Percept. Psychophys.,* 1968, *4,* 368–372.

Meiselman, H. L. Effect of presentation procedure on taste intensity functions. *Percept. Psychophys.,* 1971, *10,* 15–18.

Meiselman, H. L. Effect of response task on taste adaptation. *Percept. Psychophys.,* 1975, *17,* 591–595.

Meiselman, H. L., and Halpern, B. P. Effects of *Gymnema sylvestre* on complex tastes elicited by amino acids and sucrose. *Physiol. Behav.,* 1970, *5,* 1379–1384.

Meiselman, H. L., Bose, H. E., and Nykvist, W. E. Effect of flow rate on taste intensity responses in humans. *Physiol. Behav.,* 1972, *9,* 35–38.

Miller, I. J. Peripheral interactions among single papilla inputs to gustatory nerve fibers. *J. Gen. Physiol.,* 1971, *57,* 1–25.

Miller, I. J. Branched chorda tympani neurons and interactions among taste receptors. *J. Comp. Neurol.,* 1974, *158,* 155–166.

Moncrieff, R. W. *The Chemical Senses.* Leonard Hill, London, 1967.

Mook, D. G., and Blass, E. M. Quinine-aversion thresholds and "finickiness" in hyperphagic rats. *J. Comp. Physiol. Psychol.,* 1968, *65,* 202–207.

Morrison, G. R. Behavioral response patterns to salt stimuli in the rat. *Can. J. Psychol.,* 1967, *21,* 141–152.

Morrison, G. R. The relative effectiveness of salt stimuli for the rat. *Can. J. Psychol.,* 1969, *23,* 34–40.

Morrison, G. R., and Norrison, W. Taste detection in the rat. *Can. J. Psychol.,* 1966, *20,* 208–217.

Moskowitz, H. R. Ratio scales of sugar sweetness. *Percept. Psychophys.,* 1970, *7,* 315–320.

Moskowitz, H. R. Ratio scales of acid sourness. *Percept. Psychophys.,* 1971, *9,* 371–374.

Moskowitz, H. R. Perceptual changes in taste mixtures. *Percept. Psychophys.,* 1972, *11,* 257–262.

Moskowitz, H. R. Effects of solution temperature on taste intensity in humans. *Physiol. Behav.,* 1973, *10,* 289–292.

Moskowitz, H. R. Models of additivity for sugar sweetness. In H. R. Moskowitz, B. Scharf, and J. C. Stevens (eds.), *Sensation and Measurement: Papers in Honor of S. S. Stevens.* Reidel, Dordrecht, Netherlands, 1974*a,* pp. 379–388.

Moskowitz, H. R. Sourness of acid mixtures. *J. Exp. Psychol.,* 1974*b, 4,* 640–647.

Müller, J. *Handbuch der Physiologie des Menschen.* J. Hölscher, Coblenz, 1838.

Murray, R. G. The ultrastructure of taste buds. In I. Friedmann (ed.), *The Ultra Structure of Sensory Organs.* American Elsevier, New York, 1973, pp. 1–81.

Myers, C. S. The taste-names of primitive peoples. *Br. J. Psychol.,* 1904, *1,* 117–126.

Nachman, M. Learned aversion to the taste of lithium chloride and generalization to other salts. *J. Comp. Physiol. Psychol.,* 1963, *56,* 343–349.

Nachman, M., and Pfaffmann, C. Gustatory nerve discharge in normal and sodium-deficient rats. *J. Comp. Physiol. Psychol.,* 1963, *56,* 1007–1011.

Natanson. Analyse der Funktionen des Nervensystems. *Arch. Physiol. Heilk.,* 1844, *3,* 515–535.

Noma, A., Goto, J., and Sato, M. The relative taste effectiveness of various sugars and sugar alcohols for the rat. *Kumamoto Med. J.,* 1971, *24,* 1–9.

Norgren, R. Gustatory afferents to ventral forebrain. *Brain Res.,* 1974, *81,* 285–295.

Norgren, R. Taste pathways to hypothalamus and amygdala. *J. Comp. Neurol.,* 1976, *166,* 17–30.

Norgren, R. Gustatory neuroanatomy. In J. LeMagnen (ed.), *Olfaction and Taste VI,* in press, 1978.

Norgren, R., and Leonard, C. M. Ascending central gustatory pathways. *J. Comp. Neurol.*, 1973, *150*, 217–238.

Norgren, R., and Pfaffmann, C. The pontine taste area in the rat. *Brain Res.*, 1975, *91*, 99–117.

Norgren, R., and Wolf, G. Projections of thalamic gustatory and lingual areas in the rat. *Brain Res.*, 1975, *92*, 123–129.

Oakley, B. Microelectrode analysis of second order gustatory neurons in the albino rat. Doctoral dissertation, Brown University. University Microfilms, Ann Arbor, Mich., 1962, No. 63–1045.

Oakley, B. Altered temperature and taste responses from cross-regenerated sensory nerves in the rat's tongue. *J. Physiol. (London)*, 1967, *188*, 353–371.

Oakley, B. The role of taste neurons in the control of the structure and chemical specificity of mammalian taste receptors. In D. Schneider (ed.), *Olfaction and Taste IV*. Wissenschaftliche Verlagsgesellschaft MBH, Stuttgart, 1972, pp. 63–69.

Oakley, B. Receptive fields of cat taste fibers. *Chem. Senses Flavor*, 1975, *1*, 431–442.

Oakley, B., and Cheal, M. Regenerative phenomena and the problem of taste ontogensis. In D. A. Denton & J. P. Coghlan (eds.), *Olfaction and Taste V*. Academic Press, New York, 1975, pp. 99–105.

Ogawa, H., Yamashita, S., Noma, A., and Sato, M. Taste responses in the macaque monkey chorda tympani. *Physiol. Behav.*, 1972, *9*, 325–331.

Öhrwall, H. Untersuchungen über den Geschmackssinn. *Skand. Arch. Physiol.*, 1891, *2*, 1–69.

Öhrwall, H. Die Modalitäts- und Qualitätsbegriffe in der Sinnesphysiologie und deren Bedeutung. *Skand. Arch. Physiol.*, 1901, *11*, 245–272.

Ozeki, M., and Sato, M. Responses of gustatory cells in the tongue of rat to stimuli representing four taste qualities. *Comp. Biochem. Physiol.*, 1972, *41A*, 391–407.

Pangborn, R. M. Taste interrelationships. *Food Res.*, 1960, *25*, 245–256.

Pangborn, R. M. Sensory evaluation of foods: A look backward and forward. *Food Technol.*, 1964, *18*, 63–67.

Paton, W. D. M. A theory of drug action based on the rate of drug-receptor combination. *Proc. R. Soc. London Ser. B*, 1961, *154*, 21–69.

Pfaffmann, C. Gustatory afferent impulses. *J. Cell. Comp. Physiol.*, 1941, *17*, 243–258.

Pfaffmann, C. Gustatory nerve impulses in rat, cat and rabbit. *J. Neurophysiol.*, 1955, *18*, 429–440.

Pfaffmann, C. Taste mechanisms in preference behavior. *Am. J. Clin. Nutr.*, 1957, *5*, 142–147.

Pfaffmann, C. The sense of taste. In J. Field (ed.), *Handbook of Physiology*, Section I: *Neurophysiology*, Vol. I. American Physiological Society, Washington, D.C. , 1959, pp. 507–533.

Pfaffmann, C. Taste preference and reinforcement. In J. T. Tapp (ed.), *Reinforcement and Behavior*. Academic Press, New York, 1969, pp. 215–241.

Pfaffmann, C. Specificity of the sweet receptors of the squirrel monkey. *Chem. Senses Flavor*, 1974, *1*, 61–67.

Pfaffmann, C., and Bare, J. K. Gustatory nerve discharges in normal and adrenalectomized rats. *J. Comp. Physiol. Psychol.*, 1950, *43*, 320–324.

Pfaffmann, C., and Hagstrom, E. C. Factors influencing taste sensitivity to sugar. *Am. J. Physiol.*, 1955, *183*, 651.

Pfaffmann, C., and Powers, J. B. Partial adaptation of taste. *Psychon. Sci.*, 1964, *1*, 41–42.

Pfaffmann, C., Erickson, R. P., Frommer, G. P., and Halpern, B. P. Gustatory discharges in the rat medulla and thalamus. In W. A. Rosenblith (ed.), *Sensory Communication*, Wiley, New York, 1961, pp. 455–473.

Pfaffmann, C., Fisher, G. L., and Frank, M. K. The sensory and behavioral factors in taste preferences. In T. Hayashi (ed.), *Olfaction and Taste II*. Pergamon Press, New York, 1967.

Pfaffmann, C., Frank, M., Bartoshuk, L. M., and Snell, T. C. Coding gustatory information in the squirrel monkey chorda tympani. In J. M. Sprague and A. N. Epstein (eds.), *Progress in Psychobiology and Physiological Psychology*, Academic Press, New York, 1976, pp. 1–27.

Pfaffmann, C., Norgren, R., and Grill, H. J. Sensory affect and motivation. *Ann. N.Y. Acad. Sci.*, 1977, *290*, 18–34.

Plattig, K.-H. On the specificity of single human tongue papillae studied by electric stimulation. In D. Schneider (ed.), *Olfaction and Taste IV*. Wissenschaftliche Verlagsgesellschaft MBH, Stuttgart, 1972, pp. 323–335.

Price, S. Phosphodiesterase in tongue epithelium activation by bitter taste stimuli. *Nature (London)*, 1973, *241*, 54.

Price, S. Chemoreceptor proteins in taste cell stimulation. In T. M. Poynder (ed.), *Transduction Mechanisms in Chemoreception*. Information Retrieval, London, 1974, pp. 177–184.

Price, S., and DeSimone, J. A. Models of taste receptor cell stimulation. *Chem. Senses Flavor,* 1977, *2,* 427–456.

Price, S., and Hogan, R. M. Glucose dehydrogenase activity of a sweet-sensitive protein from bovine tongues. In C. Pfaffmann (ed.), *Olfaction and Taste III.* Rockerfeller University Press, New York, 1969, pp. 397–403.

Rapuzzi, G., and Casella, C. Innervation of the fungiform papillae in the frog tongue. *J. Neurophysiol.,* 1965, *28,* 154–165.

Renqvist, Y. Ueber den Geschmack. *Skand. Arch. Physiol.,* 1919, *38,* 97–201.

Richter, C. P. Increased salt appetite in adrenalectomized rats. *Am. J. Physiol.,* 1936, *115,* 155–161.

Richter, C. P. Salt taste thresholds of normal and adrenalectomized rats. *Endocrinology,* 1939, *24,* 367–371.

Richter, C. P., and Campbell, K. H. Taste thresholds and taste preferences of rats for five common sugars. *J. Nutr.,* 1940, *20,* 31–46.

Sato, M. The effect of temperature change on the response of taste receptors. In Y. Zotterman (ed.), *Olfaction and Taste I.* Pergamon Press, New York, 1963, pp. 151–164.

Sato, T. The response of frog taste cells (*Rana nigromaculata* and *Rana catesbeana*). *Experientia,* 1969, *25,* 709–710.

Sato, T. Site of gustatory neural adaptation. *Brain Res.,* 1971, *34,* 385–388.

Sato, T. Does an initial phasic response exist in the receptor potential of taste cells? *Experientia,* 1976, *32,* 1426–1428.

Sato, T., and Beidler, L. M. Membrane resistance change of the frog taste cells in response to water and NaCl. *J. Gen. Physiol.,* 1975, *66,* 735–763.

Schiffman, S. S., and Dackis, C. Taste of nutrients: Amino acids, vitamins, and fatty acids. *Percept. Psychophys.,* 1975, *17,* 140–146.

Schiffman, S. S., and Erickson, R. P. A theoretical review: A psychophysical model for gustatory quality. *Physiol. Behav.,* 1971, *1,* 617–633.

Scott, T. R., and Erickson, R. P. Synaptic processing of taste-quality information in thalamus of the rat. *J. Neurophysiol.,* 1971, *34,* 868–884.

Scott, T. R., and Perrotto, R. S. The pontine taste area: An analysis of neural responses in the rat. In D. H. Denton and J. P. Coghlan (eds.), *Olfaction and Taste V.* Academic Press, New York, 1975, pp. 203–211.

Shaber, G. S., Brent, R. I., and Rumsey, J. A. Conditioned suppression taste thresholds in the rat. *J. Comp. Physiol. Psychol.,* 1970, *73,* 193–201.

Shallenberger, R. S., and Acree, T. E. Chemical structure of compounds and their sweet and bitter taste. In L. M. Beidler (ed.), *Handbook of Sensory Physiology, Vol. IV: Chemical Senses, Section 2: Taste.* Springer-Verlag, New York, 1971, pp. 221–277.

Shallenberger, R. S., and Acree, T. E. Molecular theory of sweet taste. *Nature (London),* 1967, *216,* 480–482.

Shallenberger, R. S., and Lindley, M. G. A lipophilic-hydrophobic attribute and component in the stereochemistry of sweetness. *Food Chem.,* 1977, *2,* 145–153.

Shore, L. E. A contribution to our knowledge of taste sensations. *J. Physiol. (London),* 1892, *13,* 191–217.

Smith, D. V. Taste intensity as a function of area and concentration: Differentiation between compounds. *J. Exp. Psychol.,* 1971, *87,* 163–171.

Smith, D. V., and Bealer, S. L. Sensitivity of the rat gustatory system to the rate of stimulus onset. *Physiol. Behav.,* 1975, *15,* 303–314.

Smith, D. V., and Frank, M. Cross-adaptation between salts in the chorda tympani nerve of the rat. *Physiol. Behav.,* 1972, *8,* 213–220.

Smith, D. V., and McBurney, D. H. Gustatory cross-adaptation: Does a single mechanism code the salty taste? *J. Exp. Psychol.,* 1969, *80,* 101–105.

Smith, D. V., Steadman, J. W., and Rhodine, C. N. An analysis of the time course of gustatory neural adaptation in the rat. *Am. J. Physiol.,* 1975, *229,* 1134–1140.

Snell, T. C. The response of the squirrel monkey chorda tympani to a variety of taste stimuli. Unpublished Master's thesis, Brown University, 1965.

Stevens, S. S. Measurement and man. *Science,* 1958, *127,* 383–389.

Stevens, S. S. Sensory scales of taste intensity. *Percept. Psychophys.,* 1969, *6,* 302–308.

Stevens, S. S. *Psychophysics.* Wiley, New York, 1975.

Stone, H., and Oliver, S. M. Measurement of the relative sweetness of selected sweeteners and sweetener mixtures. *J. Food Sci.,* 1969, *34,* 215–222.

Storey, A. T., and Johnson, P. Laryngeal receptors initiating apnea in lambs. In J. F. Bosma and J. Showacre (eds.), *Development of Upper Respiratory Anatomy and Function*. U.S. DHEW, Bethesda, Md., 1975, pp. 184–198.

Sweeney, E. A., and Catalanotto, F. A. Salivary sodium and potassium concentrations in adrenalectomized rats. *Int. Assoc. Dent. Res. Abstr.*, 1976, No. 485.

Taglietti, V., Casella, C., and Ferrari, E. Interactions between taste receptors in the frog tongue. *Pflügers Arch.*, 1969, *312*, 139–148.

Tapper, D. N., and Halpern, B. P. Taste stimuli: A behavioral categorization. *Science*, 1968, *161*, 708–710.

Tateda, H., and Beidler, L. M. The receptor potential of the taste cell of the rat. *J. Gen. Physiol.*, 1964, *47*, 479–486.

Teeter, J., and Kare, M. R. Passive electrical properties and responses to chemical stimulation of cutaneous taste bud cells and surrounding surface cells of the catfish. *Fed. Proc.*, 1974, *33*, 416.

Vance, W. B. Oral infusion and taste preference behavior in the white rat. *Psychon. Sci.*, 1970, *18*, 133–134.

von Békésy, G. Sweetness produced electrically on the tongue and its relation to taste theories. *J. Appl. Physiol.*, 1964, *19*, 1105–1113.

von Békésy, G. Taste theories and the chemical stimulation of single papillae. *J. Appl. Physiol.*, 1966, *21*, 1–9.

von Skramlik, E. Mischungsgleichungen im Gebiete des Geschmackssinnes. *Ztschr. Psychol. Physiol. Sinnesorgane*, 1922, *53*, 36–78.

Wang, M. B. Analysis of taste receptor properties derived from chorda tympani nerve firing patterns. *Brain Res.*, 1973, *54*, 314–317.

Wang, M. B., and Bernard, R. A. Characterization and interaction of taste receptors in chorda tympani fibers of the cat. *Brain Res.*, 1969, *15*, 567–570.

Weiner, I. H., and Stellar, E. Salt preference of the rat determined by a single-stimulus method. *J. Comp. Physiol. Psychol.*, 1951, *44*, 394–401.

Wilcove, W. G. Ingestion affected by the oral evnironment: The role of gustatory adaptation on taste reactivity in the rat. *Physiol. Behav.*, 1973, *11*, 297–312.

Yackzan, K. S. Biological effects of *Gymnema sylvestre* fractions. II. Electrophysiology-Effect of gymnemic acid on taste receptor response. *Ala. J. Med. Sci.*, 1969, *6*, 455–463.

Yamaguchi, S., Yoshikawa, T., Ikeda, S., and Ninomiya, T. Studies on the taste of some sweet substances II. Interrelationships among them. *Agr. Biol. Chem.*, 1970, *34*, 187–197.

Yamamoto, T., and Kawamura, Y. An off-type response of the chorda tympani nerve in the rat. *Physiol. Behav.*, 1974, *13*, 239–243.

Yoshida, M., and Saito, S. Multidimensional scaling of the taste of amino acids . *Jap. Psychol. Res.*, 1969, *11*, 149–166.

Young, P. T., Burright, R. G., and Tromater, L. J. Preferences of the white rat for solutions of sucrose and quinine hydrochloride. *Am. J. Psychol.*, 1963, *76*, 205–217.

Zawalich, W. S. Gustatory nerve discharge and preference behavior of penicillamine treated rats. *Physiol. Behav.*, 1971, *6*, 419–423.

Zotterman, Y. The response of the frog's taste fibres to the application of pure water. *Acta Physiol. Scand.*, 1949, *18*, 181–189.

Zotterman, Y. Species differences in the water taste. *Acta Scand. Physiol.*, 1956, *37*, 60–70.

Zotterman, Y. The recording of the electrical response from human taste nerves. In L. M. Beidler (ed.), *Handbook of Sensory Physiology*, Vol. IV: *Chemical Senses*, Section 2: *Taste*. Springer-Verlag, New York, 1971, pp. 102–115.

Index